CAMPBELL'S UROLOGY
Review and Assessment

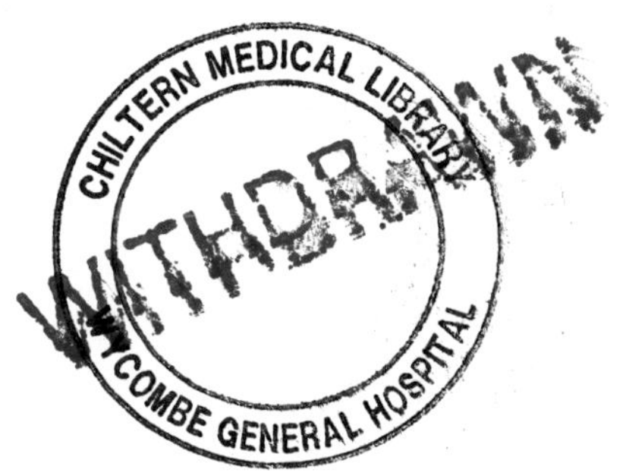

CAMPBELL'S UROLOGY
Review and Assessment

DONALD L. LAMM, M.D.
Professor and Chairman
Department of Urology
Robert C. Byrd Health Sciences Center
of West Virginia University
Morgantown, WV

ANGELO S. PAOLA, M.D.
The Bond Clinic
Department of Urology
Winter Haven, FL

FREDERICK A. PAOLA, M.D., J.D.
Assistant Professor of Medicine
S.U.N.Y. at Stony Brook
Attending Physician
Division of General Medicine
Nassau County Medical Center
East Meadow, NY

W. B. SAUNDERS COMPANY
A Division of Harcourt Brace & Company
PHILADELPHIA, LONDON, TORONTO, MONTREAL, SYDNEY, TOKYO

W. B. SAUNDERS COMPANY
A Division of Harcourt Brace & Company

The Curtis Center
Independence Square West
Philadelphia, Pennsylvania 19106

Library of Congress Cataloging-in-Publication Data

Lamm, Donald L.
Campbell's urology : review and assessment / Donald L. Lamm, Angelo S. Paola, Frederick A. Paolo. — 1st ed.
p. cm.
Based on: Campbell's urology. 6th ed. © 1992.
Includes bibliographical references.
ISBN 0-7216-5158-5
1. Urology—Examinations, questions, etc. I. Lamm, Donald L. II. Campbell's urology. III. Title.
[DNLM: 1. Urologic Diseases—examination questions. 2. Genital Diseases, Male—examination questions. WJ 18.2 L232c 1995]
RC871.C33 1992 Suppl.
616.6'0076—dc20
DNLM/DLC 95-17725

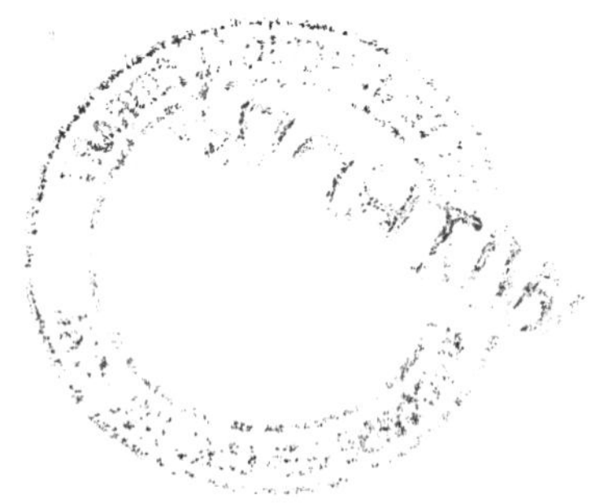

CAMPBELL'S UROLOGY: Review and Assessment ISBN 0-7216-5158-5

Printed in the United States of America.

Last digit is the print number: 9 8 7 6 5 4 3 2 1

CONTRIBUTORS

WILLIAM E. BLAYLOCK, M.D.
Resident, Department of Urology, West Virginia University School of Medicine, Morgantown, West Virginia

JOSEPH M. DEBORD, M.D.
Resident, Department of Urology, West Virginia University School of Medicine, Morgantown, West Virginia

PAUL T. ELLIS, M.D.
Chief Resident, Department of Urology, West Virginia University School of Medicine, Morgantown, West Virginia; Associate, Spartanburg Urological Associates, Spartanburg, South Carolina

NORMAN P. GEBROSKY, M.D.
Resident, Department of Urology, West Virginia University School of Medicine, Morgantown, West Virginia

J. GREG GRIFFITH, M.D.
Department of Urology, Bristol Regional Medical Center, Bristol, Tennessee

STANLEY J. KANDZARI, M.D.
Professor and Residency Program Director, Department of Urology, West Virginia University School of Medicine, Morgantown, West Virginia

JOOHYONG HENRY KIM, M.D.
Resident, Department of Urology, West Virginia University School of Medicine, Morgantown, West Virginia

STEVEN C. KOUKOL, M.D.
Adjunct Instructor, Department of Surgery/Urology Division, University of Nebraska Medical Center; Clinical Urologist, The Urology Center, Omaha, Nebraska

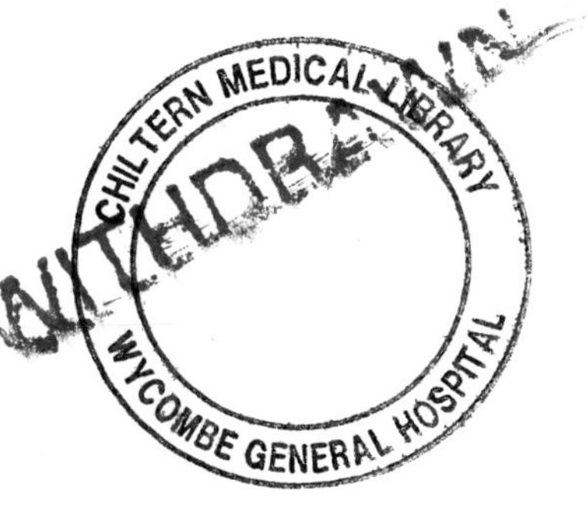

DONALD L. LAMM, M.D.
Professor and Chairman, Department of Urology, West Virginia University School of Medicine, Morgantown, West Virginia

MICHAEL W. MCDONALD, M.D.
Central Surgical Specialties, Harvard Community Health Plan, Boston, Massachusetts

UNYIME O. NSEYO, M.D.
Associate Professor, Department of Urology, West Virginia University School of Medicine, Morgantown, West Virginia

ANGELO S. PAOLA, M.D.
Department of Urology, Bond Clinic, P.A., Winter Haven, Florida

FREDERICK ADOLF PAOLA, M.D., J.D.
Assistant Professor of Medicine, SUNY at Stony Brook School of Medicine; Attending Physician, Palms of Pasadena Hospital, South Pasadena, Florida

WILLIAM F. TARRY, M.D.
Associate Professor, Department of Urology, West Virginia University School of Medicine, Morgantown, West Virginia

CHRISTIAN L. TRAYNELIS, M.S., M.D.
Resident, Department of Urology, West Virginia University School of Medicine, Morgantown, West Virginia

PREFACE

Many enter the field of urology to apply the benefits of modern surgery and medicine to an important yet circumscribed organ system, naive in the belief that the knowledge base that comprises the specialty can be mastered. The primary repository of knowledge in urology since 1952 has been *Campbell's Urology*, whose three volumes span the breadth of the field with authority and precision. Students of urology, including those who practice and those who aspire to practice the art, would be well advised to review *Campbell's Urology*, particularly when faced with a new or perplexing diagnostic problem. But what is the resident or practicing urologist to do when faced with the problem of reviewing for the certifying or recertifying examination? The breadth of the field and the detailed, comprehensive discussions which characterized *Campbell's Urology* preclude a quick review. It is hoped that this study guide will provide an efficient memory refresher for those who are studying for these examinations.

Those who have written test questions realize that the process is more difficult than one might imagine. In this text we have endeavored to cover material that is clinically or scientifically important, but many important matters do not make good test questions. In contrast, some matters which are not particularly important make excellent questions. While we have tried to limit the number of such questions, we anticipate that similar items will occur on board examinations in urology for precisely the same reason.

We are indebted to Doctors Walsh, Retik, Stamey and Vaughan, the editors of *Campbell's Urology*, and to the 134 other contributors for their outstanding review of the subject of urology on which this study guide is based. We have in general limited all comments and questions to information specifically included in the chapters reviewed, and have liberally quoted and paraphrased their work.

This study guide was first written by the residents in the Department of Urology, West Virginia University, and critiqued and rewritten by the faculty, Doctors Stanley J. Kandzari, William F. Tarry, Unyime O. Nseyo, and Michael W. McDonald. Like so much in academic medicine, this work would not have been possible without slave labor of the residents. For that reason, on their behalf, we would like to dedicate this work to residents in urology. You hold the future of the specialty in your capable hands. We hope this book will help you pass the board examination, your rite of passage, so you can get to the business of caring for patients with urological disease, teaching what you have learned, and discovering new and better ways to heal.

Donald L. Lamm
Angelo S. Paola
Frederick A. Paola

COMMENTS AND SUGGESTIONS REQUESTED

The purpose of this study guide is help the student of urology pass written board and recertification examinations. To this end we have tried to select questions which cover the important information and provide practice for the multiple choice examination format. The tests should help identify topics which need to be reviewed in more detail, and the brief answers should expedite your review. Some topics are controversial, and while we have followed the most comprehensive text on the subject of urology, we cannot, of course, guarantee that all of our answers will be the same as those on the real examination.

You will find questions on the board exam and the recertification exam which seem ambiguous. You may have information which was not available at the time the examination was written. There will be answers which you do not agree with. This study guide will be updated in the future, and we welcome your input for future editions. Your comments, suggestions, and corrections can be sent directly to the editors, in care of W.B. Saunders Company, by writing to W.B. Saunders Company, The Curtis Center, Suite 300, Independence Square West, Philadelphia, PA, 19106-3399.

CONTENTS

PART I (Chapters 1–7)

ANATOMY, PHYSIOLOGY, AND GENETICS

QUESTIONS 1

ANSWERS 12

PART II (Chapters 8–10)

THE UROLOGIC EXAMINATION AND DIAGNOSTIC TECHNIQUES

QUESTIONS 29

ANSWERS 34

PART III (Chapters 11–12)

THE PATHOPHYSIOLOGY OF URINARY OBSTRUCTION

QUESTIONS 41

ANSWERS 44

PART IV (Chapters 13–14)

NEUROGENIC BLADDER AND INCONTINENCE

QUESTIONS 49

ANSWERS 52

PART V (Chapter 15)

INFERTILITY

QUESTIONS 56

ANSWERS 58

PART VI (Chapter 16)

SEXUAL FUNCTION

QUESTIONS 62

ANSWERS 64

PART VII (Chapters 17–24)

INFECTIONS AND INFLAMMATION OF THE GENITOURINARY TRACT

QUESTIONS 67

ANSWERS 76

PART VIII (Chapter 25)
BENIGN PROSTATIC HYPERPLASIA
QUESTIONS 100
ANSWERS 102

PART IX (Chapters 26–31)
TUMORS OF THE GENITOURINARY TRACT IN THE ADULT
QUESTIONS 105
ANSWERS 117

PART X (Chapters 32–42)
EMBRYOLOGY AND ANOMALIES OF THE GENITOURINARY TRACT
QUESTIONS 149
ANSWERS 166

PART XI (Chapters 44–54)
PEDIATRIC UROLOGIC SURGERY
QUESTIONS 211
ANSWERS 224

PART XII (Chapters 55–57)
RENAL DISEASES OF UROLOGIC SIGNIFICANCE
QUESTIONS 237
ANSWERS 243

PART XIII (Chapters 58–62)
URINARY LITHIASIS
QUESTIONS 252
ANSWERS 262

PART XIV (Chapters 63–87)
UROLOGIC SURGERY
QUESTIONS 277
ANSWERS 315

PART I

ANATOMY, PHYSIOLOGY, AND GENETICS

CHAPTERS 1 THROUGH 7

DIRECTIONS: Each question below contains suggested responses. Select the ONE BEST response to each question.

1. The dorsal lumbotomy or lumbodorsal approach is made:

   A. Vertically separating the sacrospinalis and quadratus lumborum muscles
   B. Obliquely through the transverse fibers of the transversus abdominis muscle
   C. Vertically parallel to the sacrospinalis and quadratus lumborum muscle through the lumbodorsal fascia
   D. Vertically along the lateral aspects of the flank through the three anterolateral muscle layers

2. The psoas sheath is contiguous with the:

   A. External oblique muscle
   B. Transversalis fascia
   C. Transversus abdominis
   D. Rectus muscle

3. Sympathetic fibers exiting along the lumbar sympathetic trunks are:

   A. Preganglionic and synapse in ganglia within plexuses along the aorta
   B. Postganglionic
   C. Preganglionic and synapse in ganglia at the organ
   D. Highly variable

4. The genitofemoral nerve supplies all of the following EXCEPT:

   A. Sensory to genitalia
   B. Motor to dartos muscle
   C. Motor to cremaster muscle
   D. Sensory to lower thigh

5. In renal ectopia the adrenal is usually:

   A. On the opposite side
   B. In the pelvis
   C. Absent
   D. In its normal position

6. The main venous drainage of the left adrenal gland is to the:

   A. Left renal vein
   B. Inferior vena cava
   C. Inferior phrenic vein
   D. Splenic vein

7. All of the following statements are true regarding supernumery renal arteries EXCEPT:

   A. They are the most common variation in vasculature.
   B. They enter the upper pole more frequently than the lower pole.
   C. They most frequently arise from the lateral aorta.
   D. When occurring in the lower pole, they cross posterior to the ureter and may be a cause of ureteropelvic obstruction.

8. The number of papillae may vary, but the typical kidney has:

   A. 4 to 6
   B. 7 to 9
   C. 10 to 12
   D. 11 to 13

9. The narrowest point of the ureter is the:

   A. Ureteropelvic junction
   B. Mid-ureter
   C. Point of crossing of the iliac vessels
   D. Ureterovesical junction

10. Which of these statements concerning bladder sensation is *true*?

    A. Touch is carried along the sympathetic innervation.
    B. Fullness is carried along the sympathetic innervation.
    C. Pain is carried along the parasympathetic innervation.
    D. Temperature is carried along the parasympathetic innervation.

11. The main motor nerve supply to the detrusor muscle is:

    A. Sympathetic
    B. Parasympathetic
    C. Via the obturator nerve
    D. Via the pudendal nerve

12. Waldeyer's sheath:

    A. Ends at the ureterovesical junction
    B. Forms the deep trigone joined by fibers of the detrusor

C. Forms the superficial trigone joined by ureteral muscle fibers
D. Forms the superficial trigone independent of ureteral muscle fibers

13. What percentage of external sphincter muscle fibers are slow-twitch fibers?
A. 35
B. 50
C. 65
D. 80

14. The area of the prostate traversed by the ejaculatory ducts is known as the:
A. Transition zone
B. Peripheral zone
C. Central zone
D. Fibromuscular stroma

15. All the following prostate tissue is thought to originate from the urogenital sinus EXCEPT:
A. Transitional zone
B. Central zone
C. Peripheral zone
D. Periurethral glands

16. Cowper's ducts drain into the:
A. Bulbous urethra
B. Membranous urethra
C. Prostatic urethra
D. Seminal vesicles

17. The internal spermatic fascia is a continuation of the:
A. Internal oblique muscle
B. Transversus abdominis
C. Transversalis fascia
D. Internal oblique aponeurosis

18. The artery of the vas deferens arises from the:
A. Internal iliac artery
B. External iliac artery
C. Obturator artery
D. Testicular artery

19. The perineal branch of the pudendal nerve innervates all the following EXCEPT:
A. External sphincter
B. Gracilis
C. Transversus perinei
D. Levator ani

20. Which is a point of fixation for the transversalis fascia?
A. Inguinal ligament
B. Puboprostatic ligament
C. Cooper's ligament
D. Denonvilliers' fascia

21. Even without hypertension, arteriolar hyalinization and glomerulosclerosis occur, and by the 8th decade what percentage of glomeruli are lost?
A. 10
B. 25
C. 50
D. 75

22. The mesonephros might transiently produce some tubular fluid, but in the male it develops into all the following EXCEPT:
A. Efferent ductules and duct of the epididymis
B. Ductus deferens
C. Seminal vesicles
D. Ejaculatory ducts
E. Verumontanum

23. Regarding intravascular hydraulic pressure, a significant pressure drop occurs across all of the following vascular beds EXCEPT:
A. Afferent arteriole
B. Glomerular capillary
C. Efferent arteriole
D. Peritubular capillary
E. Small renal veins

24. The renal cortex receives what percentage of total renal blood flow (RBF)?
A. <40
B. 60
C. 75
D. 90

25. The principal driving force for glomerular filtration is:
A. Hydrostatic pressure in the tubule
B. Oncotic pressure of glomerular capillary pressure
C. Hydrostatic pressure at the glomerular capillary
D. Oncotic pressure of tubular fluid

26. All of the following statements about glomerular permeability are true EXCEPT:
A. The degree of filtration of a molecule is dependent on its shape, size, and electrical charge.
B. The glomerular filtration barrier is covered by sialoproteins that bear positive charges.
C. The fluid entering Bowman's space is nearly free of albumin and larger molecules.
D. Neutral dextrose is filtered more than 100 times greater than polyanionic albumin despite their similar molecular radius of 36 Å.

27. Which of the following statements regarding sodium and water transport is *true*?
A. The permeability of water in the proximal tubule is low, thus a high gradient of osmolality between tubular fluid and peritubular fluid must be established
B. The gradient in the proximal tubule is established by the Na^+,K^+-ATPase pump at the luminal aspect of the cell.
C. The proximal tubule carries a negative luminal potential, thought to be due to sodium transport.
D. The distal tubule carries a positive luminal potential, through a reverse ATPase mechanism.

28. The distal tubuloglomerular feedback phenomenon is thought to be a significant contribution to autoregulation of glomeruli filtration. The initiating signal appears to be:
A. Tubular fluid chloride
B. Tubular fluid sodium
C. Tubular fluid creatinine
D. Tubular fluid bicarbonate

29. The fractional excretion of sodium (FE_{Na} %) usually provides a reliable way to differentiate a prerenal from a renal cause of oliguria. Which of the following is true?

A. $FE_{Na}\% = C_{Cs}/C_{Na} \times 100$.
B. A value above 1 per cent favors a prerenal etiology.
C. A value lower than 1 per cent favors a renal cause.
D. A value lower than 1 per cent may be seen in nonprerenal causes.

30. The osmolality of fluid leaving the ascending loop of Henle is close to:

A. 50 mOsm/kg
B. 100 mOsm/kg
C. 500 mOsm/kg
D. 1000 mOsm/kg

31. Under the influence of antidiuretic hormone, most water reabsorption during hydropenia occurs in the:

A. Descending loop of Henle
B. Ascending loop of Henle
C. Cortical collecting tubule
D. Medullary collecting duct

32. Most of the filtered bicarbonate (HCO_3^-) is reclaimed by the:

A. Proximal tubule
B. Descending limb of the loop of Henle
C. Ascending limb of the loop of Henle
D. Distal tubule

33. The following statements about factors that can affect proximal HCO_3^- reabsorption are true EXCEPT:

A. Decrements in absolute or effective extracellular fluid enhance HCO_3^- reabsorption, whereas increments have the opposite effect.
B. Hypercapnia stimulates HCO_3^- reabsorption, whereas hypocapnia inhibits.
C. Prior potassium depletion has a slight stimulatory effect on HCO^-_3 reabsorption.
D. Parathyroid hormone stimulates HCO_3^- reabsorption.
E. Phosphate depletion inhibits reabsorption.

34. The following statements regarding net acid excretion are true EXCEPT:

A. Na^+ reabsorption in the collecting ducts creates a negative intraluminal charge that favors H^+ secretion.
B. Aldosterone can directly stimulate the H^+ pump in the collecting duct, as well as Na^+ reabsorption.
C. Intracellular and brush border carbonic anhydrase is responsible for the net acid excretion.
D. Unlike the proximal tubule, the excretion of H^+ in the collecting duct is not directly coupled to Na^+ reabsorption.
E. An adaptive ammoniagenesis is the principal mechanism for the excretion of increased acid loads.

35. The following statements about renal tubular acidosis (RTA) are true EXCEPT:

A. Hyperchloremia results from increased NaCl reabsorption stimulated by volume contraction secondary to sodium bicarbonate loss in the urine.
B. Hyperkalemia results from stimulation of the renin-angiotensin-aldosterone axis.
C. Type 2 RTA is due to a lowered reabsorptive threshold for HCO_3^- in the proximal tubule.
D. Type 1 RTA is due to an inability to excrete H^+ against a gradient.

36. The following statements are true for potassium EXCEPT:

A. More than 90 per cent of plasma K^+ undergoes glomerular filtration.
B. Most of the filtered K^+ is reabsorbed in the proximal tubule and the loop of Henle.
C. Tubular epithelial cells in the late distal tubule and cortical collecting duct secrete the K^+ by a luminal K^+, Na^+-coupled transport.
D. Mineralocorticoids stimulate K^+ secretion.

37. Calcium reabsorption is stimulated by all the following EXCEPT:

A. Hypocalcemia
B. Metabolic alkalosis
C. Hypermagnesemia
D. Phosphate loading
E. Vitamin D

38. All the following statements regarding phosphate transport are true EXCEPT:

A. Of the filtered load, 80–97 per cent is reabsorbed.
B. Tubular reabsorption can increase to nearly 100 per cent with phosphate deprivation.
C. Most reabsorption occurs in the distal tubule.
D. PTH inhibits reabsorption in the proximal tubule.

39. The following statements about organic solutes are correct EXCEPT:

A. As urine flow rates decrease, the clearance of urea may fall from 60 to 70 per cent of GFR to 10 to 20 per cent, accounting for the disproportionately high blood urea nitrogen (BUN) compared to creatinine in "prerenal azotemia."
B. Uric acid is (1) freely filtered; (2) nearly totally reabsorbed; (3) 50 per cent then secreted and; (4) 80 per cent of this then reabsorbed.
C. Glucose is freely filtered and essentially reabsorbed until the filtered load exceeds a tubular maximum reabsorption rate O(TmG), resulting in glucosuria.
D. Metabolic alkalosis inhibits citrate excretion by depleting intracellular levels, thus stimulating tubular reabsorption.

40. The following statements regarding hormonal influences on renal function are true EXCEPT:

A. The general types of receptors for hormones are (1) peptide hormone and catecholamine receptors (cell membrane receptors) and (2) steroid receptors (cell cytosol receptors).
B. Antidiuretic hormone (ADH) acts at the proximal convoluted tubule through cAMP modulation of water permeability.
C. Atrial natriuretic peptide (ANP) decreases tubular sodium resorption.

D. Insulin acts directly to decrease urinary excretion of sodium and phosphate.
E. Somatostatin induces diuresis in hydropenic animals.

41. All of the following statements about erythropoietin are true EXCEPT:

A. Its production is stimulated by the hypoxia of anemia.
B. It stimulates terminal differentiation of erythroid progenitors.
C. It is elevated in a limited number of anemias.
D. More than 85 per cent is produced by the interstitial cells and endothelial cells lining the peritubular capillaries of the cortex and outer medulla.

42. The primary site of degradation of renin is the:

A. Liver
B. Kidney
C. Lung
D. Spleen

43. All of the following statements are true of renin release with regard to perfusion EXCEPT:

A. Macula densa cells serve as baroreceptors.
B. Renin release usually occurs after an initial drop of 10 to 20 mm in the basal mean arterial pressure of 80 to 100 mm Hg.
C. Below 70 to 80 mm Hg, renin secretion responds in a steep and linear fashion.
D. Elevated perfusion pressure suppresses renin release.

44. Plasma levels of angiotensinogen are decreased in:

A. Pregnancy
B. Cushing's syndrome
C. Cirrhosis of the liver
D. Patients receiving estrogen (birth control pills)

45. The following statements regarding angiotensin-converting enzyme (ACE) are true EXCEPT:

A. ACE converts angiotensin I, a decapeptide to angiotensin II, an octapeptide.
B. ACE is a specific enzyme that cleaves only angiotensin I.
C. ACE is localized to the endothelial cells of all capillaries.
D. Drugs such as enalapril and captopril block ACE and decrease levels of angiotensin II.

46. Angiotensin II causes all of the following EXCEPT:

A. Thirst stimulation
B. Vasoconstriction of the renal vascular bed
C. Decreased sympathetic outflow in the central nervous system
D. Sodium retention

47. The preferential site of action of angiotensin II is the:

A. Afferent arteriole
B. Glomerulus
C. Efferent arteriole
D. Juxtamedullary cell

48. Angiotensin II receptors:

A. Are present only in renal tissue
B. Work by alteration of the Na^+,K^+-ATPase pump directly
C. Are intracellular
D. Increase phosphoinositide turnover and diglycerol formation

49. All of the following statements are true about urinary kallikrein EXCEPT:

A. Angiotensin II decreases its secretion.
B. It is probably secreted by connecting tubule cells.
C. Prostaglandins stimulate its secretion.
D. Mineralocorticoids increase its secretion.

50. Which of the following statements is *true*?

A. 1α-Hydroxylase of the convoluted tubule is stimulated by parathormone (PTH) and calcitonin.
B. 1α-Hydroxylase of the convoluted tubule is stimulated only by calcitonin.
C. 1α-Hydroxylase of the pars recta is stimulated only by calcitonin.
D. 1α-Hydroxylase of the pars recta is stimulated by PTH and calcitonin.

51. All of the following about 1,25-dihydroxy D_3 are true EXCEPT:

A. Its affinity for its cytosolic receptor is 10 times greater than that of 25-hydroxy D_3.
B. It stimulates 25-hydroxy-D-24-hydroxylase activity.
C. It inhibits 25-hydroxy-D-1-hydroxylase activity.
D. It is approximately 10 times more active on a weight basis than vitamin D_3 in inducing intestinal calcium transport.

52. All of the following appear to play a role in increased 1α-hydroxylase activity EXCEPT:

A. Hypocalcemia
B. Increased PTH
C. Hypophosphatemia
D. Hypernatremia

53. The following statements about insulin-like growth factor-1 (IGF-1) are true EXCEPT:

A. It has approximately 25 per cent homology to proinsulin.
B. It is localized to collecting ducts by immunohistochemistry in intact kidney.
C. It is regulated by growth hormone.
D. Its renotrophic role is suggested by elevated levels in unilateral nephrectomy.

54. Most of the important biologic eicosanoids are metabolites of:

A. Linoleic acid
B. Arachidonic acid
C. Alpha-linolinic acid
D. Beta-linolinic acid

55. All of the following regarding peptide hormones are true EXCEPT:

A. Metabolism may occur via binding to specific receptors in the basolateral membrane.
B. Removal by glomerular filtration is dependent on molecular size, shape, and charge of the molecule.
C. Once filtered, most peptides are reabsorbed in the proximal tubule.
D. Approximately 25 per cent of filtered hormones appears in the urine.

56. All of the following statements about renal metabolism of insulin are true EXCEPT:
   A. The kidney accounts for 67 per cent of the metabolic clearance of insulin.
   B. With decreasing renal mass, there is an increase in levels of immunoreactive insulin.
   C. In diabetics with renal insufficiency, insulin requirements may decrease.
   D. Renal transplantation in diabetics may increase their insulin requirements.

57. The increased carboxy terminal fragments of PTH compared to the amino terminal fragments in patients with renal failure is best explained by:
   A. The carboxy terminal fragment is filtered and relies on peritubular uptake, whereas the amino terminal fragment is filtered only.
   B. The carboxy terminal fragment is filtered only, whereas the amino terminal fragment is filtered and relies on peritubular uptake.
   C. The elevated urea binds the amino terminal fragment preferentially.
   D. The carboxy terminal fragment is degraded in the liver, but is induced by a kidney-derived molecule that is decreased with renal failure.

58. Approximately what percentage of calcitonin is cleared by the kidney?
   A. 33
   B. 50
   C. 67
   D. 75

59. All of the following statements about aldosterone are true EXCEPT:
   A. It promotes the reabsorption of sodium.
   B. It promotes the secretion of potassium.
   C. It promotes the reabsorption of hydrogen ion.
   D. Its major site of inactivation is the liver.

60. The site of the pacemaker for the ureter is:
   A. Mid-ureter
   B. Ureterovesical junction
   C. Glomerulus
   D. Proximal collecting system

61. All of the following ions contribute to the resting membrane potential (RMP) of the ureteral smooth muscle cell by ionic or concentration interactions EXCEPT:
   A. H^+
   B. Ca^{++}
   C. Na^+
   D. K^+

62. The influx of which ion is responsible for the upstroke of the action potential?
   A. H^+
   B. K^+
   C. Ca^{++}
   D. Cl^-

63. All of the following statements about smooth muscle contractions are true EXCEPT:
   A. Ca^{++} appears to act as a true activator.
   B. The concentration of Ca^{++} transiently increases from 10^{-6} M to 10^{-2} M.
   C. Ca^{++} binds to calmodulin, thus activating a calmodulin-dependent enzyme, myosin light-chain kinase.
   D. Myosin light-chain kinase catalyzes the phosphorylation of the 20,000-dalton light chain of myosin.

64. Which of the following statements regarding innervation of the ureter is *true*?
   A. Transplanted or denervated ureters are aperistaltic.
   B. The ureter contains excitatory beta-adrenergic receptors.
   C. Muscarinic cholinergic receptors are not found in the ureter.
   D. Norepinephrine increases the force of electrical-induced ureteral contractions.

65. All of the following statements about the force-length relationships of the ureter are true EXCEPT:
   A. With stretching of the ureter (lengthening), resting force (tension present when muscle is not excited) increases at a progressive rate.
   B. Ureteral resting tension is low at the length at which maximal contractile force is developed.
   C. When the ureter is stretched, resting force increases.
   D. Hysteresis refers to the variability of the resting or contractile force developed at any given length, depending on the direction and rate of change in length.

66. Which of the following statements about propulsion of the urine bolus by the ureter is *true*?
   A. Coaptation of the ureteral wall is not necessary for propulsion of the bolus.
   B. With increased flow rates, the initial response of the ureter is to increase frequency of contractions.
   C. An increase in the diameter of the ureter increases intraluminal pressure.
   D. Relaxation of the UVJ is critical to successful bolus transport.

67. All of the following statements are true of the physiology of the UPJ EXCEPT:
   A. There is a 1:1 conduction of pacemaker to ureter at low flow rates.
   B. Areas of narrowing and abnormal propagation of peristaltic waves have been implicated in UPJ obstruction.
   C. Electron microscopy has demonstrated abnormal intracellular relationships in UPJ obstruction.
   D. A closed UPJ may be a normal protective mechanism for preventing propagation of ureteral pressure to the pelvis.

68. All of the following statements are true about the UVJ EXCEPT:
   A. The UVJ does not relax.
   B. The wider and more weakly contractile the ureter, the lower the resistance at the UVJ must be in order not to interfere with bolus transport.
   C. Telescoping of the ureter within its sheath aids in decreasing UVJ resistance.
   D. Gravity does not appear to play a role in urine transport.

69. The following statements regarding ureteral obstruction are true EXCEPT:

A. There is an initial transient increase in the amplitude and frequency of peristaltic contractions.
B. After dilatation and lengthening prevent coaptation, hydrostatic forces are responsible for continued increases in pressure.
C. The ureteral pressure peaks at 1 to 2 weeks, then gradually returns to just above baseline pressure.
D. The gradual increase in ureteral length and diameter at the relatively low pressure observed in late obstruction is seen in viscoelastic structure and referred to as creep.

70. The following statements are true about renal perfusion studies EXCEPT:

A. A steady-state condition of equilibrium of inflow to outflow should be reached prior to pressure measurement.
B. The accepted flow rate of 10 ml/min is at the upper end of flow rates for usual physiologic states.
C. Fluoroscopic monitoring aids in interpretation of the data.
D. The bladder should be continuously drained to eliminate its effect on urine transport.

71. The most common etiology of reflux is:

A. UVJ abnormality
B. Impaired ureteral function
C. Inordinately high intravesical pressure
D. Trigonal abnormality

72. All of the following statements are true regarding infection and reflux EXCEPT:

A. Infection can potentiate the deleterious effects of obstruction on peristalsis.
B. *E. coli* endotoxins can inhibit ureteral activity.
C. Infection may increase the compliance of the intravesical ureter and permit reflux.
D. *E. coli* exotoxins have been shown to inhibit ureteral activity.

73. The following statements are true about ureteral function and calculi EXCEPT:

A. Hydrostatic pressure appears unimportant in stone passage.
B. Proximal peristaltic wave increases are increased in frequency.
C. There is no change in peristaltic activity distally.
D. Phentolamine, an alpha-adrenergic antagonist, has been shown to increase flow rate at the site of obstruction.

74. Factors that favor an obstructive etiology for hydronephrosis during pregnancy include all of the following EXCEPT:

A. Ureteral dilatation above but not below the pelvic brim.
B. Hydronephrosis seen in ureters not crossing the pelvic brim.
C. Normal ureteral contractile pressures seen in pregnancy.
D. Rarity of hydronephrosis in quadripeds during pregnancy.

75. During early development in the guinea pig model, there is an increase in:

A. Contractility
B. Shortening
C. Velocity
D. Work

76. Isoproterenol relaxes the ureter by:

A. Stimulating adenylyl cyclase activity, thus decreasing cyclic AMP (cAMP)
B. Inhibiting phosphodiesterase activity, thus decreasing cAMP
C. Inhibiting phosphodiesterase activity, thus increasing cAMP
D. Stimulating adenylyl cyclase activity, thus increasing cAMP

77. With regard to ureteral contractions, which of the following statements is *true*?

A. Cholinergic agonists have an inhibitory effect.
B. Alpha-adrenergic agonists have a stimulatory effect.
C. Calcium blockers have an inhibitory effect.
D. Progesterone has a stimulatory effect.

78. The following statements about the permeability of bladder mucosa are true EXCEPT:

A. Sulfated polysaccharides act as a permeability barrier to small molecules.
B. Distention or urothelial disruption increases active sodium transport.
C. Apical epithelial cells are permeable to water.
D. Various sodium transport channels exist, including those sensitive to aldosterone and those that do not respond to aldosterone.

79. Which of the following statements regarding the histology and ultrastructure of striated muscle is *true*?

A. Slow-twitch fibers have few mitochondria and thus are easily fatigued.
B. Slow-twitch fibers have numerous lipid droplets and wide Z discs compared to fast-twitch fibers.
C. Striated muscle of the distal urethra contain primarily fast-twitch fibers.
D. Striated muscle of the periurethral area contains primarily slow-twitch fibers.

80. All of the following statements are true regarding smooth muscles of the bladder and urethra EXCEPT:

A. Gap junctions are a consistent feature of smooth muscle cells of the human bladder.
B. The bladder base does not possess an anatomic sphincter.
C. In males, the smooth and striated muscles coalesce in the urethra and interdigitate with the fibrous prostatic capsule.
D. The syncytial arrangement of muscle bundles in the bladder facilitates complete evacuation.

81. The following statements regarding Ca^{++} and smooth muscles are true EXCEPT:

A. The influx of Ca^{++} required for activation of the contractile apparatus is regulated by two separate mechanisms—a voltage-sensitive channel and a receptor-operated channel.

B. A Ca^{++}-calmodulin complex binds to a myosin light-chain kinase that phosphorylates the light chain of action.
C. Three types of voltage-sensitive channels have been identified—L channels, T channels, and N channels.
D. Intracellular stores of Ca^{++}, in mitochondria and sarcoplasmic reticulum, are released via membrane-derived inositol phosphate pathways.

82. All of the following statements are true regarding the energetics of smooth muscle EXCEPT:

A. Smooth muscle maintains tone with relatively little energy expenditure.
B. A linear relationship exists between force and metabolism.
C. ATP generated from aerobic glycolysis and glucose metabolism provides energy for contraction.
D. The rate of energy expenditure to develop a bladder contraction is three times that associated with maintenance of an active contraction.

83. All of the following are characteristics of striated muscle cells EXCEPT:

A. Intermediate filaments
B. Sarcomere pattern
C. Rapid calcium influx via T-tubule
D. Disinhibition of tropomyosin responsible for contraction

84. Which of the following statements is true regarding Onuf's nucleus?

A. It is located in the sacral ventral horn.
B. It is spared in amyotrophic lateral sclerosis, which impairs somatic muscle function.
C. It is spared in Shy-Drager syndrome, which is an autonomic neuropathy.
D. It provides motor neurons to L4, L5, S1, segments.

85. All of the following statements are true of autonomic innervation of the bladder EXCEPT:

A. Parasympathetic preganglionic perikarya are arranged in a viscerotropic manner.
B. The pelvic nerve contains only preganglionic fibers.
C. The hypogastric plexus lies on the great vessels at the level of L3 to L5.
D. Sympathetic fibers that enter the pelvic plexus may interact with sacral parasympathetics or with postganglionic sympathetic fibers.

86. All of the following statments are true about cholinergic mechanisms EXCEPT:

A. Nicotinic ganglionic blockers abolish bladder contractions produced by the pelvic nerve.
B. In patients with hypotonic bladders, acetylcholinesterase staining is reduced.
C. Activation of muscarinic receptors on adrenergic terminals in the bladder and urethra inhibit norepinephrine release.
D. Cholinergic agonists produce a marked relaxation of the urethra in vivo.

87. All of the following statements are true about adrenergic mechanisms EXCEPT:

A. Adrenergic innervation is limited to the bladder base and proximal urethra.
B. Estrogens decrease the response of urethral tissues to alpha-adrenergic agonists in vitro.
C. Sympathetic pathways appear to play a minor role in normal lower urinary tract function.
D. Although propranolol increases urethral pressure, beta-adrenergic antagonists are not clinically useful in treating bladder or urethral disorders.

88. All of the following statements are true about purinergic mechanisms EXCEPT:

A. Neurons containing purine nucleotides and nucleosides have been identified by histochemical techniques.
B. Purinergic substances inhibit excitatory cholinergic transmission in the vesical ganglia.
C. Purine antagonists such as theophylline and caffeine enhance inhibition of excitatory cholinergic transmission in the vesical ganglia.
D. Electrical stimulation of the pelvic nerve produces a biphasic contraction, which is initially mediated by purines and secondly by a cholinergic component.

89. All of the following statements are true regarding peptidergic mechanisms EXCEPT:

A. Lack of specificity of the source and function of neuropeptides makes them poor markers for tracing pathways.
B. Neuropeptides are co-localized with traditional transmitters.
C. The release of neuropeptides from nerves is frequency-dependent.
D. Neuropeptides potentially released from postganglionic nerves supplying the bladder or urethra affect smooth muscle contractility.

90. Which of the following statements regarding these primarily central nervous system transmitters is *false*:

A. Gamma-aminobutyric acid (GABA) inhibits excitatory neural transmission in pelvic ganglia.
B. Serotonin (5-HT) has been shown primarily to inhibit cholinergic transmission in pelvic ganglia.
C. Serotonin (5-HT) has been shown to contract the bladder body.
D. Gamma-aminobutyric acid (GABA) is exclusively associated with small intense fluorescent (SIF) cells.

91. All of the following statements are true about afferent mechanisms EXCEPT:

A. Bladder afferents respond primarily to bladder volume.
B. Visceral afferents release transmitters capable of influencing cellular components of the immune system.
C. Afferents in the pelvic nerve respond to distention in a graded fashion.
D. Afferent nerves travel in sympathetic and parasympathetic pathways.

92. Which of the following statements regarding afferent mechanisms is *false*?

A. Pacinian corpuscles are numerous.
B. Frequency encoding has been used as a mechanism to distinguish tension from nociceptive input.

C. Lightly myelinated (A-delta) fibers conduct rapidly, up to 30 meters/second.
D. Intravesical pressure thresholds for A-delta afferents range from 5 to 15 mm Hg, corresponding to filling pressures sensed on a cystometrogram.

93. The following statements about voiding reflexes are true EXCEPT:
A. During voiding, hypogastric and pudendal neurons are excited.
B. Voiding results when mechanoreceptors in the bladder respond to a threshold tension.
C. The central mechanisms are organized as a simple on-off switching circuit.
D. Organization of central neuronal pathways allow the bladder to empty completely with a low voiding pressure.

94. Which of the following statements about voiding reflexes is *false*?
A. The spinobulbospinal micturition pathway that passes through the pons is responsible for micturition in the intact individual.
B. Voluntary voiding is abolished in humans when connections between the frontal lobe, hypothalamus, or the paralobule and the brain stem are destroyed.
C. Anterolateral cordotomies performed for chronic pain reveal that ascending routes responsible for transmitting bladder sensation and that trigger voiding travel in the dorsolateral columns.
D. The net effect of lesions rostral to the pons is often hyperactivity of the bladder.

95. The continence reflex or "guarding" refers to:
A. Increased ascending firing to the pontine micturition center with valsalva
B. Pudendal motoneuron firing when the bladder is filled near capacity
C. Hypogastric motoneuron firing when the bladder is filled near capacity
D. Increased hypogastric neuron firing with micturition

96. Which of the following statements is true about central neurotransmitters?
A. Electrical stimulation of serotonin neurons in the raphe nuclei stimulates rhythmic bladder activity.
B. Dopamine facilitates bladder storage.
C. Data suggest that urine storage may be facilitated or inhibited by cholinergic neurons in supraspinal centers.
D. Due to its depression of bladder function, intrathecal morphine is effective in the treatment of detrusor hyperreflexia.

97. Which of the following statements regarding pathologic voiding is *false*?
A. An excitatory somatobladder reflex explains "trigger voiding" in paraplegics.
B. After a supraspinal cord transection, micturition is initially lost, but is reestablished weeks to months later.
C. There is evidence of an increase in adrenergic fibers following decentralization.
D. Bladder outlet obstruction is not associated with changes in the central nervous system but is associated with peripheral changes.

98. Gonadotropin-releasing hormone (GnRH) is transmitted to the pituitary by:
A. General circulation
B. Portal venous system
C. Neuronal axons
D. Local diffusion
E. Secretory granules

99. Gonadotropin-releasing hormone stimulates synthesis and release from the pituitary of:
A. LH
B. FSH
C. Prolactin
D. LH and FSH
E. LH and prolactin

100. The normal pattern of GnRH release in adult human males is:
A. Continuous and constant
B. Continuous with varying levels
C. Pulsatile
D. Diurnal, with peaks during sleep
E. Based on a monthly cycle

101. All of the following share a common alpha subunit peptide chain EXCEPT:
A. Inhibin
B. LH
C. FSH
D. TSH
E. HCG

102. The primary control of testicular steroidogenesis is mediated by:
A. FSH
B. HCG
C. LH
D. Inhibin
E. ACTH

103. Patients with severe germinal epithelial defects with azoospermia or severe oligospermia, but with normal Leydig cell function may demonstrate:
A. Elevated FSH
B. Elevated LH
C. Elevated testosterone
D. Decreased FSH
E. Decreased LH

104. The blood supply to the testis and epididymis derives from the:
A. Internal spermatic artery
B. External spermatic artery
C. Internal and external spermatic arteries
D. Internal spermatic artery and artery to the vas deferens
E. Internal and external spermatic arteries and artery to the vas deferens

105. The cellular site of testosterone synthesis in the Leydig cell is the:
A. Ribosome
B. Golgi apparatus
C. Mitochondria

D. Endoplasmic reticulum
E. Mitochondria and endoplasmic reticulum

106. The blood-testis barrier is formed by the:

A. Capillary endothelium
B. Peritubular myxoid cells
C. Basement membrane of seminiferous tubule
D. Sertoli cells
E. Plasma membrane of spermatogenesis

107. Spermatogenesis in man requires:

A. 8 days
B. 16 days
C. 32 days
D. 64 days
E. 128 days

108. The hormonal regulation of spermatogenesis is carried out primarily by:

A. FSH
B. LH
C. Testosterone
D. GnRH
E. Seminiferous growth factor

109. Sperm transport through the epididymis is produced by all of the following EXCEPT:

A. Sperm flagellar activity
B. Flow of rete testis fluid
C. Resorption of water by ductal epithelial cells
D. Motile cilia on epithelial cells
E. Contraction of periductal cells

110. At what point during transit through the reproductive tract do spermatozoa become fully mature:

A. Rete testes
B. Efferent ductules
C. Caput epididymidis
D. Cauda epididymidis
E. Ampulla of vas

111. The portion of the spermatozoa containing enzymes and structural proteins necessary for transduction of chemical energy from ATP into mechanical movement is:

A. Acrosome
B. Connecting piece
C. Axoneme
D. Principal piece
E. End piece

112. The significant innervation of the vas deferens is by the:

A. Somatic nervous system
B. Sympathetic nervous system
C. Parasympathetic nervous system
D. Somatic and parasympathetic nervous system
E. Sympathetic and parasympathetic nervous system

113. Adenocarcinoma of the prostate arises principally from which zone of the prostate?

A. Anterior fibromuscular stroma
B. Peripheral zone
C. Central zone
D. Preprostatic tissue
E. Transition zone

114. Benign prostatic hyperplasia arises in which zone of the prostate?

A. Anterior fibromuscular stroma
B. Peripheral zone
C. Central zone
D. Pre-prostatic tissue
E. Transition zone

115. Which zone of the prostate is responsible for preventing the seminal fluid from entering the bladder during emission?

A. Anterior fibromuscular stroma
B. Peripheral zone
C. Central zone
D. Preprostatic tissue
E. Transition zone

116. Autonomic innervation of the prostate that is of clinical importance includes receptors of which type?

A. Muscarinic cholinergic
B. Nicotinic cholinergic
C. $Alpha_1$-adrenergic
D. $Alpha_2$-adrenergic
E. Beta adrenergic

117. Estrogen, when used therapeutically for metastatic prostate cancer, exerts its therapeutic effect by:

A. Activating estrogen responsive genes
B. Blocking the binding of testosterone to its receptor
C. Direct action on prostate cells
D. Inhibiting LH release
E. Blocking interaction of steroid receptor with DNA

118. The processes involved in prostate involution following androgen withdrawal are best described as:

A. Programmed cell death
B. Senescent cell death
C. Cell death by free radicals
D. Mitotic arrest
E. Cell death by metabolic failure

119. The first fraction of the ejaculate is rich in:

A. Seminal vesicle fluid
B. Fructose
C. Spermatozoa
D. Prostaglandins
E. Semenogelin

120. All of the following statements regarding zinc in the seminal plasma and sex accessory glands are true EXCEPT:

A. Zinc in seminal plasma arises from the prostate.
B. Zinc levels in BPH are normal or elevated.
C. Zinc levels in prostate tissue are higher than any other organ.
D. Zinc levels in prostate cancer tissue are elevated.
E. Prostatic fluid zinc levels are reduced in prostatitis.

121. Regarding prostatic acid phosphatase, all of the following statements are true EXCEPT:

A. Optimal enzymatic activity occurs in acid environment.
B. Prostate tissue contains more acid phosphatase than any other tissue.

C. Enzymatic activity is not inhibited by tartrate.
D. Enzymatic activity is inhibited by fluoride.
E. Thymolphthalein phosphate is most specific enzyme substrate for laboratory assay.

122. A 28-year-old man and his wife have not achieved conception after more than a year. Semen analysis reveals azoospermia. Of the following, the next step in evaluation should be:

A. Measurement of LH, FSH, and prolactin
B. Testis biopsy
C. Vasogram
D. Measurement of anti-sperm antibodies
E. Measurement of fructose in semen

123. All of the following drugs reach concentrations in prostatic secretions that approach or exceed blood concentrations EXCEPT:

A. Nitrofurantoin
B. Erythromycin
C. Tetracycline
D. Sulfamethoxazole
E. Trimethoprim

124. All of the following are found in both DNA and RNA EXCEPT:

A. Adenine
B. Thymine
C. Quanine
D. Cytosine
E. Five-carbon sugars

125. The process in which DNA is decoded and RNA produced during the first step in protein synthesis is called:

A. Transcription
B. Regulation
C. Promotion
D. Translation
E. Translocation

126. Non-coding portions of genes are known as:

A. Exons
B. Anticodons
C. Introns
D. Enhancers
E. Termination signals

127. The enzyme used by retroviruses to construct DNA is known as:

A. RNA polymerase
B. DNA polymerase
C. DNA gyrase
D. Endonuclease
E. Reverse transcriptase

128. During protein synthesis, specific amino acids are carried to the point of manufacture by:

A. Messenger RNA
B. Transfer RNA
C. Small subunit ribosomal RNA
D. Large subunit ribosomal RNA
E. Endoplasmic reticulum

129. Proto-oncogenes are normal genes that code for regulator proteins involved in:

A. Cell division
B. Protein synthesis
C. Signal transduction between cell membrane and nucleus
D. Cell growth
E. DNA synthesis

130. The genetic engineering technique in which DNA is replicated in a host cell is known as:

A. Molecular cloning
B. DNA sequencing
C. DNA linkage
D. Polymerase chain reaction
E. Gene amplification

131. The probability of detecting autosomal dominant polycystic kidney disease by renal ultrasonography in a 25-year-old affected individual is:

A. 100 per cent
B. 80 per cent
C. 60 per cent
D. 40 per cent
E. 20 per cent

132. Testicular feminization, the most common cause of male pseudohermaphroditism, is inherited in the following way:

A. Autosomal recessive
B. Autosomal dominant
C. X-linked recessive
D. Y-linked recessive
E. Variable penetrance

133. The gene (or genes) located on the Y chromosome responsible for male sex determination is called:

A. Pseudoautosomal region
B. Müllerian inhibition factor
C. Androgen receptor region
D. Sex determination factor
E. Testis-determining factor

134. The phenomenon in which a retrovirus picks up genetic information from a host cell and incorporates it into its own genome so it can be carried elsewhere is known as:

A. Transduction
B. Transfection
C. Translocation
D. Gene insertion
E. Gene amplification

135. Hypomethylation of the *myc* proto-oncogene resulting in an increase in gene product leading to malignant transformation has been associated with:

A. Renal cell carcinoma
B. Prostate adenocarcinoma
C. Testis cancer
D. Transitional cell carcinoma
E. Penile cancer

136. The *ras* family of proto-oncogenes is thought to lead to malignant transformation by:

A. Qualitative changes in gene product associated with point gene mutations
B. Chromosomal translocation
C. Gene amplifications
D. Hypomethylation
E. Gene insertion

137. Anti-oncogenes are:

A. Proteins of the immunoglobulin class

B. Tumor-suppressing genes
C. Strands of mRNA complementary to oncogenes
D. Nucleotide triplets on tRNA
E. Viral genes inserted in the human genome

138. The genitourinary tumor in which familial occurrence has been most completely investigated is:

A. Testis cancer
B. Renal cell carcinoma
C. Prostate cancer
D. Wilms' tumor
E. Transitional cell carcinoma

139. The normal diploid number of human chromosomes is:

A. 22
B. 23
C. 24
D. 46
E. 48

140. A marker chromosome is:

A. A chromosome with such abnormal morphology it can no longer be recognized.
B. The X chromosome in a photographic karyotype.
C. An autosomal chromosome carrying a dominantly inherited disease.
D. A chromosome after staining with quinacrine dye.
E. A chromosome involved in malignant transformation

141. Flow cytometry is a:

A. Urodynamic technique to measure urinary flow rate
B. Method to measure nuclear shape
C. Method to measure cell ploidy
D. Method to detect malignant cells
E. Method to measure cell size

142. Maternal genes expressed during egg maturation may help coordinate early embryonic development by:

A. Causing chemical gradients within the early fertilized egg
B. Activating homeotic genes
C. Activating segmentation genes
D. Producing estrogen receptor
E. Producing Müllerian inhibition factor

143. Androgen ablation may be therapeutic in prostate cancer because of:

A. A change in the serum estrogen/testosterone ratio
B. Increased serum levels of LH
C. Decreased availability of substrates necessary for cell division
D. Enhanced expression of a series of genes within the prostate that lead to cell death
E. Increased serum levels of prolactin

144. The most useful current method for introduction of foreign genes into target mammalian cells is by use of:

A. Transfection
B. Modified retroviral particles
C. Microinjection
D. Plasmids
E. Electroporation

145. The experimental attempt to use gene therapy to suppress cancer phenotypes in animal models of Wilms' tumor and prostate cancer by using transduction to replace missing anti-oncogenes is an example of:

A. Gene replacement
B. Gene augmentation
C. Gene modulation
D. Gene deletion
E. Antisense oligonucleotide therapy

PART I

ANATOMY, PHYSIOLOGY, AND GENETICS

CHAPTERS 1 THROUGH 7

ANSWERS

1-C *(Campbell's, p. 3)*

The dorsal lumbotomy or lumbodorsal approach is a vertical incision that parallels the lateral borders of the sacrospinalis and quadratus lumborum muscles through the lumbodorsal fascia posteromedial to the fibers of the transversis abdominis muscle.

2-B *(Campbell's, p. 12)*

The psoas sheath is contiguous with transversalis fascia.

3-A *(Campbell's, p. 18)*

Preganglionic fibers supplying the abdominal viscera exit the lumbar sympathetic trunks via the lumbar splanchnic nerves and course anteriorly over the aorta, forming autonomic nervous plexuses associated with the major branches of the abdominal aorta. They synapse with postganglionic neurons in ganglia within these plexuses.

4-D *(Campbell's, p. 18)*

The genitofemoral nerve arises from the first through the third lumbar nerves and is primarily sensory nerve to the genitalia. The genital branch of the genitofemoral nerve also supplies the cremaster and dartos muscles in the scrotum.

5-D *(Campbell's, p. 21)*

The adrenal glands are embryologically and functionally distinct from the kidneys and are physically separated from the kidneys by connective tissue septa in continuity with Gerota's fascia as well as by varying amounts of perinephric adipose tissue. Thus, in cases of renal ectopia, the adrenal usually is found in approximately its normal anatomic position and does not follow the kidney. Similarly, in cases of renal agenesis, the adrenal on the involved side is usually present.

6-A *(Campbell's, p. 22)*

The left adrenal vein is typically joined by the left inferior phrenic vein before entering the superior aspect of the left renal vein.

7-D *(Campbell's, p. 30)*

Variations of the main renal artery and vein are common and present in one quarter to one third of individuals. The most common variation is supernumerary arteries. They usually arise from the lateral aorta and may enter the hilum or directly into the parenchyma of one of the poles, the upper pole more commonly than the lower pole. Lower pole arteries must cross the urinary collecting system anteriorly and may be the cause of ureteropelvic obstruction.

8-B *(Campbell's, p. 32)*

The renal papillae may number as few as 4 or as many as 18, but 7 to 9 are present in the typical kidney. Each papilla is cupped by a corresponding minor calyx, that receives the urinary output from the collecting ducts.

9-D *(Campbell's, p. 39)*

The ureter is not of uniform caliber, with three distinct narrowings commonly present along its course. The first of these is the ureteropelvic junction, the second is the crossing of the iliac vessels, and the third is the ureterovesical junction in the pelvis. The ureter is narrowest at the ureterovesical junction and as it traverses the intramural tunnel through the bladder wall.

10-A *(Campbell's, p. 45)*

It is believed that the sensations of stretch and fullness in the bladder are carried along the pelvic parasympathetic innervation, and the sensations of pain, touch, and temperature are carried along the sympathetic innervation.

11-B *(Campbell's, p. 45)*

The motor nerve supply to the detrusor muscle is primarily the pelvic parasympathetic plexus, whereas the motor supply to the trigone and the lower end of the ureters is of sympathetic origin.

12-B *(Campbell's, p. 47)*

Waldeyer's sheath is a fibromuscular sheath originating proximal to the ureteral hiatus. Its fibers diverge at the ureteral hiatus, then fan out to form the deep trigone. Detrusor fibers join the fibers of the sheath to form the deep trigone, which ends at the level of the internal meatus.

13-A *(Campbell's, p. 50)*

Histologically the striated muscle fibers can be classified into two main groups: slow-twitch fibers and fast-twitch fibers. The slow-twitch fibers constitute about 35 per cent of the overall striated muscle mass, and the fast-twitch fibers constitute the remaining 65 per cent. Of the 65 per cent fast-twitch fibers, 50 per cent are fatigable and 15 per cent are fatigue-resistant. This mixture of muscle fibers accounts for the varied contribution of the striated sphincter to the continence mechanism.

14-C *(Campbell's, p. 54)*

After detailed anatomic and histologic study of the adult prostate, a modern nomenclature has been described. The glandular elements are now divided into two main parts; the central zone and the much larger peripheral zone. The remaining transition zone is the site of most prostatic hyperplasia but is rarely the site of malignancy. The anterior fibromuscular stroma is the remainder of the gland. The ejaculatory ducts traverse through the central zone, and it is possible that embryonic wolffian duct tissue incorporated into the prostatic gland is the origin of the central zone.

15-B *(Campbell's, pp. 54–57)*

The peripheral zone, the transition zone, and the periurethral glands form an anatomic and histologic continuum, probably reflecting their common embryonic origin—the urogenital sinus. The central zone is morphologically distinct; it is conceivable that its origin is embryonic wolffian duct tissue incorporated into the prostate gland.

REFERENCE

1. McNeal, J.E.: UICC Technical Report Series, Vol. 48, Prostate Cancer, p. 24, 1979.

16-A *(Campbell's, pp. 57–58)*

The bulbourethral, or Cowper's glands, are located in the deep perineal compartment on each side of the membranous urethra. Their ducts, however, run distally for about 3 or 4 mm into the corpus spongiosum of the penile bulb before they open into the bulbous urethra.

17-C *(Campbell's, p. 58)*

The internal spermatic fascia is a continuation of the transversalis fascia.

18-A *(Campbell's, p. 60)*

The vas deferens travels through the spermatic cord and the inguinal canal, in company with the fascia and the cremasteric muscle of the cord, as well as the testicular artery, the pampiniform plexus, the lymphatics and nerves, and the epididymis of the testis. The vas deferens, however, has its own arterial supply, which is known as the artery of the vas deferens; it is usually a branch of the umbilical or internal iliac artery.

19-B *(Campbell's, p. 63)*

The pudendal nerve, formed from the anterior branches of S2–S4, is the principal innervator of the perineal muscles, including the external sphincter, transversus perinei, and levator ani through its perineal branch.

20-C *(Campbell's, p. 65)*

Cooper's ligament is a very dense condensation on the top of the crural arch from the interior iliac tuberosity all the way to the pubic bone. It acts as a point of fixation for the transversalis fascia and forms part of the floor of the inguinal canal.

21-C *(Campbell's, p. 71)*

Approximately 50 per cent of glomeruli are lost due to arteriolar hyalinization and glomerular sclerosis even without hypertension.

REFERENCE

1. Lindeman, R.D., Tobin, J.D., and Shock, N.W.: Longitudinal studies on the rate of decline in renal function with age. J. Am. Geriatr. Soc., *33*:278, 1985.

22-E *(Campbell's, p. 71)*

In the male, the mesonephric tubules and duct (the former pronephric duct) develop into the efferent ductules of the epididymis, the duct of the epididymis, the ductus deferens, the seminal vesicle, and the ejaculatory duct.

23-B *(Campbell's, p. 72)*

The steepest axial hydraulic pressure drops occur in the afferent and efferent arterioles. No significant pressure drop has been measured along glomerular capillary beds.

24-D *(Campbell's, p. 73)*

The renal cortex receives approximately 90 per cent of the total RBF (5 to 6 ml/minute in the outer cortex), whereas the outer medullary flow is only about 1 ml/minute.

25-C *(Campbell's, p. 74)*

The principal driving force for glomerular filtration is hydrostatic pressure at the glomerular capillary as a consequence of the forces that maintain systemic blood pressure–cardiac output and systemic vascular resistance.

26-B *(Campbell's, p. 76)*

The glomerular filtration barrier is covered by sialoproteins that bear negative charges.

27-C *(Campbell's, p. 77)*

The water permeability in the proximal tubule is high, thus a small osmotic gradient is need. A negative luminal charge is seen in the proximal tubule. This is established by sodium traveling down the concentration gradient from the lumen across the apical (luminal) membrane. A low intracellular sodium concentration is maintained by Na^+, K^+-ATPase pumps on the basal and lateral membranes, representing active transport of sodium into the peritubular space to be resorbed by peritubular capillaries. A positive luminal charge in the distal tubules is thought to be established by active transport of chloride.

REFERENCES

1. Burg, M. D., and Green, N.: Function of the thick ascending limb of Henle's loop. Am. J. Physiol., *224*: 659, 1973.
2. Warnock, D. G., and Eveloff, J: NaCl entry mechanisms in the luminal membrane of the renal tubule. Am. J. Physiol., *242*:F561, 1982.

28-A *(Campbell's, p. 78)*

The initiating signal appears to be tubular fluid chloride and its reabsorption in transport by the cells of the macula densa.

REFERENCES

1. Schuermann, J., Ploth, D.W., and Hermle, M.: Activation of tubuloglomerular feedback by chloride transport. Pflugers Arch., *362*:229, 1976.
2. Wright, F.S., and Briggs, J.P.: Feedback regulation of glomerular filtration rate. Am. J. Physiol., *233*:F1, 1977.

29-D *(Campbell's, p. 78)*

A value lower than 1 per cent favors a prerenal cause, a value above 1 per cent favors a renal etiology. Although fairly specific and sensitive, FE_{Na} % values less than 1 per cent have been reported in a variety of causes of acute renal failure other than prerenal disease (e.g., myoglobinuria or hemoglobinuria, radiocontrast nephropathy, or renal azotemia superimposed on chronic prerenal failure as in hepatic cirrhosis). FE_{Na} % is calculated by the following formula: FE_{Na} % = $C_{Na}/C_{Cr} \times 100$.

REFERENCE

1. Kamel, K.S., Ethier, J.H., Richardson, R.M.A., et al.: Urine electrolytes and osmolality: When and how to use them. Am. J. Nephrol., *10*:89, 1990.

30-B *(Campbell's, p. 78)*

The ascending thick limb of the loop of Henle is impermeable to water. The reabsorption of Cl and Na separates solute from water, and the osmolality of fluid that is leaving this segment is approximately 100 mOsm/kg.

31-C *(Campbell's, p. 78)*

Most water reabsorption during hydropenia occurs in the cortical collecting tubule where hypotonic luminal fluid leaving the loop of Henle equilibrates with the isotonic interstitium of the cortex. The isotonic fluid in the cortical collecting tubule subsequently becomes hypertonic in the medullary collecting duct by osmotic equilibration with the hypertonic medullary interstitium.

32-A *(Campbell's, p. 79)*

Less than 0.1 per cent filtered HCO_3^- (normally 4500 mEq/day) appears in the final urine. Approximately 80 per cent of the filtered HCO_3^- is reclaimed by the addition of HCO_3^- to the peritubular blood as a consequence of H^+ excretion by tubular epithelial cells.

REFERENCE

1. Warnock, D.G., and Rector, F.C., Jr.: Proton secretion by the kidney. Annu. Rev. Physiol., *41*:197, 1979.

33-D *(Campbell's, pp. 79–80)*

Parathormone inhibits proximal HCO_3^- reabsorption

34-C *(Campbell's, p. 80)*

There is no brush border carbonic anhydrase in the collecting duct.

35-B *(Campbell's, pp. 81–83)*

Hypokalemia results from stimulation of the renin-angiotensin-aldosterone (due to volume contraction) axis as well as increased distal Na-K exchange occurring with the increased distal delivery of $NaHCO_3$.

36-C *(Campbell's, p. 83)*

Tubular epithelial cells take up K^+ from the peritubular fluid by a mechanism involving K^+,Na^+-ATPase. This creates an intracellular transport pool of K^+, which can travel down the concentration and electrical gradient (created by distal Na^+ reabsorption) into the luminal fluid. An active transport system may be present, but no evidence for Na^+, K^+ exchange or competition between H^+ and K^+ for tubular secretory pathways exists.

REFERENCES

1. Wright, F.S., and Giebisch, G.: Renal potassium transport: Contributions of individual nephron segments and populations. Am. J. Physiol., *235*:F515, 1978.
2. Giebish, G. and Stanton, B.: Potassium transport in the nephron. Annu. Rev. Physiol., *16*:537, 1979.

37-C *(Campbell's, p. 84)*

Reabsorption of calcium is inhibited by hypermagnesemia.

38-C *(Campbell's, p. 84)*

Most reabsorption of phosphate occurs in the proximal tubule.

39-D *(Campbell's, pp. 84–85)*

Metabolic alkalosis increases citrate excretion by increasing intracellular citrate concentration and inhibiting citrate reabsorption.

40-B *(Campbell's, pp. 85–88)*

ADH acts by binding to membrane receptors on the collecting tubule cell, activating adenylate cyclase and causing the production of cAMP. This results in phosphorylation of luminal membrane proteins and an increase in water permeability.

41-C *(Campbell's, pp. 91–92)*

Erythropoietin is a 36 kDa glycoprotein that is elevated in most amenias. Its production is stimulated by hypoxemia. It stimulates terminal differentiation of erythroid progenitors, increases cellular hemogloblin synthesis, and at high levels causes reticulocytes to enter the circulation prematurely. Greater than 85 per cent of erythropoietin is produced in the cortex and outer medulla.

REFERENCES

1. Sawada, K., Krantz, S.B., Kans, J.S., et al.: Purification of human erythroid colony-forming units and demonstration of specific binding of erythropoietin. J. Clin. Invest., *80*:357–366, 1987.
2. Spivak, J.L.: The mechanism of action of erythropoietin. Inst. J. Cell Cloning, *4*:139–166, 1986.

42-A *(Campbell's, pp. 92–93)*

The primary site of degradation of active renin (circulating half-life of 90 minutes) is the liver.

REFERENCE

1. Koury, S.T., Bondurant, M. C., and Koury, M. J.: Localization of erythropoietin synthesizing cells in murine kidneys by in situ hybridization. Blood, *71*:524–527, 1988.

43-A *(Campbell's, pp. 92–93)*

Juxtaglomerular cells (modified smooth muscle cells) function as renal baroreceptors.

REFERENCE

1. Davis, J.O., and Freeman, R.H.: Mechanisms regulating renin release. Physiol. Rev., *56*:1–56, 1976.

44-C *(Campbell's, p. 93)*

Plasma levels of angiotensinogen are increased in pregnancy, Cushing's syndrome, and patients receiving thyroid or estrogen (birth control pills), but are decreased in cirrhosis of the liver and after adrenalectomy or hepatectomy.

REFERENCES

1. Hiwada, K., Tanaka, H., and Kokubu, T.: The influence of nephrectomy, ureteral ligation and of estradiol on plasma renin substrate in unilaterally nephrectomized rats. Pflugers Arch., *365*:177–182, 1976.
2. Hasegawa, H., Nasjletti, A., Rice, K., and Masson, G.M.C.: Role of pituitary and adrenals in the regulation of plasma angiotensinogen. Am. J. Physiol., *225*: 1–6, 1973.

45-B *(Campbell's, pp. 92–93)*

ACE is a nonspecific enzyme, which also cleaves bradykinin, methenkephalin, substance P, and neurotensin.

REFERENCES

1. Erdos, E.G., and Skidgel, R.A.: The angiotensin I-converting enzyme. Lab. Invest., *56*:345–348, 1986.
2. Ondetti, M.A., and Cushman, D.W.: Enzymes of the renin-angiotensin system and their inhibitors. Annu. Rev. Biochem., *51*:183–308, 1982.

46-C *(Campbell's, pp. 92–94)*

Angiotensin II causes increased sympathetic outflow in the central nervous system.

47-C *(Campbell's, pp. 92–94)*

The role of angiotensin II seems to be designed to maintain glomerular filtration rate. Its preferential site of action is on the efferent arteriole. The vasoconstriction at this site increases intraglomerular pressure.

48-D *(Campbell's, p. 94)*

Angiotensin II receptors are on the surface of many cells, including vascular smooth muscle, adrenal glomerulosa and fasciculata cells, mesangial cells, hepatocytes, and nuclei of the CNS. Binding of the receptors increases phosphoinositide turnover and diglycerol formation, which causes transient calcium flux.

49-A *(Campbell's, pp. 94–95)*

Urinary kallikrein is primarily found in the renal cortex. It is likely synthesized by collecting tubule cells, not the intercalated cells. Angiotensin II, prostaglandins, and mineralocorticoids all stimulate its secretion.

REFERENCE

1. Omata, K., Carretero, O.A., Scicli, A.G., and Jackson, B.A.: Localization of active and inactive kallikrein (kininogenase activity) in the microdissected rabbit nephron. Kidney Inst., *22*:602, 1983.

50-C *(Campbell's, pp. 95–96)*

In animals, the renal 1α-hydroxylase located in the convoluted tubule responds only to parathormone (PTH), whereas that of the pars recta responds only to calcitonin.

REFERENCE

1. Akiba, T., Endou, H., Koseki, C., et al.: Localization of 25-hydroxyvitamin D_3-1α-hydroxylase in the mammalian kidney. Biochem. Biophys. Res. Commun., *94*: 313–318, 1980.

51-A *(Campbell's, pp. 95–96)*

The receptor for 1,25-dihydroxy D_3 has a greater than 1000-fold higher affinity for 1,25-dihydroxy D_3 than 25-hydroxy D_3 and other metabolites.

52-D *(Campbell's, pp. 95–97)*

Hypocalcemia, which induces PTH, causes an increase in 1α-hydroxylase activity, as does phosphorus deprivation.

REFERENCE

1. Portale, A.A., Halloran, B.P., Murphy, M.M., and Morris, R.C., Jr.: Oral intake of phosphorus can determine the serum concentration of 1,25-dihydroxyvitamin D by determining its production rate in humans. J. Clin. Invest., *77*:7-12, 1986.

53-A *(Campbell's, pp. 97–98)*

Both IGF-1 and IGF-2 share approximately 50 per cent homology to proinsulin.

REFERENCES

1. Anderson, G., and Jennische, E.: IGF-1 immunoreactivity is expressed by regenerating renal tubular cells after ischemic injury in the rat. Acta Physiol. Scand., *132*:453–457, 1988.
2. Bortz, J. D., Rotwein, P., DeVol, D., et al.: Focal expression of insulin-like growth factor I in rat kidney collecting duct. J. Cell Biol., *107*:811–819, 1988.

54-B *(Campbell's, pp. 98–99)*

The eicosanoids are derived from 20-carbon fatty acid precursors, including linoleic, arachidonic, and alpha-linolinic acids. Most of the important biologic eicosanoids are derived from arachidonic acid.

REFERENCE

1. Needleman, P., Turk, J., Jakschik, B.A., et al.: Arachidonic acid metabolism. Annu. Rev. Biochem., *55*:69–102, 1986.

55-D *(Campbell's, pp. 100–101)*

Less than 2 per cent of the filtered polypeptide hormones appears in the urine.

56-A *(Campbell's, pp. 101–102)*

The kidney accounts for one third of metabolic clearance of insulin; the remaining 67 per cent is removed by extrarenal organs, mainly the liver and muscles.

57-B *(Campbell's, pp. 102–103)*

The carboxy terminal fragment is exclusively degraded in the kidney by glomerular filtration, whereas the amino terminal fragment relies on filtration and peritubular uptake. Thus, even in patients with markedly decreased GFR, peritubular uptake may provide degradation of the amino terminal fragment.

REFERENCE

1. Hruska, K.A., Kopelman, R., Rutherford, W.E., et al.: Metabolism in immunoreactive parathyroid hormone in the dog: The role of the kidney and the effects of chronic renal disease. J. Clin. Invest., *56*:39–46, 1975.

58-C *(Campbell's, p. 104)*

The kidney accounts for approximately 67 per cent of the total metabolic clearance rate of calcitonin.

REFERENCE

1. Ardaillou, R., and Paillard, F.: Metabolism of polypeptide hormones by the kidney. *In* Hamburger, J., Crosnier, J. Grunfeld, J.-P., and Maxwell, M.H. (Eds.): Advances in Nephrology. Vol. 9, Chicago, Year Book Medical Publishers, 1980, pp. 247–269.

59-C *(Campbell's, pp. 104–105)*

Aldosterone promotes the secretion of hydrogen ion in the medullary collecting tubules.

REFERENCE

1. Stone, D.K., Seldin, D.W., Kokko, J.P., and Jacobsen, H.R.: Mineralocorticoid modulation of rabbit medullary collecting duct acidification. J. Clin. Invest., *72*: 77–83, 1983.

60-D *(Campbell's, pp. 111–114)*

Under normal conditions, the electrical activity initiating peristalsis originates from the pacemaker sites of the proximal urinary collecting system. In species with multiple calyces, the pacemaker cells are found near the pelvic calyceal border.

REFERENCES

1. Bozler, E.: The activity of the pacemaker previous to the discharge of the muscular impulse. Am. J. Physiol., *136*:543, 1942.
2. Constantinou, C.E.: Renal pelvic pacemaker control of ureteral peristaltic rate. Am. J. Physiol., *226*:1413, 1974.
3. Goshing, J.A., and Dixon, J.S.: Species variation in the location of upper urinary tract pacemaker cells. Invest. Urol., *11*:418, 1974.
4. Shiratori, T., and Kinoshita, H.: Electromyographic studies on urinary tract II. Electromyography study on the genesis of peristaltic movement of the dog's ureters. Tohoku J. Exp. Med., *73*:103, 1961a.
5. Tsuchida, S., and Yamaguchi, O.: A constant electrical activity of the renal pelvis correlated to ureteral peristalsis. Tohoku J. Exp. Med., *121*:133, 1977.
6. Weiss, R.M., Wagner, M.L., and Hoffman, B.F.: Localization of pacemaker for peristalsis in the intact canine ureter. Invest. Urol., *5*:42, 1967.
7. Dixon, J.S., and Gosling, J.A.: The fine structure of pacemaker cells in the pig renal calices. Anat. Rec., *175*:139, 1973.

61-A *(Campbell's, p. 112)*

The resting membrane potential (RMP) is primarily determined by K^+, although other ions, including Na^+, Ca^{++}, and possibly Cl^- are felt to have roles.

REFERENCES

1. Bennett, M. R. and Burnstock, G.: Application of the sucrose-gap method to determine the ionic basis of the membrane potential of smooth muscle. J. Physiol. (Lond.), *183*:637, 1966.
2. Hendrickx, H., Vereecken, R. L., and Casteels, R.: The influence of potassium on the electrical and mechanical activity of the guinea pig ureter. Urol. Res., *3*:155, 1975.
3. Washizu, Y.: Grouped discharges in ureter muscle. Comp. Biochem. Physiol., *19*:713, 1966.
4. Kuriyama, H.: The influence of potassium, sodium, and chloride on the membrane potential of the smooth muscle of taenia coli. J. Physiol. (Lond.), *166*:15, 1963.
5. Aickin, C.C.: Investigation of factors affecting the intracellular sodium activity in the smooth muscle of guinea-pig ureter. J. Physiol. (Lond.), *385*:483, 1987.

62-C *(Campbell's pp. 113–114)*

When the ureteral cell is excited, its membrane loses its preferential permeability to K^+ and becomes more permeable to Ca^{++} ions that move inward and give rise to the upstroke of the action potential.

REFERENCES

1. Imaizumi, Y., Muraki, K., and Watanabe, M.: Ionic currents in single smooth muscle cells from the ureter of the guinea pig. J. Physiol. (Lond.), *411*:131, 1989.
2. Kobayashi, M.: Effects Na and Ca on the generation and conduction of excitation in the ureter. Am. J. Physiol., *208*:715, 1965.
3. Kobayashi, M.: Effect of calcium on electrical activity in smooth muscle cells of cat ureter. Am. J. Physiol., *216*:1279, 1969.
4. Vereedcen, R.L., Hendrickx, H., and Casteels, R.: The influence of calcium on the electrical and mechanical activity of the guinea pig ureter. Urol. Res., *3*:149, 1975a.

63-B *(Campbell's p. 116)*

With excitation, there is a transient increase in the sarcoplasmic Ca^{++} concentration from its steady-state concentration of 10^{-8} to 10^{-7} M to a concentration of 10^{-6} or higher.

REFERENCE

1. Watterson, D.M., Harrelson, W.G., Jr., Keller, P.M., et al.: Structural similarities between the Ca^{++}-dependent regulatory proteins of 3′:5′-cyclic nucleotide phosphodiesterase and actomyosin ATPase. J. Biol. Chem., *251*:4501, 1976.

64-D *(Campbell's, pp. 117–118)*

Peristalsis may persist after transplantation or denervation of the ureter, spontaneous activity may occur in isolated in vitro ureteral segments, and normal antegrade peristalsis continues after reversal of segments of ureter in situ. The ureter contains excitatory alpha-adrenergic and inhibitory beta-adrenergic receptors. Norepinephrine increases the force of the induced ureteral contractions due to its primary alpha-adrenergic agonist activity. However, with alpha blockade, norepinephrine has been demonstrated to stimulate beta-adrenergic receptors and thus may decrease the force of ureteral contractions when administered in the presence of phentolamine. Muscarinic cholinergic receptors have been demonstrated in the ureter with receptor binding techniques. Data suggest that cholinergic agonists potentiate ureteral contractility by directly stimulating cholinergic receptors or by indirectly causing the release of catecholamines.

REFERENCES

1. McLeod, D.G., Reynolds, D.G., and Swan, K.G.: Adrenergic mechanisms in the canine ureter. Am. J. Physiol., *224*:1054, 1973.
2. Rose, J.G., and Gillenwater, J.Y.: The effect of adrenergic and cholinergic agents and their blockers upon ureteral activity. Invest. Urol., *11*:439, 1974.
3. Tindall, A.R.: Preliminary observations on the mechanical and electrical activity of the rat ureter. J. Physiol. (Lond.), *223*:633, 1972.
4. Weiss, R.M., Bassett, A.L., and Hoffman, B.F.: Adrenergic innervation of the ureter. Invest. Urol., *16*:123, 1978.
5. Latifpour, J., Morita, T., O'Hollaren, B., et al.: Characterization and autonomic receptors in neonatal urinary tract smooth muscle. Dev. Pharm. Ther., *13*:1, 1989.
6. Katifpour, J., Kondo, S., O'Hollaren, B., et al.: Autonomic receptors in urinary tract: Sex and age differences. J. Pharmacol. Exp. Ther., *253*:661, 1990.

65-B *(Campbell's, pp. 118–119)*

Ureteral resting tension is high at the length at which maximal contractile forces developed. All other statements are true.

REFERENCES

1. Weiss, R.M., Bassett, A.L., and Hoffman, B.F.: Dynamic length-tension curves of cat ureter. Am. J. Physiol., *222*:388, 1972.
2. Vereecken, R.L., Derluyn, J., and Verduyn, H.: The viscoelastic behavior of the ureter during elongation. Urol. Res., *1*:15, 1973.

66-D *(Campbell's, pp. 120–121)*

With increased flow rates, the initial response of the ureter is to increase frequency of contractions, and, after the maximum frequency is achieved, further increases in urine transport occur by means of increase in bolus volume. Coaptation of the ureteral wall is important for the bolus, and pressure generated by the contraction provides a primary component of what is recorded by intraluminal pressure measurements. An increase in the diameter of the ureter can decrease intraluminal pressure and result in inefficient urine transport. Since there is no evidence that the UVJ relaxes the relationship between ureteral intraluminal pressure and intravesical pressure is important in determining the efficacy of urine passage across the UVJ into the bladder.

REFERENCES

1. Griffiths, D.J., and Notschaele, C.: The mechanics of urine transport in the upper urinary tract: I. The dynamics of the isolated bolus. Neurourol. Urodynam., *2*:155, 1983.
2. Griffiths, D.J.: The mechanics of urine transport in the upper urinary tract: 2. The discharge of bolus into the bladder and dynamics at high rates of flow. Neurourol. Urodynam., *2*:167, 1983.
3. Weiss, R.M., and Biancani, P.: Characteristics of normal and refluxing ureterovesical junctions. J. Urol., *129*:858, 1983.
4. Briggs, M.E., Constantinou, C.E., and Govan, D.E.: Dynamics of the upper urinary tract. The relationship of urine flow rate and rate of ureteral peristalsis. Invest. Urol., *10*:56, 1972.
5. Constantinou, C.E., Grenato, J.J., Jr., and Govan, D. E.: Dynamics of the upper urinary tract: Accommodation in the rate and stroke volume of ureteral peristalsis as a response to transient alteration in urine flow rate. Urol. Int., *29*:249, 1974.
6. Morales, P.A., Crowder, C.H., Fishman, A.P., and Maxwell, M.H.: The response of the ureter and pelvis to changing urine flows. J. Urol., *67*:484, 1952.

67-A *(Campbell's, pp. 121–122)*

At low flow rates the frequency of calyceal and renal pelvic contractions is greater than that in the upper ureter, and there is a relative block of electrical activity at the UPJ. At these flows, the renal pelvis fills, and as the renal pelvic pressure rises, urine is extruded into the upper ureter, which is initially in a collapsed state. A closed UPJ may be protective of the kidney in dissipating back pressure from the ureter. As flow rates increase, the block at the UPJ ceases and a 1:1 correspondence between pacemaker and ureteral contractions then develops. Electron microscopic study has demonstrated abnormal intracellular relationships in some specimens of UPJ obstruction, and areas of narrowing and abnormal propagation of peristaltic waves have been implicated in UPJ obstructions.

REFERENCES

1. Morita, T., Ishizuka, G., and Tsuchida, S.: Initiation and progression of stimulus from the renal pelvic pacemaker in pig kidney. Invest. Urol., *19*:157, 1981.
2. Griffiths, D.J., and Notschaele, C.: The mechanics of urine transport in the upper urinary tract: I. The dynamics of the isolated bolus. Neurourol. Urodynam., *2*:155, 1983.
3. Constantinou, C.E., and Hrynczuk, J.R.: Urodynamics of the upper urinary tract. Invest. Urol., *14*:233, 1976.
4. Constantinou, C.E., and Yamaguchi, O.: Multiple-coupled pacemaker system in renal pelvis of the unicalyceal kidney. Am. J. Physiol., *241*:R412, 1981.
5. Hanna, M.K.: Some observations on congenital ureteropelvic junction obstruction. Urology, *12*:151, 1978.

68-D *(Campbell's, p. 123)*

There is evidence that gravity may assist urine transport and that the erect position may aid urine transport across the UVJ, especially in individuals with dilated upper tracts, and this suggests that bed rest may be deleterious to renal function in individuals with urinary retention and wide upper urinary tracts. All other statements are true.

REFERENCES

1. Schick, E., and Tanagho, E. A.: The effect of gravity on ureteral peristalsis. J. Urol., *109*:187, 1973.
2. Weiss, R. M., and Biancani, P.: A rationale for ureteral tapering. Urology, *20*:482, 1982.
3. Blok, C., van Venrooij, G. E. P. M., and Coolsaet, B. L. R. A.: Dynamics of the ureterovesical junction: A qualitative analysis of the ureterovesical pressure profile in the pig. J. Urol., *134*:818, 1985.

69-C *(Campbell's, pp. 123–125)*

The ureteral pressure peaks within a few hours following the onset of obstruction and then declines to a level only slightly higher than the normal baseline pressure. This occurs at a time in which dimensional changes remain stable and is attributed to a decrease in renal blood flow resulting in a decrease in glomerular filtration rate and intratubular hydrostatic pressure. All of the other statements are true.

REFERENCES

1. Biancani, P., Zabinski, M.P., and Weiss, R.M.: Bidimensional deformation of acutely obstructed in vitro rabbit ureter. Am. J. Physiol., *225*:671, 1973.
2. Vereecken, R.L., Derluyn, J., and Verduyn, H.: The viscoelastic behavior of the ureter during elongation. Urol. Res., *1*:15, 1973.
3. Weiss, R.M., Bassett, A.L., and Hoffman, B.F.: Dynamic length-tension curves of cat ureter. Am. J. Physiol., *222*:388, 1972.

70-D *(Campbell's, pp. 126–128)*

The accepted flow rate of 10 ml/min for perfusion studies is a fluid load greater than that expected during usual physiologic states, and it is theorized that if a dilated system can handle this flow rate, then it is not obstructed to such a degree that would require surgical intervention. All the other statements are correct.

REFERENCES

1. Whitaker, R.H.: Methods of assessing obstruction in dilated ureters. Br. J. Urol., *45*:15, 1973.
2. Whitaker, R.H.: Clinical assessment of pelvic and ureteral function. Urology. *12*:146, 1978.
3. Coolsaet, B.L.R.A., Griffiths, D.J., Van Mastrigt, R., and Duyl, W.A.V.: Urodynamic investigation of the wide ureter. J. Urol., *124*:666, 1980.
4. Witfield, H.N., Harrison, N.W., Sherwood, T., and Williams, D.I.: Upper urinary tract obstruction: Pres-

sure flow studies in children. Br. J. Urol., *48*:427, 1976.

71-A *(Campbell's, p. 128)*

An abnormality of the UVJ is a primary etiologic factor in most cases of reflux. Additional etiologic factors may include decreased ureteral activity and inordinately high intravesical pressure, or trigonal abnormality with bladder outlet obstruction or neurogenic bladder.

REFERENCES

1. Tanagho, E.A., Myers, F.H., and Smith, D.E.: The trigone: Anatomical and physiological considerations. 1. In relation to the ureterovesical junction. J. Urol., *100*: 623, 1968.
2. Debruyne, F.M.J., Wijdeveld, P.G.A.B., Koene, R.A.P., et al.: Ureteroneo-cystomy in renal transplantation. Is an antireflux mechanism mandatory? Br. J. Urol., *50*: 378, 1978.

72-C *(Campbell's, pp. 128–129)*

Infection may reduce the compliance of the intravesical ureter and promote reflux to occur in situations in which the UVJ is intrinsically at marginal competence. All of the other statements are true.

REFERENCES

1. Cook, W.A., and King, L.R.: Vesicoureteral reflux. *In* Harrison, J.H., Gittes, R.F., Perimutter, A.D., Stamey, T.A., and Walsh, P.C. (Eds.): Campbell's Urology. 4th ed. Philadelphia, W.B. Saunders Co., 1979, pp. 1596–1634.
2. Rose, J.G., and Gillenwater, J.Y.: Pathophysiology of ureteral obstruction. Am. J. Physiol., *225*:830, 1973.
3. Thulesius, O., and Araj, G.: The effects of uropathogenic bacteria on ureteral motility. Urol. Res., *15*:273, 1987.

73-A *(Campbell's, p. 129)*

Hydrostatic pressure appears important in stone passage and results in an increase in the proximal peristaltic wave frequency and an increase in the baseline peak and delta (peak minus baseline) pressures proximal to the site of obstruction. Distally, the peristaltic rate remains unchanged. Phentolamine, an alpha-adrenergic antagonist, has been shown to increase the flow rate at the site of obstruction and increase the ureteral lumen.

REFERENCES

1. Crowley, A.R., Byrne, J.C., Vaughan, E.D., Jr., and Marion, D.N.: The effect of acute obstruction on ureteral function. J. Urol., *143*:596, 1990.
2. Sivula, A., and Lehtonen, T.: Spontaneous passage of artificial concentrations applied in the rabbit ureter. Scand. J. Urol. Nephrol., *1*:259, 1967.
3. Peters, H.J., and Eckstein, W.: Possible pharmacological means of treating renal colic. Urol. Res., *3*:55, 1975.

74-B *(Campbell's. pp. 129–130)*

A strong case in favor of obstruction as the etiologic factor and the development of hydroureteronephrosis of pregnancy has been presented. These factors include ureteral dilation above but not below the pelvic brim; the lack of hydronephrosis in ureters that do not cross the pelvic brim, such as those in patients with urinary diversion or pelvic kidneys; normal ureteral contractile pressures seen in pregnancy (*all* of these "disfavor" hormonally-induced atony); and, finally, the rarity of hydronephrosis in quadripeds during pregnancy.

REFERENCES

1. Roberts, J.A.: Hydronephrosis of pregnancy. Urology, *8*:1, 1976.
2. Sala, N.L., and Rubi, R.A.: Ureteral function in pregnant women. II. Ureteral contractility during normal pregnancy. Am. J. Obstet. Gynecol., *99*:228, 1967.
3. Traut, H.F., and Kuder, A.: Inflammation of the upper urinary tract complicating the preproductive period of woman. Collective review. Int. Abst. Surg., *67*:568, 1938.

75-A *(Campbell's, p. 130)*

The increase in force that develops between 3 weeks and 3 months of age in the guinea pig model seems to be attributable to an increase in contractility, since there is an associated increase in active stress (force per unit area of muscle). The increase in force that develops between 3 months and 3 years of age can be explained by an increase in mass alone because there is no change in active stress between these two age groups. Although ureteral contractility increases during early development, no significant change is apparent in shortening, velocity, work, or power.

REFERENCES

1. Hong, K.W., Biancani, P., and Weiss, R.M.: Effect of age on contractility of guinea pig ureter. Invest. Urol., *17*:459, 1980.
2. Biancani, P., Onyski, J.H., Zabinski, M.P., and Weiss, R.M.: Force-velocity relationships of the guinea pig ureter. J. Urol., *131*:988, 1984.

76-D *(Campbell's, pp. 131–132)*

Studies have shown that isoproterenol stimulates adenylyl cyclase activity and phosphodiesterase activity. Both of these thus increase the cyclic AMP levels and cause relaxation of ureteral smooth muscle.

REFERENCE

1. Weiss, R.M., Vuliemoz, Y., Verosky, M., et al.: Adenylate cyclase and phosphodiesterase activity in rabbit ureter. Invest. Urol., *15*:15, 1977.

77-C *(Campbell's, pp. 133–136)*

Cholinergic agonists in general have been observed to have a stimulatory effect on ureteral function. Both alpha-adrenergic agonists and progesterone have an inhibitory effect, as do calcium channel blockers.

REFERENCES

1. Barastegui, C.A.: Motility of the rat ureter in vitro. Responses to cholinergic drugs. Rev. Esp. Fisiol., *33*: 1, 1977.
2. Boatman, D.L., Lewin, M.L., Culp, D.A., and Flocks, R.H.: Pharmacologic evaluation of ureteral smooth muscle: A technique of monitoring ureteral peristalsis. Invest. Urol., *4*:509, 1967.
3. Golenhofen, K., and Lammel, E.: Selective suppression of some components of spontaneous activity in various types of smooth muscle by iproveratril (verapamil). Pfluegers Arch., *331*:233, 1972.
4. Hundley, J.M., Jr., Diehl, W.K., and Diggs, E.S.: Hormonal influences upon the ureter. Am. J. Obstet. Gynecol., *44*:858, 1942

78-C *(Campbell's, pp. 142–143)*

Because the mammalian bladder functions as a reservoir for hypertonic urine, it must be impermeable to water. Although apical epithelial cells in the bladder are impermeable to water, they actively transport sodium by means of various channels, including some that are sensitive to aldosterone and others that are not. Distention or urothelial disruption increases the active transport of sodium. Sulfated polysaccharides covering apical cells have been shown to act as an epithelial permeability barrier to small molecules.

REFERENCES

1. Donaldson, P.J., Chen, L.K., and Lewis, S.A.: Effects of serosal axion composition of the permeability properties of rabbit urinary bladder. Am. J. Physiol., *256*: F1125, 1989.
2. Eaton, G.C., Hamilton, K.L., and Johnson, K.E.: Intracellular acidosis blocks the basolateral Na-K pump in rabbit urinary bladder. Am. J. Physiol., *247*:946, 1984.
3. Hanarahan, J.W., Alles, W.P., and Lewis, S.A.: Single anionselective channels in basolateral membrane of a mammalian tight epithelium,. Proc. Natl. Acad. Sci. U.S.A., *82*:7791, 1985.
4. Lewis, S.A.: A reinvestigational of the function of the mammalian urinary bladder. Am. J. Physiol., *232*: F187, 1977.
5. Parsons, C.L., Boychuk, D., Jones, S., et al.: Bladder surface glycosaminoglycans: An epithelial permeability barrier. J. Urol., *143*:139, 1990.

79-B *(Campbell's, p. 145)*

On electron microscopy, slow-twitch myofibrils are observed to have numerous mitochondria, abundant lipid droplets, and wide Z discs compared with fast-twitch fibers. The slow-twitch fibers are fatigue resistant, whereas fast-twitch fibers may be fatigable or fatigue-resistant, depending on the amount of oxidative enzyme activity. Histochemical evidence in humans indicates that striated muscle within the distal urethra is composed primarily of slow-twitch myofibrils in contrast to the periurethral striated muscles of the pelvic floor that contain fast-twitch and slow-twitch fibers.

REFERENCES

1. Padykula, H.A., and Gather, G.F.: The ultrastructure of the neuromuscular junctions of mammalian red, white and intermediate skeletal muscle fibers. J. Cell Biol., *46*:27, 1967.
2. Gosling, J.A., Dixon, J.S., Critchley, O.D., and Thompson, S.A.: A comparative study of the human external sphincter and periurethral levator ani muscles. Br. J. Urol., *53*:35, 1981.

80-A *(Campbell's, pp. 143–144)*

Gap junctions are a class of cellular connections that occur in smooth muscle. They are associated with cells demonstrating electrical coupling. Gap junctions are not found in bladder smooth muscle of humans, but they are present in other species. Although the bladder base does not posses an anatomic sphincter, the predominantly circular orientation of muscle bundles in the deep muscle layer in the bladder base provides a functional basis for its role as a sphincter. Examinations of adult and fetal specimens show that striated and smooth muscles coalesce in the urethra and interdigitate with the fibrous prostatic capsule. The spherical geometry of the bladder maintains a relatively low tension during increases in urine volume, whereas the syncytial arrangement of muscle bundles facilitates complete evacuation.

REFERENCES

1. Wein, A.J., and Barrett, D.B.: Voiding function: Relevant anatomy, physiology, and pharmacology. *In* Gillenwater, J. Y., Howards, S., and Duckett, J. (Eds.): Textbook of Adult and Pediatric Urology, 1987, pp. 880–862.
2. Dixon, J., and Gosling, J.: Structure and innervation of human bladder. *In* Torrens, M., and Morrison J.F.B. (Eds.): The Physiology of the Lower Urinary Tract. Berlin, Springer-Verlag, 1987, pp. 3–22.
3. Oerlich, T.M.: The urethral sphincter muscle in the male. Am. J. Anat., *158*:229, 1980.

81-B *(Campbell's, pp. 145–148)*

It is hypothesized that a Ca^{++}-calmodulin complex binds to a myosin light-chain kinase (MLCK) that phosphorylates the light-chain of myosin. Phosphorylated myosin allows actin to activate a myosin Mg^{++}ATPase that provides the energy for cross-bridging between thick and thin filaments, with subsequent smooth muscle contraction. The influx of Ca^{++} required for activation of the contractile apparatus is regulated by two separate mechanisms—a voltage-sensitive channel and a receptor-operated channel. Three types of voltage sensitive channels have been identified: (1) channels susceptible to classic antagonists, referred to as L channels, (2) small transient current or T channels, and (3) channels found on neurons termed N channels. In addition to the influx of extracellular Ca^{++}, Ca^{++} is released from intracellular stores, such as mitochondria and sarcoplasmic reticulum. This release involves membrane-derived inositol phosphates.

REFERENCES

1. Andersson, K.-E., Fovaeus, M., Hedlund, H., and Sundler, R: Muscarinic receptor stimulation of phosphoinositide hydrolysis in human urinary bladder. J. Urol., *141*:324A, 1989.
2. Mostwin, J.L.: Receptor operated calcium stores in smooth muscle of the guinea pig bladder. J. Urol., *133*: 900, 1985.
3. Miller, R.J.: Multiple calcium channels and neuronal function. Science, *235*:46, 1987.
4. Kamm, K.E., and Stull, J.T.: Regulation of smooth muscle contractile elements by second messengers. Annu. Rev. Physiol., *51*:299, 1989.
5. Kamm, K.E., and Stull, J.T.: The function of myosin and myosin light chain kinase phosphorylation in smooth muscle. Annu. Rev. Pharmacol. Toxicol., *25*: 593, 1985.

82-D *(Campbell's, p. 148)*

Smooth muscle maintains tone with relatively little expenditure of energy. Studies have shown that a linear relationship exists between force and metabolism in bladder smooth muscle. ATP generated from aerobic glycolysis and glucose metabolism provides the energy required for a bladder contraction. The rate of energy expenditure to develop a bladder contraction is only one half that associated with maintenance of an active contraction.

REFERENCES

1. Wendt, I.R., and Gibbs, C.L.: Energy expenditure of longitudinal smooth muscle of rabbit urinary bladder. Am. J. Physiol., *252*:C88–C96, 1987.
2. Levin, R.M., Haugaard, N., Ruggieri, M.R., and Wein, A.J.: Biochemical characterization of the rabbit urinary bladder. J. Urol., *137*:782, 1987.

83-A *(Campbell's, pp. 147–148)*

The contractions of striated muscles are regulated by the rapid Ca^{++} influx by the T-tubule which is responsible for the disinhibition of tropomyosin. The ultrastructure reveals the sarcomere pattern and no evidence of intermediate filaments. These are seen, however, in smooth muscle cells.

REFERENCES

1. Brading, A.: Physiology of bladder smooth muscle. *In* Torrens, M., and Morrison, J.F.B. (Eds.): The Physiology of the Lower Urinary Tract. Berlin, Springer-Verlag, 1987, pp. 161–191.
2. Tao, T., Gonj., B.-J., and Leavis, P.C.: Calcium-induced movement of troponin ± relative to actin in skeletal muscle thin filaments. Science, 247:1339, 1990.

84-B *(Campbell's, pp. 149–150)*

Striated muscle of the external urethral sphincter is innervated by the pudendal nerve that contains motor axons from the second, third, and fourth segments of the sacral spinal cord. The somatic motoneurons are located anterior to bladder preganglionics in a region termed Onuf's nucleus. Cells within Onuf's nucleus are unique and their properties more closely resemble autonomic neurons than other somatic motoneurons within the spinal cord. For example, Onuf's nucleus is spared in amyotrophic lateral sclerosis, which impairs somatic muscle function, but is affected in an autonomic neuropathy known as Shy-Drager syndrome.

REFERENCES

1. Beattie, M.S., Li, Q., Leedy, M.G., and Bresnahan, J.C.: Motoneurons innervating the external anal and urethral sphincters of the female cat have different patterns of dendritic arborization. Neurosci. Lett., *111*: 69, 1990.
2. Sakuta, M., Nakanishi, T., and Toyokura, Y.: Anal muscle electromyography difference in amyotrophic lateral sclerosis and Shy-Drager syndrome. Neurology, *28*:1289, 1978.

85-B *(Campbell's, pp. 149–150)*

Parasympathetic preganglionic perikarya and their dendrites are organized in a viscerotropic manner within the sacral spinal cord. A viscerotropic configuration probably represents a mechanism for coordinating visceral and somatic function during voiding, defecation, penile erection, ejaculation, and lower limb movement. The sacral preganglionic axons projecting to the bladder are conveyed by the pelvic nerve, which also contains postganglionic sympathetic fibers from the chain ganglia. Synaptic connections between axons in the pelvic nerve and ganglion cells innervating the bladder occur in the pelvic plexus and on the surface of the bladder in humans. The sympathetic fibers that enter the pelvic plexus may interact with sacral parasympathetic pathways or with postganglionic neurons from the sympathetic chain. The hypogastric plexus lies on the great vessels at the level of the third lumbar to first sacral vertebrae and gives rise to the left and right hypogastric nerves.

REFERENCE

1. Keast, J.F., and De Groat, W.C.: Immunocytochemical characterization of pelvic neurons which project to the bladder, colon, or penis in rats. J. Comp. Neurol., *288*: 387, 1989.

86-D *(Campbell's, pp. 150–152)*

Nicotinic ganglionic blockers abolish contractions of the bladder produced by electrical stimulation of the pelvic nerve. It is noted that in patients with idiopathic hypertonic bladders, acetylcholinesterase staining is reduced, and this finding has been interpreted as a reduction of cholinergic innervation. Activation of muscarinic receptors on adrenergic terminals in the bladder and urethra inhibit norepinephrine release and therefore can influence transmitter release as well as the contractility of bladder smooth muscle. Cholinergic innervation to the urethra is supported by histochemical identification of acetylcholinesterase staining fibers and this finding has lead to the assumption that efferent stimulation produces urethral relaxation. However, cholinergic agonists do not produce relaxation of the urethra when given in vivo and actually may produce a very weak contraction, thus providing evidence that parasympathetic pathways mediating urethral relaxation rely on a noncholinergic transmitter.

REFERENCES

1. Ek, A., Alan, P., Hendersson, K.E., and Persson, C.G.: Adrenergic and cholinergic nerves of the human urethra and urinary bladder: A histochemical study. Acta Physiol. Scand., *99*:345, 1987.
2. Yalla, S.V., Rossier, A.B., Fam, B.A., et al.: Functional contribution of autonomic innervation to urethral striated sphincter: Studies with parasympathomimetic, parasympatholytic, and alpha-adrenergic blocking agents in spinal cord injury and control male subjects. J. Urol., *117*:494, 1977.
3. Mattiasson, A., Andersson, K.-E., Elbadawi, A., et al.: Interaction between adrenergic and cholinergic nerve terminals in the urinary bladder of rabbit, cat, and man. J. Urol., *137*:1017, 1987.
4. Learmonth, J.R.: A contribution to the neurophysiology of the urinary bladder in man. Brain, *54*:147, 1931.
5. Kinn, A.-C., Alm, P., Lundgren, G., and Negardh, A.: Changes in cholinergic innervation and neuropharmacological properties in idiopathic hypotonic urinary bladders. Scand. J. Urol. Nephrol., *21*:17, 1987.

87-B *(Campbell's, pp. 152–154)*

Adrenergic innervation in the human bladder and urethra compared to that of other species is sparse and limited to the bladder base and proximal urethra. Estrogens increase the response of urethral tissues to alpha-adrenergic agonists in vitro, and some clinicians combined these agents in vivo in order to elevate urethral pressure in patients with stress incontinence. However, the clinical efficacy of this method has been questioned. Although propanolol increases urethral pressure after sacral root stimulation, unfortunately, beta-adrenergic antagonists are not clinically useful in treating bladder or urethral disorders. Sympathetic pathways appear to play a minor role in normal lower urinary tract function. However, denervation, decentralization, and smooth muscle hypertrophy trigger changes in adrenergic mechanisms that regulate the bladder and urethra; that is, there is up-regulation of cholinergic receptors in the bladder and urethra in response to injury.

REFERENCES

1. Castleden, C.M., and Morgan, B.: The effect of beta-adrenoceptor agonists on urinary incontinence in the elderly. Br. J. Clin. Pharmacol., *10*:619, 1980.
2. Naglo, A.S., Negardh, A., and Boreus, L.O.: Influence of atropine and isoprenaline on detrusor hyperactivity in children with neurogenic bladder. Scand. J. Urol. Nephrol., *15*:97, 1981.
3. Walter, S., Wolfe, H., Barlebo, H., et al.: Urinary incontinence in post-menopausal women treated with estrogens: A double blind clinical trial. Urol. Int., *33*: 135, 1978.
4. Wilson, P.D., Faraher, B., and Butler, B.: Treatment with piperazine oestrone sulphate for genuine stress incontinence in postmenopausal women. Br. J. Obstet. Gynaecol., *84*:568 1987.
5. Benson, G.S., McConnell, J.A., and Wood, J.G.: Adrenergic innervation of the human bladder body. J. Urol., *122*:189, 1979.
6. Ek, A., Alan, P., Hendersson, K.E., and Persson, C.G.: Adrenergic and cholinergic nerves of the human urethra and urinary bladder: A histochemical study. Acta Physiol. Scand., *99*:345, 1977.
7. Kluck, P.: The autonomic innervation of the human urinary bladder, bladder neck, and urethra, a histochemical study. Anat. Rec., *198*:439, 1980.
8. Sundin, T., Dahlstrom, A., Norlen, L., and Svedmyr, N.: The sympathetic innervation and adrenoreceptor function of the human lower urinary tract in the normal state and after parasympathetic denervation. Invest. Urol., *14*:322, 1977.

88-C *(Campbell's, p. 154)*

Purinergic substances have been shown to inhibit excitatory cholinergic transmission in the vesical ganglia. Purine antagonists such as theophylline and caffeine block the inhibition of excitatory cholinergic transmission in the vesical ganglia. Purine nucleotides and nucleosides have been identified by histochemical techniques. Electrical stimulation of the pelvic nerve produces a biphasic contraction. The initial portion of the contraction is mediated by purines, and the second component is cholinergic.

REFERENCES

1. Senba, E., Daddona, P.F., and Nagy, J.I.: A subpopulation of preganglionic parasympathetic neurons in the rat containing adenosine deaminase. Neuroscience, *20*: 487, 1987.
2. Aksau, T., Shinnick-Gallagher, P., and Gallagher, J.P.: Adenosine mediates a slow hyperpolarizing synaptic potential in autonomic neurones. Nature, 311:62, 1984.
3. Theobold, R.J. and de Groat, W.C.: The effects of purine nucleotides on transmission in vesical parasympathetic ganglia of the cat. J. Auton. Pharmacol., *9*: 167, 1989.

89-A *(Campbell's, pp. 154–155)*

Neuropeptides are co-localized with traditional transmitters. The release of neuropeptides from nerves is frequency-dependent, and the neuropeptides potentially released from postganglionic nerves supplying the bladder or urethra affect smooth muscle contractility. The specificity of the source of neuropeptides make them potential markers for tracing pathways that could be clinically useful because some substances are exclusively found in efferent pathways, whereas others are confined to afferent pathways.

REFERENCES

1. Dail, W.G., Minorsky, N., Moll, M.A., Manzanares, K.: The hypogastric nerve pathway to penile erectile tissue and histochemical evidence supporting a vasodilatory role. J. Auton. Nerv. Syst., *15*:341, 1986.

2. Schmidt, R.A.: Advances in genitourinary neurostimulation. Neurosurgery, *18*:1041, 1986.
3. Tanagho, E.A., Schmidt, R.A., and Orivs, B.R.: Neural stimulation for control of voiding dysfunction: Preliminary report in 22 patients with serious neuropathic voiding disorders. J. Urol., *142*:340, 1989.
4. de Groat, W.C., and Kawatani, M.: Neural control of the urinary bladder: Possible relationship between peptidergic inhibitory mechanisms and detrusor instability. Neurourol. Urodynam. *4*:285, 1984.

90-D *(Campbell's, pp. 155–156)*

Gamma-aminobutyric acid (GABA) has been associated with small intensely fluorescent (SIF) cells as well as serotonin (5-HT). 5-HT has been shown primarily to inhibit cholinergic transmission in pelvic ganglia. It has also been shown to contract the bladder body and relax the bladder neck.

REFERENCES

1. Karhula, T., Happola, O., Joh, T., and Wu, J.-Y.: Localization of L-glutamate decarboxylase immunoreactivity in the major pelvic ganglion and in the coeliac-superior mesenteric ganglion complex of the rat. Histochemistry, *90*:255, 1988.
2. Nishimura, T., Yoshida, M., Nagatsu, I., and Akasu, T.: Frequency-dependent inhibition of nicotinic transmission by serotonin in vesical pelvic ganglia of the rabbit. Neurosci. Lett., *103*:179, 1989.
3. Erspamer, V., Ronzoni, G., and Erspamer, F.: Effects of active peptides on the isolated muscle of the human urinary bladder. Invest. Urol., *18*:302, 1981.
4. Hills, J., Meldrum, L., and Klarskov, P.: A novel non-adrenergic, non-cholinergic nerve mediated relaxation of the pig bladder neck: An examination of possible neurotransmitter candidates. Eur. J. Pharmacol., *99*: 287, 1984.

91-A *(Campbell's, p. 156)*

Visceral afferents are capable of local transmitter release, which influences cellular components of the immune system, vascular permeability, smooth muscle contractility, and neural transmission. Afferent nerves to the bladder travel in sympathetic and parasympathetic pathways. Afferents in the pelvic nerve respond to bladder distention in the graded fashion. Bladder afferents respond primarily to tension rather than to bladder volume.

REFERENCES

1. de Groat, W.C.: Neuropeptides in pelvic afferent pathways. Experientia, *43*:801, 1987.
2. Maggi, C.A., and Meli, A. The role of neuropeptides in the regulation of the micturition reflex. J. Auton. Pharmacol, *6*:133, 1986.
3. Iggo, A.: Tension receptors in the stomach and the urinary bladder. J. Physiol. (Lond.), *128*:593, 1955.
4. McMahon, S.B.: Sensory-motor integration in urinary bladder function. *In* Cervero, F., and Morrison, J.F.B. (Eds.): Visceral Sensation. Amsterdam, Elsevier Science Publ., 1986, pp. 245–283.
5. Janig, W., and Morrison, J.F.B.: Functional properties of spinal visceral afferents supplying abdominal and pelvic organs, with special emphasis on visceral nociception. *In* Cervero, F., and Morrison, J.F.B. (Eds.): Visceral Sensation. Amsterdam, Elsevier Science Publications, 1986, pp. 87–114.

92-A *(Campbell's, pp. 156–157)*

The intravesical pressure thresholds for A-delta afferents range from 5 to 15 mm Hg, corresponding to pressures at which humans sense filling on a cystometrogram. Frequency in coding has been proposed as a mechanism to distinguish tension from nociceptive input. Alternatively, some afferent neurons of the bladder may be unimodal and achieve specificity by varying the frequency of firing or the type of chemical transmitter. Lightly myelinated (A-delta) fibers conduct rapidly up to 30 meters/second, whereas unmyelinated fibers (C-fiber) conduct much more slowly at approximately 0.3 meters/second. Pacinian corpuscles are rarely seen in the bladder, whereas free nerve endings in the bladder wall are felt to represent afferent terminals.

REFERENCES

1. Abrams, P., Fineley, R., and Torrens, M.J.: Urodynamics. Berlin, Springer-Verlag, 1983, p. 229.
2. Fletcher, T.F., and Bradley, W.D.: Afferent nerve endings in the urinary bladder of the cat. Am. J. Anat., *128*:147, 1968.
3. de Groat, W.C.: Nervous control of the urinary bladder in the cat. Brain Res., *87*:201, 1975.

93-A *(Campbell's, p. 160)*

During voiding, hypogastric neurons are inhibited. Voiding results when mechanoreceptors in the bladder respond to threshold tension. Central mechanisms are organized as a simple on-off switching circuit with a reciprocal relationship between the bladder and its outlet. Organization of central neuronal pathways allow the bladder to empty completely with low voiding pressure.

REFERENCES

1. de Groat, W.C.: Nervous control of the urinary bladder in the cat. Brain Res., *87*:201, 1975.
2. de Groat, W.C., and Steers, W.D.: Autonomic regulation of the urinary bladder and sexual organs. In Loewy, A.D., and Spyer, K.M. (Eds.): Central Regulation of the Autonomic Functions. Oxford, Oxford University Press, 1990, pp. 313–333.
3. Kuru, M.: Nervous control of micturition. Physiol. Rev., *45*:425, 1965.
4. Morrison, J.F.B.: Reflex control of the lower urinary tract. *In* Torrens, M., and Morrison, J.F.B. (Eds.): The Physiology of the Urinary Bladder. Berlin, Springer-Verlag, 1987a, pp. 194–235.
5. Iggo, A.: Tension receptors in the stomach and the urinary bladder. J. Physiol. (Lond.), *128*:593, 1955.
6. Garry, R.C., Roberts, T.D.M., and Todd, J.K.: Reflexes involving the external urethral sphincter in the cat. J. Physiol. (Lond.), *149*:653, 1959.
7. Okada, H., Yamane, M., and Orchi, K.: The reciprocal activity between the pelvic nerves and external ure-

thral sphincter muscles during micturition reflex in the dog. J. Auton. Nerv. Syst., *12*:178, 1975.

94-C *(Campbell's, pp. 160–163)*

Anterolateral cordotomies performed for chronic pain reveal that ascending routes responsible for transmitting bladder sensation and that trigger voiding travel in the lateral spinothalamic tract. Lesioning studies have shown that destruction of the neuraxis above the pons does not eliminate involuntary micturition. However, voluntary voiding in humans is abolished when connections between the frontal lobe hypothalamus or paralobule and brain stem are destroyed. A spinobulbospinal micturition pathway that passes through the pons is responsible for micturition in the intact individual. Voiding following spinal cord transection results from a reorganization of spinal micturition reflex pathways. The roles of the basal ganglion, parietal frontal cortex, and cerebellum in micturition have been inferred from urodynamic studies following selective lesioning, cerebellar vascular accident, epilepsy, intracranial aneurysms, and tumors. Excitatory inhibitory effects have been described from many sites within the brain; however, the net effect of a lesion rostral to the pons is often hyperactivity of the bladder.

REFERENCES

1. Barnett, H.I., and Hyland, H.H.: Tumors involving the brain stem. Q. J. Med., *21*:265, 1952.
2. Tshida, S., Noto, H., Yamaguchi, O., and Itoh, M.: Urodynamic studies on hemiplegic patients after cerebrovascular accident. Urology, *21*:315, 1983.
3. Zhan, A.: Predictive correlation of urodynamic dysfunction and brain injury after cerebrovascular accident. J. Urol., *126*:86, 1981.
4. Nathan, P.W.: The central nervous connectives of the bladder. *In* Williams, D.I., and Chisholm, G.D. (Eds.): Scientific Foundations of Urology. London, Heineman, 1976, pp. 51–58.
5. Nathan, P.W., and Smith, M.C.: The centrifugal pathway for micturition within the spinal cord. J. Neurol. Neurosurg. Psychiatry, *21*:177, 1958.
6. Pool, J.L.: The visceral brain of man. J. Neurosurg., 11:45, 1954.
7. de Groat, W.C., and Steer, W.D.: Autonomic regulation of the urinary bladder and sexual organs. *In* Loewy, A.D., and Spyer, K.M. (Eds.): Central Regulation of the Autonomic Functions. Oxford, Oxford University Press, 1990, pp. 313–333.
8. Thor, K., Kawatani, M., and de Groat, W.C.: Plasticity in reflex pathways to the lower urinary tract of the cat during postnatal development and following spinal cord injury. *In* Goldberger, A.G., and Murray, M. (Eds.): Development and Plasticity of the Mammalian Spinal Cord. Padova, Liviana Press, 1986, pp. 65–80.

95-B *(Campbell's, p. 163)*

Urodynamic and electromyographic (EMG) data indicate that a rise in maximal urethral pressure corresponds to increased EMG activity of the striated muscles of the pelvic floor. Pudendal motoneuron firing occurs when the bladder is filled near capacity or following a sudden increase in intravesical pressure. This phenomenon has been termed the "guarding" or continence reflex and represents a somatic mechanism for increasing urethral resistance.

96-C *(Campbell's, pp. 164–167)*

Data suggest that urine storage may be facilitated or inhibited by cholinergic neurons in supraspinal centers primarily. Due to the development of tolerance with continuous intrathecal morphine administration, it is not effective in the treatment of detrusor hyperreflexia, although initially it does significantly suppress bladder activity and increase external urethral sphincter function. Dopamine has not been shown to facilitate voiding, whereas electrical stimulation of serotonin neurons in the raphe nuclei inhibit rhythmic bladder activity.

REFERENCES

1. Herman R.M., Coombs, D.W., Saunders, R., and Wellscher, M.D.: Intrathecal clonidine induces inhibition of micturation reflexes and spasticity in spinal cord patients made tolerant to spinal morphine. Abstr. Soc. Neurosci., 14:537, 1988.
2. Benson, G.S., Wein, A.J., Raezer, D.M., and Corriere, J.N.: Adrenergic and cholinergic stimulation and blockade of the human bladder base. J. Urol., *116*: 174, 1976.
3. Christmas, T.J., Chapple, C.R., Kempster, P.A., et al.: The role of subcutaneous apomorphine in the treatment of parkinsonian voiding dysfunction. J. Urol., *141*:327A, 1989.
4. Ryall, R.W., and de Groat, W.C.: The microiontophoretic administration of noradrenaline, 5-hydroxytryptamine, acetylcholine, and glycine on parasympathetic preganglionic neurones. Brain Res., *37*:345, 1972.

97-D *(Campbell's, pp. 167–169)*

Bladder outlet obstruction has been associated with neuroanatomic and electrophysiologic changes in the central and peripheral neuropathways in response to partial urethral obstruction in the rat. It has also been shown to induce hypertrophy of afferent and efferent neurons and increased labeling of afferent spinal projections in experimental models. There is evidence of an increase in adrenergic fibers following decentralization as well as in a peripheral nerve injury. After supraspinal cord transection, micturition is initially lost but is reestablished weeks to months later. Paraplegics are sometimes able to exploit a somatobladder reflex for "trigger voiding." This is seen in many newborn animals where the mother stimulates micturition by licking or stimulating the perineum, and if this is not performed these neonatal animals will go into urinary retention. This reflex is lost as the neonate matures.

REFERENCES

1. Thor, K., Kawatani, M., and de Groat, W.C.: Plasticity in reflex pathways to the lower urinary tract of the cat during postnatal development and following spinal cord injury. *In* Goldberg, A.G., and Murray, M. (Eds.): Development and Plasticity of the Mammalian Spinal Cord. Padova, Liviana Press, 1986, pp. 65–80.

2. Elbadawi, A., and Atta, M.A., and Hanno, A.: Intrinsic neuromuscular defects in the neurogenic bladder: VII. Effects of unilateral pelvic and pelvic plexus neurectomy on ultrastructure of the feline bladder base. Neurol. Urodynam., *7*:77, 1988.
3. Dundin, T., Dahlstrom, A., Norlen, L., and Svedmyr, N.: The sympathetic innervation and adrenoreceptors function of the human lower urinary tract in the normal state and after parasympathetic denervation. Invest. Urol., *14*:322, 1977.
4. Steers, W.D.: Future of neurourology. *In* Future of Urology Symposium. Orlando, FL, American Urological Association, January 1989. pp. 157–173.
5. Steers, W.D., and de Groat, W.C.: Effect of bladder outlet obstruction on micturition reflex pathways in the rat. J. Urol., *140*:864, 1988.

98-B *(Campbell's, p. 177)*

GnRH is transmitted from the hypothalamus to the pituitary by a portal system, i.e., a system of vessels that begins with venules and ends in venules. This portal system connects the hypothalamus with the pituitary.

99-D *(Campbell's, pp. 177, 180)*

GnRH stimulates synthesis and release from the pituitary of both FSH and LH, which are secreted into the general circulation and carried to the testis.

100-C *(Campbell's, p. 180)*

GnRH is released into the portal circulation in pulses occurring every 70 to 90 minutes. GnRH has a very short half-life of 2–5 minutes. Paradoxically, continuous exposure of the pituitary to GnRH results in inhibition of LH and FSH release, a fact that has been exploited therapeutically by use of GnRH analogues as treatment for prostate cancer.

101-A *(Campbell's, p. 181)*

LH, FSH, TSH, and HCG share a common alpha-peptide chain, and differ from each other in the structure of their beta subunits. Production of HCG-like substance by neoplasms like testicular choriocarcinoma is detected by use of the beta-HCG assay, which measures the beta subunit of HCG, and does not cross-react with LH.

102-C *(Campbell's, p. 184)*

LH acts via a specific receptor on Leydig cells to promote testosterone production. FSH may indirectly affect testosterone synthesis through its action on Sertoli cells and on spermatogenesis.

103-A *(Campbell's, pp. 183, 186)*

FSH is thought to be partly controlled by a negative feedback loop involving inhibin, a peptide produced by Sertoli cells in the germinal epithelium. Decreased inhibin formation in conditions associated with germinal epithelial defects leads to increased FSH.

104-E *(Campbell's, p. 191)*

The blood supply to the testis and epididymis is derived from the internal spermatic artery arising from the aorta, the artery to the vas deferens arising from the inferior vesical artery, and the external spermatic or cremasteric artery.

105-D *(Campbell's, p. 193)*

Testosterone synthesis begins when cholesterol is transported to the mitochondria where it is acted on by cholesterol side-chain cleavage enzymes to form pregnenolone. Pregnenolone is transported to the endoplasmic reticulum where it is converted into testosterone. Testosterone diffuses across the cell membrane and is trapped in blood by testosterone-binding globulin.

106-D *(Campbell's, pp. 197, 198)*

The blood testis barrier is formed primarily by tight junctions between Sertoli cells that subdivide the seminiferous epithelium into basal, intermediate, and adluminal compartments. Developing spermatocytes are isolated for a time in the intermediate compartment by Sertoli-Sertoli cell tight junctions that are located both above and below. When the tight junctions located above the spermatocytes break down, the spermatocytes enter the adluminal compartment.

107-D *(Campbell's, p. 201)*

The entire process of spermatogenesis in man requires approximately 64 days. Type A spermatogonia divide at intervals of 16 days to form type B spermatogonia, which will divide to form primary spermatocytes, located in the adluminal compartment behind the blood-brain barrier. Primary spermatocytes undergo meiosis to form spermatids, which then mature gradually into spermatocytes.

108-C *(Campbell's, pp. 201, 202)*

The primary hormonal regulation of spermatogenesis is by testosterone, which probably acts via an effect on the Sertoli cell. FSH appears to have little effect on the maintenance of spermatogenesis, but probably plays a role in initiation of spermatogenesis at puberty and reinitiation of spermatogenesis in hypophysectomized animals after complete regression of the germinal epithelium.

109-A *(Campbell's, p. 206)*

Spermatozoa are immotile in the epididymis and depend for transport through the ductal system on other mechanisms like the flow of rete testis fluid into the epididymis facilitated by resorption of water by epithelial cells, motile cilia, and rhythmic contraction of cells surrounding the epididymal duct.

110-D *(Campbell's, pp. 208, 210)*

The ability to fertilize eggs is gradually acquired as spermatozoa migrate to the distal epididymal duct in the cauda epididymidis. Complex molecular and biochemical changes are involved in this maturation. Some clinical experience, however, such as fertility achieved after vasoepididymostomy to the level of the caput epididymidis and in vitro fertilization using spermatozoa from the caput epididymidis suggest that some maturation is possible without completely transecting the ductal epididymidis.

111-C *(Campbell's, p. 212)*

The axoneme, in the middle, principal, and end pieces of the spermatozoa, consists of nine peripheral and two central microtubules. Outer dense fibers rich in disulfide bonds surround the axoneme in the middle and principal pieces and provide the rigidity necessary for progressive motility.

112-B *(Campbell's, pp. 213–214)*

Although nerves from both the sympathetic and parasympathetic systems supply the vas deferens, only the sympathetic innervation is of significance. During sexual stimulation adrenergic neurotransmitters cause propulsion of spermatozoa from the cauda epididymidis and proximal ductus deferens into the urethra, along with the secretions from the seminal vesicles and prostate that make up seminal fluid.

113-B *(Campbell's, p. 226)*

The peripheral zone is the largest anatomic subdivision of the prostate and contains 75 per cent of the total glandular tissue. Almost all carcinomas arise in this region, and it is the site sampled in most random biopsies.

114-E *(Campbell's, p. 227)*

The transition zone arises from a small group of ducts, arising at a single point at the junction of the proximal and distal urethral segments of the prostatic urethra. The transition zone and other periurethral glands are the exclusive site of origin of benign prostatic hyperplasia. At times, adenocarcinoma can arise from the transition zone.

115-D *(Campbell's, pp. 226, 227)*

The preprostatic tissue consists of a cylinder of smooth muscle surrounding the anterior-directed prostatic urethra proximal to the verumontanum, which acts as a sphincter during ejaculation to prevent seminal fluid from entering the bladder. Periurethral glands within the area surrounded by the sphincter make up about 1 per cent of prostate glandular tissue and can grow proximally toward the bladder neck.

116-C *(Campbell's, p. 228)*

Alpha$_1$-adrenergic receptors are found on smooth muscle cells in the prostate and appear to be involved in the mechanism that closes the proximal prostatic urethra to prevent retrograde passage of seminal fluid during ejaculation. Long-acting alpha$_1$-adrenergic blockers like terazosin have been used clinically to decrease smooth muscle tone in the prostate and improve voiding in men with BPH.

117-D *(Campbell's, pp. 230–235)*

Estrogen activates the negative feedback mechanism that stops LH release from the pituitary, thereby stopping testosterone production by the Leydig cells. Estrogen may also reduce free testosterone levels by increasing testosterone binding globulin. There may also be some direct action of estrogen on prostate cells.

118-A *(Campbell's, pp. 250–251)*

Androgen withdrawal appears to initiate a chain of events within prostate cells, including the synthesis of specific proteins and the influx of calcium that activates calcium-dependent DNAase, which is called programmed cell death. Apoptosis is a name given for the formation of a clear zone in the perinuclear area seen early in programmed cell death.

119-C *(Campbell's pp. 251–253, 256)*

The first fraction of the ejaculate is rich in spermatozoa and prostatic secretions. Seminal vesicle secretions make up later fractions of the ejaculate. Prostaglandins, despite the origin of their name, are secreted primarily by the seminal vesicle. Semenogelin is a seminal vesicle product important in clotting of the ejaculate. In men with higher than normal volumes of ejaculate and resultant low sperm concentration, use of the split ejaculate technique (penile withdrawal after the first part of ejaculation) may result in higher concentrations of spermatozoa in the seminal fluid and improved fertility.

120-D *(Campbell's, pp. 253–254)*

Zinc levels are decreased in prostate cancer tissue. Zinc may play a protective bactericidal role in prostatic fluid; zinc levels have been found to be decreased in prostatic fluid from patients with prostatitis.

121-C *(Campbell's, p. 255)*

Although development of PSA has reduced interest in the use of acid phosphatase as a marker for prostate cancer, it can still be clinically useful in some circumstances. Measuring acid phosphatase at the time of original diagnosis of prostate cancer may aid in staging, since an elevated level almost always means metastatic disease. The acid phosphatase found in the prostate is inhibited by tartrate and fluoride, and thymolphthalein is the optimal synthetic substrate. Use of these laboratory assay methods can help distinguish acid phosphatase elevations of prostate origin from other causes of elevation, for example, Paget's disease.

122-E *(Campbell's, p. 257)*

Fructose is produced in the seminal vesicles. Men with congenital absence of the seminal vesicles and vas deferens, one cause of azoospermia, will not have fructose in the semen. The simple office laboratory test for fructose should be done for all men with azoospermia. Obstruction of the ejaculatory ducts will also cause azoospermia and absence of fructose.

123-A *(Campbell's, p. 258)*

Nitrofurantoin is not a useful antibiotic for prostate infection because it does not achieve useful levels in prostate secretions. Drugs like erythromycin, tetracycline, sulfonamides, chloramphenicol, and trimethoprim appear to be trapped in prostate fluid by a process of pH-dependent ionization. Drugs with basic pK are ionized in the acidic environment of prostatic fluid and not able to diffuse back across the prostate cell membrane. This mechanism is complex, however, since prostate fluid may have a more basic pH when inflammation is present.

124-B *(Campbell's, pp. 268–270)*

In RNA, uracil replaces thymine. Both RNA and DNA have five-carbon sugars; deoxyribose in DNA and ribose in RNA.

125-A *(Campbell's, p. 268)*

Transcription refers to production of messenger RNA and translation to the conversion of messenger RNA nucleotide sequences into protein amino acids.

126-C *(Campbell's, p. 272)*

The purpose of the noncoding sequences known as introns remains unclear. Exons are the coding sequences of genes.

127-E *(Campbell's, p. 272)*

Retroviral particles, such as HIV, use reverse transcriptase to construct DNA from their RNA genome.

128-B *(Campbell's, pp. 272–274)*

Anticodon nucleotide triplets on transfer RNA molecules specific for each amino acid are complementary to messenger RNA codons and help determine proper sequencing of amino acids during protein synthesis in the ribosomes.

129-C *(Campbell's, p. 276)*

Current theories of carcinogenesis hold that proto-oncogenes normally controlling proteins involved in signal transduction are altered to become oncogenes, resulting in malignancy.

130-A *(Campbell's, pp. 277–279)*

Polymerase chain reaction refers to the technique of amplification of DNA by chemical proliferation, rather than by biologic replication in a host cell, as in molecular cloning.

131-B *(Campbell's, p. 285–286)*

DNA linkage analysis using polymorphic markers located near the gene for autosomal dominant polycystic kidney disease on chromosome 16 can detect this disease with 95 per cent accuracy.

132-C *(Campbell's, p. 286)*

An abnormality in a gene for the androgen receptor on the long arm of the X chromosome causes an abnormality in the steroid-binding region of the receptor protein that leads to androgen insensitivity.

133-E *(Campbell's, pp. 289–290)*

The testis-determining factor gene apparently encodes a DNA-binding protein that regulates transcription, resulting eventually in Sertoli cell formation from cells that would be follicle cells in the ovary.

134-A *(Campbell's, p. 290)*

Discovery of transduction in the case of the Rous sarcoma virus led to the concept of proto-oncogenes and oncogenes.

135-D *(Campbell's, p. 291)*

Hypomethylation of proto-oncogene cytosine residues is thought to result in increased transcription of genes and has been correlated with the stage and grade of bladder cancer.

136-A *(Campbell's, pp. 291–292)*

Point mutations in the *ras* proto-oncogene can result in changes in its gene product, a protein with 189 amino acids that functions as a part of the membrane signal-transducing GTP-binding system.

137-B *(Campbell's, p. 292)*

The inactivation of anti-oncogenes, which are present in the normal genome, is thought to be another mechanism of malignant transformation, and is likely involved in hereditary malignancy.

138-D *(Campbell's, p. 293)*

Although heredity may be involved in many tumors, to date Wilms' tumor is the genitourinary neoplasm in which malignant transformation due to inherited loss of anti-oncogene activity has been most clearly documented.

139-D *(Campbell's, p. 294)*

The haploid number (n) of chromosomes is 22 autosomes plus a single sex chromosome, X or Y; the diploid number is 2n.

140-A *(Campbell's, p. 295)*

Chromosomal morphology can become abnormal as a result of deletions, duplications, and translocations occurring during mitosis.

141-C *(Campbell's, p. 296)*

Variations in cell ploidy (the number of chromosomes as a simple or complex multiple of the haploid state) have been correlated with the clinical prognosis of a number of urologic neoplasms.

142-A *(Campbell's, p. 297)*

Maternal gene products may form gradients within the early fertilized egg that determine spatial relationships in embryologic development.

143-A *(Campbell's, p. 298)*

A developing theory holds that normal homeostasis may be a balance between programmed cell senescence leading to death and malignant transformation. Understanding how to activate built-in cellular programs for cell death could have major therapeutic benefit for cancer.

144-B *(Campbell's, p. 299)*

Retroviral particles modified to prevent viral replication have been successfully used to introduce foreign genes into mammalian cells in a technique that could eventually be used for gene replacement therapy.

145-B *(Campbell's, pp. 298–299)*

Gene replacement refers to the site-specific replacement of an abnormal gene with a normal copy; gene augmentation is the addition of a normal gene to the genome, but at a random location. Gene replacement has not yet been successfully accomplished.

PART II

THE UROLOGIC EXAMINATION AND DIAGNOSTIC TECHNIQUES

CHAPTERS 8 THROUGH 10

DIRECTIONS: Each question below contains suggested responses. Select the ONE BEST response to each question.

146. All of the following statements regarding pain in the genitourinary tract are true EXCEPT:

A. Pain associated with malignancies is usually a late manifestation and a sign of advanced disease.
B. Gastrointestinal symptoms of renal pain occur because of reflex stimulation of the pelvic ganglia.
C. Constant suprapubic pain that is unrelated to urinary retention is seldom of urologic origin.
D. Ureteral pain may be referred to the scrotum or labium.

147. With terminal hematuria, bleeding usually occurs:

A. In the bladder
B. At the prostatic urethra
C. In the kidney
D. At the bladder neck

148. The symptom which is *least* specific for bladder outlet obstruction is:

A. Hesitancy
B. Intermittency
C. Nocturia
D. Post-void dribbling

149. Which form of incontinence is usually treated pharmacologically initially?

A. Continuous
B. Stress
C. Urgency
D. Overflow

150. Which of the following statements regarding male sexual dysfunction is *false*?

A. Preservation of emission occurs when loss of libido is due to hypogonadism.
B. For erections to occur, neurogenic, arterial, and venous mechanisms must be intact.
C. The absence of orgasm with normal libido and erectile function is almost always due to a psychiatric disorder.

151. Which of the following statements is *true*?

A. Hematospermia usually results from malignancy of the prostate.
B. Pneumaturia is most frequently due to gas-forming infections in diabetic patients with high concentrations of urinary sugar.
C. A thick, purulent, profuse urethral discharge is usually seen in nongonococcal urethritis.
D. Cloudy urine most commonly results from phosphate crystal precipitation in alkaline urine.

152. The following statements are true about the physical examination of the urinary tract EXCEPT:

A. The left kidney is generally palpable in men.
B. Transillumination of the kidney may be helpful in children younger than 1 year of age.
C. The adult bladder cannot usually be palpated or percussed until there is 150 ml of urine in it.
D. Bimanual examination of the bladder to assess tumor extent is best done under anesthesia.

153. Which of the following statements about abnormal physical findings of the penis is *false*?

A. In children under 5 years of age, it is abnormal for the foreskin to be unretractable.
B. Priapism usually presents with a rigid and mildly tender penis and firm rigid glans.
C. Paraphimosis is frequently iatrogenic.
D. Carcinoma of the penis is almost exclusively seen in uncircumcised men.

154. Which of the following statements about scrotal and testicular problems is *true*?

A. Torsion of the testis is seen most commonly between the ages of 20 and 30.
B. Hydrocele is diagnosed by transillumination, thus if any portion transilluminates, malignancy is ruled out.
C. A right-sided varicocele is slightly less common than a left-sided lesion.
D. A painless testicular mass in a man aged 20 to 35, which is incidentally found when bathing, is the most common presentation of testicular tumor.

155. Which of the following statements about urinalysis is *true*?

A. The inability to acidify one's pH below 5.0, despite fasting or acid load, is indicative of renal tubular acidosis.
B. VB1 refers to the first 50 ml of void urine.
C. Dipstick reagents are more sensitive to albumin than to globulins, Bence-Jones protein, or mucoproteins.

D. Urobilinogen is not normally excreted in the urine.

156. False-positive determination of urinary ketones can be caused by all of the following EXCEPT:

A. Dilute alkaline urine
B. Levodopa metabolites
C. 2-Mercaptoethane sulphonate sodium (MESNA)
D. Sulfhydryl-containing compounds

157. Causes of false-negative results for nitrite detection in urine include all of the following EXCEPT:

A. Organisms that further reduce nitrite to urea
B. Dilute urine
C. Alkaline urine
D. Large dietary intake of vitamin C

158. Factors that can cause false-negative results for leukocyte esterase include all of the following EXCEPT:

A. Glycosuria
B. Dilute urine
C. Large dietary intake of vitamin C
D. Presence of urobilinogen

159. All of the following statements about urinary dipstick for blood are true EXCEPT:

A. The amounts of color change and oxidant are directly related to the amount of hemoglobin.
B. Vitamins and food high in oxidants can cause false-negative results.
C. Normal individuals excrete approximately 1000 erythrocytes per milliliter of urine.
D. The most common cause of false-positive results is contamination of urine in menstruating women.

160. All of the following statements about epithelial cells are true EXCEPT:

A. They are frequently seen in the urine.
B. Transitional cells with multiple nuclei are usually malignant.
C. Transitional cells from the renal pelvis and ureter have larger cytoplasmic granules than those in the bladder.
D. Squamous cells line the trigone of postpubertal females.

161. Which of the following is typically seen microscopically in a normal expressed prostatic secretion?

A. Macrophages
B. Clumps of leukocytes
C. Oval fat macrophages
D. Secretory granules

162. In institutionalized patients with incontinence, which method is preferable?

A. Indwelling urethral catheter
B. Diaper
C. Intermittent catheterization
D. Urinary diversion

163. Which of the following statements regarding urethral dilation is *false*?

A. Urethral stricture in females is commonly encountered.
B. Repeated dilation can result in urethral trauma, which may ultimately worsen the stricture disease.
C. No objective data support the practice of urethral dilation in females for voiding dysfunction or recurrent infections.
D. An angioplasty balloon can be placed over a wire and inflated under fluoroscopic guidance as a method of ureteral stricture dilation.

164. All of the following statements are true regarding retrograde pyelography EXCEPT:

A. A scout film should be routinely performed.
B. Ureteral catheterization should be performed gently without force.
C. Flushing of air bubbles is important to the quality of the study.
D. Cytologies may be obtained from ureters at any point in the study.

165. The apposition of tissues of different densities creates a/an:

A. Coupling medium
B. Focal point
C. Acoustic interface
D. Acoustic shadow

166. The peripheral zone makes up what percentage of the glandular tissue in a normal prostate of a young adult?

A. 30
B. 50
C. 70
D. 90

167. Approximately what percentage of prostate cancer originates in the peripheral zone?

A. 90
B. 70
C. 50
D. 30

168. At low power, the peripheral zone appears similar to the:

A. Central zone
B. Transition zone
C. Anterior fibromuscular stroma
D. Seminal vesicles

169. Calculi associated with benign prostatic hyperplasia (BPH) tend to cluster:

A. In the periurethral tissue
B. At the junction of the transition zone and peripheral zone
C. In the central zone
D. In the anterior fibromuscular tissue

170. Which of the following statements regarding ultrasound and prostatitis is *false*?

A. No sonographic pattern for acute prostatitis is diagnostic.
B. Acute prostatitis may cause a change in the shape of the gland and patchy areas of decreased echogenicity.
C. Chronic prostatitis may have an echo-free or low-amplitude halo surrounding a slightly echogenic central area.
D. Granulomatous prostatitis often produces hyperechoic foci diagnostic of the entity.

171. With digital rectal examination as the mainstay of diagnosis, what percentage of patients present with metastatic cancer of the prostate?

A. 10
B. 30
C. 50
D. 70

172. Extracapsular extension of prostate cancer tends to occur:

A. Along the ejaculatory ducts to the seminal vesicles.
B. Anteriorly at the apex.
C. At the posterolateral margin along the perforating branches.
D. Through small micrometastases.

173. Prostate cancer is hypoechoic on ultrasound in what percentage of cancer (when viewing the largest focus of cancer in the specimen)?

A. 30
B. 50
C. 70
D. 90

174. Although it is well known that prostate cancer tends to be multifocal, ultrasonography usually identifies only the "index" or principal cancer. Reasons for nonvisualization of accessory foci include all of the following EXCEPT:

A. They tend to be isolated close to the "index" lesion.
B. They are usually smaller.
C. They are probably better differentiated.
D. They tend to grow in an infiltrative pattern among normal glands.

175. All of the following statements are true regarding prostate cancer EXCEPT:

A. Tumor volume correlates strongly with pathologic stage.
B. The higher the grade, the more likely the cancer is to be detected by ultrasound.
C. The prevailing pattern of hypoechoic appearance is thought to be due to the decrease in sonographically detectable interfaces in the tissue.
D. Hematomas from prior biopsies are rarely confused with possible cancer.

176. Ultrasonography detects nonpalpable cancers in about 5 per cent of men studied in a urologist's office. By what percentage does ultrasonography increase the number of cancers detected in this population compared to rectal examination alone?

A. 0 to 5
B. 10 to 15
C. 20 to 25
D. 30 to 35

177. Significant bleeding and infection requiring further treatments is encountered in what percentage of patients undergoing transrectal needle biopsy of the prostate?

A. 1
B. 4
C. 7
D. 10

178. All of the following features are true descriptions of the ultrasound appearance of the prostate in localized cancer EXCEPT:

A. Diffusely hetereogenous echoes
B. Symmetric, semilunar, flattened shape
C. Boundary echo intact and well defined
D. Symmetric seminal vesicles with fluid-filled lumen

179. The presence of a hypoechoic lesion adjacent to the boundary echo in prostate cancer increases the probability of extracapsular extension to approximately what percentage?

A. 25
B. 45
C. 65
D. 85

180. Three types of seminal vesicle invasion have been described. The most common is:

A. Extension along ejaculatory ducts
B. Invasion "from outside" after extracapsular penetration
C. Invasion "from outside" after invasion through the bladder neck

181. Transrectal ultrasound of the seminal vesicles or ejaculatory duct complex is useful in evaluating some patients with infertility. All of the following statements are true EXCEPT:

A. They are best visualized in the transaxial plane.
B. The vesicles appear saccular, filled with seminal fluid.
C. Visualization of the vas is indicative of pathology.
D. Ejaculatory duct cysts are sometimes seen in patients with infertility.

182. Testicular cysts may occur in 10 per cent of cases. Approximately what percentage of the more rare testicular carcinoma may have cystic components?

A. 15
B. 25
C. 35
D. 45

183. All of the following statements are true about ultrasound determination of bladder volume EXCEPT:

A. It requires careful training and is highly operator-dependent.
B. It is quick.
C. There is no significant risk of infection.
D. Patient position has no effect on accuracy.

184. All of the following statements are true about duplex ultrasonography evaluation of impotence EXCEPT:

A. It involves two kinds of ultrasound: real-time imaging and Doppler ultrasonography.
B. Real-time imaging is especially important in focusing Doppler ultrasonography for determining blood velocity values.
C. The average dilatation of the cavernosal arteries is 75 to 130 per cent of the preinjection diameter.
D. It is effective in identifying arteriovenous lesions.

185. Ionic contrast media activates all of the following anaphylactic mediators EXCEPT:

A. Leukotrienes
B. Histamine
C. Bradykinin
D. Complement C3a
E. Complement C5a

186. The advantages of the drip infusion when delivering contrast media as compared to bolus injection includes all of the following EXCEPT:

A. There is a markedly prolonged nephrogram.
B. An intense initial vascular nephrogram is obtained.
C. Enhanced diuresis fully distends the collecting system and ureters.
D. The collecting system is visualized for a longer period of time.
E. Ureteral compression need not be used because excellent ureteral visualization is usually obtained.

187. Which of the following urologic conditions and preferred radiographic triage examinations is *incorrect*?

A. Blunt abdominal trauma with hematuria — CT scan
B. Urolithiasis—intravenous urography
C. Renal failure—ultrasonography
D. Pseudotumor—CT scan
E. Adult male with pyelonephritis—intravenous urography

188. Patients receiving beta-blockers, who are suffering anaphylaxis from administration of contrast media refractory to epinephrine, should be given:

A. Repeated doses of epinephrine
B. Atropine
C. Isoproterenol
D. Antihistamines
E. Corticosteroids

189. The most characteristic abnormality during excretory urography in patients with renovascular hypertension is:

A. Poor visualization of collecting system
B. Extrinsic vascular impression
C. Enlarged kidney
D. Delayed excretion of contrast
E. Early excretion of contrast

190. The urogram is a physiologic study that permits a rough assessment of renal function. Which of the following physiologic changes is *not* generally seen with intravenous urography?

A. Increased serum osmolality
B. Transient hypotension
C. Peripheral vasodilatation
D. Tachycardia
E. Decreased cardiac output

191. The procedure of choice to define anatomic details of the calyces, pelvis, and ureter is:

A. Intravenous urography
B. Ultrasonography
C. CT scan
D. Nuclear renogram
E. Retrograde pyelography

192. All of the following statements regarding cystourethrography are true EXCEPT:

A. Clinically significant narrowing of the anterior urethra is infrequently associated with proximal distention.
B. The retrograde urethrogram is not a physiologic examination.
C. 30–50 per cent of children with urinary tract infections will demonstrate reflux on VCU.
D. The main indication for a retrograde urethrogram in women is a suspected urethral diverticulum.
E. Excluding trauma, retrograde urethrography is of little value in evaluating the posterior urethra.

193. Ultrasonography has many advantages in uroradiology, which include all of the following EXCEPT:

A. It is safe and does not use ionizing radiation.
B. It allows discrimination between pseudotumor and true lesions.
C. The study is not affected by renal function.
D. It requires little or no pre-procedural preparation.
E. It is relatively inexpensive, rapid, and mobile.

194. Ultrasound is routinely used to identify and exclude hydronephrosis. The most important sign in discriminating between parenchymal cysts and hydronephrosis is:

A. Echo-free
B. Smooth-walled
C. Posterior acoustic enhancement
D. Small sinus in the center of the kidney
E. Inability to connect the cystic structures

195. Ultrasound is used in patients with renal failure to exclude obstructive uropathy. Which of the following conditions may lead to obstructive uropathy without obvious urinary tract dilatation?

A. Retroperitoneal fibrosis
B. Ureteral stricture
C. BPH
D. Ureteral calculi
E. Posterior urethral valves

196. A 48-year-old female is undergoing right upper quadrant ultrasound due to biliary colic. Sonographic views of the right kidney reveal a very bright, highly reflective mass. The most likely diagnosis is:

A. Simple cyst
B. Renal calculus
C. Renal cell carcinoma
D. Angiomyolipoma
E. Septum of Bertin

197. All of the following lesions may be highly reflective on ultrasound EXCEPT:

A. Renal cell carcinoma
B. Angiomyolipoma
C. Renal abscess
D. Renal infarct
E. Hemorrhagic pyelonephritis

198. Homogeneous enlargement of the transition zone during transrectal ultrasound of the prostate is usually seen with:

A. Chronic prostatitis

B. BPH
C. Prostatic carcinoma
D. Prostatic calculi
E. Prostatic abscess

199. Transrectal ultrasound can be useful in the evaluation of all of the following conditions EXCEPT:

A. Teratozoospermia
B. Ejaculatory duct obstruction
C. Pyospermia
D. Azoospermia
E. A low-volume ejaculate

200. CT scan is capable of detecting tissue density differences of less than:

A. 10 per cent
B. 15 per cent
C. 5 per cent
D. 8 per cent
E. 1 per cent

201. Imaging features of benign renal lesions on contrast-enhanced CT scan include:

A. Thick or nodular walls
B. Chunky, irregular calcification
C. No enhancement
D. Heterogeneous attenuation
E. Ill-defined margin with normal parenchyma

202. The "gold standard" for detection and characterization of renal mass is:

A. MRI
B. Ultrasound
C. Intravenous urography
D. CT scan
E. Angiography

203. MRI has the following advantages over CT scans EXCEPT:

A. It has greater resolving power.
B. Images can be obtained in any plane.
C. No ionizing radiation is required.
D. It is easily performed in patients with marginal renal function.
E. Excellent vascular detail may be obtained.

204. Color Doppler sonography of the testis is helpful in differentiating testicular torsion from:

A. Tumor
B. Epididymo-orchitis
C. Cysts
D. Fracture of the testis
E. Hydrocele

PART II

THE UROLOGIC EXAMINATION AND DIAGNOSTIC TECHNIQUES

CHAPTERS 8 THROUGH 10

ANSWERS

146-B *(Campbell's, p. 308)*

All of the statements are true except B. Gastrointestinal symptoms of renal pain occur due to the reflex stimulation of the celiac ganglion and the proximity of adjacent organs (liver, pancreas, duodenum, gallbladder, and colon).

147-D *(Campbell's, p. 309)*

In terminal hematuria, bleeding usually occurs at the bladder neck at the termination of micturition. Initial hematuria usually occurs from the anterior or prostatic urethra. Total hematuria is associated with bleeding from the bladder or upper tracts.

148-C *(Campbell's, pp. 309–310)*

Obstructive symptoms include hesitancy, decreased force of stream, intermittency, and post-void dribbling. Those are usually secondary to benign prostatic hyperplasia, urethral stricture, or neurogenic bladder, and less commonly due to malignant prostatic obstruction, urethral carcinoma, or a foreign object. Nocturia is an irritative symptom secondary to increased urine output or decreased capacity.

149-C *(Campbell's, p. 310)*

Urgency incontinence is typically treated pharmacologically. It is the precipitous loss of urine preceded by a strong urge to void. Continuous incontinence in the absence of prior injury to the sphincter indicates a fistula or ectopic ureter until proven otherwise. Stress incontinence refers to leakage with increased intra-abdominal pressure. Overflow or paradoxical incontinence is due to advanced retention when intravesical pressure finally overcomes outlet resistance.

150-A *(Campbell's, pp. 310–311)*

All of the statements are true except A. Since the testosterone required to maintain libido is usually less than the amount to maintain full stimulation of the prostate and seminal vesicles, absence of emission occurs when the loss of libido is due to hypogonadism.

151-D *(Campbell's, p. 311)*

The most common cause of cloudy urine is secondary to alkaline pH, which causes the precipitation of phosphate crystals, although it may occur in the presence of infection. Although hematospermia can occur with malignancies, it is usually due to nonspecific inflammation of the prostate or seminal vesicles. Pneumaturia is almost always due to a fistula between the intestine and bladder. In rare instances it is due to infection with gas-forming organisms in diabetic patients. Urethral discharge is the most common symptom of venereal infection. A purulent, thick, profuse discharge is commonly seen with gonococcal urethritis, whereas a scant and watery discharge is generally associated with nonspecific urethritis.

152-A *(Campbell's, p. 312)*

All of the statements are true except A. The left kidney is almost always impalpable in men unless it is abnormally enlarged.

153-B *(Campbell's, p. 315)*

All of the statements are true except B. Priapism is a prolonged painful erection that is not related to sexual activity. Physical examination reveals a rigid and mildly tender penis with a glans that is usually flaccid.

154-D *(Campbell's, pp. 315–316)*

A painless testicular mass is the most common presentation of a testicular tumor. It typically occurs from ages 20 to 35, and is frequently discovered by the patient while bathing. Torsion of the testis is usually seen between ages 10 and 20, and less frequently in the first year of life. Varicocele almost always occurs on the left side. A right-sided varicocele in a patient raises the suspicion of a retroperitoneal neoplasm.

155-C *(Campbell's, pp. 317–319)*

Protein dipstick reagents are more sensitive to albumin than to globulins, Bence-Jones protein, or mucoproteins. They are sensitive to levels of 10 mg/dl or less. The first 5 to 8 ml represent the urethral specimen (VB1). The inability to lower the urinary pH less than 5.5 with fasting or acid load is indicative of renal tubule acidosis. Urobilinogen is normally excreted in urine.

REFERENCE

1. Jones, E.A., and Berk, P.D.: Chemical and immunological tests in the evaluation of liver disease. *In* Brown, S.S., Mitchell, F.L., and Young, D.S. (Eds.): Chemical Diagnosis of Disease. Amsterdam, Elsevier, 1979, pp. 525–662.

156-A *(Campbell's, p. 319)*

False-positive determinations of urinary ketones are sometimes seen with very acidic urine with high specific gravity (dehydration). Other causes include abnormally colored urine, levodopa metabolites, MESNA, and other sulfhydryl-containing compounds.

REFERENCE

1. Csako, G.: False positive results for ketone with the drug MESNA and other free-sulhydryl compounds. Clin. Chem., *33*:289, 1987.

157-C *(Campbell's, pp. 319–320)*

False-negative results for nitrite detection in random urine samples can occur in 40 to 50 per cent of patients with urinary tract infections. Causes can include nonnitrate-reducing organisms, organisms that further reduce nitrites to ammonia, acid urine, large dietary intake of vitamin C, and the presence of urobilinogen. Current data indicate a positive Griess test is significant, but a negative test does not indicate that bacteria are not present.

158-B *(Campbell's, p. 320)*

False-negative results for leukocyte esterase can be seen with increased specific gravity, glycosuria, presence of urobilinogen, medications that alter urine color (rifampin, nitrofurantoin, phenazopyridine), and large intake of vitamin C.

REFERENCES

1. Gillenwater, J.Y.: Detection of urinary leukocytes by chemstrip. J. Urol., *125*:383, 1981.
2. Smalley, D.L., and Dittman, A.N.: Use of leukocyte esterase-nitrate activity as predictive assays of significant bacteriuria. J. Clin. Microbiol., *18*:1256, 1983.

159-B *(Campbell's, pp. 320–321)*

All of the statements are true except B. Various vitamins and foods with high concentrations of oxidants can cause false-positive readings.

REFERENCES

1. Addis, T.: The number of formed elements in the urinary sediment of normal individuals. J. Clin. Invest., 2:409, 1926.
2. Larcom, R.C., and Carter, G.H.: Erythrocytes in urinary sediment: Identification and normal limits with a note on the nature of granular cast. J. Lab. Clin. Med., *33*:875, 1948.
3. Leonards, J.: Single test for hematuria compared with established tests. JAMA, *179*:807, 1962.

160-B *(Campbell's, pp. 328–329)*

All of the statements are true except B. It is not uncommon for normal transitional cells to have multiple nuclei. Malignant cells have altered nucleus size and morphology. Sediment stained with the Papanicolaou stain can help identify malignant urothelial cells.

REFERENCE

1. Papanicolaou, G.N., and Marshall, V.F.: Urine sediments smears as a diagnostic procedure in cancers of the urinary tract. Science, *101*:519, 1945.

161-D *(Campbell's, p. 329)*

In normal prostatic fluid, there should be few, if any, leukocytes but numerous secretory granules of various sizes. Macrophages and clumps of leukocytes are indicators of inflammation. Oval fat macrophages characterize postinfection prostatic fluid.

162-C *(Campbell's, p. 331)*

Clean intermittent catheterization or condom catheter drainage is preferable to manage patients with urinary incontinence in the institutional setting due to risk of infection with long-term indwelling urethral catheters.

163-A *(Campbell's, pp. 333–335)*

All of the statements are true except A. True urethral strictures in the female are uncommon without a history of prior urethral or bladder neck surgery.

164-D *(Campbell's, pp. 337–338)*

Ureteral cytologies should be obtained prior to injection of hyperosmolar contrast to avoid poorly preserved cytologic specimens. All of the other statements are correct.

165-C *(Campbell's, pp. 342–343)*

The apposition of tissues of different densities creates an acoustic interface. The poor transmission of sound through gas makes it necessary to use a coupling medium, either a water-filled balloon or gel, to provide good transmission from the transducer to the body. A characteristic dark streak distal to the high-density object that reflects ultrasound waves is referred to a point where the cross-sectional area is at a minimum and the intensity is at a maximum.

166-C *(Campbell's, p. 343)*

The glandular portion of the prostate is divided into the peripheral zone, the central zone, and the transition zone, which comprise approximately 70, 20, and 10 per cent, respectively, in a normal young adult prostate.

REFERENCES

1. McNeal, J.E.: Regional morphology and pathology of the prostate. Am. J. Clin. Pathol., *49*:347, 1968.

2. McNeal, J.E.: The zonal anatomy of the prostate. Prostate, *2*:35, 1981.
3. McNeal, J.E.: Normal histology of the prostate. Am. J. Surg. Pathol., *12*:619, 1988.

167-B *(Campbell's, p. 343)*

The peripheral zone is the most frequent site of origin of prostate cancer, accounting for about 70 per cent. The central zone is the least common site, approximately 10 per cent, with the transition zone accounting for the remaining 20 per cent.

REFERENCE

1. McNeal, J.E., Redwine, E.A., Freiha, F.S., and Stamey, T.A.: Zonal distribution of prostatic adenocarcinoma: Correlation with histologic pattern and direction of spread. Am. J. Surg. Pathol., *12*:897, 1988b.

168-A *(Campbell's, p. 344)*

Because the peripheral and the central zones appear similar at low power, they are difficult to distinguish sonographically.

REFERENCE

1. Stamey, T.A., and Hodge, K.K.: Ultrasound visualization of prostate anatomy and pathology. Monogr. Urol., *9*:55, 1988.

169-B *(Campbell's, p. 347)*

Multiple small calculi are often seen in the periurethral glandular tissue and are distinct from the large calculi associated with BPH. These tend to cluster at the junction of the transition and peripheral zones.

170-D *(Campbell's, p. 350)*

All of the statements are true except D. Granulomatous prostatitis often produces prominent hypoechoic foci on ultrasound. There may be an accompanying elevated PSA and a palpable, nontender nodule that makes it difficult to distinguish from cancer.

REFERENCES

1. Harada, B., Friedrich, M., and Kilami, A.: Ultrasound imaging in Peyronie's disease. Urology, *28*:540, 1986.
2. Peeling, W.J., and Griffiths, G.J.: Ultrasonic imaging of the prostate. *In* Fitzpatrick, J.M., and Krane, R.J. The Prostate. Edinburgh, Churchill Livingstone, 1989, p. 281.

171-B *(Campbell's, p. 352)*

With digital rectal examination as the mainstay of diagnosis, 30 per cent of prostate cancers present with metastatic disease and 30 per cent present with locally advanced disease as nodal metastases at the time of diagnosis.

172-C *(Campbell's, pp. 353–355)*

Extracapsular extension of prostate cancer tends to occur at the posterolateral margin, over the neurovascular bundles, along the perforating branches.

REFERENCE

1. Villers, A., McNeal, J.E., Redwin, E.A., Freiha, F.S., and Stamey, T.A.: The role of perineural space invasion in the local spread of prostatic adenocarcinoma. J. Urol., *142*:763, 1989.

173-C *(Campbell's, p. 355)*

In a series of 147 specimens, the largest or "index" focus of cancer appeared hypoechoic in 71.3 per cent, isoechoic in 27.4 per cent, and hyperechoic in only 1.3 per cent.

REFERENCE

1. Eqawa, S., Flanagan, W., Greene, D.R., Wheeler, T.M., and Scardino, P.T.: Transrectal Ultrasonography in stage A prostate cancer: Detection of residual tumor after TURP. J. Urol., in press, 1995.

174-A *(Campbell's, p. 357)*

Although prostate cancer tends to be multifocal, ultrasonography seldom detects the small accessory foci of cancer, even when the "index" cancer is apparent. These foci tend to be smaller, more diffused, better differentiated, and they tend to grow in a infiltrative pattern among the normal glands of the prostate compared to the "index" cancer.

REFERENCES

1. Carter, H.B., Hamper, U.M., Sheth, S., Sanders, R.C., Epstein, J.I., and Walsh, P.C.: Evaluation of transrectal ultrasound in the early detection of prostate cancer. J. Urol., *142*:1008, 1989.
2. Shinohara, K., Wheeler, T.W., Scardino, P.T.: The appearance of prostate cancer on transrectal ultrasonography: Correlation of imaging and pathological examinations. J. Urol., *142*:76, 1989b.
3. Shinohara, K., Scardino, P.T., and Wheeler, T.W.: The pathologic basis of the sonographic appearance of the normal and malignant prostate. Urol. Clin. North Am., *16*:674, 1989b.

175-D *(Campbell's, pp. 357–360)*

All of the statements are true except D. Perhaps the most frequently encountered artifact simulating prostate cancer is hematoma from recent biopsy. It appears hypoechoic, is in the peripheral zone, and may even cause bulging of the boundary echo, reminiscent of a cancer penetrating the capsule.

REFERENCES

1. Andriole, G.L., Coplen, D.E., Mikkelsen, D.J., and Catalona, W.J.: Sonographic and pathologic staging of

patients with localized prostate cancer. J. Urol., *142*: 1259, 1989.
2. McNeal, J.E., Kindrachuk, R.A., Freiha, F.S., Bostwick, D.G., Redwine, E.A., and Stamey, T.A.: Patterns of progression in prostate cancer. Lancet, *1*:60, 1986.
3. Shinohara K., Wheeler, T., and Scardino, P.T.: The appearance of prostate cancer on transrectal ultrasonography: Correlation of imaging and pathological examinations. J. Urol., *142*:76, 1989a.

176-C *(Campbell's, p. 360)*

Ultrasonography increases the number of cancers detected in men in a urologist's office by 20 to 25 per cent compared to rectal examination alone.

REFERENCES

1. Cooner, W.H., Mosley, B.R., Rutherford, C.L., Jr., Beard, J.H., Pond, H.S., Terry, W.J., Igel, T.C., and Kidd, D.D.: Prostate cancer detection in a clinical urological practice by ultrasonography, digital rectal examination, and prostate specific antigen. J. Urol., *143*: 1146, 1990.
2. Shabsigh, R., Carter, S. St., C., Egawa, S., Wright, C.D., Carlton, C.E., Jr., and Scardino, P.T.: Transrectal ultrasound and/or digital guided biopsy of the prostate (abstr. 449). J. Urol., *141*:282A, 1989a.

177-A *(Campbell's, p. 363)*

Bleeding and infection requiring further treatment is seen in 1 per cent of patients undergoing transrectal needle biopsy of the prostate with ultrasound guidance. Broad-spectrum antibiotics and enemas are routinely used.

REFERENCES

1. Hodge, K.K., McNeal, J.E., and Stamey, T.A.: Ultrasound-guided transrectal core biopsies of the palpably abnormal prostate. J. Urol., *142*:66, 1989a.
2. Torp-Pederson, S.T., and Lee, F.: Transrectal biopsy of the prostate guided by transrectal ultrasound. Urol. Clin. North Am., *16*:703, 1989.

178-A *(Campbell's, pp. 365–368)*

All of the descriptions are true except A. The typical ultrasound appearance of a localized cancer is generally homogeneous with possible hypoechoic foci indicative of cancer.

REFERENCE

1. Scardino, P.T., Shinohara, K., Carter, S. St. C., and Wheeler, T.M.: Staging of prostate cancer: The value of ultrasonography. Urol. Clin. North Am., *16*:713, 1989.

179-C *(Campbell's, p. 369)*

The presence of a hypoechoic lesion adjacent to the boundary echo increases the probability of extracapsular extension of cancer at that site from 18 to 64 per cent.

REFERENCES

1. Scardino, P.T., Shinohara, K., Carter, S. St. C., and Wheeler, T.M.: Staging of prostate cancer: The value of ultrasonography. Urol. Clin. North Am., *16*:713, 1989.
2. Shinohara, K., Wheeler, T.M., Cantini, M., and Scardino, P.T.: Ultrasonic detection of extracapsular extension: A clinicopathologic study of localized prostate cancer (abstr. 555). J. Urol., *137*:242A, 1987.

180-A *(Campbell's, p. 370)*

Three types of seminal vesicle invasion have been described. The most common is Type I, invasion along the ejaculatory ducts. The most important ultrasound clue is a large hypoechoic lesion at the base of the prostate adjacent to the seminal vesicles. Type II refers to extracapsular penetration and invasion of the seminal vesicles "from outside." There is a loss of the hyperechoic fat pad on the involved side. Type III is due to micrometastases.

REFERENCES

1. Wheeler, T.M.: Anatomical consideration in carcinoma of the prostate. Urol. Clin. North Am., *16*:30, 1989.
2. McNeal, J.E., and Bostwick, D.G.: Intraductal dysplasia: A premalignant lesion of the prostate. Hum. Pathol., *17*:64, 1986.
3. Greene, D.R., and Scardino, P.T.: Transrectal ultrasonography for prostate cancer. Principles and Practice of Oncology Updates, *4*:1–15, 1990.
4. Scardino, P.T., Shinohara, K., Carter, S. St. C., and Wheeler, T.M.: Staging of prostate cancer: The value of ultrasonography. Urol. Clin. North Am., *16*:713, 1989.
5. Shinohara, K., Wheeler, T.M., and Scardino, P.T.: Ultrasonic detection of nonpalpable seminal vesicle invasion: A clinicopathologic study (abstr. 603). J. Urol., *139*:313A, 1988.

181-C *(Campbell's, pp. 373–374)*

All of the statements are true except C. Frequently the vas can be visualized on either side as it passes inward and posterior to the seminal vesicles. This is a normal finding.

182-B *(Campbell's, p. 377)*

Although testicular tumors are much less common than cysts, 24 per cent of tumors have cystic components.

REFERENCE

1. Dähnert, W.F., Hamper, U.M., Eggleston, J.C., Walsh, P.C., and Sanders, R.C.: Prostatic evaluation by transrectal sonography with histopathologic correlation: The echogenic appearance of early carcinoma. Radiology, *158*:97, 1986.

183-A *(Campbell's, pp. 380–381)*

Bladder ultrasonography of volume dependence is quick, painless, harmless, and easily repeatable. Patient position has no effect on accuracy. A highly significant correlation between measurements by trained examiners and inexperienced examiners indicates little "operator dependence."

REFERENCES

1. Cardenas, D.D., Kelly, E., Krieger, J.N., and Chapman, W.H.: Residual urine volumes in patients with spinal cord injury: Measurement with portable ultrasound instrument. Arch. Phys. Med. Rehabil., *69*:514, 1988.
2. Massagli, T.L., Cardenas, D.D., and Kelly, E.W.: Experience with portable ultrasound equipment and measurement of urine volumes: Inter-user reliability and factors of patient position. J. Urol., *142*:969, 1989.

184-D *(Campbell's, pp. 386–389)*

All of the statements are true except D. Duplex scanning is not effective in identifying arteriovenous lesions. A rigid erection after vasoactive agent administration which is improved or maintained by exercise rules out a significant vascular lesion. An erection that is lost with exercise, then returns after rest, indicates pelvic steal syndrome.

REFERENCES

1. Shabsigh, R., Fishman, I.J., Quesada, E.T., Seale-Hawkins, C.K., and Dunn, J.K.: Evaluation of vasculogenic erectile impotence using penile duplex ultrasonography. J. Urol., *142*:1469, 1989b.
2. Mueller, S.T., and Lue, T.F.: Evaluation of vasculogenic impotence. Urol. Clin. North Am., *15*:65, 1988.

185-A *(Campbell's, p. 406)*

The precise pathogenesis of systemic reactions to contrast media is incompletely understood. Histamine, bradykinin, and leukotrienes are well-accepted mediators of anaphylaxis, and vasoactive prostaglandins and the complement factors C3a and C5a are considered likely mediators. Ionic contrast media have been reported to liberate or activate all of these with the exception of the leukotrienes. Because of the complex interactions between these substances, it is easy to understand why it is so difficult to isolate critical or unique initiating and sequential activation factors.

186-B *(Campbell's, pp. 413–418)*

Although the bolus injection of contrast is the most commonly used method, certain variations may be helpful. The advantages of the drip infusion as compared to bolus injection are as follows: (1) there is a markedly prolonged (not more intense) nephrogram; (2) enhanced diuresis from the additional contrast material and water more fully distends the collecting systems and ureters; (3) no significant increase in reactions occurs; (5) ureteral compression need not be used because excellent ureteral visualization is usually obtained; and (6) administration is easy.

The disadvantages of the drip infusion include the following: (1) it overloads the normal patient with more iodine than necessary; (2) calyceal blunting may be produced; (3) it may lead to pyelosinus extravasation and significant pain in patients with partial obstruction; (4) the increased diuresis produced may decrease visualization if there is a low fixed specific gravity; (5) drip infusion may occasionally produce cardiac compensation; and (6) an initial vascular nephrogram is not obtained.

187-D *(Campbell's, pp. 431–433)*

When evaluating patients with urologic complaints, it is of utmost importance to answer the questions posed by the clinician. With significant trauma to the abdomen, CT is the triage examination of choice. The urogram is still the study of choice for calculi. It can readily be performed on an emergency basis and is the procedure of choice when anatomic details of the calyces, pelvis, or ureter are desired. If pseudotumor is suspected, nuclear medicine is the triage of choice. In infection, the urogram is the best for visualizing calyceal distortion, and CT is the preferred choice if a mass is revealed. The triage examination of choice for renal failure is ultrasonography and is usually performed to rule out hydronephrosis.

188-C *(Campbell's, p. 409)*

For severe contrast media reactions, immediate assurance of an open airway with oxygen supplementation, initiation of intravascular physiologic fluids, and monitoring of blood pressure and heart rate should be undertaken.

Antihistamines are the most frequent drugs used to treat reactions; however, Goldberg pointed out that, in fact, antihistamines are probably of little value during severe contrast-induced reactions. Corticosteroids given in customary dosages shortly before contrast material challenge failed to confer any protection against reactions. Patients given corticosteroids for acute asthmatic attacks did not gain appreciable help until 4 to 6 hours after corticosteroid administration. Epinephrine is the first line of defense in acute anaphylactic reactions, but if a patient is receiving beta-blockers, repeated doses may generate unwanted alpha-effects. This may lead to a dominance of cholinergic activity and possibly a secondary bradycardia. In such circumstances, patients undergoing anaphylaxis refractory to increased doses of epinephrine should be given isoproterenol, a beta-agonist. The precise role of atropine in patients suffering contrast-induced anaphylaxis with associated bradycardia remains to be defined.

REFERENCES

1. Goldberg, M.: Sytemic reactions to intravascular contrast media: A guide for the anesthesiologist. Anesthesiology, *60*: 46–56, 1984.
2. Morris, H.G.: Mechanisms of action and therapeutic role of corticosteroids in asthma. J. Allergy Clin. Immunol., *75*:1–113, 1985.

189-D *(Campbell's, p. 430)*

The hypertensive urogram, with a rapid sequence of films taken during the first 4 minutes after contrast injection, has been used as a screening test for renovascular hypertension. Positive findings include decreased renal size, delayed excretion of contrast, and hyperconcentration of contrast on delayed films because of increased absorption of water. A high false-negative rate has reduced the use of this test.

190-C *(Campbell's, p. 431)*

After administration of contrast medium, which, for all practical purposes, is excreted solely by glomerular filtration with currently used agents, significant fluid and ionic shifts occur. Serum osmolality rapidly increases, causing influx of water from interstitial space into the blood stream, and blood volume increases as much as 16 per cent. Concurrently, cardiac output *increases*. Hemodynamic changes consist of transient hypotension, peripheral vasodilatation, increased pulmonary artery pressure, and tachycardia. These cardiovascular effects are much less pronounced with nonionic contrast agents than with the ionic ones.

191-A *(Campbell's, p. 431)*

Intravenous urography is the procedure of choice when anatomic details of the calyces, pelvis, or ureter are desired. If function is sufficient, the urogram localizes the obstruction. Its primary use today appears to be in the areas of known or suspected calculi, ureteral obstruction, congenital anomalies, infection, and intraluminal tumors. It is the study of first choice in patients with unexplained hematuria or pyuria and in those requiring thorough screening of the entire urinary tract.

192-A *(Campbell's, pp. 438–447)*

The retrograde urethrogram is not a physiologic study. Contrast material is often injected under pressure to overcome resistance. The main indications for retrograde urethrogram in men are trauma to the urethra or urethral stricture; in women the main indication is a suspected urethral diverticulum. Except in patients with trauma, retrograde urethrography is of little or no value in evaluating the posterior urethra. In addition, clinically significant narrowing is almost always associated with proximal distention.

The main indication for VCU in children is urinary tract infection. It usually occurs in girls, and the VCU in childhood is performed in girls under 6 years of age. The incidence of reflux in children with urinary tract infection is between 30 and 50 per cent.

193-B *(Campbell's, pp. 449–451)*

Ultrasonography has become the most commonly performed examination for evaluating the urinary tract. The performance of the ultrasound study is not affected by renal function, and it is, therefore, the procedure of choice in patients with renal failure. Ultrasonography is safe, rapid, mobile, inexpensive, and does not require any preparation. It is of less value in applications that take advantage of renal function, such as discriminating between pseudotumor and true lesions.

194-E *(Campbell's, pp. 451–453)*

When evaluating for hydronephrosis, it may be difficult to discriminate between renal parenchymal cysts and urinary tract dilatation. The most important sign that one is observing parenchymal cysts is the inability to connect the cystic structures. Parapelvic cysts may completely mimic hydronephrosis on ultrasonography.

195-A *(Campbell's, p. 453)*

Ultrasound is appropriately used in patients with chronic renal failure to exclude destructive uropathy as the cause. In general, only retroperitoneal fibrosis leads to chronic renal failure due to obstruction, without obvious urinary tract dilatation. Occasionally with staghorn calculi, significant hydronephrosis may be absent behind the stone when it is responsible for renal failure without associated dilatation.

196-D *(Campbell's, p. 462)*

The angiomyolipoma is a mass that typically is very bright. The high reflectivity of this lesion is a strong clue to the presence of fat and should lead one to obtain a CT scan to confirm the lesion. A cyst is generally echo-free and has a smooth back wall. Renal cell carcinoma may produce either an echo-poor mass or an echogenic mass. A septum of Bertin is similar to the normal parenchyma, and nephrolithiasis reveals an echogenic focus that may be associated with acoustic shadowing.

197-A *(Campbell's, pp. 459–462)*

Renal cell carcinoma may produce either an echo-poor mass or an echogenic mass. The typical findings of a solid mass will be seen with none of the artifacts of fluid. The angiomyolipoma is a mass that is typically very bright and reflective. Renal abscesses may be echo-free, may contain low level echoes, or may be highly reflective. Blood within the renal parenchyma is of variable echogenicity, but at some stage it is highly reflective. Therefore, hemorrhagic pyelonephritis and an acute renal infarct can produce highly reflective images.

198-B *(Campbell's, pp. 475–476)*

The region of the prostate and seminal vesicles is well visualized transabdominally, but is seen to even better advantage transrectally. Benign prostatic hyperplasia leads to symmetric enlargement of the gland, usually due to selective enlargement of the transition zone, whereas prostatic carcinoma usually appears as a hypoechoic mass in the peripheral zone.

199-A *(Gilbert, B., Schlegel, P., and Goldstein, M.: AUA Update Series, Vol. XIII, Lesson 9)*

Indications for TRUS in evaluating the subfertile male include: (1) azoospermia; (2) abnormal digital rectal examination; (3) retrograde ejaculation; (4) suspicion of partial obstruction; and (5) hematospermia or pyospermia. In the azoospermic patient, seminal vesicle and ejaculatory duct obstruction can be documented. Partial obstruction of the ejaculatory duct can be diagnosed, as well as abnormalities of the seminal vesicles. In patients with pyospermia, the characteristic findings associated with acute and chronic prostatic infections can be assessed.

200-E *(Campbell's, p. 482)*

CT scans depict the anatomy of the upper urinary tract and surrounding structures in unsurpassed detail. CT functions by comparing the specific gravity of tissues. CT is much more sensitive to small differences in contrast density than in conventional radiographic film technique. CT scans can demonstrate density differences of 1 per cent or less, whereas x-ray film cannot demonstrate density differences of less than 10 per cent in contiguous structures.

201-C *(Silverman, S., Bloom, D., Seltzer, S.: AUA Update Series, Vol. XIII, Lesson 1)*

Key features of CT scans of benign renal lesions include low attenuation, no enhancement, imperceptible wall, sharply marginated, no calcification, small, border-forming calcifications, thin septation, and fatty elements.

202-D *(Silverman, S., Bloom, D., Seltzer, S.: AUA Update Series, Vol. XIII, Lesson 1)*

A carefully performed CT, with and without intravenous contrast-enhanced scans, remains the "gold standard" for the detection and characterization of renal masses. CT yields several key features that determine the probable diagnosis. These include attenuation before and after administration of contrast media, margin with the surrounding kidney, the presence and type of calcification, and the type and presence of cyst wall or septation.

203-A *(Silverman, S., Bloom, D., Seltzer, S.: AUA Update Series, Vol. XIII, Lesson 1)*

Like CT, MRI is a tomographic technique; however, MR images can be obtained in any plane. MRI appears to be safe, and no ionizing radiation is required. It is not necessary to use iodinated contrast materials in MRI; therefore, the examinations may be easily performed in patients with marginal renal function. In addition, MRI is remarkably sensitive to blood flow, so excellent vascular detail may be obtained. However, the approach to renal mass evaluation using MRI is still based on macroscopic structural analyses. Therefore CT, because of its greater resolving power, continues to be the primary modality in renal mass characterization.

204-B *(King, B., Hattery, R.: AUA Update Series, Vol. XII, Lesson 21)*

The application of color Doppler sonography has had a most dramatic impact in the evaluation of patients with acute scrotal pain. The clinical question of torsion versus epididymo-orchitis can be difficult to distinguish. Epididymo-orchitis will always result in increased blood flow to the epididymis and testis. Torsion results in decreased or total lack of color flow to the affected testis. Because there is a companion testis for comparison, the relative degree of increased or decreased blood flow can be easily determined. Doppler sonography is a useful, noninvasive, quick, and harmless examination in the evaluation of patients with acute scrotal pain in helping to differentiate acute torsion of the testis from epididymo-orchitis.

PART III

THE PATHOPHYSIOLOGY OF URINARY OBSTRUCTION

CHAPTERS 11 AND 12

DIRECTIONS: Each question below contains suggested responses. Select the ONE BEST response to each question.

205. The finding on a renal biopsy pathognomonic of urinary tract obstruction is:
   A. Tamm-Horsfall protein casts within Bowman's space of glomeruli
   B. Eosinophilic infiltration
   C. Interstitial fibrosis
   D. Glomerulosclerosis
   E. Mononuclear cell infiltration

206. Which statement regarding pathologic changes associated with complete ureteral obstruction is *false*?
   A. Pathologic changes in the glomerulus first appear after 28 days of obstruction.
   B. Ultrastructural changes include thickening of glomerular basement membranes and obliteration of filtration slits.
   C. Renal tissue atrophy causes a decrease in the kidney weight during the first few weeks of obstruction.
   D. By the 28th day of obstruction, renal medullary thickness decreases by 50 per cent.
   E. Polar regions of the kidney are initially damaged.

207. All of the following statements concerning renal lymphatics are true EXCEPT:
   A. Renal lymph volume normally approximates that of urine flow.
   B. Renal lymphatic drainage occurs via hilar and capsular lymphatics.
   C. Acute renal lymphatic obstruction causes diuresis, natriuresis, and decrease in renal blood flow and GFR.
   D. Ligation of both the renal lymphatics and ureter produces severe renal damage with necrosis and destruction in several days.
   E. Pyelocanalicular and pyelosinus backflow preserve renal function in the hydronephrotic kidney.

208. How long can the human kidney be completely obstructed before sustaining enough damage to prevent any recovery of function after release of obstruction?
   A. 7 days
   B. 14 days
   C. 28 days
   D. 42 days
   E. 69 days

209. All aspects of renal function are impaired in the hydronephrotic kidney EXCEPT:
   A. Urinary concentrating ability
   B. Ammonia excretion
   C. Renal blood flow
   D. Urinary dilution
   E. Glomerular filtration rate

210. The normal renal pelvic pressure measured with percutaneous puncture is:
   A. 1.0 mm Hg
   B. 2.5 mm Hg
   C. 6.5 mm Hg
   D. 10.5 mm Hg
   E. 15.0 mm Hg

211. Which statement regarding the different physiologic changes associated with unilateral versus bilateral ureteral obstruction in experimental animals is *true*?
   A. Natriuresis and diuresis occur after release of both unilateral and bilateral obstruction.
   B. Renal blood flow and single nephron GFR are similar after release of 24 hours of unilateral or bilateral obstruction.
   C. Distal tubular pressures are elevated in unilateral and bilateral ureteral obstruction.
   D. In bilateral obstruction, vasoconstriction of afferent arterioles causes a reduction in renal blood flow and GFR.
   E. In unilateral obstruction, vasoconstriction of efferent arteriole and increased proximal tubular pressure causes a reduction in renal blood flow and GFR.

212. Which of the following statements concerning postobstructive diuresis is *false*?
   A. It is rare and occurs after release of bilateral ureteral obstruction or solitary kidney obstruction.
   B. Pathologic diuresis results from impaired sodium reabsorption, impaired urine concentrating ability, and solute diuresis due to retained urea and glucose.
   C. Parenteral fluid replacement therapy with 0.9 per cent NS at 100 per cent of urine flow is re-

quired to correct excessive water and sodium loss in pathologic diuresis.
D. Alert, conscious patients undergoing mild physiologic diuresis do not require parenteral fluid administration and can be monitored with daily weights, orthostatic blood pressure measurements, and urine flow determination.
E. Usually, postobstructive diuresis is mild, self-limiting, and physiologic with excretion of retained sodium and water.

213. Of the following, which statement is *not* true concerning renal metabolism?
A. The major metabolic substrate used in the renal cortex is fatty acids.
B. The environment of the inner medulla is anaerobic, and the major substrate is keto acids
C. The kidney extracts only 1.5 ml of O_2 from each 100 ml of arterial blood.
D. After 2 weeks of ureteral obstruction, the hydronephrotic kidney demonstrates decreased utilization of α-ketoglutarate, oxygen, and carbon dioxide, decreased citrate production, and increased respiratory quotient indicating a shift towards anaerobic metabolism.
E. The major biochemical reactions in the renal cortex include fatty acid oxidation, Krebs's cycle oxidations, and gluconeogenesis.

214. Arterial anomalies causing obstruction of the ureter are most common:
A. In the upper third of the ureter
B. In the middle third of the ureter
C. In the lower third of the ureter
D. At the ureterovesical junction (UVJ)

215. All of the following statements are true of abdominal aortic aneurysms EXCEPT:
A. Severe abdominal and low back pain of sudden onset are the symptoms associated most often with an acute or dissecting aneurysm.
B. The ureter is affected in 10 per cent of cases.
C. The left ureter is usually deviated laterally.
D. Hemosiderin-laden macrophages are found frequently in fibrous tissue, which supports the theory of scarring due to multiple small leaks.

216. All of the following statements are true of diagnostic studies for evaluation of extrinsic ureteral obstruction EXCEPT:
A. Ultrasound provides an economical safe method for routinely, precisely pinpointing the site of obstruction.
B. Intravenous urography (IVU) can identify the presence and often the site of obstruction with delayed films.
C. Computed tomography (CT) scans with intravenous contrast often clearly delineate the point of obstruction and frequently the retroperitoneal or intra-abdominal disorder that may be causing the obstruction.
D. Magnetic resonance imaging provides detailed imaging of the vascular system but has a limited role in the assessment of extrinsic ureteral obstruction.

217. The most common cause of postoperative ureteral obstruction following reconstructive vascular surgery is:
A. Retroperitoneal fibrosis secondary to surgery
B. Infection
C. Development of new vascular lesion
D. Neoplasm

218. The following statements about the ovarian vein syndrome are true EXCEPT:
A. Usually it is noted in pregnancy in a multiparous patient.
B. It has been convincingly argued that this entity is a myth.
C. The left ureter is usually involved.
D. Symptoms are not infrequently worse during menses.

219. Which of the following statements about postpartum ovarian vein thrombophlebitis is *true*?
A. 75 per cent are bilateral.
B. It is more common in multiparous women.
C. Ureteral obstruction is uncommon.
D. When unilateral, the left side is more commonly involved.

220. The embryologic developmental abnormality usually responsible for the retrocaval ureter is:
A. Abnormal regression of the posterior cardinal vein
B. Abnormal persistence of the supracardinal vein
C. Abnormal regression of the subcardinal vein
D. Abnormal persistence of the posterior cardinal vein

221. What is the approximate percentage of right-sided predominance of hydroureteronephrosis in pregnancy?
A. 50
B. 65
C. 80
D. 95

222. The most benign pelvic mass to cause ureteral obstruction is:
A. Uterine fibroids
B. Ovarian cysts
C. Ovarian fibromas
D. Hydrometrocolpos

223. The most common site of obstruction of the ureter by a benign pelvic mass is at the:
A. Ureteropelvic junction
B. Mid-ureter
C. Point where ureters cross iliac vessels
D. Ureterovesical junction

224. The incidence of hydroureteronephrosis associated with tubo-ovarian abscesses is approximately what percentage?
A. 25
B. 40
C. 55
D. 70

225. The most common site of urinary tract involvement with endometriosis is:
A. Kidney
B. Ureter

C. Bladder
D. Urethra

226. The most common sites of damage to the ureter in the female during surgery include all of the following EXCEPT:

A. In the ovarian fossa
B. In the infundibulopelvic ligament
C. Where the ureter crosses dorsal to the uterine artery
D. Where the ureter crosses the iliac vessels

227. Ureteral obstruction due to Crohn's disease is:

A. Rarely reported
B. Usually bilateral
C. More common on the left
D. More common on the right

228. Ureteral obstruction due to diverticulitis is:

A. Commonly seen
B. Seen on the left more often than the right
C. Seen on the right more often than the left
D. Usually bilateral

229. All of the following statements about retroperitoneal fibrosis are true EXCEPT:

A. Encasement of the ureters leads to hydronephrosis and varying degrees of renal failure.
B. Arterial obstruction is frequently seen.
C. The middle third of the ureter is displaced toward the midline in one half to two thirds of patients.
D. Occasionally the fibrous process invades the psoas muscles and the ureters.

230. Approximately what portion of patients with retroperitoneal fibrosis have a nonfunctioning kidney at presentation?

A. One third
B. Two thirds
C. One half
D. One fourth

231. All of the following statements are true of the treatment of retroperitoneal fibrosis EXCEPT:

A. Steroids can be helpful in certain instances.
B. Although desirable, ureteral catheters can rarely be placed due to extrinsic compression of ureters.
C. Ureterolysis is usually accomplished with relative ease if the appropriate plane is found.
D. Ureterolysis and transposition, transplantation, or omental wrapping are advocated bilaterally, even in the presence of unilateral disease.

232. All of the following are true of radiation-induced ureteral obstruction EXCEPT:

A. The ureter is relatively radioresistant.
B. The most common site of obstruction is at the site of crossing of the uterine vessels.
C. Chronic obstruction usually becomes evident 1 to 3 years following completion of radiation therapy.
D. One half of late obstructions are due to recurrent cancer.

233. Which of the following is *not* one of the three most common tumors to cause ureteral obstruction:

A. Ovary
B. Cervix
C. Prostate
D. Bladder

234. All of the following statements are true about pelvic lipomatosis EXCEPT:

A. It occurs more frequently in blacks.
B. The lipomatous tissue is composed of mature fatty cells with or without inflammation.
C. Intravenous urography (IVU) demonstrates characteristic lateral displacement of the distal ureters.
D. There is an increased incidence of cystitis glandularis in patients with pelvic lipomatosis.

PART III

THE PATHOPHYSIOLOGY OF URINARY OBSTRUCTION

CHAPTERS 11 AND 12

ANSWERS

205-A *(Campbell's, p. 500)*

A renal biopsy revealing Tamm-Horsfall protein within Bowman's space of the glomerulus is pathognomonic of urinary tract obstruction. Other findings associated with obstructive nephropathy include interstitial fibrosis, glomerulosclerosis, interstitial inflammation, and glomerulocystic changes. Infiltration of mononuclear cells into the renal parenchyma has also been demonstrated in the urinary tract of rabbits following chronic obstruction. In addition, in experimental animals, significant numbers of eosinophils are found in obstructive kidneys.

206-C *(Campbell's, pp. 500–501)*

Although renal tissue atrophies following complete ureteral exclusion, the weight of the kidney increases during the first few weeks secondary to progressive dilation of the renal pelvis and perirenal and periureteral edema. After 4 to 8 weeks, there is a decrease in parenchyma weight because the atrophy of the tissue is greater than the intrarenal edema. Grossly, the obstructive kidney will appear dark blue with scattered areas of ischemia, wedges of congestion, necrosis, and some frank infarcts. Histologic changes include atrophy of the collecting tubules by the seventh day of obstruction. By 14 days, atrophy is noted in the proximal tubular epithelial cells. There is a 50 per cent decrease in medullary thickness by 28 days of obstruction. The glomerulus is last to be damaged, and pathologic changes are first noted after 28 days of complete ureteral obstruction. Ultrastructural changes noted by electron microscopy include thickening of the glomerular basement membrane and obliteration of the filtration slits. Obstruction has been noted to damage the polar regions of the kidneys initially.

207-C *(Campbell's, pp. 501–502)*

Renal lymphatic drainage is through both hilar and capsular lymphatic vessels. Renal lymph volumes are between 0.25 and 0.5 ml/minute in each kidney, and thus the normal kidney produces a lymph volume similar to the volume of urine output. Acute obstruction of renal lymphatics has no significant effect on renal blood flow or glomerular filtration rate; however, there is an increase in the excretion of sodium, chloride, and water. Studies have also shown that in a state of hydronephrosis renal function is preserved by pyelolymphatic backflow, pyelovenous backflow, and extravasation into the perirenal space. Initially, with low pressures most of the fluid enters the lymphatics by pyelocanalicular and pyelosinus backflow. With higher renal pelvis pressures, however, the egress of urine is mainly by pyelovenous backflow and extravasation from traumatic rupture of the calyceal fornix. The ligation of both renal lymphatics and the ureter causes severe renal damage with necrosis and destruction in several days as opposed to several months.

208-E *(Campbell's, pp. 505–506)*

The human kidney can recover function after release of periods of obstruction up to 69 days. Return of function also depends on other factors, such as absence of infection, presence of intrarenal or extrarenal pelvis in the obstructive kidney, or the degree of pyelolymphatic and pyelovenous backflow.

209-D *(Campbell's, pp. 506–508)*

Impairment of all aspects of renal function except urinary dilution has been demonstrated in the hydronephrotic kidney of humans. Impairment of urinary concentrating ability is probably the first derangement of physiologic function that occurs with obstructive uropathy. Impairment of urinary acidification, including ammonia excretion, titratable acidity, and bicarbonate absorption, has been demonstrated in the hydronephrotic kidney. Furthermore, the postobstructive kidney exhibits a reduction in glomerular filtration rate and renal blood flow.

210-C *(Campbell's, pp. 508–509)*

The pressure in the renal pelvis slightly exceeds the intraperitoneal and bladder pressures. Normal renal pelvic pressure measured via the percutaneous puncture method is 6.5 mm of mercury. Ureteral obstruction causes an elevation in the renal pelvic pressure. With obstruction secondary to calculi, baseline pressures have been measured to be elevated to 20 to 25 mm of mercury. Pressures as high as 50 to 70 mm of mercury have been recorded in patients experiencing pain from obstruction.

211-B *(Campbell's, pp. 516–519)*

Significant differences in physiologic changes have been observed in experimental animals depending on whether the ureteral obstruction was bilateral or unilateral. Proximal tubular pressure is lower than normal in unilateral ureteral obstruction but significantly increased in bilateral ureteral obstruction. On the other hand, distal tubule pressure is significantly increased in bilateral ureteral obstruction but is normal in unilateral obstruction. Natriuresis and diuresis occur after release of bilateral but not unilateral obstruction. Renal blood flow and single nephron glomerular filtration rate are 33 per cent of control values after release of 24 hours of bilateral and unilateral ureteral obstruction. Total renal blood flow and GFR are reduced in both unilateral and bilateral obstruction; however, different mechanisms account for these changes. In unilateral obstruction there is vasoconstriction of the afferent arteriole reducing blood flow and GFR. On the other hand, in bilateral ureteral obstruction, proximal tubular pressure and efferent arteriole resistance are increased.

212-C *(Campbell's, pp. 519–521)*

Postobstructive diuresis is rare and usually occurs after release of bilateral ureteral obstruction or solitary kidney obstruction. Usually the diuresis is mild, self-limiting, and physiologic with excretion of retained excess amounts of sodium and water. Rarely, however, pathologic diuresis can occur when there is significant impaired sodium reabsorption, impaired urine concentrability, and solute diuresis due to retained urea or glucose. Since the majority of patients experience mild diuresis and natriuresis that are physiologic, total fluid replacement is unnecessary. Patients that are alert and conscious can usually be monitored with daily weight, orthostatic blood pressure measurements, and hourly urine volume measurements. The normal thirst mechanisms serve to restore fluid volume in these mild cases. In rare cases where the diuresis is pathologic and the patient is unconscious, close monitoring is necessary and replacement with half-normal saline or Ringer's lactate solution at 50 to 60 per cent of urine output is usually necessary.

213-B *(Campbell's, pp. 522–524)*

The kidneys receive 25 per cent of the cardiac output and consume 8 to 10 per cent of the body's oxygen. Despite the high blood flow per gram of tissue, the kidneys extract only 1.5 ml of oxygen from each 100 ml of arterial blood. The metabolism in zones of the kidney differ significantly. In the renal cortex, which is an aerobic environment, the major substrate used in biochemical reactions is fatty acids. The primary reactions that occur are fatty acid oxidation, Krebs's cycle oxidations, and gluconeogenesis. The outer medullary zone has a mixed environment where the major substrates are glucose and keto acids and the major biochemical reactions are Krebs's cycle oxidations and glycolysis. The inner medullary zone has an anaerobic environment where the major substrate is glucose and the major biochemical reaction is glycolysis. Ureteral obstruction causes significant impairment of renal metabolism. In vivo studies have shown that following 2 weeks of total ureteral obstruction there is decreased utilization of α-ketoglutarate, oxygen, and carbon dioxide, decreased citrate production, and elevated respiratory quotient indicating a shift towards anaerobic metabolism. Furthermore, there is an increase in the lactate to pyruvate ratio, indicating a shift toward anaerobic metabolism. Beyond 6 weeks of obstruction, there are marked and probable irreversible changes in renal metabolic function.

214-C *(Campbell's, pp. 537–538)*

There are a number of vascular anomalies that rarely cause ureteral obstruction. Although obstruction may occur at any level, it is more frequently in the lower third of the ureter. Treatment of a significant obstructive vascular anomaly requires surgical exploration, at which time the surgeon must decide whether to resect the ureter or the offending vessel.

REFERENCE

1. Quattlebaum, R., and Anderson, A. IV: Ureteral obstruction secondary to a patient umbilical artery in a 79-year-old man: A case report. J. Urol., *134*:347, 1985.

215-D *(Campbell's, p. 536)*

All the statements are true except D. Two theories exist for the development of perianeurysmic fibrosis and retroperitoneal scarring. One is that small leaks develop at the weakest points of the aneurysm. If this theory were true, the fibrous tissue should contain hemosiderin-laden macrophages, which have not been identified. The second explanation relates to the generalized atherosclerotic process involving the formation aneurysm. This is often associated with desmoplastic inflammation and is felt to be a likely explanation for the significant scarring.

REFERENCES

1. Abbott, D.L., Skinner, D.G., Yalowitz, P.A., and Mulder, D.: Abdominal aortic aneurysms: An approach to management. J. Urol., *109*:987, 1973.
2. Peck, D.R., Bhatt, G.M., and Lowman, R.M.: Traction displacement of the ureter: A sign of aortic aneurysm. J. Urol., *109*:983, 1973.

216-A *(Campbell's, p. 534)*

All of the other statements are correct except A. Ultrasound provides an economical and safe method for detecting hydronephrosis and if significant ureteral obstruction is present, hydroureters can be detected as well. The study usually has little value in precisely pinpointing the site of obstruction, but it may be useful in detecting its cause.

217-A *(Campbell's, p. 538)*

Retroperitoneal fibrosis secondary to surgical procedures is the most common cause of ureteral obstruction. It is likely secondary to bleeding or excessive dissection with resultant fibrosis, but other causes include direct surgical injury (ligation, ischemia), pseudoaneurysm formation, and compression from an anteriorly placed graft.

REFERENCES

1. Bergqvist, D., and Takolander, R.: Ureteral obstruction as a complication in aorto-iliac reconstructive surgery. Scand. J. Urol. Nephrol., *17*:391, 1983.
2. Sant, G.R., Heaney, J.A., Parkhurst, E.C., and Blaivas, J.G.: Obstructive uropathy: A potentially serious complication of reconstructive vascular surgery. J. Urol., *129*:16, 1983.

218-C *(Campbell's, p. 539)*

Ovarian vein syndrome is an entity not entirely acknowledged by all investigators. Convincing arguments against it exists. It is usually described in the right ureter of multiparous women, and symptoms are not infrequently worse during menses.

REFERENCES

1. Melnick, R.G., and Bramwit, D.M.: Bilateral ovarian vein syndrome, Am. J. Roentgenol. Radium. Ther. Nucl. Med., *113*:309, 1971
2. Dure-Smith, P.: Ovarian vein syndrome: Is it a myth? Urology, *13*:355, 1979.

219-B *(Campbell's, p. 540)*

Postpartum ovarian vein thrombophlebitis should be differentiated from ovarian vein syndrome. This phenomenon occurs in 1 in 600 deliveries. It is more common in multiparous women, approximately 10 per cent of the cases are bilateral, and the right side is more commonly involved than the left side. Ureteral obstruction is not uncommon.

REFERENCE

1. Dure-Smith, P.: Ovarian vein syndrome: Is it a myth? Urology, *13*:355, 1979.

220-D *(Campbell's, p. 540)*

The usual embryologic developmental abnormality responsible for the retrocaval ureter is due to the abnormal persistence of the posterior cardinal vein. Normally the posterior cardinal vein undergoes complete regression caudal to the renal vein behind the ureter to assume a normal position ventral to the developing inferior vena cava, which is from the supracardinal vein. The subcardinal vein remains as a tributary to the inferior vena cava, the gonadal vein. This anomaly develops almost exclusively on the right side except in patients with situs inversus.

REFERENCE

1. Lepage, V.R., and Baldwin, G.N.: Obstructive periureteric venous ring. Radiology, *104*:313, 1972.

221-C *(Campbell's, p. 541)*

Experience has demonstrated that unilateral or bilateral obstruction occurs by the third trimester in 90 to 95 per cent of asymptomatic pregnant women, and in more than 80 per cent of the patients right-sided hydroureteronephrosis predominates.

222-A *(Campbell's, p. 542)*

Benign pelvic masses may cause deviation and extrinsic obstruction of the ureter. Uterine fibroids are the most common of these benign tumors to result in extramural ureter obstruction. Years ago, the reported incidence of ureteral involvement due to benign pelvic masses was as high as 50 to 65 per cent. Although the incidence may be less today, it is generally known that ureteral obstruction is a frequent finding with benign masses of the uterus and ovary.

REFERENCE

1. Ney, C., and Friendenberg, R.M.: Gastrointestinal and obstetric gynecologic conditions relating to the urinary system. *In* Radiographic Atlas of the Genitourinary System, 2nd ed. Philadelphia, J. B. Lippincott, 1981, Chapter 12.

223-C *(Campbell's, p. 543)*

The most common site of obstruction is at the point where the ureter crosses the iliac vessels. Uterine fibroids most commonly affect the right side, but they may cause deviation or obstruction of the left ureter or both ureters. The ureteral obstruction and hydronephrosis are generally relieved following treatment with pelvic laparotomy and excision of the mass.

224-B *(Campbell's, p. 543)*

Hydroureteronephrosis is frequently found in the association with tubo-ovarian abscesses with an incidence of ureteral obstruction approaching 40 per cent.

REFERENCE

1. Phillips, J.C.: Spectrum of radiologic abnormalities due to tubo-ovarian abscess. Radiology, *110*:311, 1974.

225-C *(Campbell's, p. 544)*

A variable incidence of urinary tract involvement of up to 24 per cent in women afflicted with endometriosis has been reported. Involvement of the ureter is much less frequent than that of the bladder.

REFERENCE

1. Williams, T.J.: The role of surgery in the management of endometriosis. Mayo Clin. Proc., *50*:198, 1975.

226-D *(Campbell's, p. 547)*

After its descent into the true pelvis, the ureter lies in intimate proximity with the female genital organs, making it subject to injury during surgery. Most commonly the ureter is damaged: (1) in the ovarian fossa during excision of large tumors or cysts; (2) in the infundibulopelvic ligament, when this is taken during hysterectomy; (3) where the ureter crosses dorsal to the uterine artery as the artery is ligated and divided; and (4) in the vesicovaginal space, during the process of reperitonealization.

REFERENCE

1. Persky, L., and Hoch, W.H.: Genitourinary tract trauma. Curr. Probl. Surg., September 1972, 1.

227-D *(Campbell's, pp. 547–548)*

The association of ureteral obstruction in Crohn's disease was first reported in 1943. Using radioactive renography as a sensitive index of ureteral stasis, Schofield and associates found stasis in 50 per cent of patients with regional enteritis. Extrinsic compression of the ureter appears to be caused by the retroperitoneal extension of the severe inflammatory process. Since the predominant area of involvement is the terminal ileum, the proximity of the latter to the right retroperitoneum is responsible for the occurrence of extrinsic ureteral compression on the right side in most reported cases.

REFERENCES

1. Schofield, P.F., Staff, W.G., and Moore, T.: Ureteral involvement in regional ileitis (Crohn's disease). J. Urol., *99*:412, 1968.
2. Hyams, J.A., Weinberg, S.R., and Alley, J.L.: Chronic ileitis with concomitant ureteritis: Case report. Am. J. Surg., *61*:117, 1943.

228-B *(Campbell's, pp. 549–550)*

Diverticulitis is the most frequent complication of diverticulosis. Diverticulosis affects approximately 5 per cent of the population. Urologic complications are found in approximately 20 per cent of patients with diverticulitis; the most frequent is colovesical fistula. Although rare, there have been reports of ureteral obstruction occurring secondary to diverticulitis. The left ureter is involved more often than the right.

REFERENCES

1. Hafner, C.D., Ponka, J.L., and Brush, B.E.: Genitourinary manifestations of diverticulitis of the colon: A study of 500 cases. JAMA, *179*:76, 1962.
2. Kubota, Y., Kawamura, S., Ishii, N., et al.: Ureteral obstruction secondary to sigmoid diverticulitis. Urol. Int., *43*:359, 1988.

229-B *(Campbell's, p. 550)*

Retroperitoneal fibrosis appears as an exuberant mass of tan to white, woody, fibrous tissue covering the retroperitoneal structures. The fibrous process envelops the ureter, tending to drag the middle third of the ureter toward the midline in one half to two thirds of patients. Fibrous encasement of ureters eventually leads to hydronephrosis and varying degrees of renal failure. Although there is generally extensive involvement overlying the great vessels, significant arterial obstruction is rare. Venous obstruction is more common, apparently because of the greater compressibility of the thin-walled veins. Reports have emphasized the occasional invasion of the psoas muscle and the ureters by the fibrous process.

REFERENCES

1. Persky, L., and Huus, J.C.: Atypical manifestations of retroperitoneal fibrosis. J. Urol., *111*:340, 1974.
2. Abdel-Dayem, H.M., Mathew, C.V., Sahwell, A., and El-Sayed, M.: Inferior vena caval obstruction secondary to retroperitoneal fibrosis causing abnormal venous return to left lower limb to portal circulation. Clin. Nucl. Med., *9*:635, 1984.
3. Utz, D.C., and Henry, J.D.: Retroperitoneal fibrosis. Med. Clin. North Am., *50*:1091, 1966.

230-A *(Campbell's, p. 553)*

One third of patients have a nonfunctioning kidney at presentation due to the long-standing obstruction. The obstruction is usually bilateral, but it may be asymmetric and unilateral. The cause of obstruction has been debated but is believed to be due to an interference with ureteral peristalsis by the periureteral inflammatory process.

REFERENCES

1. Baker, L.R.I., Mallinson, W.J.W., Gregory, M.C., et al.: Idiopathic retroperitoneal fibrosis: A retrospective analysis of 60 cases. Br. J. Urol., *60*:497, 1988.
2. Feinstein, R.S., Gatewood, O.M.B., Goldman, S.M., et al.: Computed tomography in the diagnosis of retroperitoneal fibrosis. J. Urol., *126*:255, 1961.

231-B *(Campbell's, p. 554)*

All of the statements are true except B. Despite marked hydronephrosis and significant extrinsic ureteral compression, ureteral catheters of sufficient size, or possibly double J catheters, usually can be passed to the renal pelves. Drainage via percutaneous nephrostomy may also be helpful. Steroids have been found to be helpful in certain incidences, and in select patients the need for major surgery possibly may be averted. Ureterolysis is usually accomplished with relative ease if the appropriate plane is found. After the ureters are completely lysed, they are managed in one of several ways: (1) they may be transplanted into an intraperitoneal position; (2) they may be transposed laterally, interposing retroperitoneal fat between the ureters and the fibrosis; or (3) they may be wrapped with omental fat. The procedure should be performed bilaterally, even in the presence of unilateral disease because later involvement of the contralateral ureter is almost inevitable.

REFERENCES

1. Barnhill, D., Hoskins, W., Bruke, T., et al.: The treatment of retroperitoneal fibromatosis with medroxyprogesterone acetate. Obstet. Gynecol., *70*:502, 1987.
2. Higgins, P.M., Bennett-Jones, D.N., Naish, P.F., and Aber, G.M.: Nonoperative management of retroperitoneal fibrosis. Br. J. Surg., *75*:593, 1988.
3. Ross, J.C., and Goldsmith, H.J.: The combined surgical and medical treatment of retroperitoneal fibrosis. Br. J. Surg., *58*:422, 1971.
4. Tiptaft, R.C., Costello, A.J., Paris, A.M.I., and Blandy, J.P.: The long-term follow-up of idiopathic retroperitoneal fibrosis. Br. J. Urol., *54*:620, 1982.

232-D *(Campbell's, pp. 555–556)*

All of the statements are true except D. The ureter is relatively resistant to radiation, and studies have demonstrated that radiation-induced stricture is unlikely in a normal ureter administered up to 600 rad. The most common point of ureteral obstruction is where the ureter and uterine arteries cross, which is 3 to 6 cm above the ureterovesical junction and 2 cm from the cervical os. Acute ureteral obstruction may become evident near the end of the course of radiation but usually resolves within 3 to 4 months. Chronic obstruction usually becomes evident 1 to 3 years following completion of radiation therapy, although it has been seen as soon as 6 months following completion and up to 10 years or more following completion of radiation therapy. Approximately 90 per cent of late ureteral obstructions following radiation therapy are secondary to recurrent cancer.

233-A *(Campbell's, p. 560)*

Tumors that spread to the retroperitoneum by direct extension usually involve the lower third of the ureter. Typically, these include tumors of cervix, endometrium, bladder, prostate, sigmoid colon, and rectum. The tumor may simply compress the ureteral wall, but it also can invade the serosa to involve the muscularis and mucosa. In decreasing order of frequency, the tumors that cause extrinsic obstruction of the ureter include the cervix, prostate, bladder, colon, ovary and uterus, and stomach.

234-C *(Campbell's, pp. 563–565)*

All of the statements are true except C. Pelvic lipomatosis is rare, fewer than 100 cases have been reported in the literature. Only 4 of these cases have been in females. An unexplained but definite racial predominance has also been noted, with about one half of reported cases occurring in black patients. On pathologic examination, the lipomatous tissue is found to be composed of mature fatty cells with or without inflammation. An increased incidence of edema of the bladder in cystitis glandularis has been noted in association with pelvic lipomatosis. The intravenous urogram IVP usually demonstrates normal upper tracts, but on occasion there may be severe hydroureteronephrosis or, more often, mild distal ureterectasia. Characteristically, the distal ureters are displaced medially.

REFERENCES

1. Yalla, S.V., Duker, M., Burkos, H.M., and Dorey, F.: Cystitis glandularis with perivesical lipomatosis: Frequent association of two unusual proliferative conditions. Urology, *5*:383, 1975.
2. Joshi, W.G., and Wise, H.A. II: Pelvic lipomatosis: 8-year follow-up in a woman. J. Urol., *129*:1233, 1983.

PART IV

NEUROGENIC BLADDER AND INCONTINENCE

CHAPTERS 13 AND 14

DIRECTIONS: Each question below contains suggested responses. Select the ONE BEST response to each question.

235. Which statement is *true* in reference to urethral sphincters?
   A. Internal sphincter is composed of striated muscle.
   B. Internal sphincter is an anatomic entity.
   C. External sphincter is extramural only.
   D. External sphincter extends above the urogenital diaphragm.
   E. Both internal and external sphincters are under voluntary control.

236. Low-pressure storage of urine and continence are a result of all the following conditions EXCEPT:
   A. Viscoelastic properties of the bladder
   B. Cortical inhibition of sacral parasympathetics
   C. Stimulation of beta-adrenergic receptors in the smooth musculature of the bladder body
   D. Inhibition of motor neurons in the sacral cord by pudendal afferents generated by receptors in the striated sphincter
   E. Active and passive urethral wall tension

237. The organizational center for the micturition reflex is:
   A. Pelvic nerve
   B. Basal ganglia
   C. Cerebral cortex
   D. Brain stem
   E. Sacral spinal cord

238. Voluntarily induced micturition results from all the coordinated neural components EXCEPT:
   A. Parasympathetic outflow through the pudendal nerve from the sacral cord
   B. Ascending and descending spinal cord pathways
   C. Cortical facilitory and inhibitory influences
   D. Inhibition of somatic efferents to sphincter
   E. Inhibition of spinal sympathetic reflex

239. Involuntary contractions are most commonly seen in association with:
   A. Inflammation of bladder
   B. Bladder outlet obstruction
   C. Neurologic disease or injury
   D. Indwelling catheters
   E. Urethral hypermobility

240. The bulbocavernosus reflex involves the:
   A. External anal sphincter
   B. Internal anal sphincter
   C. External urethral sphincter
   D. Ischiocavernosus and bulbocavernosus muscles
   E. Levator ani

241. A closed bladder neck on a VCUG will be seen in all the following EXCEPT:
   A. Smooth sphincter dyssynergia
   B. Detrusor areflexia during attempted voiding
   C. External sphincter dyssynergia
   D. Normal resting state

242. In the absence of neurologic disease, uninhibited contractions are referred to as:
   A. Detrusor instability
   B. Detrusor hyperreflexia
   C. Rises in detrusor pressure of >15 cm H_2O
   D. Involuntary bladder contraction
   E. Rises in detrusor pressure of <15 cm H_2O

243. Upper tract deterioration is likely to occur when intravesical pressures are greater than:
   A. 15 cm H_2O
   B. 25 cm H_2O
   C. 40 cm H_2O
   D. 60 cm H_2O

244. A positive bethanechol supersensitivity test results when intravesical pressure rises greater than ___ cm H_2O at ___ cc volume after ___ mg bethanechol IM:
   A. 25, 100, .035
   B. 25, 100, 2.5
   C. 10, 300, .035
   D. 15, 100, .035
   E. 15, 100, 2.5

245. The normal female voiding pressure is:
   A. 10–120 cm H_2O
   B. < 40 cm H_2O
   C. 40–160 cm H_2O
   D. > 60 cm H_2O
   E. The same as seen in males

246. In the Lapides classification, a suprasacral spinal cord injury patient would have an:
   A. Sensory neurogenic bladder
   B. Motor paralytic bladder

C. Uninhibited neurogenic bladder
D. Reflex neurogenic bladder
E. Autonomous neurogenic bladder

247. Urinary tract dysfunction after a cerebrovascular accident is characterized by:

A. Loss of the sensation of fullness
B. Detrusor instability
C. Detrusor hyperreflexia
D. External sphincter dyssynergia
E. Internal sphincter dyssynergia

248. Voluntary contraction of the external sphincter in response to an uninhibited contraction is called:

A. Sacral reflex
B. External sphincter dyssynergia
C. Autonomic dysreflexia
D. Pseudodyssenergia
E. Internal sphincter dyssynergia

249. Which of the following does not have detrusor hyperreflexia when voiding dysfunction occurs?

A. Dementia
B. Concussion
C. Myasthenia gravis
D. Normal pressure hydrocephalus
E. Brain tumor

250. Cerebral palsy patients most commonly will have the following urodynamic findings:

A. Normal urodynamics
B. Detrusor hyperreflexia
C. Detrusor areflexia
D. Striated sphincter dyssynergia
E. Detrusor instability

251. Bladder outlet obstruction can be distinguished from voiding dysfunction in Parkinson's patients with video-urodynamics after the administration of:

A. L-Dopa
B. Apomorphine
C. Ditropan
D. Minipress
E. Urocholine

252. Shy-Drager syndrome is associated with all of the following EXCEPT:

A. Orthostatic hypotension
B. Anhydrosis
C. Incontinence
D. Open bladder neck on VCUG
E. Increased outlet resistance

253. Voiding dysfunction is the first symptom in what percentage of multiple sclerosis patients?

A. 1 per cent
B. 10 per cent
C. 30 per cent
D. 75 per cent
E. 90 per cent

254. All of the following statements are true of spinal shock EXCEPT:

A. It generally lasts 1–12 weeks.
B. Autonomic and somatic activity is absent.
C. An areflexic bladder exists.
D. May last 1–12 years.
E. Retention is the rule.

255. Autonomic hyperreflexia occurs with spinal injuries above which vertebral level:

A. S2
B. T12
C. T10
D. T6
E. C7

256. An areflexic bladder can be seen in all of the following EXCEPT:

A. Poliomyelitis
B. Disc disease
C. Nonneurogenic neurogenic bladder
D. Herpes
E. Pelvic surgery

257. Oxybutynin has all the following properties EXCEPT:

A. Anticholinergic
B. Strong musculotropic relaxant
C. Local anesthetic activity
D. Cannot be given intravesically
E. Can be taken orally

258. Imipramine acts on the bladder primarily by:

A. Anticholinergic action
B. Smooth muscle relaxation
C. Alpha-adrenergic action
D. Beta-adrenergic action
E. Local anesthetic-like action

259. The heaviest concentration of alpha-adrenergic receptors is found in:

A. Membranous urethra
B. Trigone
C. Bladder body
D. External sphincter
E. Bladder neck and proximal urethra

260. A Credé maneuver is relatively contraindicated with:

A. Vesicoureteral reflux
B. Increased outlet resistance
C. Urinary tract infection
D. Neurogenic bladder
E. Coagulopathy

261. Electrical stimulation:

A. Is most effective at the spinal cord level
B. To the ventral nerve roots results in best bladder emptying
C. To the dorsal nerve roots results in best bladder emptying
D. Cannot be delivered directly to the bladder wall
E. Does not result in successful bladder contraction

262. External sphincterotomy can be achieved by all of the following EXCEPT:

A. Endoscopic sphincterotomy
B. Botulinum A toxin injection
C. Urethral overdilatation
D. Pudendal neurectomy
E. Dorsal rhizotomy

263. Synchronous sphincter relaxation and detrusor contraction is coordinated by the:

A. Sacral cord
B. Pelvic plexus

C. Pudendal nucleus
D. Pontine micturition center
E. Cerebral cortex

264. All the following are physiologic changes associated with aging EXCEPT:

A. Increased bladder capacity
B. Increased prevalence of uninhibited contractions
C. Increased post-void residual
D. Body fluid excreted more at night
E. Prostatic hypertrophy

265. Transient incontinence is responsible for incontinence in what percentage of community-dwelling incontinent patients?

A. 10 per cent
B. 25 per cent
C. 33 per cent
D. 50 per cent
E. 67 per cent

266. The most common cause for incontinence in the elderly is:

A. Stool impaction
B. Polypharmacy
C. Outlet obstruction
D. Urethral hypermobility
E. Detrusor overactivity

267. Stress leakage occurs in all of the following EXCEPT:

A. Urethral instability
B. Detrusor hyperactivity with impaired contractility
C. Urethral hypermobility
D. Type III stress incontinence
E. Urinary retention

268. The sensation of precipitant urination or urgency is seen in what percentage of patients with detrusor hyperactivity?

A. 100 per cent
B. 80 per cent
C. 50 per cent
D. 40 per cent
E. 20 per cent

269. One of the most valuable pieces of historical data about incontinence is:

A. Number of past urinary tract infections
B. Quantification of leakage
C. Sexual habits
D. Voiding record
E. Bowel function

270. What part of the physical examination reveals the most about bladder and urethral function?

A. Simple cystometry
B. Video-urodynamics
C. Voiding cystourethrogram
D. Marshall or Bonney test
E. Observed voiding

271. The best treatment for detrusor overactivity is:

A. To provide a bedside commode or urinal
B. Behavioral therapy
C. Anticholinergic therapy
D. Smooth muscle relaxants
E. Indwelling catheter

272. Leakage around an indwelling catheter is best treated by:

A. Removing the catheter
B. Antibiotic suppression
C. Changing the catheter
D. Anticholinergic/bladder suppressants
E. Placing a larger catheter

PART IV

NEUROGENIC BLADDER AND INCONTINENCE

CHAPTERS 13 AND 14

ANSWERS

235-D *(Campbell's, p. 574)*

The internal sphincter is composed of smooth muscle of the bladder neck and the proximal urethra. This has physiologic function but is not present anatomically. The classic external sphincter was a portion of striated muscle within the leaves of the urogenital diaphragm. This concept has been expanded to also include an intramural portion that extends up to the bladder neck in females and to the apex of the prostate in males. Therefore, answer D is the correct response. The external sphincter can be voluntarily controlled, but the internal sphincter is under involuntary control.

236-B *(Campbell's, p. 575)*

Bladder filling is the result of viscoelastic properties of the bladder wall, and relaxation of the smooth body musculature by stimulation of beta-adrenergic receptors. The inhibition of the motor neurons in the sacral cord is by pudendal afferents generated by receptors in the striated sphincter. The sympathetics may have an inhibitory affect on the cholinergic ganglionic transmission. There is also the creation of active and passive urethral wall tension by alpha-adrenergic stimulation, as well as the bulk of the elastic collagenous tissue and the mucosa and submucosal tissue.

237-D *(Campbell's, pp. 575–576)*

The stimulus responsible for initiating voluntary bladder contraction is increased intravesical pressure. This is sensed by the cortex, and the organizational center for the micturition reflex is in the brain stem. The parasympathetic outflow to the bladder originates in the sacral spinal cord and travels out through the pelvic nerve to the detrusor musculature.

238-A *(Campbell's, pp. 575–576)*

Voluntarily induced voiding requires parasympathetic outflow through the pelvic nerves from the sacral cord. There are cortical facilitory and inhibitory influences that are mediated through the ascending and the descending spinal cord pathways. Inhibition of the somatic efferents to the external sphincter through the pudendal nerve and also inhibition of the spinal sympathetic reflex to relax the internal sphincter must also occur. The pudendal nerve, however, does not carry the motor fibers to the bladder, and therefore selection A is a false statement.

239-C *(Campbell's, p. 576)*

Involuntary contractions are most commonly seen in association with neurologic disease or injury. They can also be seen with inflammatory conditions of the bladder, bladder outlet obstruction, indwelling catheters, or urethral hypermobility. They may also be due to idiopathic reasons where no etiology can be identified.

240-D *(Campbell's, p. 578)*

The bulbocavernosus reflex results from contraction of the bulbocavernosus and the ischiocavernosus muscles due to stimulation of the glans or corpora and also with stimulation of the urethral and bladder mucosa. It is mediated by the pudendal nerve, both afferent and efferent, and is thought to involve S2–S4 activity. It can be demonstrated in 98 per cent of normal male patients and 81 per cent of normal female patients. Absence of this reflex in the male suggests neurologic lesions involving the sacral spinal cord. However, presence of the bulbocavernosus reflex in either sex does not rule out the possibility that a significant lesion may still exist.

241-C *(Campbell's, p. 580)*

Radiographic studies can help complement the work-up of neuromuscular voiding dysfunction. A closed bladder neck is seen in the normal resting state while the bladder is filling. It is also seen in cases of detrusor areflexia during attempted voluntary micturition and with smooth sphincter dyssynergia. An open bladder neck would be seen with external sphincter dyssynergia as well as during normal voiding or in patients with a nonfunctional bladder neck or proximal urethra. This stresses the importance of incorporating both the historical and the urodynamic findings when interpreting radiologic findings.

242-A *(Campbell's, p. 586)*

Uninhibited contractions are referred to as detrusor hyperreflexia when neurologic disease is present. When there is no neurologic process ongoing, it is referred to as detrusor instability. Another term for an uninhibited contraction would be an involuntary bladder contraction, which occurs in neurologic and nonneurologic conditions. A contraction can be clinically significant if it is greater or even less than 15 centimeters of water. The International Continence Society originally defined these as only two consistent spikes greater than 15 centimeters of water above baseline.

243-C *(Campbell's, pp. 587)*

Adequate storage at low intravesical pressure will prevent upper urinary tract deterioration in patients with neurogenic bladders. McGuire and others found that upper tract deterioration is much more likely to occur when intravesical storage pressures are greater than 40 centimeters of water. This is commonly referred to as the "leak point" measured during urodynamic study.

244-E *(Campbell's, p. 588)*

The bethanechol supersensitivity test is positive in patients with a motor paralytic bladder. First, an average baseline pressure is obtained, and then 2.5 mg of bethanechol chloride is injected IM and pressure readings taken again at 10, 20, and 30 minutes at 100 ml volume. In heavier patients, it has been recommended to administer bethanechol in the dose of .035 mg/kg. A rise of greater than 15 cm H_2O above baseline pressure is consistent with a positive bethanechol supersensitivity test. This is suggestive of an interruption in the peripheral, neural, and/or distal spinal pathways to and from the bladder.

245-B *(Campbell's, p. 588)*

The normal adult male generally voids with a pressure of between 40 and 60 centimeters of water. The normal female voids at a much lower pressure. Many women will void with almost no detectable rise in detrusor pressure. This is mostly due to a much lower outlet resistance. The range may vary in women and generally would be less than 40 centimeters of water. Therefore, selection B is more correct than selection A.

246-D *(Campbell's, p. 598)*

In the Lapides classification, sensory neurogenic bladder results from disease processes that interrupt sensory fibers between the bladder and the spinal cord or the afferent tracts to the brain. Diabetes mellitus, tabes dorsalis, and pernicious anemia are the most common etiologies. The motor paralytic bladder results from destruction of the parasympathetic motor innervation to the bladder. This is seen in conditions such as pelvic surgery, trauma, or herpes zoster. An uninhibited neurogenic bladder is commonly seen in patients with cerebral cortex abnormalities and disruption of the corticoregulatory fibers. A reflex neurogenic bladder is seen after complete interruption of the sensory and motor pathways between the sacral spinal cord and the brain stem. This is typified by no bladder sensation and inability to initiate voluntary micturition with detrusor hyperreflexia and striated sphincter dyssynergia. An autonomous neurogenic bladder results from complete motor and sensory separation of the bladder from the sacral spinal cord and results in an areflexic bladder.

247-C *(Campbell's, p. 601)*

After an acute cerebrovascular accident, urinary retention may occur. The long-term voiding dysfunction is characterized by detrusor hyperreflexia. Sensation is generally intact. The uninhibited contraction is coordinated with the external sphincter. Internal sphincter dyssynergia does not occur after cerebrovascular accidents. The patients will experience urgency with the uninhibited contractions and may be able to suppress the urge consciously by contracting their external sphincter.

248-D *(Campbell's, p. 602)*

Voluntary contraction of the external sphincter in response to an uninhibited contraction is called pseudodyssynergia. The patient is consciously aware of the uninhibited contraction and feels the urgency and has the ability to voluntary contract his sphincter to avoid leakage and incontinence.

249-C *(Campbell's, p. 602)*

Disease processes involving the cerebral cortex will be associated with detrusor hyperreflexia and usually synergic striated and smooth sphincter activity. Dementia, concussions, brain tumors, cerebrovascular accidents, cerebellar ataxia, normal pressure hydrocephalus, and any other primary cerebral processes will manifest detrusor hyperreflexia as the most common urodynamic finding. Many of these patients with these disease processes will have normal voiding function.

250-A *(Campbell's, pp. 602–603)*

Patients with cerebral palsy usually have total urinary control with normal filling and storage and normal emptying. Control may not be gained until adulthood due to the delayed development. When they do have voiding dysfunction, 75 per cent will manifest detrusor hyperreflexia with coordinated sphincters. Spinal cord damage can also occur and striated sphincter dyssynergia or an areflexic bladder could potentially be seen.

251-B *(Campbell's, p. 603)*

Parkinson's disease is associated with voiding dysfunction in 25–75 per cent of the patients. The most common urodynamic finding is detrusor hyperreflexia. Around 8 to 10 per cent of patients may actually have detrusor areflexia. This group of patients is very difficult to determine whether or not they will benefit from relief of coexistent bladder outlet obstruction. The apomorphine is a dopamine receptor agonist and can rapidly reverse Parkinsonian symptoms. Sophisticated video urodynamic studies obtained during the motor improvement after administration of the apomorphine can help distinguish between bladder outlet obstruction secondary to prostatic hypertrophy or bladder dysfunction secondary to the Parkinson's disease itself.

252-E *(Campbell's, p. 604)*

Shy-Drager syndrome is a rare disorder characterized by orthostatic hypotension, anhydrosis, cerebellar dysfunction, impotence, and voiding dysfunction. Detrusor hyperreflexia occurs in about one third of the patients and decreased compliance without phasic interruption appears to be just as common. The patients are unable to generate a voluntary detrusor contraction, and many exhibit evidence of external sphincter denervation. An open bladder neck can often be seen on a VCUG. Because of the autonomic insufficiency they will have decreased smooth or internal sphincter function, and, coupled with the external sphincter weakness, this results in decreased outlet resistance.

253-B *(Campbell's, p. 604)*

Multiple sclerosis is a demyelinating process which most commonly involves the posterior and lateral columns of the cervical spinal cord. Involvement of the lumbar and sacral cord occurs in 40 and 18 per cent of patients, respectively. At some time during the disease process, 50 to 80 per cent of the patients will have voiding symptoms. Lower urinary tract involvement may be the initial complaint in around 10 per cent of the patients and is usually in the form of acute urinary retention or an acute onset of urgency and frequency. Detrusor hyperreflexia is the most common urodynamic abnormality seen on urodynamics and is seen in 50 to 90 per cent of cases; 30 to 65 per cent will also have coexistent striated sphincter dyssynergia. The smooth sphincter is generally synergic.

254-A *(Campbell's, pp. 605–606)*

Spinal shock is seen after acute injury of the spinal cord and is due to a period of decreased excitability of the cord segments below the injury. Autonomic as well as somatic activity is suppressed, and the bladder is usually acontractile and areflexic. Generally, it lasts 6–12 weeks but may last up to 1 to 2 years.

255-D *(Campbell's, p. 608)*

Autonomic hyperreflexia is an exaggerated sympathetic response to stimuli below the level of the lesion. Sympathetic outflow comes out primarily through T10–L1 nerve roots. The level of the vertebral body above which this comes out is T6.

256-C *(Campbell's, pp. 609–612)*

An areflexic bladder due to motor nerve involvement is seen in 4 to 42 per cent of patients with poliomyelitis. Disc disease most commonly occurs at L4-L5 and L5-S1 interspaces, and voiding dysfunction can be seen in 1 to 18 per cent of patients. A laminectomy may not improve bladder function. Interruption of the pelvic plexus is most commonly seen in abdominal perineal resections and hysterectomies. Neurologic dysfunction can be seen in 10 to 60 per cent of these patients, and in 15 to 20 per cent of them the dysfunction is permanent. Herpes zoster can involve the sacral spinal nerves and will produce urinary retention and detrusor areflexia. Nonneurogenic/neurogenic bladder is the presence of urodynamic evidence of involuntary obstruction at the striated sphincter level in the absence of any demonstrable neurologic disease. Etiology is uncertain.

257-D *(Campbell's, p. 616)*

Ditropan is a moderately potent anticholinergic agent with strong musculotropic relaxant activity and also local anesthetic properties in the bladder. It is usually given orally at 5 mg three times a day and has recently been given in an intravesical preparation as well.

258-B *(Campbell's, p. 618)*

Imipramine has very strong systemic anticholinergic effects, but only weak antimuscarinic effects on the bladder. It has a very strong direct inhibitory effect on bladder smooth muscle, and this is the main action of imipramine. It also has an enhanced alpha-adrenergic effect on the smooth muscle in the bladder base and proximal urethra. This is the main reason why it increases urethral resistance. It has some local anesthetic-like action as well. There is no beta-adrenergic action of imipramine.

259-E *(Campbell's, p. 623)*

The heaviest concentration of alpha-adrenergic receptors is found in the bladder neck and the proximal urethra. Beta-adrenergic receptors are more preponderant in the bladder body.

260-A *(Campbell's, p. 628)*

The Credé maneuver is relatively contraindicated in vesicoureteral reflux. This would transmit high pressures to the upper urinary tract and generally result in more rapid deterioration. The other factors mentioned are not contraindications.

261-B *(Campbell's, pp. 631–632)*

Electrical stimulation can be used to help achieve bladder emptying. Initial results when applied directly to the cord resulted in both contraction of the bladder muscle as well as the external sphincter. Selective stimulation of the ventral roots coupled with a dorsal rhizotomy helps to achieve maximal detrusor stimulation and minimal external sphincter activity. Transurethral intravesical electrotherapy has also been used with some success. It is theorized that as the motor activity in a neurogenic bladder is stimulated, vegetative afferentation begins, and new pathways are stimulated.

262-E *(Campbell's, p. 635)*

External sphincterotomy can be achieved by endoscopic incision at the 12 o'clock position. Botulinum A toxin can also be injected into the sphincter and is given once a week for 3 weeks and can have a duration of up to 2 months. In females, urethral overdilatation of 40–50 Fr. is equivalent to an external sphincterotomy in the male. Pudendal neurectomy will result in non-function of the external sphincter but is also associated with a high incidence of fecal incontinence and impotence. Dorsal rhizotomy interrupts the sensory nerves to the bladder.

263-D *(Campbell's, pp. 643–644)*

The pontine micturition center mediates synchronous sphincter relaxation and detrusor contraction. The cerebral cortex, basal ganglia, and cerebellum all exhibit some inhibitory and facilatory effects. Detrusor relaxation is accomplished by central nervous system inhibition of parasympathetic tone. Sphincter closure is mediated by reflex increase in alpha-adrenergic and pudendal somatic activity. The other choices conduct impulses, but they are not involved in the coordination as is the pontine micturition center.

264-A *(Campbell's, p. 644)*

Aging affects the lower urinary tract in many ways, which may predispose elderly people to incontinence. None of these changes cause incontinence, but each one predisposes to it. The bladder capacity, the ability to postpone voiding, and urinary flow rate probably decline in both sexes. Therefore A is the desired selection, as aging is not associated with increased bladder capacity. In women the maximal urethral closure pressure and urethral length decrease. Uninhibited contractions appear more commonly in elderly patients even in the absence of neurologic disease. The post-void residual generally increases but often to no more than 50 to 100 ml. Elderly patients who are healthy often excrete the bulk of their daily fluid intake during the night. Prostatic hypertrophy in men also changes the voiding pattern. These are all normal responses, and there are certainly many pathologic conditions that will exacerbate these changes or create symptoms of their own.

265-C *(Campbell's, pp. 644–645)*

Transient incontinence is responsible for one third of the cases of community-dwelling incontinent individuals. It is also responsible for up to half of hospitalized patients who are incontinent. The mnemonic DIAPPERS is used to help remember the causes. This stands for delirium, infections, atrophic vaginitis, pharmaceuticals, psychologic, excess of urine output, restricted mobility, and stool impaction. There are many different classes of drugs that may cause voiding dysfunction, including sedatives, hypnotics, diuretics, anticholinergic agents, adrenergic agents, calcium channel blockers, and vincristine.

266-E *(Campbell's, pp. 646–648)*

Established incontinence is responsible for two thirds of incontinence in elderly individuals. Of these, detrusor overactivity is the leading cause in older individuals. Stool impaction is a reversible cause of incontinence that is responsible for up to 10 per cent of the cases of incontinence. Polypharmacy in itself does not increase incontinence unless the medication profile involves medications that affect voiding mechanisms. Outlet obstruction is a common cause of incontinence in men, but, overall, most obstructed men are not incontinent. Urethral hypermobility is also seen in elderly patients and is the leading cause of incontinence in middle-aged women and the second most common cause in older women. This should be managed in the same manner as in a younger individual.

267-B *(Campbell's, p. 647)*

Stress leakage will be seen in patients with both urethral hypermobility and Type 3 stress incontinence in elderly patients as well as in younger patients. Urinary retention is an uncommon cause of stress-associated leakage, but a full bladder will leak when intra-abdominal pressure overcomes the outlet pressure. Urethral instability is a condition where the sphincter abruptly and paradoxically relaxes in the absence of any detrusor contractions. This is an uncommon cause of stress leakage. Detrusor hyperactivity with impaired contractility will not result in stress incontinence. It can, however, be very difficult to differentiate this as a cause without more sophisticated urodynamic evaluation.

268-B *(Campbell's, pp. 648–649)*

Detrusor hyperactivity classically causes urge incontinence. This is an abrupt sensation that the patient must urinate, whether or not leakage occurs. About 20 per cent of patients will not experience a feeling of urgency with uninhibited contractions. In demented patients this number is even higher. Therefore, the correct answer is that only 80 per cent of patients will experience urgency.

269-D *(Campbell's, p. 650)*

The voiding record is one of the most valuable historical aids. This should be recorded for a period of 24–72 hours and information recorded every 2 hours. The volume voided and the frequency of voiding as well as incontinent episodes should all be a part of this record. This may give important insight and subtle clues to factors associated with the patient's incontinence, which might otherwise be overlooked. All the other statements are also portions of the history that should be obtained, although by themselves would rarely or never be as helpful as a well-documented voiding record.

270-E *(Campbell's, pp. 651–652)*

Observed voiding is a very important component of the physical examination and will reveal more about bladder and urethral functions than any other portion. Volume voided and observing for evidence of straining, force of the stream, and inability to interrupt stream can provide important clues to the etiology of incontinence. Post-void residual at the end of this examination will provide important information as to how well the patient empties. Adding the post-void residual volume to the voided volume provides an estimate for total bladder capacity.

271-B *(Campbell's, p. 652)*

Detrusor overactivity should be initially evaluated so that reversible causes can be identified and treated. If there are no treatable reversible causes, then behavioral therapy is the cornerstone of treatment. Bedside urinals can be very successful in some cases. By extending the intervoiding interval with a bladder training regimen, the patient can extend the dry period for longer intervals. Once they are dry during the day, then they generally become dry at night as well. If the patient is demented, then prompted voiding can be used. It can reduce the frequency of incontinence by 25 to 45 per cent. Usually within the first 1 to 2 days 75 per cent of nursing home patients who will respond to prompted voiding can be identified. Patients with more than four incontinent episodes per 12-hour period will not usually become totally dry and need further therapy. Anticholinergics or smooth muscle relaxants can help, although they usually do not completely suppress the contractions, and toileting schedules must be incorporated. Indwelling catheters are not a good choice and will usually exacerbate uninhibited contractions.

272-D *(Campbell's, p. 655)*

Leakage around an indwelling urethral catheter or suprapubic tube is usually secondary to uninhibited contractions due to mucosal irritation of the catheter. Catheters with small balloons of small caliber are best to use because they are less irritating. If the catheter must be left indwelling, an anticholinergic or bladder suppressant medication is indicated. Placing larger catheters will usually exacerbate the problem and will also dilate the suprapubic tract or increase urethral complications. Antibiotic suppression with long-term catheter drainage usually results in development of bacterial resistance.

PART V

INFERTILITY

CHAPTER 15

DIRECTIONS: Each question below contains suggested responses. Select the ONE BEST response to each question.

274. Of the 15 per cent of infertile couples, how often is the subfertility due to the male factor?
   A. 10 per cent
   B. 20 per cent
   C. 33 per cent
   D. 50 per cent
   E. 67 per cent

275. Which lubricant does not impair sperm motility?
   A. K-Y jelly
   B. Keri Lotion
   C. Saliva
   D. Lubifax
   E. Petroleum jelly

276. The optimal frequency of intercourse to conceive is:
   A. Twice daily during the mid-menstrual cycle
   B. Once a day during the mid-menstrual cycle
   C. Every 2 days during the mid-menstrual cycle
   D. On the day of ovulation
   E. Weekly

277. Azoospermia with a history of frequent respiratory infections is seen in:
   A. Klinefelter's syndrome
   B. Young's syndrome
   C. Kartagener's syndrome
   D. Kallmann's syndrome
   E. Immotile cilia syndrome

278. Subclinical varicoceles:
   A. Are visible in the supine position
   B. Do not increase intrascrotal/testicular temperatures
   C. Are seen in only 10 per cent of infertile men
   D. Are best identified by venography
   E. Have not been shown to definitively improve pregnancy rates when fixed

279. With regard to nonliquefaction or hyperviscosity of semen:
   A. It is always a significant factor.
   B. A postcoital test should be performed.
   C. FSH, LH, and testosterone levels should be ordered.
   D. Seminal vesicles are hypertrophic.
   E. A post-ejaculate urine should be evaluated.

280. Patients with obstructed or congenitally absent seminal vesicles manifest which of the following conditions?
   A. Semen pH > 7
   B. Normal semen fructose
   C. Bilateral absence of vas deferens
   D. Normal ejaculate volume
   E. Hyperviscous semen

281. Minimally adequate semen parameters include all the following EXCEPT:
   A. Volume of 1.5–5.0 ml
   B. Total sperm count >20 million
   C. Motility ≥60 per cent
   D. Morphology ≥60 per cent
   E. Forward progression >2

282. White blood cells can be differentiated from other round cells in semen by:
   A. Light microscopy
   B. Phase contrast microscopy
   C. Electron microscopy
   D. H & E stains
   E. Immunohistochemical stains

283. The most common cause for an abnormal postcoital test is:
   A. Anatomic abnormalities
   B. Antisperm antibodies
   C. Anovulation
   D. Inappropriate timing of test
   E. Inappropriately performed intercourse

284. Antisperm antibodies should be investigated in all the following situations EXCEPT:
   A. Impaired motility
   B. Sperm agglutination
   C. >10–15 round cells/hpf
   D. Abnormal postcoital test
   E. Unexplained infertility

285. The gold standard for validation of the sperm penetration assay (SPA) is:
   A. Postcoital test
   B. Hemizona assay
   C. Immunobead assay
   D. In vitro fertilization
   E. Micromanipulation

286. Distal ductal obstruction of the vas is ruled out as a cause of azoospermia if:
   A. TRUS reveals nondilated seminal vesicles
   B. Semen fructose levels are normal
   C. Bilateral vasography is normal
   D. Retrograde vasography is normal
   E. Unilateral vasography is normal

287. In patients with bilateral atrophic testes and markedly elevated FSH, testicular biopsy usually shows:

A. Absence of Sertoli cells
B. Absence of germ cells
C. Tubular sclerosis
D. Hypospermatogenesis
E. Maturation arrest

288. Crystalloids of Reinke are seen in:

A. Yolk sac tumors
B. Sertoli cells
C. Leydig cells
D. Spermatogonia
E. Macrophages

289. The most common histologic finding on a testicular biopsy done for infertility is:

A. Normal testes
B. Hypospermatogenesis and maturation arrest
C. Germinal aplasia
D. Fetal pattern
E. End-stage testes

290. The diagnosis of retrograde ejaculation may be made when:

A. The patient is anejaculatory
B. A low semen volume exists
C. There are >5–10 sperm/hpf in a postejaculate urine
D. Azoospermia and anejaculatory states coexist
E. Infertility occurs after RPLND for testis tumor

291. To initiate spermatogenesis in the hypogonadotropic hypogonadism patient, you must give:

A. Testosterone enanthate 200 mg IM every other week
B. hCG 2000 U IM 3 times per week
C. FSH 75 IU IM 3 times per week
D. Pergonal 1/2 vial 3 times per week
E. Oral testosterone supplementation

292. Fertile eunuchs characteristically have:

A. Low FSH levels
B. High FSH levels
C. Low LH levels
D. High LH levels
E. Atrophic testes

293. The most common etiology for infertility seen in most large series is:

A. Varicocele
B. Endocrine
C. Antisperm antibodies
D. Testicular failure
E. Idiopathic

294. Hypogonadotropic hypogonadism is seen in all the following syndromes EXCEPT:

A. Prader-Willi syndrome
B. Kallmann's syndrome
C. Laurence-Moon-Bardet-Beidl syndrome
D. Klinefelter's syndrome
E. Fertile eunuch syndrome

295. Excess of all the following may produce infertility EXCEPT:

A. FSH
B. Prolactin
C. Androgens
D. Estrogens
E. Glucocorticoids

296. Infertility may be seen with the following karyotype:

A. XX
B. XY
C. XYY
D. XXY
E. All the above

297. Testicular dysfunction is not seen in:

A. Intra-abdominal testes
B. Inguinal cryptorchidism
C. Vanishing testis syndrome
D. Ectopic testes
E. All the above

298. Which of the following statements regarding varicoceles is *false*?

A. Varicoceles are found in about 30 per cent of infertile males.
B. Oligospermia is the most common semen finding.
C. Seminal parameters are improved in 70 per cent of patients after repair.
D. Intrascrotal temperatures are 0.6°C higher in patients with varicoceles.
E. Conception rates are 40–50 per cent after repair.

299. All of the following can improve fertility in patients with antisperm antibodies EXCEPT:

A. Semen processing
B. Corticosteroids — high-dose regimen
C. Intrauterine insemination
D. In vitro fertilization
E. Corticosteroids — intermediate cyclic regimen

300. Which of the following agents has shown great promise in treating idiopathic male infertility?

A. Clomiphene citrate
B. hCG
C. Pergonal
D. GnRH
E. None of the above

301. Epididymal obstruction may be caused by all EXCEPT:

A. Tuberculous epididymitis
B. Young's syndrome
C. Chlamydia
D. Cystic fibrosis
E. Smallpox

PART V

INFERTILITY

CHAPTER 15

ANSWERS

274-D *(Campbell's, p. 661)*

Fifteen per cent of couples are unable to achieve conception within a 1-year period of time. Data have shown that about 20 per cent of these cases are due to a male factor alone. An additional 30 per cent of cases involve both male and female factors. This means that one half of infertility problems involve the male factor as the direct cause or as a contributing cause.

275-E *(Campbell's, pp. 661–662)*

Unless absolutely necessary, lubricants should not be used for intercourse. Lubifax, K-Y Jelly, Keri Lotion, Surgilube, and saliva all adversely affect sperm motility. Peanut oil, safflower oil, vegetable oil, petroleum jelly, and raw egg whites have been demonstrated to not impair sperm motility in vitro.

276-C *(Campbell's, p. 661)*

The ovulatory period is during the mid-menstrual cycle. Sperm remain viable within the cervical mucus and crypts for about 48 hours. Intercourse every 2 days ensures that viable sperm are present during the 12- to 24-hour period in which the oocyte is within the fallopian tube and is capable of being fertilized. Intercourse that is too frequent may cause inadequate concentrations of sperm, and, obviously, too infrequent intercourse will often miss the time interval when fertilization is possible.

277-B *(Campbell's, p. 662)*

Young's syndrome is associated with azoospermia and frequent respiratory infections. Epididymal obstruction often occurs due to inspissation of secretions. Klinefelter's syndrome is also associated with azoospermia but is not associated with any respiratory infections. Immotile cilia syndrome and Kartagener's syndrome have sperm present, but they are immotile. They also have a history of frequent respiratory infections, and Kartagener's syndrome is associated with situs inversus. Kallmann's syndrome is hypogonadotropic hypogonadism and is associated with anosmia.

278-E *(Campbell's, pp. 663–664)*

Varicoceles occur commonly in both fertile and infertile men. Grade I varicoceles are palpable only during a Valsalva maneuver; moderate-sized varicoceles are palpable in the standing position; and large varicoceles are visible through the scrotal skin. Subclinical varicoceles are identified by other methods and are not grossly demonstrated. Doppler studies, scrotal thermography, and venography are able to identify subclinical varicoceles. With use of these techniques, up to 91 per cent of patients with idiopathic infertility may have subclinical varicoceles. There are no definitive studies that show repairing subclinical varicoceles is associated with improved pregnancy rate.

279-B *(Campbell's, p. 666)*

Nonliquefaction or hyperviscosity of semen is of uncertain significance in regard to infertility. When it is present, a postcoital test should be performed. If normal numbers of sperm are penetrating the cervical mucus, then you can disregard the hyperviscosity or nonliquefaction. If the postcoital test demonstrates few sperm in the mucous, then a cross-mucus hostility test or an in vitro cervical mucous-sperm interaction test may be employed.

280-C *(Campbell's, p. 667)*

Semen pH is normally between 7.05 and 7.8. The pH of seminal vesicle secretions is greater than 7 and that of prostatic secretions is usually less than 7. Therefore, in congenitally absent or obstructed seminal vesicles the pH would be less than 7. Fructose is produced by seminal vesicles and normal concentrations in the semen are 120 to 450 mg/dl. You would expect to see low concentrations with obstructed or absent seminal vesicles. Bilateral absence of the vas deferens is usually seen with obstructed or absent seminal vesicles. The ejaculate volume is usually low and the semen usually does not coagulate due to the absence of the substances from the seminal vesicle responsible for coagulation.

281-B *(Campbell's, pp. 666, 669)*

Normal ranges for semen analysis parameters include a volume of 1.5 to 5.0 ml, and total sperm count of greater than 50 to 60 million. Therefore, response B is false. Normal motility and morphology should be noted in greater than 60 per cent of the spermatozoa, and this should have a forward progression of greater than 2. There should also be minimal agglutination and normal viscosity in the semen specimen.

Forward progression is noted as zero for no motility, 1 for sluggish or nonprogressive movement, 2 for slow meandering forward progression, 3 for movement in a reasonably straight line with moderate speed, and 4 for movement in a straight line with high speed.

282-E *(Campbell's, p. 670)*

Round cells in semen represent either immature germ cells or leukocytes. Pyospermia or the presence of more than 10 to 15 round cells per high-powered field or more than 1 to 3 million round cells per milliliter is abnormal and should be further evaluated with a white blood cell stain. PAP stains can be used to differentiate white cells from immature germ cells, but requires a very trained observer. Immunohistochemical techniques have been developed, which stain leukocytes red-brown and make them easy to differentiate from immature germ cells. Peroxidase can also be used to stain white blood cells dark brown but this does not stain macrophages. Patients with pyospermia should be evaluated for genital tract infection with appropriate cultures.

283-D *(Campbell's, p. 671)*

Postcoital tests assesses the interaction of sperm with the cervical mucus. It should be performed just prior to ovulation when the cervical mucus becomes clear and thin with the highest percentage of water. The cervical mucus is usually obtained several hours after the couple has intercourse, although it could also be obtained the following day. A normal test result is defined as one where more than 10 to 20 sperm are identified per high-powered field. The majority of the sperm should have good motility. A postcoital test should be performed in cases of hyperviscous semen, unexplained infertility, low-volume or high-volume semen specimens with good sperm density, and abnormal anatomy of the penis.

Inappropriate timing of the postcoital test is the most common cause for abnormal results. Other causes also include anatomic abnormalities, antisperm antibodies in the semen or cervical mucus, inappropriately performed intercourse, and abnormal semen.

284-C *(Campbell's, pp. 672–673)*

Antisperm antibodies are associated with infertility. Available tests include a mixed agglutination reaction using red blood cells, sperm, and antihuman antiserum; an ELISA using sperm, antihuman antibody bound to an enzyme, and a substrate; the Immunobead Assay with washed spermatozoa; and micrometer sized polyacrylamide beads linked with antihuman antibodies.

Antisperm antibodies are higher in patients with ductal obstruction, postvasectomy, history of epididymo-orchitis, history of torsion, cryptorchidism, and with varicoceles. Antisperm antibodies should be tested for in patients with those risk factors, impaired sperm motility, sperm agglutination, abnormal postcoital test, or with unexplained infertility.

285-D *(Campbell's, pp. 673–674)*

In vitro fertilization is the gold standard for validation of the sperm penetration assay. A sperm penetration assay is performed by combining sperm with a hamster oocyte after the removal of the zona pellucida. Sperm must be able to undergo capacitation, the acrosome reaction, fusion with the oolemma, and incorporation in the ooplasm. It does not test for penetration through the zona pellucida. It should be performed in patients with unexplained infertility. It is a somewhat controversial test in regard to its utility and interpretation.

286-E *(Campbell's, p. 674)*

Radiologic evaluation of the ductal system of the genital tract is indicated in patients with azoospermia and normal spermatogenesis on testicular biopsy. Absence of fructose from the semen is indicative of an obstruction below the seminal vesicles but will not rule out vasal obstructions. Transrectal ultrasound can be helpful to diagnose obstruction distal to the seminal vesicles, noting enlarged seminal vesicles on evaluation. Vasography should be performed to rule out vasal obstructions. A normal unilateral vasogram rules out distal obstruction. Although response C is also correct, there is no need to do bilateral vasograms and risk injuring both vasa deferentia. Retrograde vasography is contraindicated because it may rupture the epididymal tubule and result in subsequent epididymal obstruction. Azoospermia with a normal testicular biopsy and nonobstructed vasography is indicative of obstruction in the epididymis.

287-B *(Campbell's, pp. 674–676)*

Bilateral atrophic testes with a markedly elevated FSH usually reveal absence of germ cells or Sertoli cell-only syndrome on testicular biopsy. Biopsies revealing tubular sclerosis generally also have atrophic and firm testes. These are classically seen in patients with Klinefelter's syndrome. This is known as end-stage testes. The testes in the Sertoli cell-only syndrome are generally soft. Hypospermatogenesis is when a reduction in the number of all germinal elements is present with thinner layers of germ cells. Maturation arrest is either early or late and may be partial or complete. Findings are of a progression to one stage of maturation with no differentiation beyond that point.

288-C *(Campbell's, p. 674)*

Crystalloids of Reinke are seen in Leydig cells. They are also seen in one third of cells in Leydig cell tumors.

289-B *(Campbell's, pp. 674–676)*

The most common abnormality found on a testicular biopsy for infertility is hypospermatogenesis and maturation arrest. Testicular biopsy is, however, rarely pathognomonic of a single etiology. Germinal aplasia is also known as Sertoli cell-only syndrome. Normal testes are usually found in azoospermia patients with distal obstruction. Fetal pattern is noted in cases of hypogonadotropic hypogonadism where the seminiferous tubules are very small with absence of germ cells and Leydig cells. End-stage testes are seen in Klinefelter's syndrome or other similar processes with peritubular sclerosis and absence of germ cells from the sclerotic semeniferous tubules. Leydig cells may be absent or decreased in numbers.

290-C *(Campbell's, pp. 676–677)*

Retrograde ejaculation may be diagnosed when there are greater than 5 to 10 sperm per high-power field in a postejaculatory urine. Low volume or anejaculatory states could also be due to obstruction. Retrograde ejaculation should only occur in a small percentage of patients after a bonafide nerve-sparing retroperitoneal lymph node dissection. Other patients with testis cancer commonly have impaired fertility due to abnormalities in the remaining testis.

291-D *(Campbell's, pp. 677–678)*

Hypogonadotropic hypogonadism is impaired or absent gonadotropin secretion with otherwise normal pituitary function. It is otherwise known as Kallmann's syndrome. A failure of GnRH secretion by the hypothalamus is responsible for the majority of these. It has an association with anosmia and is thought to be inherited by autosomal dominant inheritance from male to male with variable penetrance. Anosmia can be seen without hypogonadotropism and you can get hypogonadotropism without anosmia. Delay in pubertal development is the hallmark of this syndrome. The first sign of puberty is usually testicular growth. Patients with Kallmann's syndrome will not have a rise in LH when given clomiphene citrate, whereas early pubertal males will respond with a rising LH level after clomiphene. After priming with GnRH they will have rises in both FSH and LH similar to prepubertal boys. Giving doses of 5000 international units of hCG to prepubertal boys demonstrated larger rises in testosterone levels as compared to the patients with Kallmann's syndrome.

Androgen replacement with testosterone or hCG in teenagers will result in virilization. Treatment with exogenous androgens will suppress intratesticular testosterone production. Therefore spermatogenesis and testicular growth will not occur. Gonadotropin therapy (FSH) is required for the initiation of spermatogenesis. hCG given 2000 international units IM three times per week will initiate spermatogenesis in most patients. However, completion of spermiogenesis will only occur in 20 per cent of them. Addition of FSH is required and is commonly given after 6 months of hCG therapy. FSH is usually given as Pergonol, which is 75 international units of FSH and 75 international units of LH per vial given 1/2 vial three times per week. This will stimulate testicular growth as well as complete spermatogenesis. The patients usually have ogliospermia but often are able to conceive with this low density. GnRH given either subcutaneously or by an infusion pump can offer excellent results in these patients as well.

292-C *(Campbell's, p. 678)*

Fertile eunuch syndrome is an isolated LH deficiency. Patients have normal FSH levels. These men have a eunuchoid habitus, large testes, but small ejaculates that may contain only a few spermatozoa. Sufficient intratesticular testosterone is produced for testicular growth and to support spermatogenesis, but inadequate peripheral androgen levels result in a lack of virilization.

293-A *(Campbell's, p. 678; Table 15–5)*

The most common etiology for infertility as seen in most large series has been associated with varicoceles. Between 21 and 39 per cent had a diagnosis of varicocele as the etiology. Idiopathic was the next most common, ranging from 5.4 to 66 per cent. Testicular failure was seen in 6.6 to 25 per cent, and obstruction was seen in 6.1 to 8.5 per cent.

294-D *(Campbell's, pp. 679–680)*

Hypogonadotropic hypogonadism is seen in Prader-Willi syndrome, which is associated with a chromosome 15 abnormality. LH and FSH are deficient because of the lack of GnRH. Kallmann's syndrome also demonstrates a lack of GnRH, as does Laurence-Moon-Bardet-Biedl syndrome; fertile eunuch syndrome involves isolated LH deficiency. Klinefelter's syndrome is usually associated with elevated FSH and either normal or elevated LH.

295-A *(Campbell's, pp. 679–680)*

Elevated FSH is often associated with infertility, but is secondary to primary testicular Sertoli cell failure. Elevated prolactin commonly causes infertility and impotence. Most elevations are only mild in nature and are associated with normal LH and testosterone. Markedly elevated levels are usually associated with a secreting macroadenoma of the pituitary. Cases of idiopathic hyperprolactinemia are treated with bromocriptine. Large macroadenomas can be treated with bromocriptine but sometimes need radiation therapy. Microadenomas are also treated with bromocriptine. Androgens and estrogens will cause negative inhibitory feedback on gonadotropin production, which will secondarily result in underdeveloped testes and impaired fertility. Treatment is directed at the cause. Glucocorticoid excess will suppress LH secretion, resulting in androgen deficiency and testicular dysfunction.

296-E *(Campbell's, pp. 680–681)*

Chromosomal abnormalities are seen in 6 per cent of infertile men. It is seen in 21 per cent of azoospermia patients. The majority of these are Klinefelter's syndrome or XXY with a classic triad of small firm testes, gynecomastia, and elevated urinary gonadotropins; this occurs in 1 in 600 males. They have azoospermia and markedly elevated FSH levels. LH may be elevated or normal. The XYY syndrome is associated with aggressive and criminal behavior and tall stature. Semen analysis usually shows severe ogliospermia or azoospermia. FSH, LH, and testosterone levels are usually normal. The patients with an XX karyotype may have the sex reversal syndrome, and these patients often carry the portion of the Y chromosome needed for male development. Findings are similar to patients with Klinefelter's syndrome. Noonan syndrome has a 46 XY karyotype and a similar phenotypic appearance to Turner's syndrome. Patients have hypertelorism, short stature, and webbed neck. Cryptorchidism and testicular atrophy are common with elevation of gonadotropins.

297-D *(Campbell's, pp. 681–682)*

Testicular dysfunction is commonly seen in problems of testicular descent. The most extreme situation is the vanishing testis syndrome where no testicular tissue can be found, which is probably due to an in-utero event. Low testosterone and elevated gonadotropin levels are seen with this. Any other forms of cryptorchidism are associated with impaired fertility. Sperm concentrations below 12 to 20 million per milliliter are seen in 50 per cent of patients with bilateral cryptorchidism and 30 per cent of patients with unilateral cryptorchidism. Neither ectopic testes nor retractile testes are associated with any testicular dysfunction.

298-B *(Campbell's, pp. 682–683)*

Varicoceles are seen in 30 per cent of infertile males and 9.4 per cent of asymptomatic males. Intratesticular temperatures have been found to be elevated. Theories center around increased temperature, reflux of renal and adrenal metabolites, decreased blood flow, and hypoxia in order to account for the varicocele effect on fertility. True etiology is not entirely known. Decreased motility is the most common finding present in 90 per cent of semen analyses. Sperm concentrations are less than 20 million per milliliter in 65 per cent of patients. Morphologic changes are also common. The stress pattern described by McCloud consists of increased numbers of amorphous cells and immature germ cells as well as more than 15 per cent tapered forms of sperm. Varicoceles are recommended to be repaired in adolescents with grade II or III varicoceles associated with ipsilateral testicular growth retardation, and of any clinically detected varicocele in infertile couples associated with an abnormal semen analysis, as long as the female partner has been evaluated and found to be normal.

299-A *(Campbell's, pp. 686–687)*

Infertility associated with antisperm antibodies can be improved with corticosteroid therapy with pregnancy rates anywhere between 30 and 40 per cent. Both high-dose cyclic, low-dose continuous, and intermediate cyclic regimens have been tried, and the currently recommended regimen is an intermediate cyclic steroid dose. Semen-processing techniques have not been able to remove the antibodies or increase fertility rates. These patients should be encouraged to consider intrauterine insemination or in vitro fertilization as viable options.

300-E *(Campbell's, pp. 688–691)*

Idiopathic male infertility, counts for up to 25 per cent of patients in whom no etiology can be found for their abnormal semen analysis. There has been no effective therapy found for the treatment of this group of patients. A trial of pharmacologic therapy may be tried for a 3 to 6 month period empirically, and if this is unsuccessful, then assisted reproductive techniques are usually recommended. An anti-estrogens such as clomiphene work because it has estrogenic as well as antiestrogenic activity. It binds with the estrogen receptor in the hypothalamus to prevent feedback inhibition of GnRH. Therefore, GnRH levels are increased, and then you see an elevated FSH and LH. Pregnancy rates are usually less than 30 per cent with this method. Tamoxifen is a similar agent to clomiphene. Aromatase inhibitors have been tried without much significant success; they work by decreasing the peripheral conversion of testosterone to estrogen. Both estrogens and androgens will decrease the production of LH, and therefore intratesticular testosterone levels will not be high enough for spermatogenesis. Human chorionic gonadotropin has LH-like activity, and Pergonol is a combination of LH and FSH. Kallikreins have also been used in Europe.

301-C *(Campbell's, pp. 691–692)*

Ductal obstruction is responsible for about 7 per cent of infertile patients. Congenital absence of the vas is seen in anywhere from 11 to 50 per cent of cases of congenital ductal obstruction. Low-volume azoospermia ejaculates with normal-size testes are characteristic of these patients. Many achieve pregnancy by aspiration of epididymal sperm and in vitro fertilization. Epididymal obstruction can be caused by gonococcal and tuberculous epididymitis, smallpox and filariasis, Young's syndrome, and cystic fibrosis. It is not common in chlamydia infections.

PART VI

SEXUAL FUNCTION

CHAPTER 16

DIRECTIONS: Each question below contains suggested responses. Select the ONE BEST response to each question.

302. The cavernosal artery is a branch of:
   A. Hypogastric artery
   B. Obturator artery
   C. External iliac artery
   D. Internal pudendal artery
   E. Inferior gluteal artery

303. The superficial dorsal vein drains into the:
   A. Saphenous vein
   B. Internal pudendal vein
   C. Santorinus plexus
   D. Obturator vein
   E. Inferior epigastric vein

304. The highest intracavernosal pressures occur during which phase?
   A. Latent
   B. Tumescence
   C. Full erection
   D. Rigid erection
   E. Refractory period

305. The cavernosal nerves are at which positions at the level of the apex of the prostate?
   A. 12 o'clock
   B. 6 o'clock
   C. 5 and 7 o'clock
   D. 3 and 9 o'clock
   E. 1 and 11 o'clock

306. Tumescence is mediated by:
   A. Sacral sympathetics
   B. Sacral parasympathetics
   C. Thoracolumbar sympathetics
   D. Pudendal efferents
   E. Pudendal afferents

307. All the following neurotransmitters are involved in tumescence EXCEPT:
   A. Neuropeptide Y
   B. Acetylcholine
   C. Nitric oxide
   D. VIP
   E. Prostacycline

308. Reflexogenic erection cannot be produced in patients with:
   A. Cervical cord injuries
   B. Thoracolumbar cord injury
   C. Sacral cord injury
   D. Normal men
   E. Parkinson's disease

309. Yohimbine enhances sexual performance because it is a/an:
   A. $Alpha_1$-antagonist
   B. $Alpha_1$-agonist
   C. $Alpha_2$-antagonist
   D. $Alpha_2$-agonist
   E. Dopamine agonist

310. All of the following are associated with erectile dysfunction EXCEPT:
   A. Inderal
   B. Minipress
   C. Spironolactone
   D. Lasix
   E. Digoxin

311. The most common etiology for priapism in children is:
   A. Idiopathic
   B. Sickle-cell disease
   C. Leukemia
   D. Traumatic
   E. Medications

312. In priapism, tissue ischemia begins after:
   A. 1–2 hours
   B. 2–4 hours
   C. 4–6 hours
   D. 12–18 hours
   E. 24-48 hours

313. Drugs associated with priapism include all the following EXCEPT:
   A. Pseudofed
   B. Chlorpromazine
   C. Trazodone
   D. Alcohol
   E. Hydralazine

314. Treatment of priapism that has lasted longer than 36–48 hours usually requires:
   A. Aspiration of intracorporeal blood
   B. Aspiration of blood and irrigation with an alpha-agonist
   C. Injection of an alpha-agonist
   D. Amyl nitrite
   E. Shunting procedure

315. Which of the following statements regarding the anatomy of the emissary veins from the penis is most correct in explaining their role in trapping of blood during erection?
   A. Venous pollsters are activated to occlude blood flow.

B. Venous constriction is mediated by neurogenic mechanisms.
C. Emissary veins have no role in trapping of blood.
D. Emissary veins are occluded by shearing forces of the tunica albuginea.
E. Valves within the emissary veins act to trap blood.

316. Blood gas measurements of penile blood demonstrate:

A. Arterial values in both the flaccid and erect state
B. Venous values in both the flaccid and erect state
C. Arterial values in the erect state and venous values in the flaccid state
D. Venous values in the erect state and arterial values in the flaccid state
E. No consistent relationship to erection

317. Which of the following statements regarding blood flow and intracavernous pressure during full rigid erection is correct?

A. Blood flow is increased, pressure is equal to systolic pressure.
B. Blood flow is decreased, pressure is less than systolic.
C. Blood flow is decreased, pressure is greater than systolic.
D. Blood flow is increased, pressure is greater than systolic.
E. Blood flow is increased, pressure is less than systolic.

318. Active detumescence occurring after ejaculation is thought to be mediated by:

A. Norepinephrine
B. Acetylcholine
C. Nitric oxide
D. Vasoactive intestinal polypeptide
E. Prostaglandins

319. Which of the following agents is thought to inhibit sexual drive?

A. Serotonin
B. L-Dopa
C. Amphetamine
D. Yohimbine
E. Apomorphine

320. Cigarette smoking may reduce erectile function by:

A. Decreasing testosterone levels
B. Increasing estrogen levels
C. Causing vasoconstriction and venous leaking
D. Decreasing libido via central effects
E. Causing hypoxia

321. Which of the following has not been associated with decreasing serum testosterone and decreased libido?

A. Diabetes mellitus
B. Digoxin
C. Marijuana
D. Hyperprolactinemia
E. Chronic alcoholism

322. Which of the following statements regarding erectile function in spinal cord injury patients is most correct?

A. Spinal cord injury patients cannot obtain erections.
B. Spinal cord injury patients obtain psychogenic but not reflexogenic erection.
C. Most patients with sacral cord injuries obtain reflexogenic but not psychogenic erection.
D. Most patients with suprasacral cord lesions obtain reflexogenic erections; some patients with sacral cord lesions obtain psychogenic erections.
E. Most patients with sacral cord injury obtain psychogenic erections; some patients with suprasacral cord lesions obtain reflexogenic erections.

323. The class of drugs most often associated with priapism is:

A. Antipsychotics
B. Antidepressants
C. Antihypertensives
D. Amphetamines
E. Narcotics

PART VI

PHYSIOLOGY OF ERECTION AND PATHOPHYSIOLOGY OF IMPOTENCE

CHAPTER 16

ANSWERS

302-D *(Campbell's, p. 709)*

The cavernosal artery is are a branch of the internal pudendal artery. Occasionally accessory arteries exist and may arise from the external iliac or obturator and be the dominant blood supply to the corpora cavernosa. Collaterals exist among the cavernosal arteries, the bulbourethral arteries, and the dorsal arteries.

303-A *(Campbell's, pp. 710–711)*

The superficial dorsal vein drains into the saphenous vein. The venous drainage of the rest of the penis starts in the sinusoids of the corpora cavernosa, which then drain into venules that travel in the trabeculae between the tunica and the peripheral sinusoids to form the subtunical venular plexus before exiting as the emissary veins. Emissary veins will then join the deep dorsal vein dorsally, or laterally to the circumflex veins, which then ultimately will drain into the deep dorsal veins. Proximal corpora and the crura will drain into the internal pudendal vein along with the urethral veins.

304-D *(Campbell's, pp. 711–713)*

Intracavernosal pressures are highest during the rigid erection phase. A full erection has pressures of around 100 mm Hg. Further increased pressure up to 200 mm Hg occurs during the rigid erection phase; this occurs when the stimulus triggers the bulbocavernosus reflex, which will initiate contraction of the ischiocavernosus and bulbocavernosus muscles. Pressure within the glans and the corpus spongiosum are also increased during erection, but only one third to one half that of the corpora cavernosa. Because of their thinner tunica coverings (there is no venous occlusion mechanism as in and the corpora cavernosa), they do not achieve pressures as high.

305-C *(Campbell's, p. 714)*

The cavernosal nerves are branches of the pelvic plexus just lateral to the pedicle of the seminal vesicle. They course along the posterolateral aspect of the prostate and at the apex of the prostate are at the 5 and 7 o'clock positions, lateral to the membranous urethra at 3 and 9 o'clock, and then they come anterior to the bulbous urethra at 1 and 11 o'clock before entering the penis.

306-B *(Campbell's, p. 714)*

Tumescence is mediated by the sacral parasympathetics. These originate in the second, third, and fourth sacral spinal cord segments. Preganglionic nerves enter the pelvic plexus where they are joined by sympathetic nerves from the hypogastric plexus and continue as the cavernous nerves. The sympathetic nerves originate from T11 to L2 and descend through the preaortic plexus, then through the superior and inferior hypogastric plexuses, and then communicate in the pelvic plexus to form the cavernous nerves. The sympathetic pathway is primarily responsible for detumescence.

307-A *(Campbell's, p. 715)*

Acetylcholine is thought to be the main neurotransmitter effecting smooth muscle relaxation during erection. Investigation has shown that there are multiple other neurotransmitters that also play a role. Endothelium-derived relaxing factor, which has been identified to be nitric oxide, causes muscle relaxation by stimulating guanylate cyclase, which results in increased levels of cyclic GMP. Vasointestinal peptide and prostacyclines also have been found to play a role in vasodilatation. Neuropeptide Y has a vasoconstrictive property and plays a role in detumescence, but not tumescence.

308-C *(Campbell's, p. 716)*

Reflexogenic erection is provided by stimulation to the genitalia. Impulses travel as pudendal afferents to the spinal erection center in S2–S4 and T10–L2. The anatomic nuclei then reflexively send impulses to induce the erectile process. Ascending tracts will result in sensory perception and make the subject aware of the stimuli. Psychogenic erections originate from audiovisual stimuli and result from signals descending from the brain to the spinal erection center. It is not well known what causes nocturnal erections. Patients with suprasacral spinal cord injuries are able to have reflexogenic erections. Obviously, normal men can do so as well. Cortical lesions have not been found to affect the ability to have reflexogenic erection.

309-C *(Campbell's, p. 717)*

Yohimbine is an $alpha_2$ antagonist, and it has been found to increase sexual behavior. Experience suggests that its main function may be to increase sex drive rather than actually improving erection.

310-D *(Campbell's, pp. 717–718)*

Many medications are often implicated in causing erectile dysfunction. Some reviews show that up to 25 per cent of cases may be associated with drug-induced etiologies. Excessive alcohol intake, cigarette smoking, antihypertensive and antidepressant medications, and psychotropics may all play a role. Propanolol (Inderol), prazosin (Minipress), spironolactone, and digoxin are all associated with some degree of erectile dysfunction, but furosemide (Lasix) has not been incriminated. Antihypertensives that are least likely to cause impotence would be direct smooth muscle relaxants, calcium channel blockers, and ACE inhibitors.

311-B *(Campbell's, p. 723)*

Priapism is defined as persistence of an erection without sexual desire. There is primary priapism or idiopathic priapism that is secondary to other causes. There can be low-flow or ischemic states and high-flow or nonischemic states. The most common etiology in children is sickle cell disease, which in some studies was responsible for 63 per cent of cases. Leukemic infiltrates are also relatively common causes in children; the other causes are less common. Treatment for priapism associated with sickle cell disease in children is hydration, alkalinization, analgesia, and hypertransfusion to a hemoglobin greater than 10 mg/dl and to reduce hemoglobin concentration to less than 30 per cent. Many episodes of priapism are preceded by stuttering attacks. If priapism does not respond to these conservative measures, then intracavernous injection of an alpha-adrenergic agent is indicated.

312-C *(Campbell's, p. 723)*

Tissue ischemia begins around 4 to 6 hours after the onset of priapism, and this is when pain is first recognized. Usually, if patients are treated within 24 hours they will not have any irreversible effects. If therapy is delayed for more than 36 to 48 hours, then marked tissue damage is likely to occur. with fibrosis and organ failure.

313-A *(Campbell's, p. 724)*

Medications are associated with priapism in up to 21 per cent of adult cases. The most common agents are antihypertensive drugs such as hydralazine, guanethidine, and prazosin. Antipsychotic drugs of the phenothiazine group, especially clorpromazine, also cause priapism. Trazodone is an antidepressant that has been implicated in many cases. These all seem to cause some sort of alpha-adrenergic blockade. Other agents not in these categories have also been associated with priapism.

314-E *(Campbell's, p. 725)*

Treatment of priapism should be initiated as early as possible. Aspirating the blood to reduce intracavernous pressure is the safest method in patients who have severe cardiac disease. If this alone is not successful, then injecting alpha-adrenergic agents intracorporally after aspirating blood can be effective. This can be repeated every 5 minutes. If therapy is delayed longer than 36 to 48 hours, then tissue injury will often occur and will not respond to these more conservative methods. A shunting procedure, such as a corporoglanular or corporospongiosal shunt, may be necessary. Amyl nitrite has occasionally been used to cause detumescence, however, it is associated with hypotension. Alpha-adrenergic agents commonly used would be 10 to 20 μg of epinephrine or 100 to 500 μg of phenylephrine. Ephedrine or norepinephrine can be used.

315-D *(Campbell's, p. 710)*

Unlike arterial and nerve branches that traverse the tunica albuginea, which are surrounded by sheaths of loose areolar tissue, the emissary veins are in direct contact with the tunica albuginea and are occluded by the shearing action of tunica layers during erection.

316-C *(Campbell's, p. 710)*

In the flaccid state, the blood slowly diffuses from the central to the peripheral sinusoids of the corpora cavernosa and blood gas levels are similar to venous blood. Rapid inflow of blood during erection changes the blood gas value to that of arterial blood.

317-C *(Campbell's, p. 712)*

During full rigid erection, the ischiocavernosus and bulbocavernosus muscles compress the already engorged corpora resulting in an increase of corpora cavernosa pressure to levels well above systolic and decreased flow relative to the flaccid state.

318-A *(Campbell's, p. 715)*

The large amounts of norepinephrine released during the sympathetic discharge occurring at ejaculation is probably responsible for active detumescence. Passive detumescence after interruption of sexual stimulation may be mediated by intrinsic smooth muscle tone, tonic discharge of the sympathetic system, and/or release of vasoconstrictors like endothelin.

319-A *(Campbell's, pp. 716–717)*

In general, central dopaminergic and adrenergic receptors are thought to increase, and serotonin receptors to decrease, sexual drive. However, $alpha_1$ and $alpha_2$ receptors may mediate different effects. Prazosin, an $alpha_1$-antagonist, and clonidine, an $alpha_2$-agonist, seem to suppress sexual drive in animal experiments, whereas yohimbine, an $alpha_2$-antagonist, increases sexual drive. Apomorphine is a direct-acting dopamine agonist that increases sexual drive.

320-C *(Campbell's, p. 717)*

The contractile effect of cigarette smoking on cavernous smooth muscle may cause vasoconstriction and venous leakage. Alcohol, marijuana, cocaine, and narcotics can also reduce erectile function after long-term use.

321-A *(Campbell's, pp. 717–721)*

Diabetes is the most common endocrine cause of impotence, but impairment results from neurogenic and vascular disease, rather than hormonal causes directly. Hyperprolactinemia from pituitary adenoma, medications, or chronic renal failure can decrease serum testosterone, as can chronic alcoholism and marijuana use. Digoxin also can cause decreased testosterone, probably because of its similar chemical structure to sex steroids.

322-D *(Campbell's, pp. 719–720)*

Patients with suprasacral cord lesions have an intact sacral spinal cord, which is the most important erectile center. Ninety-five per cent of these patients are able to obtain reflexogenic erections. About 25 per cent of patients with sacral cord lesions are able to obtain psychogenic erections because of the preserved thoracolumbar pathways.

323-C *(Campbell's, p. 724)*

The antihypertensive drugs hydralazine, guanethidine, and prazosin have been commonly implicated in patients with priapism, but it has also been caused by other drugs, including phenothiazines and antidepressants. Total parenteral nutrition with fat emulsion is another therapy that can cause priapism.

PART VII

INFECTIONS AND INFLAMMATION OF THE GENITOURINARY TRACT

CHAPTERS 17 THROUGH 24

DIRECTIONS: Each question below contains suggested responses. Select the ONE BEST response to each question.

324. The most common cause of unresolved bacteriuria during treatment of UTI is:
   A. Bacterial resistance to the drug selected for treatment
   B. Development of resistance from initially susceptible bacteria
   C. Rapid reinfection with a new, resistant species
   D. Presence of more than one species of bacteria
   E. Persistence of bacteria within renal calculi

325. What is the threshold for significant bacteriuria in dysuric women?
   A. ≥ 10 CFU/ml
   B. $\geq 10^2$ CFU/ml
   C. $\geq 10^3$ CFU/ml
   D. $\geq 10^4$ CFU/ml
   E. $\geq 10^5$ CFU/ml

326. Which of the following statements regarding localization of urinary tract infections is *false*?
   A. Ureteral catheter localization can reliably determine unilateral renal bacteriuria.
   B. The Fairley bladder washout test is unreliable in patients with vesicoureteral reflux.
   C. C-reactive protein appears immediately in the serum of patients with pyelonephritis.
   D. Antibody-coated bacteria can reliably localize infection to the kidneys in adults.
   E. A fever greater than 38°C is a reliable indication of pyelonephritis in children.

327. Which of the following agents has *not* been shown to be effective as single-dose therapy for uncomplicated cystitis?
   A. Amoxicillin
   B. Trimethoprim-sulfamethoxazole
   C. Ampicillin
   D. Sulfisoxazole
   E. Cefalexin

328. The most common etiologic organism in emphysematous pyelonephritis is:
   A. *P. mirabilis*
   B. *E. coli*
   C. *P. aeruginosa*
   D. *S. faecalis*
   E. *S. aureus*

329. Which of the following statements regarding asymptomatic bacteriuria is *false*?
   A. Treatment with antibiotics for 7 days results in improved long-term cure rates.
   B. One third of these patients will develop acute symptoms within 12 months if untreated.
   C. Infection from *Proteus* species should be eradicated.
   D. Pregnant women with bacteriuria have a higher incidence of complications.
   E. The incidence of bacteriuria is the same in pregnant and nonpregnant women.

330. A 47-year-old diabetic female presents with a 2-day history of fever and right flank pain. An IVP reveals an enlarged right nephrogram with cortical striations. The most likely diagnosis is:
   A. Pyonephrosis
   B. Xanthogranulomatous pyelonephritis
   C. Perirenal abscess
   D. Acute pyelonephritis
   E. Emphysematous pyelonephritis

331. The most common organism associated with xanthogranulomatous pyelonephritis is:
   A. *P. mirabilis*
   B. *E. coli*
   C. *P. aeruginosa*
   D. *S. faecalis*
   E. *S. aureus*

332. Which of the following statements is true regarding xanthogranulomatous pyelonephritis?
   A. Incision and drainage is usually curative.
   B. The diagnosis can be made by CT scan in most cases.
   C. It is a precancerous lesion.
   D. The resulting parenchymal damage frequently leads to azotemia.
   E. About one third of patients present with negative urine cultures.

333. Michaelis-Gutmann bodies are pathognomonic for:

A. Xanthogranulomatous pyelonephritis
B. Malacoplakia
C. Emphysematous pyelonephritis
D. *Mycobacterium tuberculosis* infection
E. *Chlamydia trachomatis* infection

334. The best technique for diagnosing chronic pyelonephritis is:

A. Intravenous urogram
B. Computed tomography
C. DMSA renal scan
D. Renal ultrasound
E. Indium 111 scan

335. All of the following are findings on intravenous urogram suggestive of chronic pyelonephritis EXCEPT:

A. An atrophic kidney
B. Focal coarse renal scarring
C. Calyceal clubbing
D. Calcification of renal papillae
E. The presence of pseudotumors

336. A 63-year-old man presents with right flank pain and chills. Physical examination shows a blood pressure of 80/40 mm Hg, pulse 128, temperature 40°C and right flank tenderness. Ultrasound shows a fluid-debris level with dependent echoes in a dilated right renal pelvis. Broad-spectrum IV antibiotics are started. The best next step in treatment is:

A. Observation
B. Right ureteral catheter placement
C. Right nephrectomy
D. Right percutaneous nephrostomy placement
E. Right pyeloplasty

337. All of the following antibiotics have been shown to be effective in prophylaxis of recurrent UTIs EXCEPT:

A. Trimethoprim
B. Nitrofurantoin
C. Cephalexin
D. Norfloxacin
E. Sulfamethoxazole

338. The greatest obstacle in the treatment of perinephric abscess is the:

A. Inability to obtain positive cultures in many patients
B. Presence of comorbid diseases in many patients
C. Low sensitivity in currently available radiologic imaging techniques
D. Delay in diagnosis due to nonspecific symptoms
E. Poor cure rate with percutaneous drainage

339. The most common etiologic factor for recurrent UTIs in women is:

A. The presence of abnormal vaginal biologic flora
B. Personal hygiene habits that place them at risk
C. The presence of structural urinary tract abnormalities
D. Noncompliance with treatment regimens
E. Increased virulence of fecal flora

340. Which of the following statements regarding prophylaxis against recurrent UTIs with nitrofurantoin is *true*?

A. Urinary tract infection is prevented by eliminating Enterobacteriacae from the fecal flora.
B. Bacterial resistance usually develops when therapy is continued for more than 6 months.
C. The risk of an adverse reaction increases with increasing patient age.
D. Liver damage is the most common adverse drug reaction.
E. There is minimal absorption of nitrofurantoin in the intestinal tract.

341. All of the following statements regarding bacterial adherence are true EXCEPT:

A. Type 1 pili are found in most strains of *E. coli.*
B. Strains of *E. coli* with P pili are more common in pyelonephritis than in cystitis.
C. Bacterial cells can alternate between piliated and nonpiliated forms.
D. There is increased epithelial receptivity for *E. coli* in patients with recurrent UTI.
E. Epithelial receptivity for bacteria decreases after menopause.

342. Women with screening bacteriuria:

A. Are at increased risk of developing symptomatic infections
B. Comprise about 25 per cent of sexually active women
C. Should undergo treatment to eradicate the bacteriuria
D. Are at increased risk of developing hypertension
E. Are at increased risk of progressive renal scarring

343. A 24-year-old female in the third trimester of pregnancy is undergoing treatment of acute pyelonephritis with broad spectrum antibiotics. After 3 days of treatment she remains febrile and symptomatic. The most appropriate management is:

A. Obtain a renal ultrasound
B. Obtain an abbreviated intravenous urogram
C. Continue the present antibiotics
D. Change the antibiotic regimen
E. Obtain a renal scan

344. Which of the following antibiotics is safe and effective during all phases of pregnancy?

A. Fluoroquinolones
B. Trimethoprim
C. Nitrofurantoin
D. Cephalosporins
E. Sulfonamides

345. A 57-year-old man presents with urinary frequency, dysuria, and pelvic discomfort. Physical examination reveals a temperature of 37°C and a tender prostate. Expressed prostatic secretions show 20 WBC per high-power field with macrophages containing oval bodies. The most likely diagnosis is:

A. Granulomatous prostatitis
B. Acute bacterial prostatitis
C. Chronic bacterial prostatitis
D. Prostatodynia
E. Nonbacterial prostatitis

346. All of the following have a role in the treatment of nonbacterial prostatitis EXCEPT:

A. Nonsteroidal anti-inflammatory agents
B. 6 to 8 weeks of empiric antibiotic treatment
C. Normal sexual activity
D. Hot sitz baths
E. Anticholinergics

347. All of the following are common urodynamic findings in patients with prostatodynia EXCEPT:

A. Decreased urinary flow rates
B. High urethral closure pressures
C. Uninhibited bladder contractions
D. Incomplete relaxation of the prostatic urethra
E. Incomplete relaxation of the bladder neck

348. Bacterial prostatitis is usually caused by:

A. Hematogenous infection
B. Gram-positive pathogens
C. Anaerobic pathogens
D. A single pathogen
E. Direct invasion by rectal bacteria

349. Chronic bacterial prostatitis is best diagnosed by:

A. Histologic examination of prostatic tissue
B. History and physical examination
C. Examination of expressed prostatic secretions
D. Segmented urine cultures
E. Semen culture

350. The prostatic fluid in men with chronic bacterial prostatitis has:

A. Increased pH
B. At least 10^5 CFU/ml of bacteria
C. Increased specific gravity
D. Increased acid phosphatase concentration
E. Increased citric acid concentration

351. All of the following statements are true regarding prostatic calculi EXCEPT:

A. They usually cause no symptoms or harm.
B. Infected calculi cannot be sterilized by medical therapy.
C. Intraprostatic reflux of urine probably plays an important role in their formation.
D. They are seen in about 50 per cent of elderly men on transrectal ultrasound.
E. They are seen most commonly in the peripheral zones of the prostate.

352. All of the following statements are true regarding the diagnosis and treatment of acute bacterial prostatitis EXCEPT:

A. Acute urinary retention is best managed with a suprapubic catheter.
B. Antibiotic treatment should be continued orally for 30 days.
C. The pathogen is usually identified by urine culture.
D. Preferred initial therapy is trimethoprim-sulfamethoxazole, either orally or intravenously.
E. The prostatic expressate should be examined to confirm the diagnosis.

353. Which of the following statements regarding the role of zinc in prostatitis is *true*?

A. Prostatic zinc levels are usually elevated in nonbacterial prostatitis.
B. Zinc is bacteriocidal to most pathogens that cause urinary tract infections.
C. Low prostatic zinc levels have been shown to predispose to bacterial prostatitis.
D. Prostatic zinc levels can be increased with oral zinc preparations.
E. Zinc and prostate antibacterial factor (PAF) act synergistically to prevent bacterial prostatitis.

354. All of the following are predisposing factors for the development of prostatic abscess EXCEPT:

A. Diabetes
B. Urethral instrumentation
C. Indwelling urethral catheter
D. AIDS
E. Prostatic calculi

355. A 37-year-old male presents with a high fever and urinary retention. Physical examination reveals an enlarged, firm prostate. Routine urine and blood cultures are negative. Peripheral blood smear shows significant eosinophilia. The most likely diagnosis is:

A. Prostatic abscess
B. Gonococcal prostatitis
C. Granulomatous prostatitis
D. Mycotic prostatitis
E. Tuberculous prostatitis

356. The most sensitive test for detecting *Trichomonas vaginalis* is:

A. Saline wet mount examination of secretions
B. Addition of KOH to vaginal secretions
C. Culture of secretions
D. Direct fluorescent antibody testing
E. Aquadine orange staining of secretions

357. Which of the following statements regarding gonococcal urethritis is *true*?

A. The incubation period is 1 to 3 days.
B. Around 50 per cent of the contacts of patients with known gonorrhea are asymptomatic.
C. Gram stain of the urethral swab has low sensitivity in confirming the diagnosis.
D. The current recommended treatment includes tetracycline to eradicate resistant strains of gonorrhea.
E. Strains of gonorrhea that cause systemic disease are more common in whites than blacks.

358. A patient is treated with ceftriaxone and tetracycline for urethritis. Symptoms return in 4 weeks despite abstaining from sexual activity. The organism most likely to be cultured from a urethral swab is:

A. *Ureaplasma urealyticum*
B. *Chlamidya trachomatis*
C. *Trichomonas vaginalis*
D. *Gardnerella vaginalis*
E. *Neisseria gonorrhoeae*

359. All of the following are indicated in a 65-year-old man with bacteriuria and epididymitis EXCEPT:

A. Scrotal elevation
B. Quinolone antibiotics
C. IVP
D. Cystoscopy
E. Prednisone

360. Which of the following diseases can be reliably diagnosed by the appearance of the lesions alone?

A. Lymphogranuloma venereum
B. Syphilis
C. Chancroid
D. Donovanosis
E. Herpes simplex

361. All of the following statements are true regarding herpes simplex infection EXCEPT:

A. HSV types I and II produce primary infections of equal severity.
B. The clinical illness of primary infection tends to be more severe in men.
C. Dysuria is present in most women with primary infection.
D. Virus isolation by culture is the most sensitive diagnostic technique.
E. Acyclovir is currently the most effective treatment.

362. *Primary* syphilis is best diagnosed by:

A. Fluorescent treponemal antibody absorption test (FTA-ABS)
B. Examination of chancre scrapings by dark-field microscopy
C. Microhemagglutination assay for antibody to *Treponema pallidum* (MHATP)
D. Venereal Disease Research Laboratory (VDRL) test
E. Rapid plasma reagin (RPR) test

363. The preferred treatment for primary syphilis is:

A. Benzathine penicillin G, 2.4 million units IM, one dose
B. Doxycycline, 100 mg orally BID for 2 weeks
C. Tetracycline, 500 mg orally QID for 2 weeks
D. Erythromycin, 500 mg orally QID for 2 weeks
E. Ceftriaxone, 250 mg IM, one dose

364. A painful genital ulcer with a deep undermined border is most consistent with:

A. Chancroid
B. Lymphogranuloma verereum
C. Herpes
D. Primary syphilis
E. Granuloma inguinale

365. All of the following are generally accepted indications for HIV testing EXCEPT:

A. Pneumococcal pneumonia
B. Positive hepatitis B markers
C. Gonococcal urethritis
D. Active tuberculosis
E. Unexplained elevated levels of hepatic enzymes

366. At any given time, the majority of patients with HIV infection:

A. Have a mononucleosis-type syndrome
B. Have generalized adenopathy
C. Are asymptomatic
D. Have a secondary infectious disease
E. Have a negative ELISA for HIV antibodies

367. All of the following meet the criteria for the diagnosis of AIDS EXCEPT:

A. *Pneumocystis carinii* pneumonia in a patient without another cause of immune deficiency
B. Kaposi's sarcoma in a patient younger than 60 with no other cause of immune deficiency
C. Documented HIV infection and generalized adenopathy
D. Documented HIV infection and wasting syndrome
E. Documented HIV infection and encephalitis

368. The prevalence of HIV within semen:

A. Decreases with zidovudine therapy
B. Does not change significantly with the stage of infection
C. Increases as CD4+ T-lymphocyte counts decrease
D. Increases with symptomatic infection
E. Increases as CD8+ T-lymphocyte counts decrease

369. AIDS-associated renal disease:

A. Is more prevalent in homosexual AIDS patients
B. Is caused by HIV infection of the renal parenchyma
C. Is characterized by interstitial nephritis
D. Closely resembles heroin-associated nephropathy
E. Is usually seen early in the course of HIV infection

370. There is a direct relationship between AIDS and all of the following malignancies EXCEPT:

A. Kaposi's sarcoma
B. Testicular carcinoma
C. B-cell lymphoma
D. Non-Hodgkin's lymphoma
E. Central nervous system lymphoma

371. The risk of acquiring HIV by receiving a single unit of blood is estimated to be approximately:

A. 1 in 1,000
B. 1 in 10,000
C. 1 in 100,000
D. 1 in 1,000,000
E. 1 in 10,000,000

372. The most effective therapy for essential pruritus is:

A. Topical nonsteroidal antipruritic lotion
B. Topical steroidal cream
C. Oral antidepressant
D. Oral sedating antihistamine
E. Oral anxiolytic

373. The products most often documented as etiologic agents in contact dermatitis are:

A. Topically applied medications
B. Clothing dyes
C. Detergents
D. Antistatic products
E. Toilet papers

374. Pruritus is a prominent symptom in all of the following skin conditions EXCEPT:

A. Atopic dermatitis
B. Contact dermatitis
C. Intertrigo
D. Psoriasis
E. Seborrheic dermatitis

375. The most commonly encountered genital lesion in Reiter's syndrome is:

A. Lichen nitidus
B. Lichen planus
C. Erythema multiforma
D. Balanitis circinata
E. Vitiligo

376. The term for squamous cell carcinoma in situ occurring on the glans penis is:

A. Erythroplasia of Queyrat
B. Bowen's disease
C. Paget's disease
D. Bowenoid papulosis
E. Behçet's disease

377. The organisms most commonly associated with balanoposthitis are:

A. *Pseudomonas* species
B. *Candida* species
C. *Streptococcus* species
D. *Staphylococcus* species
E. *Trichophyton* species

378. A 47-year-old man presents with a bright red, moist patch on the inner prepuce measuring 2 cm in diameter that has not changed in appearance for 2 years. Biopsy reveals a marked plasma cell infiltrate but no evidence of malignancy. The primary treatment of choice is:

A. Topical nystatin
B. Circumcision
C. Topical steroids
D. Topical tretinoin
E. Topical neomycin

379. All of the following statements are true regarding balanitis xerotica obliterans (lichen sclerosis) EXCEPT:

A. Topically applied 2 per cent testosterone is the primary treatment in women.
B. The lesions are characteristically sharply marginated white patches.
C. Lesions occur most commonly on the glans in men.
D. Lesions occur most commonly on the vulvar vestibule and perianal area in women.
E. Surgical excision of involved tissue is usually curative in men.

380. All of the following are consistent with the diagnosis of hidradenitis suppurativa EXCEPT:

A. The presence of multiple lesions at the same time.
B. A history of repeatedly recurring lesions
C. Confinement of lesions to the groin and axillae
D. Bacterial culture with heavy growth of *Staphylococcus* species
E. Tender, fluctuant lesions

381. The etiologic organism in erythrasma is:

A. *Corynebacterium minutissimum*
B. *Pseudomonas aerginosa*
C. *Trichophyton rubrum*
D. *Staphylococcus aureus*
E. *Candida albicans*

382. A 63-year-old diabetic presents with a 5-cm red plaque with an overlying pustule on the scrotum. There is moderate surrounding edema. The most appropriate management is:

A. Oral dicloxacillin and observation
B. Intravenous broad-spectrum antibiotic and observation
C. Needle aspiration culture of pustule and antibiotic coverage based on sensitivities
D. Intravenous broad spectrum antibiotics and soft tissue radiographs to rule out gas gangrene
E. Intravenous broad spectrum antibiotics and a deep stab incision through the pustule.

383. All of the following statements are true regarding tinea cruris EXCEPT:

A. The recurrence rate is high.
B. Response is usually seen with topical nystatin.
C. The lesions rarely involve the scrotum and penis.
D. The most active portion of the lesion occurs as a thin, red ring at the periphery.
E. The causative organisms are *Trichophyton* and *Epidermophyton* species.

384. A 27-year-old presents with closely set white papules about 1 mm in diameter, each of which encircles the penile corona in an aligned row. The most appropriate management of this patient is:

A. Biopsy of the lesions
B. No treatment
C. Circumcision
D. Topical steroids
E. Laser of the lesions

385. Which of the following statements regarding angiokeratomas of Fordyce is *false*?

A. Treatment is rarely necessary.
B. They appear as minute red or violaceous lesions.
C. Usually 10 to 50 lesions are present.
D. They are more common in women than men.
E. They may represent varices.

386. Which of the following statements regarding the life cycle of *Schistosoma haematobium* is true?

A. Human infection is acquired by exposure to infested fresh and salt waters.
B. The intermediate host is the mosquito.
C. The cercariae penetrate unbroken skin.
D. Extensive clotting and inflammation occur around adult worm pairs.
E. The estimated mean life span is 3 to 6 months.

387. Which of the following statements regarding the epidemiology of schistosomiasis is true?

A. The percentage of severe infections increases as the prevalence increases.
B. Southeast Asia has the highest prevalence of infection.
C. Infection rarely leads to clinical uropathy.
D. The severity of disease is not related to tissue egg burden.
E. Resistance to repeated infection is stronger in men than women.

388. Schistosomal disease results *directly* from:

A. Adult worms in the urinary tract
B. Host response to adult worms in the urinary tract

C. Schistosome eggs in the urinary tract
D. Host response to schistosome eggs in the urinary tract
E. Excretion of schistosome eggs into the urine

389. The classic clinical presentation of "active" schistosomiasis is:

A. Hematuria and dysuria
B. Fever and lymphadenopathy
C. Pelvic pain
D. Azotemia
E. Pruritic rash

390. Which of the following statements regarding diagnostic tests for schistosomiasis is *false*?

A. Serologic tests do not differentiate active and inactive disease.
B. Dipstick proteinuria has high sensitivity for detecting schistosomiasis in endemic areas.
C. Dipstick hematuria has high sensitivity for detecting schistosomiasis in endemic areas.
D. The schistosome species can be confirmed by Ziehl-Nielson staining of biopsy specimen.
E. Urinary egg excretion accurately estimates infection intensity in both active and inactive stages.

391. Which of the following statements regarding the medical management of schistosomiasis is *true*?

A. Successful treatment requires elimination of all worm pairs.
B. Metrifonate is the treatment of choice for *S. haematobium* in its endemic setting.
C. Due to high toxicity, treatment should be limited to symptomatic infections.
D. Relapses are common following treatment.
E. Medical treatment is not indicated after sequelae of late infection occur.

392. The most common bladder cancer seen in patients with schistosomiasis is:

A. Adenocarcinoma
B. Transitional cell carcinoma
C. Leiomyosarcoma
D. Squamous cell carcinoma
E. Rhabdomyosarcoma

393. Which of the following statements regarding bilharzial bladder cancer is *false*?

A. The most common site of tumor is the posterior wall.
B. Most tumors are exophytic.
C. Patients can be effectively screened for cancer using urinary cytology.
D. Bladder cancers are more common in patients with higher urinary tract egg burdens.
E. Necrotouria is more frequent than in nonschistosomal bladder cancer.

394. Which of the following statements regarding schistosomal obstructive uropathy (SOU) is *true*?

A. The most common site of obstruction is at the ureteral orifice.
B. There is a marked increase in pyelonephritis in patients with severe SOU.
C. Hydronephrosis usually precedes hydroureter.
D. Functional obstruction is more common than anatomic obstruction in late chronic active and inactive infection.
E. Recurrent stenosis following mechanical dilation of ureteral lesions is uncommon.

395. The organism responsible for the majority of human lymphatic filariasis is:

A. *Brugia malayi*
B. *Brugia timori*
C. *Onchocerca volvulus*
D. *Strongyloides stercoralis*
E. *Wuchereria bancrofti*

396. The most common location of lymphatic filariae in man is the:

A. Tail of the epididymis
B. Testis
C. Inguinal lymphatics
D. Cisterna chyli
E. Thoracic duct

397. Which of the following statements regarding the life cycle of lymphatic filariasis is *false*?

A. Microfilariae live for several months after release from adult females.
B. All lymphatic filariae are transmitted by mosquitoes.
C. Infective larvae can cross the normal conjunctiva or buccal mucosa.
D. Multiple infections over a prolonged period are necessary to produce disease.
E. Most patients with microfilaremia develop pathologic sequelae.

398. The treatment of choice for scrotal and penile elephantiasis secondary to filarial infection is:

A. Surgical excision and plastic reconstruction
B. Oral diethylcarbamazine
C. Oral ivermectin
D. Inguinal lymphadenectomy
E. Inguinal radiation

399. Which of the following statements regarding hydatid disease is *true*?

A. Biopsy is required to establish the diagnosis.
B. Treatment, if warranted, is by surgical excision.
C. The most frequent urologic presentation is hematuria.
D. The most frequent site of hydatid cysts is the renal parenchyma.
E. Cysts are acquired by humans who inhale the particulate eggs.

400. Which statement concerning fungi is *false*?

A. Fungi are eukaryotic organisms.
B. Cholesterol is the principle sterol in fungal cell membranes.
C. They belong to the kingdom Eumycetes.
D. Fungi can reproduce asexually.
E. Fungi can reproduce sexually.

401. Which of the following statements regarding blastomycosis is *true*?

A. Genitourinary involvement occurs in the majority of patients with systemic blastomycosis.
B. The fungus has a predilection for dry soil with high salinity.
C. Clinical manifestations of Cushing's syndrome are seen in patients with adrenal blastomycosis.
D. Ketoconazole is the treatment of choice for systemic blastomycosis.

E. Genitourinary blastomycosis most commonly involves the epididymis and prostate.

402. A 35-year-old migrant farm worker in Arizona has obstructive voiding symptoms and complains of perineal discomfort. The prostate is tender and boggy on examination. A CXR reveals granulomas, but a tuberculin skin test is negative. What is the most likely causative organism?

A. *Coccidioides immitis*
B. *Mycobacterium tuberculosis*
C. *Cryptococcus neoformans*
D. *Aspergillus fumigates*
E. *Geotrichum candidum*

403. A 60-year-old farmer develops acute adrenal insufficiency after renovating his chicken coops under poorly ventilated conditions. A CXR reveals multiple granulomas but a tuberculin skin test is negative. What is the most likely causative organism?

A. *Candida albicans*
B. *Histoplasma capsulatum*
C. *Torulopsis glabrata*
D. *Mycobacterium tuberculosis*
E. *Aspergillus fumigates*

404. What is the treatment of choice for the condition in question 403?

A. Isoniazid and rifampin
B. Oral ketoconazole
C. IV amphotericin B
D. Fluconazole
E. Miconazole

405. Genitourinary aspergillosis most commonly affects the:

A. Seminal vesicles
B. Testes
C. Bladder
D. Prostate
E. Kidney

406. A 35-year-old male with AIDS develops a severe headache, nuchal rigidity, and prostatitis. India ink stains of the CSF and urine reveal budding yeasts with capsules. What is the etiologic agent?

A. *Candida albicans*
B. *Histoplasma capsulatum*
C. *Aspergillus fumigates*
D. *Torulopsis glabrata*
E. *Cryptococcus neoformans*

407. Which of the following urinary candidal counts (clean catch) is indicative of a candidal infection rather than colonization?

A. 10^1
B. 10^2
C. 10^3
D. 10^4
E. 10^5

408. An elderly, debilitated female has persistent candiduria despite removal of an indwelling catheter. She is asymptomatic and has negative candidal antigen titers. What is the most appropriate treatment?

A. Intravesical irrigation with amphotericin B
B. Observation
C. Systemic amphotericin B therapy
D. Oral ketoconazole
E. Systemic miconazole

409. Which statement concerning amphotericin B is *false*?

A. The primary route of elimination is hepatic.
B. It is poorly absorbed from the GI tract.
C. It exerts its antifungal effect by interfering with fungal DNA and protein synthesis.
D. Hemodialysis does not affect plasma levels.
E. There is minimal CSF penetration.

410. Which of the following is not an adverse effect of amphotericin B?

A. Fever, chills, rigors
B. Headaches
C. Hyperkalemia
D. Thrombophlebitis
E. Nephrotoxicity

411. Which statement concerning flucytosine (5-FC) is *false*?

A. Elimination is primarily via the biliary tract.
B. Bone marrow depression is a potentially dangerous side effect.
C. It is well absorbed by the GI tract.
D. Flucytosine requires enzymatic conversion to active metabolites.
E. Flucytosine has good CSF penetration.

412. The most serious adverse effect of ketoconazole therapy is:

A. Seizures
B. Cardiac arrhythmia
C. Aplastic anemia
D. Nephrotoxicity
E. Hepatotoxicity

413. A premature infant treated with broad-spectrum antibiotics for pneumonia becomes anuric. Renal sonography reveals hydronephrosis and multiple fungal accretions. The treatment of choice is:

A. Nephrectomy
B. Cystoscopy and placement of ureteral stent
C. Systemic amphotericin B
D. Percutaneous nephrostomy with regional and systemic amphotericin B
E. Intravesical amphotericin B irrigation

414. Which of the following statements regarding the epidemiology of tuberculosis is *true*?

A. The majority of patients with tuberculosis have the genitourinary form of the disease.
B. In developed countries, the incidence of tuberculosis is decreasing.
C. In developing countries, the incidence of tuberculosis is decreasing.
D. Vaccination programs decrease the incidence of tuberculosis in the elderly.
E. In developed countries, the disease tends to infect adolescents and young adults, whereas in developing countries, the elderly are primarily infected.

415. All of the following are features of *M. tuberculosis* EXCEPT:

A. It is more prone than most bacteria to developing antibiotic resistance.
B. A proportion of the organisms are able to become dormant for many years.
C. It is slower growing than most bacteria.

D. It is more resistant to intracellular killing mechanisms than most bacteria.
E. Its cytoplasm differs considerably from most other bacteria.

416. In which of the following organs does tuberculosis infection usually result directly from the hematogenous spread of organism:
A. Testis
B. Bladder
C. Epididymis
D. Ureter
E. Urethra

417. Which of the following statements regarding tuberculosis of the kidney is *true*?
A. Most metastatic lesions within the kidney become clinically significant.
B. Polymorphonuclear leukocytes are the predominant cells in granulomas.
C. When the organisms reach the kidney they usually settle in the renal papillae.
D. Most small calcified lesions remain unchanged for many years.
E. There is no evidence that renal tuberculosis can cause hypertension.

418. Tuberculosis of the prostate:
A. Is usually caused by seeding from another focus in the urinary tract
B. Is best treated by transurethral resection of the prostate
C. Is usually associated with intense perineal pain, dysuria and high fever
D. Can be confused with carcinoma of the prostate on palpation
E. Commonly leads to perineal sinuses

419. The most common symptom in patients with genitourinary tuberculosis is:
A. Urinary urgency
B. Urinary frequency
C. Gross hematuria
D. Flank pain
E. Anorexia

420. Which of the following statements regarding laboratory investigations for tuberculosis is *false*?
A. Serial erythrocyte sedimentation rate (ESR) determinations give an indication of response to treatment.
B. A positive tuberculin test indicates active tuberculous disease.
C. The response in the tuberculin test is cell-mediated through the T-lymphocyte mediator.
D. The longer the urine remains in contact with organisms the less likely it is that the organisms will grow.
E. *M. tuberculosis* is strictly aerobic, *M. bovis* partially anaerobic.

421. All of the following cystoscopic findings can be assumed to be secondary to tuberculosis in a patient with known renal tuberculosis EXCEPT:
A. Velvety, erythematous mucosa
B. Bullous edema obscuring a ureteral orifice
C. A dilated, "golf-hole" ureteral orifice
D. A solitary ulcer on the trigone
E. A solitary erythematous patch on the dome

422. Which of the following statements regarding chemotherapy of genitourinary tuberculosis is *false*?
A. Treatment should include isoniazid, rifampicin and pyrazinamide.
B. Adding streptomycin adds little to the three drugs above.
C. Treatment should continue for at least 12 months.
D. There is no evidence that steroids influence the sterilizing activity of standard regimens.
E. Completely dormant organisms are not affected by any of the recommended antimicrobials.

423. Which of the following statements regarding the toxicity of antituberculosis drugs is *true*?
A. Toxicity most commonly occurs after several months of treatment.
B. Pyrazinamide should be stopped and not restarted if jaundice occurs.
C. Should a severe allergic reaction occur, the offending drug should be stopped and not restarted.
D. Isoniazid should be stopped and not restarted if neurologic symptoms occur.
E. Toxicity leading to termination of one or more drugs is uncommon.

424. Which of the following is not an indication for nephrectomy in renal tuberculosis?
A. A localized polar lesion that is slowly increasing in size despite medical treatment
B. A nonfunctioning kidney without calcification
C. A nonfunctioning kidney with extensive calcification
D. Extensive renal disease associated with hypertension
E. Renal disease with coexisting renal carcinoma

425. Ureteric strictures resulting from tuberculosis:
A. Most commonly occur at the ureteropelvic junction
B. Most commonly occur in the middle third of the ureter
C. Are best managed by dilation
D. Should be managed surgically if no improvement is seen after 6 weeks of appropriate medical treatment
E. Are best managed by nephrectomy if longer than 10 cm and associated with renal calcification.

426. Augmentation cystoplasty in patients with tuberculosis of the bladder:
A. Is contraindicated in the presence of renal insufficiency
B. Is contraindicated in patients with incontinence
C. Should be preceded by excision of as much inflamed tissue as possible
D. Should be performed using a stomach patch for best results
E. Should be performed using an ileal patch for best results

427. The syndrome of interstitial cystitis is defined by all of the following EXCEPT:
A. Characteristic histologic findings
B. Sterile urine
C. Cytologically negative urine
D. Characteristic cystoscopic findings
E. Chronic irritative voiding symptoms

428. Which of the following is characteristic of patients with interstitial cystitis?

A. They tend to have a higher number of sexual partners than the general population.
B. They tend to be single.
C. Their symptoms rarely progress after the first few years.
D. They are usually better educated than the general population.
E. They are usually diagnosed within 1 to 2 years of developing symptoms.

429. Which of the following is *least* likely to play a role in the etiology of interstitial cystitis?

A. Psychoneurosis
B. Inflammation
C. Neuropathy
D. Deficiencies in the bladder lining
E. Toxic substances in the urine

430. The most common cystoscopic finding in interstitial cystitis is:

A. Reduced bladder capacity
B. Hunner's ulcers
C. Pinpoint petechial hemorrhages after hydrodistention
D. Erythematous patches of mucosa
E. Trabeculations

431. The most common histologic abnormality in interstitial cystitis is:

A. Increased mast cell density in the muscularis
B. Submucosal edema and vasodilation
C. Patchy submucosal vasculitis
D. Perineural inflammation
E. Intraepithelial deposition of Tamm-Horsfall protein

432. In patients being evaluated for interstitial cystitis, urodynamic studies are helpful in all of the following settings EXCEPT:

A. Patients with urgency incontinence
B. Patients suspected of having reduced bladder capacity
C. Patients who are to undergo "bladder training"
D. Patients who do not have pain
E. Patients who are to undergo cystolysis

433. Which of the following systemic agents is the most effective in the treatment of interstitial cystitis?

A. Oral antihistamines
B. Oral amitriptyline
C. Subcutaneous heparin
D. Oral prednisone
E. Oral ibuprofen

434. Which of the following statements regarding DMSO therapy of interstitial cystitis is *false*?

A. Continuous treatment is usually required to obtain long-term symptomatic improvement.
B. DMSO has been shown to have anti-inflammatory properties.
C. Satisfactory subjective improvement is noted in 50 to 80 per cent of patients.
D. DMSO has been shown to have analgesic properties.
E. Endoscopic improvement is noted in most patients with symptomatic improvement.

435. The most effective open surgery for interstitial cystitis patients with severe pain is:

A. Presacral neurectomy
B. Augmentation cystoplasty
C. Cystolysis
D. Urinary diversion
E. Sacral rhizotomy

436. Which of the following statements regarding the evaluation of patients with interstitial cystitis is *true*?

A. Most patients complain of dysuria.
B. Bladder distention should be performed initially without anesthesia to determine if symptoms can be reproduced
C. Carcinoma in situ can be ruled out by history and endoscopic findings
D. Most patients should undergo extensive gynecologic evaluation
E. The severity of symptoms rarely correlates with the degree of endoscopic findings

437. All of the following statements are true regarding the natural history and treatment of interstitial cystitis EXCEPT:

A. Interstitial cystitis does not pose a risk to health or life.
B. There is usually no progression of the disease.
C. At least 10 per cent of patients will have lasting, spontaneous remissions
D. Most patients will not have relief of symptoms with nonsurgical means
E. One fourth of patients require no further treatment after a single hydraulic distention and one chlorpactin WCS-90 instillation

438. Which of the following statements regarding the urethral syndrome is *true*?

A. There is no evidence to support a psychogenic etiology.
B. There is an increased incidence in patients who have had multiple episodes of *Chlamydia* infections.
C. Urethral biopsies should be performed to rule out malignancy.
D. Cobblestoning and erythema of the urethra confirm the diagnosis.
E. There is no evidence to support an anatomically obstructive etiology.

439. A 37-year-old female with a history of prior recurrent UTIs presents with urinary frequency and dysuria. Urinalysis, urine culture, urethral cultures, urine cytology and cystoscopy with hydrodistention are all negative. The best initial therapy is:

A. Psychotherapy
B. A course of long-term, low-dose nitrofurantoin
C. Intravesical DMSO instillation
D. Urethral dilation
E. A course of terazosin

PART VII

INFECTIONS AND INFLAMMATION OF THE GENITOURINARY TRACT

CHAPTERS 17 THROUGH 24

ANSWERS

324-A *(Campbell's, pp. 734–735; Table 17–1)*

All of the answers listed can be a cause of unresolved bacteriuria during therapy; however, the most common cause is the presence of organisms that are resistant to the antimicrobial agent selected to treat the infection. These resistant strains of organisms usually develop in the fecal flora of patients that have recently received antimicrobial therapy. This underscores the importance of susceptibility testing, especially in patients who have a recent history (3 months or less) of antimicrobial therapy. Development of resistence in a previously susceptible population of bacteria is less common, but can occur within 42 to 78 hours of starting therapy. In mixed infections, treatment of the dominant organism can unmask the presence of a second strain that is resistant to the antimicrobial agent chosen. Fortunately, most reinfections, even in highly susceptible females, do not occur quickly. Giant staghorn calculi are rare; however, they represent a situation in which susceptible bacteria can continue to cause an unresolved bacteriuria in the presence of proper antimicrobial therapy.

325-B *(Campbell's, p. 735)*

A cutoff of 10^5 colony forming units per millimeter (CFU/mm) had traditionally been used to define significant bacteriuria. However, in numerous studies, it has been shown that 20 to 40 per cent of women with symptomatic urinary tract infections present with bacteria counts below this cutoff level. A threshold of $\geq 10^2$ colony forming units per millimeter of a known pathogen is therefore recommended for defining significant bacteriuria in dysuric women. Most of these patients will have pyuria on urinalysis in addition to symptoms of a urinary tract infection. Over diagnosis of a urinary tract infection using this lower cutoff level can be avoided by obtaining a noncontaminated specimen. The two means for accomplishing this include suprapubic aspiration and urethral catheterization. Bladder aspiration, while neither painful or dangerous, is unpleasant for most patients, and therefore urethral catheterization is more commonly used. The risk of introducing a urinary tract infection by urethral catheterization can be signficantly reduced by administration of 1 or 2 doses of oral antibiotics.

REFERENCES

1. Kraft J.K., and Stamey, T.A.: The natural history of symptomatic recurrent bacteriuria in women. Medicine, *56*:55, 1977.
2. Kunz, H.H., Siebert, H.G., Freiberg, J., et al.: Zur Bedeutung der Blasenpunktion für den sicheren Nachweiss einer Bacteriurie. Dtsch. Med. Wochenschr., *100*:2252, 1975.
3. Mabeck, C.E.: Studies in urinary tract infections: I. The diagnosis of bacteriuria in women. Acta Med. Scand., *186*:35, 1969a.
4. Stamm, W.E., Counts, G.W., Running, K.R., et al.: Diagnosis of coliform infection in acutely dysuric women. N. Engl. J. Med., *307*:463, 1982.

326-E *(Campbell's, pp. 737–740)*

There are several methods for attempting to localize the site of a urinary tract infection. The ureteral catheter technique initially described by Stamey, although somewhat invasive, can reliably localize unilateral renal bacteria. The Fairley bladder washout test can distinguish between an upper tract origin and a bladder origin; however, it cannot lateralize the site of an upper tract infection and is unreliable in patients with reflux. The C-reactive protein is an acute-phase susbstance that usually appears immediately in the serum of patients with pyelonephritis; however, this is a nonspecific test and has not proven highly accurate in localizing infection. Antibody-coated bacteria is an immunofluorescent technique for separating renal from bladder infection. This has been shown to correspond with the Fairley washout method in some studies; however, false positive findings have been seen in children as well as with prostatitis and hemorrhagic cystitis.

Although fever has been generally accepted as a sign of renal infection, the observation that bladder bacteriuria in children causes production of antibody may be reason for caution in this assumption. In addition, aggressive localization studies have shown substantial incidences of fever and flank pain in bacteriuric patients in whom infection was localized to the bladder.

REFERENCES

1. Stamey, T.A., Govan, D.E., and Palmer J.M.: The localization and treatment of urinary tract infections: The role of bactericidal urine levels as opposed to serum levels. Medicine *44*:1, 1965.
2. Hellerstein, S., Kennedy, E., and Nusbaum, L., et al.: Localization of the site of urinary tract infections by

means of antibody-coated bacteria in the urinary sediments. J. Pediatr., *8*:188, 1978.
3. Forsum, U., Hjelm, E., and Jonsell, G.:Antibody-coated bacteria in the urine of children with urinary tract infections. Acta Paediatr. Scand., *65*:639, 1976.
4. Busch, R., and Huland, H.: Correlation of symptoms and results of direct bacterial localization in patients with urinary tract infections. J. Urol., *132*:282, 1984.

327-E *(Campbell's, p. 744)*

Single-dose therapy for acute cystitis is effective in 85 to 100 per cent of episodes and is preferable to 7-day therapy because it is equally efficacious, allows better compliance, is associated with fewer side effects, is less expensive, and may decrease emergence of resistant flora within the gut. Several agents have been used effectively as a single-dose therapy, including amoxicillin, trimethoprim-sulfamethoxazole, ampicillin, and sulfisoxazole. Reports on single-dose cephalosporin therapy have been less promising, with a cure rate less than 50 per cent in ambulatory symptomatic women.

REFERENCES

1. Brumfitt W., Faiers, M.C., and Franklin, I.N.: The treatment of urinary infection by means of a single dose of cephaloridine. Postgrad. Med. J., *46*:65, 1970.
2. Greenberg, R.N., Sanders, C.V., Lewis, A.C., et al.: Single-dose cefaclor therapy of urinary tract infection. Evaluation of antibody-coated bacteria test and C-reactive protein assay as predictors of cure. Am. J. Med., *71*:841, 1981.

328-B *(Campbell's, pp. 757–758)*

Emphysematous pyelonephritis is an uncommon complication of acute pyelonephritis that is characterized by the appearance of intraparenchymal gas. This gas is thought to be generated by bacterial fermentation of glucose in the necrotic, infected tissue. *E. coli* is the most common etiologic organism, but any of the lactose fermenters may be involved. This condition is almost exclusively seen in diabetic patients and carries an overall mortality of 43 per cent.

REFERENCE

1. Freiha F.S., Messing, E.M., and Gross, D.M.: Emphysematous pyelonephritis. J. Contin. Educ. Urol., *18*:9, 1979.

329-A *(Campbell's, pp. 748, 791–794)*

While 80 per cent of patients with asymptomatic bacteriuria can be cured with a 7-day course of oral antimicrobial therapy, long-term cure rates are no better than placebo therapy because of reinfections in treated patients and spontaneous cures in untreated patients. Even though one third of patients with asymptomatic bacteria develop acute symptoms within 12 months if untreated, a sound argument can be made against treating an asymptomatic infection just to achieve no growth in the urine for a short period of time. Infection from *Proteus* species should be eradicated to prevent struvite stones, and bacteriuria in pregnancy should be treated to prevent the increased risk of pyelonephritis and its possible sequelae in these patients.

REFERENCES

1. Asscher, A.W., Sussman, M., Waters, W.E., et al.: Asymptomatic significant bacteriuria in the non-pregnant woman. J. Infect. Dis., *120*:17, 1969b.
2. Lindberg, U., Claesson, I., Hanson, L.A., et al.: Asymptomatic bacteriuria in schoolgirls. VIII. Clinical course during a 3-year follow-up. J. Pediatr., *92*:194, 1978.
3. Savage, D.C.L., Howie, G., Adler, K., et al.: Controlled trial of therapy in covert bacteriuria of childhood. Lancet, *1*:358, 1975.

330-D *(Campbell's, pp. 758–767)*

About one fourth of patients with acute pyelonephritis will have characteristic changes on their intravenous urogram. These changes include generalized or focal renal enlargement, impaired contrast secretion, dilation of the ureter and renal pelvis without obstruction, and cortical striations in the nephrogram. Perinephric abscess is much less common and is characterized by decreased function on the involved side, calyectasis or calycele stretching, calculi and renal displacement. Pyonephrosis refers to infected hydronephrosis. A renal mass and renal calculi are the most common IVP findings in xanthogranulomatous pyelonephritis. As mentioned previously, the hallmark finding in emphysematous pyelonephritis is intraparenchymal gas.

REFERENCES

1. Little, P.J., McPherson, D.R., and Wardener, H.E.: The appearance of the intravenous pyelogram during and after acute pyelonephritis. Lancet, *1*:1186, 1965.
2. Silver, T.M., Kass, E.M., Thornbury, J.R., et al.: The radiological spectrum of acute pyelonephritis in adults and adolescents. Radiology, *118*:65, 1976.
3. Anhalt, M.A., Cawood, C.D., and Scott, R.Jr.: Xanthogranulomatous pyelonephritis: A comprehensive review with report of 4 additional cases. J. Urol., *105*: 10, 1971.
4. Malek, R.S., and Elder, J.S.,: Xanthrogranulomatous pyelonephritis. Br. J. Urol., *44*:296, 1972.

331-A *(Campbell's, pp. 765–766)*

Proteus species are the most common organisms involved with xanthogranulomatous pyelonephritis; however, *E. coli* is also common. Approximately 10 per cent of patients have mixed urine cultures and in about one third of patients, no growth will be detected in the urine at presentation.

REFERENCES

1. Anhalt, M.A., Cawood, C.D., and Scott, R. Jr.: Xanthogranulomatous pyelonephritis: A comprehensive review with report of 4 additional cases. J. Urol., *105*: 10, 1971.
2. Tolia, B.M., Iloreta, A., Freed, S.Z., et al.: Xanthogranulomatous pyelonephritis: Detailed analysis of 29

cases and a brief discussion of atypical presentations. J. Urol., *126*:437, 1981.

332-E *(Campbell's, pp. 765–767)*

The high rate of negative urine cultures in xanthogranulomatous pyelonephritis is probably related to the fact that many patients have recently taken or are currently taking antimicrobials when cultures are obtained. CT usually demonstrates a large reniform mass with the renal pelvis tightly surrounding a central calcification and multiple water density masses along with abcess cavities filled within the parenchyma. These findings, although distinctive, often cannot differentiate between xanthogranulomatous pyelonephritis and renal cell carcinoma and subsequently the diagnosis is made postoperatively in most patients. There is no evidence that this is a precancerous lesion; however, incision and drainage is usually not curative and either partial or total nephrectomy is usually required. The lesions are almost always unilateral and therefore azotemia or frank renal failure is uncommon.

REFERENCES

1. Goldman, S.M., Hartman, D.S., Fishman, E.K., et al.: CT of xanthogranulomatous pyelonephritis. Radiologic-pathologic correlation. AJR, *141*:963, 1984.
2. Malek, R.S., and Elder, J.S.: Xanthogranulomatous pyelonephritis: A critical analysis of 26 cases and of the literature. J. Urol., *119*:589, 1978.
3. Goodman, M., Curry, T., and Russell, T.: Xanthogranulomatous pyelonephritis (XGP): A local disease with systemic manifestations: Report of 23 patients and review of the literature. Medicine, *58*:171, 1979.

333-B *(Campbell's, pp. 767–768)*

Malacoplakia is an unusual inflammatory disease that most commonly affects the genitourinary tract but can also affect other organ systems. It is characterized by mucosal plaques or nodules, and the diagnosis is made by biopsy. Michaelis-Gutmann bodies are pathognomonic of malacoplakia and are seen as small basophilic, extracytoplasmic, or intracytoplasmic calculospherules. A coliform infection can be documented in 90 per cent of patients. It is hypothesized that bacteria or bacterial fragments form the nidus for the calcium phosphate crystals that laminate the Michaelis-Gutmann bodies.

REFERENCE

1. Stanton, M.J., and Maxted, W.: Malacoplakia: A study of the literature and current concepts of pathogenesis, diagnosis, and treatment. J. Urol., *125*:139, 1981.

334-A *(Campbell's, pp. 760–761; Figs. 17–1, 17–2)*

In contrast to the patient with clinical acute pyelonephritis, the patient with chronic pyelonephritis is diagnosed by radiologic and pathologic means. The intravenous urogram is the best technique for diagnosing chronic pyelonephritis. The involved kidneys are usually atrophic. Focal course renal scarring with clubbing of the underlying calyx is characteristic. Localized areas of normal renal tissue within a scarred kidney may undergo a compensatory hypertrophy suggesting a renal mass or what is referred to as a pseudotumor. The scarring and atrophy most commonly affect the renal poles.

REFERENCE

1. Witten, E.M., Meyers, G.H., and Utz, D.G.: Emmett's Clinical Urography. Philadelphia, W.B. Saunders Co., 1977.

335-D *(Campbell's, p. 761)*

Atrophic kidneys with focal course renal scarring and clubbing of the underlying calyces are the characteristic urogram findings in patients with chronic pyelonephritis. Pseudotumors represent areas of normal renal tissue within a scarred kidney that undergo compensatory hypertrophy. Calcification of renal papillae is not usually seen in chronic pyelonephritis.

REFERENCE

1. Witten, E.M., Meyers, G.H., and Utz, D.G.: Emmett's Clinical Urography. Philadelphia, W.B. Saunders Co., 1977.

336-B *(Campbell's, p. 763)*

The clinical picture presented here is consistant with pyonephrosis. This refers to infected hydronephrosis associated with suppurative destruction of the parenchyma of the kidney. Rapid diagnosis and treatment of pyonephrosis are essential to avoid permanent loss of renal function and to prevent sepsis. The treatment is initiation of appropriate antimicrobial drugs and drainage of the infected pelvis. A ureteral catheter can be passed to drain the kidney, but if the obstruction prevents this, a percutaneous nephrostomy tube can be placed. Neither nephrectomy nor pyeloplasty would be indicated in the acute setting. The renal ultrasound is the most useful procedure to diagnosis pyelonephritis and may show 1 of 4 patterns: (1) persistent echoes from the inferior portion of the collecting system, (2) a fluid-debris level with dependent echoes that shift when the patient changes position, (3) strong echoes with acoustic shadowing from air and the collecting system, or (4) weak echoes throughout a dilated collecting system.

REFERENCES

1. Camunez, F., Echenagusia, A., Prieto, M.L., et al.: Percutaneous nephrostomy in pyonephrosis. Urol. Radio., *11*:77, 1989.
2. Coleman, B.G., Arger, P.H., Mulhern, C.B. Jr., et al.: Pyonephrosis: Sonography in the diagnosis and management. Am. J. Roentgenol., *137*:939, 1981.

337-E *(Campbell's, pp. 786–788; Table 17–3)*

The success of prophylaxis depends in large part on the effect an antimicrobial agent has on the introital and fecal resevoirs of pathogenic bacteria. Antimicrobial agents that eliminate pathogenic bacteria from these sites and/or do not cause bacterial resistance at the sites can be effective for prophylaxis of urinary tract infections. All of the listed antibiotics except sulfamethoxazole (used as a single agent) have been shown to be effective prophylactic agents. Trimethoprim and the fluoroquinolones prevent infection by eliminating the pathogens from the fecal flora, whereas nitrofurantoin and cephalexin do not alter the gut flora but act by repeated elimination of bacteria from the urine.

REFERENCES

1. Svensson, R., Larsson, P., and Lincoln, K.: Low dose trimethoprim prophylaxis in long term control of chronic recurrent urinary infection. Scand. J. Infect. Dis., *14*:139, 1982.
2. Fairley, K.F., Hubbard, M., and Whitworth, J.A.: Prophylactic long-term cephalexin in recurrent urinary infection. Med. J. Aust., *1*:318, 1974.
3. Nicolle, L.E., Harding, G.K.M., Thompson, M., et al.: Prospective, randomized, placebo-controlled trial of norfloxacin for the prophylaxis of recurrent urinary tract infection in women. Antimicrob. Agents Chemother., *33*:1032, 1989.
4. Martinez, F.C., Kindrachuk, R.W., Stamey, T.A., et al.: Effect of prophylactic, low dose cephalexin on fecal and vaginal bacteria. J. Urol., *133*:994, 1985.
5. Nord, C.E.: Effect of new quinolones on the human gastrointestinal microflora. Rev. Infect. Dis., *10*: (Suppl.):193, 1988.

338-D *(Campbell's, pp. 763–765)*

The high mortality rate from perinephric abscess is due in large part to the long delay in making the diagnosis. The diagnosis is difficult to make from a patient's history and physical and examination alone because the findings are nonspecific. Two factors that help to distinguish perinephric abscess from acute pyelonephritis are duration of symptoms for longer than 5 days before hospitalization, and presence of a fever for longer than 4 days after appropropiate antimicrobial agents are started. Once a perinephric abscess is suspected, the diagnosis can usually be confirmed using ultrasound and CT. Urine and blood cultures are frequently negative; however, the delay in diagnosis is more commonly due to misdiagnosis as uncomplicated acute urinary tract infection. Percutaneous drainage of abscesses has been shown to be successful; however, it is less effective in draining larger abscess cavities filled with thick purulent fluid.

REFERENCES

1. Thorley, J.D., Jones, S.R., and Sanford, J.P.: Perinephric abscess. Medicine, *53*:441, 1974.
2. Haaga, J.R., and Weinstein, A.J.: CT guided percutaneous aspiration and drainage of abscesses. Am. J. Roentgenol., *135*:1187, 1980.

339-A *(Campbell's, pp. 773–776)*

It has been demonstrated that bacteriuria is preceded by colonization of the vaginal introitus with the responsible organism, and that the biology of the vagina of women susceptible to urinary tract infections is different from that in normal control women who never have infections. The etiology for this increased colonization of vaginal mucosa with fecal pathogens in women susceptible to urinary tract infections has been a matter of considerable investigation. Stamey and associates have reported that women resistant to urinary tract infections carry specific vaginal antibody against their own *E. coli*, whereas those who are susceptible have substantially less vaginal antibody. It has also been shown that vaginal epithelial cells in patients susceptible to reinfection have a higher affinity for *E. coli* adherence, which is thought to be due to an increase in receptor sites for *E. coli.*

REFERENCES

1. Shaeffer, A.J., and Stamey, T.A.: Studies of introital colonization in women with recurrent urinary tract infections: IX. The role of antimicrobial therapy. J. Urol., *118*:221, 1977.
2. Stamey, T.A., and Sexton, C.C.: The role of vaginal colonization with Enterobacteriaceae in recurrent urinary infections. J. Urol. *113*:214, 1975.
3. Stamey, T.A., Wehner, N., Mihara, G., et al.: The immunologic basis of recurrent bacteriuria; role of cervicovaginal antibody in enterobacterial colonization of the introital mucosa. Medicine, *57*:47, 1978.
4. Fowler, J.E. Jr., and Stamey, T.A.: Studies of introital colonization in women with recurrent urinary infections. VII. The role of bacterial adherence. J. Urol., *117*:472, 1977.
5. Schaeffer, A.J., Jones, J.M., Duncan, J.L., et al.: Adhesion of uropathogenic *Escherichia coli* to epithelial cells from women with recurrent urinary tract infection. Infection. *10*:186, 1982.

340-C *(Campbell's, p. 787)*

Nitrofurantoin is either completely absorbed or degraded in the intestinal tract and therefore very little of the active drug reaches the colon. Because of this, nitrofurantoin does not alter gut flora and produce minimal fecal resistance. The drug is present in the urine for brief periods at high concentrations and leads to repeated elimination of bacteria, presumably interfering with bacterial initiation of infection. The most common adverse drug reactions are acute pulmonary reactions and allergic reactions. The risk of an adverse reaction increases with age, with the greatest number occurring in patients over 50 years of age.

REFERENCES

1. Stamey, T.A., Condy, M., and Mihara, G.: Prophylactic efficacy of nitrofurantoin macrocrystals and trimethoprim-sulfamethoxazole in urinary infections; Biologic effects on the vaginal and rectal flora. N. Engl. J. Med., *296*:780, 1977.
2. Holmberg, L., Boman, G., Bottiger, L.E., et al.: Adverse reactions to nitrofurantoin: Analysis of 921 reports. Am. J. Med., *69*:733, 1980.

341-E *(Campbell's, pp. 780–783)*

It has been shown that pyelonephritic strains of *E. coli* have an increased adhesive ability and that this ability is related to the presence of P pili. Reid and associates found that uropathogens attached in larger numbers to uroepithelial cells from women older than 65 years of age than to cells from premenopausal women. Type 1 pili are found in most strains of *E. coli*, and their role in urinary tract infections is less clear. Envirnomental growth conditions can produce rapid changes in pilus expression, wherein cells switch back and forth between piliated and nonpiliated phases. This process is called phase variation and may account for the fact that strains isolated from different sites in the urogenital tract can show variation in the state of piliation.

REFERENCES

1. Svanborg, Eden, C., Hanson, L.A., Jodal. V., et al.: Variable adherence to normal human urinary-tract epithelial cells of *Escherichia coli* strains associated with various forms of urinary tract infection. Lancet, 2:490, 1976.
2. Kallenius, G., and Mollby, R.: Adhesion of *Escherichia coli* to human periurethral cells correlated to mannose-resistant agglutination of human erythrocytes. FEMS Microbiol. Lett., *5*:295, 1979.
3. Reid, G., Zorzitto, M.L., Bruce, A.W., et al.: Pathogenesis of urinary tract infection in the elderly: The role of bacterial adherence to uroepithelial cells. Corr. Microbiol., *11*:67, 1984.
4. Eisenstein, B.I.: Phase variation of type-1 fimbriae in *Escherichia coli* is under transcriptional control. Science, *214*:337, 1981.

342-A *(Campbell's, pp. 783–786)*

When bacteriuria is detected by screening survey, it is conveniently called screening bacteriuria. About 3 to 6 per cent of sexually active women of child-bearing age are bacteriuic on screening surveys, and the majority of these women have had irritative symptoms within a year before their bacteriuria was detected. It has been shown that the probablility of acquiring a symptomatic infection is 7 times greater in women with known screening bacteriuria than those without. There is, however, no evidence that the bacteriuria leads to an increased risk of hypertension, azotemia, or progressive renal cortical destruction. In addition, it has been shown that successful therapy in screening bacteriuria was little different in the long run from the natural history of spontaneous remissions. All of these issues lead to the conclusion that the physician should focus on diagnosis, treatment, and assessment of the renal risk to the symptomatic patient, rather than screening and treating asymptomatic populations with bacteriuria.

REFERENCES

1. Asscher, A.W., Chick, S., Radford, N., et al.: Natural history of asymptomatic bacteriuria (ASB) in nonpregnant women. *In* Bromfitt, W., and Asscher, A.W., (Eds.): Urinary Tract Infection. London, Oxford University Press, 1973, p. 51.
2. Gaymans, R., Haverkorn, M.J., Valkenburg, H.A., et al.: A prospective study of urinary-tract infections in a Dutch general practice. Lancet, 2:674, 1976.
3. Asscher, A.W., Sussman, M., Waters, W.E., et al.: The clinical significance of asymptomatic bacteriuria in the nonpregnant woman. J. Infect. Dis., *120*:17, 1969b.

343-B *(Campbell's, p. 793)*

If a pregnant women has acute clinical pyelonephritis that is unresponsive to antimicrobial treatment within 48 to 72 hours, radiographic evaluation is needed. Unfortunately, renal ultrasound, which is ordinarily useful for detecting urinary tract obstruction, is inadequate for detecting obstruction in pregnancy because normal pregnancy is accompanied by hydronephrosis. An abbreviated intravenous urogram—consisting of an initial abdominal plain film, 15-minute film, and then a third film at 1 hour if the collecting system was not visualized at 15 minutes—limits radiation of the fetus and is usually sufficient to determine the site and cause of obstruction. The low radiation exposure might make renal nuclear scans useful for locating obstruction; however; little is written about the use of these studies in pregnancy.

REFERENCE

1. Waltzer, W.C.: The urinary tract in pregnancy. J. Urol., *125*:271, 1981.

344-D *(Campbell's, pp. 793–794)*

Only the penicillins and cephalosporins, given orally or parenterally, are thought to be safe and effective during all phases of pregnancy. The fluoroquinolones are contraindicated during pregnancy because of potential adverse effects on cartilage formation. Trimethoprim should be avoided during the first trimester of pregnancy because of its potential teratogenic activity. The nitrofurantoins, a group of oxidizing drugs, can cause hemolytic anemia in fetuses with a glucose-6 phosphate dehydrogenase deficiency. Sulfa preparations should be avoided in the third trimester of pregnancy because they compete for fetal bilirubin-binding sites on albumin and can cause neonatal hyperbilirubinemia and kernicterus.

REFERENCE

1. Gerstner, G.J., Muller, G., and Nahler, G.: Amoxicillin in the treatment of asymptomatic bacteriuria in pregnancy: A single dose of 3 g amoxicillin versus a 4-day course of 3 doses 750 mg amoxicillin. Gynecol. Obstet. Invest., *27*:84, 1989.

345-E *(Campbell's, pp. 814–819)*

The clinical presentation is consistant with either chronic bacterial prostatis or nonbacterial prostatis. Nonbacterial prostatis is, however, the most common prostatitis syndrome exceeding bacterial prostatis in incidence by 8-fold. Acute bacterial prostatitis is characterized by the sudden onset of moderate to high fever, chills, low back, and perineal pain along with variable degrees of bladder outlet obstruction. Granulomatous prostatitis is rare and can be distinguished from the other entities by the presence of an enlarged, firm prostate that feels malignant. Prostatodynia cannot be distinguished from nonbacterial prostatis by symptoms alone. It is, however, less common, and patients with prostatodynia have normal prostatic secretions.

REFERENCE

1. Shaeffer, A.J., Jones, J.M., and Dunn, J.K.: Association of in vitro *Escherichia coli* adherence to vaginal and buccal epithelial cells with susceptibility of women to recurrent urinary-tract infections. N. Engl. J. Med., *304*:1062, 1981.

346-B *(Campbell's, pp. 816–817)*

Since the cause of nonbacterial prostatis is unknown, an effective clinical management is often difficult to achieve. The main treatment plan is to control symptoms and to relieve anxieties and concerns. Painful symptomatic episodes are often relieved by hot sitz baths or short courses of anti-inflammatory agents, for example, Ibuprofen, 600 mg orally 4 times daily. Irritative voiding dysfunction usually respondes to the use of anticholinergics, for example, oxybutynin chloride, 5 mg orally 3 times daily. Some patients may benefit from normal sexual activity and dietary restrictions if spicy foods or alcoholic beverages appear to cause or aggravate the symptoms. A 14-day course of tetracycline or erythromycin may be reasonable if infection with *U. urealyticum* or *C. trachomatis* infection is suspected. Once other forms of prostatis are excluded, the diagnosis of nonbacterial prostatis is established, and antibacterial agents are neither effective nor indicated at that point.

347-C *(Campbell's, p. 818; Table 18–6)*

Clinical and video-urodynamic studies of prostatodynia patients demonstrate that most have "spastic" dysfunction of the bladder neck and prostatic urethra. The principal findings are depressed urinary flow rates, incomplete relaxation of the bladder neck and prostatic urethra and abnormally high maximum urethral closure pressures at rest. Normal relaxation of the external urinary sphincter during voiding is typical of these patients, and uninhibited bladder contractions are unusual. The symptoms probably result from nonrelaxation of the internal urinary sphincter and nonrelaxation of the pelvic floor striated muscles leading to elevated prostatic urethral pressures and intraprostatic urinary reflux. Accordingly, most patients respond to alpha blocking agents, for example, prazosin.

REFERENCES

1. Barbalias, G.A., Meares, E.M. Jr., and Sant, G.R.: Prostatodynia: Clinical and urodynamic characteristics. J. Urol., *130*:514, 1983.
2. Meares, E.M. Jr.: Prostatodynia: Clinical findings and rationale for treatment. *In* Weidner, W., Brunner, H., Krause, W., Ruthage, C.F. (Eds.): Therapy of Prostatitis. Munich, W. Zuckswerdt Verlag, 1986a, pp. 207–212.
3. Blacklock, N.J.: Urodynamic and psychometric observations and their implication in the management of prostatodynia. *In* Weidner, W., Brunner, J., Krause, W., Ruthage, C.F. (Eds.): Therapy of Prostatitis. Munich, W. Zuckswerdt Verlag, 1986, pp. 201–206.

348-D *(Campbell's, pp. 807–808)*

Most prostatic infections are caused by a single pathogen, and the causative organisms are similar in type and incidence to those responsible for UTI. Strains of *E. coli* clearly predominate, followed by species of *Proteus, Klebsiella, Enterobacter, Pseudomonas, and Serratia.* Gram-positive bacteria and anaerobic pathogens are felt to occur only rarely. Most evidence points to ascending urethral infection or reflux of infected urine into prostatic ducts as the etiology for bacterial prostatitis rather than direct invasion by rectal bacteria or hematogenous infection.

REFERENCES

1. Meares, E.M. Jr.: Acute and chronic prostatitis: Diagnosis and treatment. Infect. Dis. Clin. North Am., *1*:855, 1987.
2. Mårdh, P.-A., and Colleen, S.: Search for urogenital tract infections in patients with symptoms of prostatitis. Studies on aerobic and strictly anaerobic bacteria, mycoplasmas, fungi, trichomonads, and viruses. Scand. J. Urol. Nephrol., *9*:8, 1975.
3. Sutor, D.J., and Wooley, S.E.: The crystalline composition of prostatic calculi. Br. J. Urol., *46*:533, 1974.
4. Rameriz, C.T., Ruiz, J.A., Gomez, A.Z., et al.: A crystallographic study of prostatic calculi. J. Urol., *124*: 840, 1980.
5. Kirby, R.S., Lowe, D., Bultitude, M.I., and Shuttleworth, K.E.D.: Intra-prostatic urinary reflux: An aetiological factor in a bacterial prostatitis. Br. J. Urol., *54*:729, 1982.

349-D *(Campbell's, pp. 808–811)*

The diagnosis of bacterial prostatis is confirmed when quantitative bacteriologic cultures clearly localize pathogenic bacteria to the prostate. Segmented urine cultures are the best technique for localizing bacteria to the prostate. The counts of pathogenic bacteria in the prostatic specimen (VB3) should exceed by tenfold or more the counts in the urethral (VB1) and bladder (VB2) specimens.

Histologic changes seen in chronic bacterial prostatis are not sufficiently specific to confirm a bacterial etiology of the inflammation. The findings of excessive leukocytes and macrophages suggest prostatic inflammation but are also seen in nonbacterial prostatis. Semen contains fluids from several accessory glands and can be easily contaminated by urethral organisms of nonprostatic origin as it passes through the urethra.

REFERENCES

1. Meares, E.M., and Stamey, T.A.: Bacteriologic localization patterns in bacterial prostatitis and urethritis. Invest. Urol., *5*:492, 1968.
2. Kohnen, P.W., and Drach, G.W.: Patterns of inflammation in prostatic hyperplasia: A histologic and bacteriologic study. J. Urol., *121*:755, 1979.

350-A *(Campbell's, p. 811; Table 18–4)*

Significant alterations in the secretory products of the prostate occur in patients with documented chronic bacterial prostatitis and are sufficiently inclusive to suggest generalized secretory dysfunction of the prostate. The best recognized of these changes is the increase in the pH value. Because prostatitis is a focal, not diffuse, tissue infection, no absolute count of bacteria is diagnostic. In addition to elevated pH, elevations in LDH isoenzyme 5 and immunoglobulins have been noted. The decreased levels of citric acid and acid phosphatase are usually seen along with decreases in specific gravity, zinc, spermine, and cholesterol.

REFERENCES

1. Anderson, R.U., and Fair, W.R.: Physical and chemical determinations of prostatic secretion in benign hyperplasia, prostatitis, and adenocarcinoma. Invest. Urol., *14*:137, 1976.
2. Pfau, A., Perlberg, S., and Shapira, A.: The pH of the prostatic fluid in health and disease: Implications of treatment in chronic bacterial prostatitis. J. Urol., *119*: 384, 1978.
3. Fair, W.R., Crane, D.B., Schiller, N., and Heston, W.D.W.: A reappraisal of treatment in chronic bacterial prostatitis. J. Urol., *121*,437, 1979.

351-D *(Campbell's, pp. 815–816)*

Prostatic calculi are seen in almost 100 per cent of elderly men on transrectal prostatic ultrasound. These stones are typically small but tend to occur in clusters. Multiple large calculi are seen most often in men who have chronic bacterial infections of the prostate. Uninfected prostatic calculi usually cause no symptoms or apparent harm; however, in men who have bacterial prostatitis, prostatic stones can become infected and serve as a source of bacterial persistence and relapsing UTI. Intraprostatic reflux of urine and ductal obstruction are two factors that have been implicated in the etiology of prostatic calculi. Although appropriate antimicrobial therapy usually controls symptoms and prevents bacteriuria, infected prostatic calculi cannot be sterilized by medical therapy. The peripheral zones of the prostate contain the greatest foci of infection and stones.

REFERENCE

1. Peeling, W.B., and Griffiths, G.J.: Imaging of the prostate by ultrasound. J. Urol., *132*:217, 1984.
2. Eykyn, S., Bultitude, M.I., Mayo, M.E., et al.: Prostatic calculi as a source of recurrent bacteriuria in the male. Br. J. Urol., *46*:527, 1974.
3. Blacklock, N.J.: Anatomical factors in prostatitis. Br. J. Urol., *46*:47, 1974.
4. Meares, E.M. Jr.: Chronic bacterial prostatitis: Role of transurethral prostatectomy (TURP) in therapy. *In* Weidner, W., Brunner, H., Krause, W., Rothauge, C.F. (Eds.): Therapy of Prostatitis. Munich, W. Zuckschwerdt Verlag, 1986c, pp. 193–197.

352-E *(Campbell's, pp. 814–815)*

The diagnosis of acute bacterial prostatis can usually be made by the combination of the distinctive symptoms and an exquisitely tender, swollen prostate on digital rectal examination. Prostatic massage to express secretions is not recommended as it is very painful for the patient and may lead to bacteremia. Because bacteriuria usually accompanies acute bacterial prostatitis, the pathogen is generally identified by culture of the voided urine.

Preferred initial therapy in the nonallergic patient is trimethoprim-sulfamethoxazole, either orally or intravenously until culture and sensitivity test results are known. If the pathogen is susceptible and the clinical response is satisfactory, treatment is continued orally for 30 days to prevent chronic bacterial prostatitis. Transurethral catheters are tolerated poorly in this setting and may lead to complications. Acute urinary retention, therefore, is best managed by temporary placement of a punch suprapubic tube under local anesthesia.

353-B *(Campbell's, pp. 811–812)*

It has been shown that the prostatic fluid contains a potent antibacterial factor (PAF) that is bactericidal to most pathogens that commonly cause urinary tract infections. Potent antibacterial factor has been identified as free zinc. Since zinc concentrations are low in the prostatic fluid of men who have chronic bacterial prostatitis, clinicians believe that zinc may serve as a natural defense against ascending urinary tract infections in normal men. Whether men become infected because their prostatic secretions contain inadequate levels of zinc, however, or whether zinc is depressed as a consequence of prostatic infection remain unanswered questions. Fair and coworkers have demonstrated that depressed levels of zinc in prostatic secretions remain unaltered during therapy with oral zinc preparations.

REFERENCES

1. Parrish, R.F., Perinetti, E.P., and Fair, W.R.: Evidence against a zinc binding peptide in pilocarpine-stimulated canine prostatic secretions. Prostate, *4*:189, 1983.
2. Fair, W.R., Couch, J., and Wehner, N.: Prostatic antibacterial factor. Identity and significance. Urology, *7*: 169, 1976.

354-E *(Campbell's, p. 820)*

Ascending urethral infection and the intraprostatic reflux of infected urine are thought to initially cause acute bacterial prostatitis, which then leads to prostatic abscess. Men especially prone to prostatic abscess include those who are diabetic, those who are on maintenance dialysis, those who are immunocompromised for various reasons, and those who undergo urethral instrumentation or require indwelling urethral catheters. Prostatic calculi, as mentioned previously, are very common and have not been demonstrated to predispose to prostatic abscess.

REFERENCES

1. Weinberger, M., Cytron, S., Servadio, C., et al.: Prostatic abscess in the antibiotic era. Rev. Infect. Dis., *10*:239, 1988.
2. Meares, E.M. Jr.: Prostatic abscess (editorial). J. Urol., *136*:281, 1986d.

355-C *(Campbell's, p. 819)*

Granulomatous prostatis occurs in two forms: a nonspecific variety and an eosinophilic variety. The eosinophilic variety occurs almost exclusively in patients with allergies, especially in asthmatics. Generally, affected patients become severely ill and high fevers develop. Hemograms of the peripheral blood typically show significant eosinophilia. The prostate gland typically becomes markedly enlarged and indurated, and complete urinary retention often develops. Prostatic abscesses can also present with high fever and urinary retention as well as an enlarged firm prostate on rectal examination. Urine cultures are usually positive, however, and there is no associated eosinophilia with prostatic abscesses.

REFERENCE

1. Towfighi, J., Sadeghee, S., Wheller, J.E., et al.: Granulomatous prostatitis with emphasis on the eosinophilic variety. Am. J. Clin. Pathol., *58*:630, 1972.

356-C *(Campbell's, p. 833)*

The diagnosis of *T. vaginalis* is usually made from history and physical examination. Women commonly present with vaginal itching, dysuria, and discharge. The findings on physical examination include vulvar and vaginal erythema and colpitis macularis ("strawberry cervix"). Wet mount evaluation of vaginal secretions may confirm the diagnosis; however, it has been shown to be relatively insensitive. Culture is the most sensitive technique, detecting 95 per cent or more of infections. The best culture media to use are Diamond's Medium or Feimberg-Whittington's Medium.

REFERENCES

1. Wolner, H.P., Krieger, J.N., and Stevens, C.E.: Clinical manifestations of vaginal trichomoniasis. JAMA, *261*: 571, 1989.
2. Bennett, J.R., Barnes, W.G., and Coffman, S.: The emergency department diagnosis of *Trichomonas* vaginitis. Ann. Emerg. Med., *18*:564, 1989.
3. Clay, J.C., Veeravahu, M., and Smyth, R.W.: Practical problems of diagnosing trichomoniasis in women. Genitourin. Med., *64*:115, 1988.

357-B *(Campbell's, pp. 825–826)*

Gonococcal urethritis may be asymptomatic in 40 to 60 per cent of the contacts of partners with known gonorrhea. These asymptomatic patients may remain infected; therefore, all sexual contacts of symptomatic patients should be treated. The CDC currently recommends treatment with ceftriaxone 250 mg intramuscularly as the drug of choice for all gonococcal infections. Tetracycline should be added to this regimen because about 30 per cent of men with gonococcal urethritis also will be infected with *Chlamydia trachomatis*, which is not sensitive to ceftriaxone.

The incubation period for gonococcal urethritis varies from 3 to 10 days, but exceptions are very common. Gram staining of urethral swabs has been shown to be highly specific and sensitive in diagnosing gonorrhea. The strains of gonorrhea that cause systemic disease are more common in blacks than whites.

REFERENCES

1. Crawford, G., Knapp, J.S., Hale, J., et al.: Asymptomatic gonorrhea in men. Science, *196*:1352, 1937.
2. John, J., and Donald, W.H.: Asymptomatic urethral gonorrhea in men. Br. J. Vener. Dis., *54*:322, 1978.
3. Portnoy, J., Mendelson, J., Clecner, B., et al.: Asymptomatic gonorrhea in the male. Can. Med. Assoc. J., *110*:169, 1974.
4. Granato, P.A., Schneible-Smith, C., and Weiner, L.B.: Use of New York City medium for improved recovery on *N. gonorrhoeae* from clinical specimens. J. Clin. Microbiol., *13*:963, 1981.
5. Knapp, J.S., Thornsberry, C., Schoolnik, G.K., et al.: Phenotypic and epidemiologic correlates of auxotype in *Neisseria gonorrhoeae*. J. Infect. Dis., *138*:160, 1978.

358-A *(Campbell's, pp. 826–829; Table 19–4)*

Resistance of *N. gonorrhoeae* to ceftriaxone is rare as is resistance of *C. trachomatis* to tetracycline, however, *U. urealyticum* can be isolated in 20 to 30 per cent of men at the time of recurrence. *Trachomatis* and *Gardnerella* species are found only rarely on urethral cultures in these patients. Treatment with erythromycin for 1 to 2 weeks is recommended to erradicate tetracycline-resistant *U. urealyticum* in patients with recurrent or persistant nongonococcal urethritis.

REFERENCE

1. Bowie, W.R., Alexander, E.R., Stimson, J.B., et al.: Therapy for nongonococcal urethritis: Double-blind randomized comparison of two doses and two durations of minocycline. Ann. Intern. Med., *95*:306, 1981.

359-E *(Campbell's, pp. 831–832)*

Epididymitis is usually caused by spread of infection from the urethra or bladder and as such usually responds to the same antibiotics commonly used to treat UTIs. Bed rest with scrotal elevation improves lymphatic drainage. Oral nonsteroidal anti-inflammatory drugs may be of symptomatic benefit; however, prednisone has been found to be of no value as an adjunct to antibiotic therapy. Younger boys and older men who have epididymitis secondary to bacteriuria often have structural urologic abnormalities and should undergo radiographic and cystoscopic evaluation.

REFERENCE

1. Moore, C.A., Lockett, B.L., Lennox, K.W., et al.: Prednisone in the treatment of acute epididymitis: A cooperative study. J. Urol., *106*:578, 1971.

360-E *(Campbell's, pp. 834–837)*

Vesicles grouped on an erythematous base that do not follow a neural distribution are essentially pathognomonic for genital herpes. The only other conditions that can be reliably diagnosed by presentation alone include fixed drug eruptions and traumatic genital lesions.

REFERENCE

1. Krauss, S.J.: Evaluation and management of acute genital ulcers on sexually active patients. Urol. Clin. North Am., *11*:155, 1985.

361-B *(Campbell's, p. 837)*

The clinical illness of primary genital herpes tends to be more severe in women. Dysuria is present in 83 per cent of women as opposed to only 44 per cent of men and is thought to be secondary to a true urethritis in most of these patients. HSV types I and II produce primary genital infections of equal severity; however, recurrences are more frequent with primary HSV type II infections. As mentioned previously, the presentation is often pathognomonic; however, virus isolation by culture is the most sensitive of techniques for confirming the diagnosis of herpes virus infections. Acyclovir is the only drug that has shown efficacy in the treatment of genital herpes. Oral acyclovir (200 mg 5 times per day for 5–10 days) appears to be more effective than topical therapy in the treatment of both primary and recurrent herpes. To have maximal effect, the drug must be given during the prodrome.

REFERENCES

1. Corey, L., Benedetti, A., Critchlow, C., et al.: Treatment of primary first-episode genital herpes simplex virus infections with acyclovir: Results of topical, intravenous and oral therapy. J. Antimicrob. Chemother., *12*(Suppl. B):79, 1983a.
2. Goldstein, L.C., Corey, L., McDougall, J., et al.: Monoclonal antibodies to herpes simplex viruses: Use in antigenic typing and rapid diagnosis. J. Infect. Dis., *147*:829, 1983.

362-B *(Campbell's, p. 839)*

Presumptive diagnosis of primary syphilis may be made on the basis of serologic tests for *Treponema* with the fluorescent treponemal antibody absorption test (FTA-ABS) and the microhemagglutination assay for antibody to *Treponema pallidum* (MHATP) or the nontreponemal tests, such as Veneral Disease Research Laboratory (VDRL) and rapid plasma reagin (RPR). None of these tests is sufficient for diagnosis, which requires visualization of the spirochete by dark-field or fluorescent antibody microscopy of the scrapings taken from the base of the chancre.

363-A *(Campbell's, p. 839)*

All of the antibiotics listed are effective treatment for primary syphilis; however, the single IM dose of benzathine penicillin G is the preferred treatment for primary syphilis, as it is the most cost effective. Treatment failures occur with all regimens, and patients need to be reexamined serologically at 3 and 6 months. If the primary antibodies have not declined by 4-fold within 6 months of treating early syphilis, patients should undergo cerebrospinal fluid examination for CNS syphilis and be retreated appropriately.

364-A *(Campbell's, pp. 834–840)*

Chancroid must be considered in the differiental diagnosis in any man with a painful genital ulcer. The ulcer typically has a deep undermined border, and the base of the lesion is often friable and bleeds easily. All of the other diseases listed, with the exception of herpes, classically present as painless lesions. Herpes usually presents as vesicles grouped on an erythematous base and not as an ulcer.

The definitive diagnosis of chancroid can be made from gram-stain smear at the base of the lesion or by using selective cultures for *Haemophilus ducreyi.*

365-A *(Campbell's, pp. 856–858)*

While the pneumococcal vaccine is recommend for all persons infected with HIV, the presence of pneumococcal pneumonia is not an indication for HIV testing. Most experts agree that persons at risk for HIV infection should be tested routinely. Such persons include those with an STD, including hepatitis B and gonococcal urethritis. In addition, patients with a history of sexual contact with homosexual men, multiple unsafe heterosexual contacts, and any history of needle sharing or use of IV drugs should be tested. Testing is also encouraged for those patients with a history of disease that might be associated with HIV infection (such as lymphopenia), unexplained elevated levels of hepatic enzymes, or positive status for hepatitis B markers.

The CDC has also recommended that HIV testing be done for all patients with active tuberculosis. Because a large fraction of persons infected with HIV eventually develop AIDS, those with positive tuberculin test results should receive isoniazid prophylaxis unless there are major contraindications. This therapy should be instituted as soon as possible because active tuberculosis may be the first sign of HIV-related disease.

REFERENCE

1. Rhame, F.S., and Maki, D.G.: The case for wider use of testing for HIV infection. N. Engl. J. Med., *320*: 1248, 1989.

366-C *(Campbell's, pp. 852–853)*

The CDC system classifies HIV-infected persons into four categories: class I: acute infection; class II: asymptomatic sero-positive infection; class III: persistent generalized lymphadenopathy; class IV: symptomatic HIV disease. Acute infection is represented by a mononuculosis-like syndrome that is believed to occur in approximately one third to two thirds of the persons who acquire HIV infection. After becoming HIV-positive, approximately 50 to 70 per cent of infected persons develop persistent generalized lymphadenopathy. Currently, however, at any given time most patients with HIV infection are totally asymptomatic (class II). The ELISA for HIV antibodies generally becomes positive 2 to 3 months after infection.

REFERENCES

1. Chaisson, R.E., and Volberding, P.A.: Clinical manifestations of HIV infection. *In* Mandell, G.L., Douglas, R.G. Jr., and Bennett, J.E. (Eds.): Principles and Practice of Infectious Diseases. New York, Churchill Livingstone, 1990.

367-C *(Campbell's, pp. 851–852; Table 19–15)*

HIV infection results in a wide range of clinical presentations, ranging from totally asymptomatic carriage of the virus to life-threatening opportunistic infections and malignancies. Documented HIV infection with generalized adenopathy defines a class III HIV infection using the CDC system. This does not, however, meet the CDC criteria for the definition of AIDS. A useful functional definition of AIDS is the occurrence of certain systemic infections or malignancies in a patient with no other cause or defective cell-mediated immunity. In addition, a presumptive diagnosis of AIDS can be made with the confirmation of HIV infection and the presence of encephalopathy or wasting syndrome.

REFERENCES

1. Chaisson, R.E., and Volberding, P.A.: Clinical manifestations of HIV infection. *In* Mandell, G.L., Douglas, R.G. Jr., and Bennett, J.E. (Eds.): Principles and Practice of Infectious Diseases. New York, Churchill Livingstone, 1990.
2. Centers for Disease Control: Current trends: Classification system for human T lymphotropic virus type III/lymphadenopathy associated virus infections. MMWR, *35*:334–339, 1986.
3. Centers for Disease Control: Revision of the CDC surveillance case definition for acquired immunodeficiency syndrome. MMWR *36*(S)(1): 35–95, 1987c.

368-B *(Campbell's, p. 857)*

It has been shown that semen is clearly important for sexual transmission of HIV. Kreiger and coworkers have evaluated the stage of infection and antiviral chemotherapy on isolation of cultural HIV from semen. HIV was isolated in culture from 36 per cent of semen specimens from 18 asymptomatic patients and from 29 per cent of semen specimens from 18 AIDS patients. Isolation of HIV did not correlate with either CD4+ or CD8+ T-lymphocyte counts and zidovudine therapy did not effect the isolation from patients with AIDS. These results are consistent with the concepts that HIV may invade the male genital tract early in the course of infection and that virus excretion in the semen may be independent of the clinical stage of HIV infection. These observations support recommendations for safe sexual practices by all patients infected with HIV regardless of the stage of infection or concurrent antiviral chemotherapy.

REFERENCES

1. Curran, J.W., Jaffee, H.W., Hardy, A.M., et al.: Epidemiology of HIV infection and AIDS in the United States. Science, *239*:610–616, 1988.
2. Peterman, T.A., Stoneburner, R.L., Allen, J.R., et al.: Risk of human immunodeficiency virus transmission from heterosexual adults with transfusion-associated infections. JAMA, *259*:55–58, 1988.
3. Krieger, J.N., Coombs, R.W., Collier, A.Z., et al.: Recovery of human immunodeficiency virus from semen: Minimal impact of stage of infection and current antiviral chemotherapy. J. Infect. Dis., *163*:386–388, 1991a.

369-D *(Campbell's, p. 857)*

Rao and others described a series of AIDS patients with renal disease. These patients had a disease characterized by proteinuria, elevated serum creatinine levels, and focal and segmental glomerulosclerosis on biopsy. Although this disorder closely resembles heroin-associated nephropathy, only half the patients had a history of drug abuse. Whether there is a specific "AIDS-associated nephropathy" is still debateable. The problem is that many patients with AIDS are at high risk for renal disease because of concomitant factors, such as hepatitis B infection, treatment with toxic drugs, fluid and electorolyte abnormalities, opportunistic infections, and malignancies, that have all been associated with renal disorders. Renal disease has been described as a "late syndrome" in patients with AIDS, and is not usually seen early in the course of HIV infection. The etiology for this AIDS-associated nephropathy is presently unclear. It appears more frequently in the eastern United States where there are large numbers of patients who have AIDS associated with IV drug abuse. In contrast, there are large numbers of patients with AIDS in San Francisco, Seattle, and other cities who have had little renal involvement compared with patients in New York and Miami. The clinical course of AIDS-associated nephropathy is variable. Patients with other causes of renal dysfunction, such as nephrotoxic drugs or acute tubular necrosis, may improve. Others experience rapidly progressive clinical deterioration.

REFERENCES

1. Rao, T.K.S., Filippone, E.J., Nicastri, A.D., et al.: Associated focal and segmental glomerulosclerosis in the acquired immunodeficiency syndrome. N. Engl. J. Med. *310*:669–673, 1984.
2. Chaisson, R.E., and Volberding, P.A.: Clinical manifestations of HIV infection. *In* Mandell, G.L., Douglas, R.G. Jr., and Bennett, J.E. (Eds.): Principles and Practice of Infectious Diseases. New York, Churchill Livingstone, 1990.

370-B *(Campbell's, p. 857)*

A broad range of malignancies has been described in patients with AIDS and other HIV infections. These malignancies include squamous cell carcinomas in various sites, malignant melanoma, testicular cancers of all histologic types, Hodgkin's disease, and primary hepatocellular carcinoma. With the possible exception of Hodgkin's disease, there is minimal evidence that any of these cancers is caused by the HIV-induced immunologic deficits. However, there is a direct relationship between AIDS and Kaposi's sarcoma, primary central nervous system, non-Hodgkin's lymphoma, and high grade peripheral B-cell lymphomas. These malignancies are now diagnostic of AIDS in patients with HIV infections. Although the cause of these AIDS-associated malignancies has not been clearly defined, most authorities believe that deficient immune surveillance is the key factor, perhaps combined with viral activation.

REFERENCES

1. Volberding, P.A.: AIDS-related malignancies. *In* Holmes, K.K., Mårdh, P.-A., Sparling, P.F., et al. (Eds.): Sexually Transmitted Diseases, 2nd ed. New York, McGraw-Hill, 1990.
2. Centers for Disease Control: Update: Revised Public Health Service definition of persons who should re-

frain from donating blood and plasma—United States. MMWR, *34*:547–548, 1985.

371-C *(Campbell's, p. 855)*

It is possible for an infected donor to transmit HIV during the "window" period prior to the development of the HIV antibiodies. This "window" period is generally estimated to be 3 months or less. Because screening cannot detect every infectious unit, all blood centers have established policies for self-referral of donors who think that they may be at risk for HIV infection. But it is still possible for an infected unit to be transfused, and this does occur. It is estimated that the number of such infected units being transfused ranges from 70 to 460 per year in the United States, for a risk of 1 in 40,000 to 1 in 250,000 transfused units. Since approximately 60 per cent of blood in blood components are used for people who do not survive the condition for which they are hospitalized, a worst-case scenario is that the risk of acquiring HIV by receiving a single unit of blood is less than 1 per 100,000. This risk should not deter anyone who needs a unit of blood from receiving it.

REFERENCE

1. Peterman, T.A., Stoneburner, R.L., Allen, J.R., et al.: Risk of human immunodeficiency virus transmission from heterosexual adults with transfusion-associated infections. JAMA, *259*:55–58, 1988.

372-D *(Campbell's, p. 861)*

The term essential pruritis describes the presence of itching without any recognizable primary skin lesions. There is usually no rash visible at the time the itching occurs and examination by the clinician reveals normal tissue with the possible exception of a slight, mild redness or a few excoriations secondary to the scratching itself. Environmental factors, including both too much and too little moisture can play a role in the etiology. In addition anxiety, depression, and obsessive compulsive traits are commonly present and may play an etiologic role.

The single most effective therapy is the use of sedating-type antihistamines such as hydroxyzine. Effective treatment also requires a reduction in the patient's sweat retention and the application of standard hand creams or lotions after gentle bathing. Topically applied nonsteroidal antipruritic agents and nonsedating antihistamines may also be used; however, their effectiveness is somewhat marginal. Steroid creams are not helpful in the absence of inflammation. Rarely, anxiolytic or antidepressant agents are required.

REFERENCES

1. Hanno, R., and Murphy, P.: Pruritis ani. Dermatol. Clin. *5*:811, 1987.
2. Verbov, J.: Pruritis ani and its management—A study and reappraisal. Clin. Exp. Dermatol. *9*:46, 1984.

373-A *(Campbell's, p. 862)*

Medications, whether purchased over the counter or obtained by prescription, are the products most often documented as etiologic agents in contact dermatitis. Topically applied analgesics, antipruritic agents, or antibiotics are rather frequent offenders; preservatives and stablizers used in these and other medications also may be troublesome. Clothing dyes, detergents, antistatic products, and toilet paper are often suspected but are rarely proved to be etiologic agents.

REFERENCE

1. Goette, D.K., and Odom, R.B.: Vaginal medications as a cause for varied widespread dermatitides. Cutis, *26*: 406, 1980.

374-D *(Campbell's, pp. 861–863)*

All of the skin conditions listed, except psoriasis, are classifed as eczematous diseases. Psoriasis, a very common condition, is a papulosquamous disease. Other papulosquamous lesions include balanitis circinata, lichen planus, Darier's disease, and Hailey-Hailey disease. Both eczematous lesions and papulosquamous lesions occur as red patches or plaques. Two features help to distinguish between papulosquamous and eczematous lesions. First, the papulosquamous lesions are very sharply marginated, whereas eczematous lesions are poorly marginated. Second, pruritis is more notable in the eczematous diseases. The presence of excoriations, which result from pruritis, strongly suggests eczematous disease.

REFERENCE

1. Horan, D.B., Redman, J.F., and Jansen, G.T.: Papulosquamous lesions of glans penis. Urology, *23*:1, 1984.

375-D *(Campbell's, p. 864)*

Reiter's syndrome is characterized by the triad of arthritis, urethritis, and inflammatory disease of the eye. Cutaneous diseases, when present, are clinically and histologically identical to those of pustular forms of psoriasis. The most commonly encountered genital lesion is that of balanitis circinata. This lesion begins as one or more small red papules on the glans penis that subsequently enlarge centrifugally. The larger lesions may take on an anular or ring-like shape. Scale, when discernable, often has a yellow hue because of the many neutrophils that are found in the outer layers of the affected epithelium.

The cause of Reiter's syndrome is unknown, but its occurrence following nongonococcal urethritis or *Shigella* dysentery suggests that infectious agents play some role, possibly by way of triggering an immune reaction, which then cross-reacts against "self" antigens.

REFERENCE

1. Keat, A.: Reiter's syndrome and reactive arthritis in perspective. N. Engl. J. Med., *309*:1606, 1983.

376-A *(Campbell's, p. 870)*

Both Bowen's disease and erythroplasia of Queyrat represent squamous cell carcinoma in situ of the penis. They both occur as sharply marginated, erythematous plaques and thus mimic the appearance of the papulosquamous diseases. The differentiation of Bowen's disease from erythroplasia of Queyrat is semantic. Bowen's disease refers to lesions on keratinizing surfaces, whereas erythroplasia of Queyrat refers to lesions occurring on the glans and inner aspects of the prepuce. The lesions of Bowen's disease often have discernible scale; those of erythroplasia do not. Bowenoid papulosis, another form of carcinoma in situ, are sharply marginated dusky red, brown, or even black papules and small plaques on nonmucosal genital tissue. The genital ulcers in Behçet's disease are similar in appearance to those of the common cold sore in that they are painful, deep, sharply marginated, and have a clean, usually white, base. The lesions of extramammary Paget's disease mimic the appearance of psoriasis and some of the eczematous diseases.

377-B *(Campbell's, p. 872)*

Candida species can be cultured, as a colonizing agent, from most forms of balanitis or, alternatively, may be the sole cause of inflammation. In men, the combination of retained heat and moisture under the foreskin provides an extremely favorable habitat for growth. *Candida* organisms also can be acquired from a sexual partner's infected vagina.

The most common cause of balanoposthitis, however, is simply poor hygiene. When the foreskin is not regularly retracted and cleaned, a buildup of desquamated cells and retention of moisture lead to maceration and irritation.

REFERENCE

1. Sobel, J.D.: Vulvovaginal candidiasis—What we do and do not know. Ann. Intern. Med., *101*:390, 1984.

378-B *(Campbell's, p. 872)*

The scenario presented here is consistant with plasma cell balanitis (Zoon's balanitis). Although the number of reported cases is small, plasma cell balanitis is not terribly rare. This condition seems to occur only in uncircumcised men. The clinical appearance is that of a bright red, moist patch 2 cm or more in diameter that occurs on the glans or inner prepuce. The appearance is strikingly like that of candidal balanitis, although plasma cell balanitis has sharper margination, lacks pustules, is less symptomatic, and is stable in size and location over months to years. Diagnosis can be confirmed by biopsy which reveals marked plasma cell infiltrate.

The primary treatment is circumcision. In many instances, this procedure alone results in resolution. Topical applications of tretinoin (Retin-A) also may improve the condition, but the inflammation produced by application of this product may be more troublesome than the disease itself. There have been reports of successful treatment with laser surgery.

REFERENCES

1. Souteyrand, P., Wong, E., and MacDonald, D.M.: Zoon's balanitis circumscripta plasmacellularis. Br. J. Dermatol., *105*:195, 1981.
2. Sonnex, T.S., Dawber, R.P.R., Ryan, T.J., et al.: Zoon's (plasma cell) balanitis: Treatment by circumcision. Br. J. Dermatol., *106*:585, 1982.
3. Baldwin, H.E., and Geronemus, R.G.: The treatment of Zoon's balanitis with the carbon dioxode laser. J. Dermatol. Surg. Oncol., *15*:491, 1989.

379-E *(Campbell's, pp. 872–873)*

Treatment of balanitis xerotica obliterans is problematic. In males, circumcision is appropriate and may be sufficient. Topically applied steroids and anticandidal therapy also can be used. Topically applied 2 per cent testosterone in petrolatum is the time-honored approach to therapy in women. Surgical excision of involved tissue should be avoided, as it may lead to further scarring and, more importantly, because of the high recurrence rate. A few reports exist regarding the beneficial effect of orally administered retinoids, but the number of patients treated is small and the length of follow-up has been short.

The clinical appearance of classic BXO is that of a sharply marginated white patch on the glans that often surrounds or even involves the urethral meatus. Lesions on the shaft of the penis or elsewhere on the trunk are rare. In women, lichen sclerosis is mostly commonly found in the vulvar vestibule and perianal area. The disease is usually asymptomatic in men. In women, itching is usually quite severe, and pain, expecially dyspareunia, is common.

REFERENCE

1. Thomas, R.H.M., Ridley, C.M., and Black, M.M.: Clinical features and therapy of lichen sclerosus et atrophicus affecting males. Clin. Exp. Dermatol., *12*: 126, 1987.

380-D *(Campbell's, pp. 874, 877)*

The differentiation of hidradenitis suppurativa from recurrent furunculosis sometimes can be quite difficult. In both conditions lesions begin as inflammatory papules that enlarge, become quite tender and fluctuant, and eventually rupture through to the surface. Hidradenitis suppurativa can be simplistically considered as cystic acne of those areas of skin containing hair follicles with attached apocrine glands. Current opinion suggests that the lesions arise because of keratin blockage in the hair follicle at the pont where the duct of the apocrine gland enters into it. Clinical features favoring the diagnosis of hidradenitis suppurativa are (1) history of repeatedly recurring lesions, (2) the presence of multiple lesions at the same time, (3) a poor response to conventional antibiotic therapy, (4) the confinement of lesions to the groin and axillae, and (5) the presence of nearby comedones. In addition, bacterial culture reveals light growth of multiple diverse organisms instead of the expected heavy growth of *Staphylococcus* species.

REFERENCE

1. Yu, C.C., and Cook, M.G.: Hidradenitis suppurativa: A disease of follicular epithelium, rather than apocrine glands. Br. J. Dermatol., *126*:763, 1990.

381-A *(Campbell's, p. 874)*

Erythrasma is a common condition caused by the gram-positive bacillus *Corynebacterium minutissimum.* The lesions of erythrasma occur as sharply marginated, slightly scaling, dusky red patches on the upper, inner thighs. These lesions differ from those of tinea cruris in that the latter are brighter red and have annular borders. Correct identification of erythrasma is easily accomplished by examination in a darkened room with a Wood's lamp. These hand-held lights are filtered so as to admit light in the UVA part of the ultraviolet light spectrum. The presence of porphyrins as part of the metabolic pathway in *Corynebacterium* species results in a distinct rose or pink fluorescence over the involved areas. Culture of the bacterium is difficult to obtain with routine media; for that reason, a suspected diagnosis is confirmed clinically by a rapid response to orally administered erythromycin or by the topical application of standard antibiotics.

382-E *(Campbell's, p. 875)*

The presence of yellow or purpuric fluid in a blister overlying an area of cellulitis is almost pathognomonic of underlying necrotizing fasciitis (Fournier's gangrene). This is one of the few settings in which an apparently simple dermatologic process can develop into a life-threatening illness within a matter of hours. Thus, when the clinical picture is even the least bit suggestive for the presence of necrotizing fasciitis, a deep stab incision should be made through the center of the lesion. If gray, purulent fluid emerges from the site, the diagnosis is established. A probe should be inserted if no fluid is noted. Easy movement of the tip of the probe suggests necrotizing tissue destruction in the subcutaneous plane. Cultures, including those for anaerobic organisms, should be taken from the incision. Definitive treatment requires wide débridement and appropriate intravenous administration of antibiotics. Patients with diabetes, alcoholism, morbid obesity, and various types of immune suppression are predisposed to this kind of infection.

REFERENCE

1. Radaelli, F., Volpe, A.D., Columbi, M., et al.: Acute gangrene of the scrotum and penis in four hematologic patients. Cancer, *60*:1462, 1987.

383-B *(Campbell's, pp. 875–876)*

Treatment of tinea cruris is easily accomplished through the use of naftifine (Naftin) or any of the other topical antifungal agents effective against candidal skin infections. However, it should be noted that dermatophyte fungal infections do not respond at all to nystatin and respond rather poorly to many of the over-the-counter antifungal agents that are well advertised. Regardless of the treatment, however, the recurrences are common and repeated courses of therapy are almost inevitable.

The organisms most often responsible for these infections are *trichophyton rubrum, Trichophyton mentagrophytes,* and *Epidermophyton floccosum.* The classic lesions of tinea cruris are dusky red-brown patches on the upper inner thighs. The most active portion of the lesion occurs as a thin, red ring at the periphery of the plaque. This border accounts for the colloquial term "ringworm." Extension of the infection onto the buttocks occurs with some frequency, but for reasons that are not apparent these fungal infections rarely involve the scrotum and penis.

REFERENCES

1. Lesher, J.L., and Smith, J.G.: Antifungal agents in dermatology. J. Am. Acad. Dermatol., *17*:383, 1987.
2. Elewski, B.E., and Hazen, P.G.: The superficial mycoses and dermatophytes. J. Am. Acad. Dermatol., *21*: 655, 1989.

384-B *(Campbell's, pp. 879–880)*

Pearly penile papules are found on the corona of the glans penis as closely set, but not confluent, papules about 1 mm in diameter. They may be white, pink, or red. The papules generally encircle the corona in carefully aligned rows. Histologically, the lesions are fibrovascular papillomas and should be considered as variants of normal tissue. No treatment is needed. Patients and clinicians alike may confuse these lesions with genital warts. The location, alignment, and invariability (monotony) in appearance from one lesion to the next helps to identify pearly penile papules correctly.

REFERENCES

1. Rehbein, H.M.: Pearly penile papules: Incidence. Cutis, *19*:54, 1977.
2. Tanenbaum, M.H., and Becker, S.W.: Papillae of the corona of the glans penis. J. Urol., *93*:391, 1965.

385-D *(Campbell's, p. 880)*

Angiokeratomas of Fordyce are found in at least 20 per cent of adult men. They also occur in women but at a much lower prevalence. In men, the lesions appear on the scrotum as red or violaceous, minute (1 to 2 mm) papular hemangiomas. The number of lesions is highly variable; most commonly, 10 to 50 are present. It is thought that these angiokeratomas might represent varices. The lesions are usually asymptomatic, although occasionally one bleeds following trauma. Treatment is rarely necessary, but individual lesions can be destroyed with electrosurgery or laser therapy.

REFERENCE

1. Novick, N.L.: Angiokeratoma vulvae. J. Am. Acad. Dermatol., *12*:561, 1985.

386-C *(Campbell's, pp. 884–885; Fig. 21–1)*

Schistosoma haematobium is a digenic trematode whose life cycle consists of a sexual reproductive phase (egg laying) and asexual reproduction (sporocyst development). Sporocysts develop within the intermediate host, snails of the *Bulinus* species. Sporocysts give rise to the cercariae, which infest fresh (not salt) water and penetrate unbroken skin of the human host. Schistosomula develop from cercariae within the dermis and migrate to the gut and bladder via the portal venous system. Although worm pairs attach to the endothelia, no clotting or inflammation occurs around them while they produce and deposit 200 to 500 eggs per day over a mean life span of 3–6 years. About 20 per cent of the eggs erode into the lumina of the hollow viscera in which they are laid and are excreted into the urine and feces; the rest are either microembolized or remain where deposited.

REFERENCES

1. Butterworth, A.E., Fulford, A.J., Dunne, D.W., et al.: Longitudinal studies on human schistosomiasis. Phil. Trans. R. Soc. Lond. (Biol.), *321*:495, 1988.
2. Wilkins, H.A., Goll, P.H., Marshall, T.F.C., and Moore, P.J.: Dynamics of *Schistosoma haematobium* infections in a Gambian community: III. Acquisition and loss of infection. Trans. R. Soc. Trop. Med. Hyg., *78*:227, 1984.
3. Cheever, A.W., and Anderson, L.A.: Rate of destruction of *Schistosoma mansoni* eggs in the tissues of mice. Am. J. Trop. Med. Hyg., *20*:62, 1971.

387-A *(Campbell's, pp. 886–887)*

In both clinical and autopsy studies, the prevalence of infection and its intensity are related. Severe uropathy is uncommon when the frequency of infection in a population is below 30 per cent but increases linearly after this threshold is exceeded. Tissue egg burden, in turn, is related to severity of disease and to the frequency of complications. What proportion of infections is sufficiently heavy to cause clinical urinary schistosomiasis is uncertain, but some series indicated that 60 per cent demonstrate schistosomal obstructive uropathy. Transmission of *S. haematobium* occurs throughout the African continent and in southwest Asia. Outside these zones, all diagnosed cases have been imported. In endemic settings, first exposure usually occurs in preschool children and resistance to repeated infection arises between 10 and 15 years of age. This resistance is stronger in women than in men.

REFERENCES

1. Smith, J.H., Torky, H., Mansour, N., and Cheever, A.W.: Studies on egg excretion and tissue egg burden in urinary schistosomiasis. Am. J. Trop. Med. Hyg., *23*:163, 1974b.
2. Edington, G.M., von Lichtenberg, F., Nwabuebo, I., et al.: Pathologic effects of schistosomiasis in Ibadan, Western State of Nigeria: I. Incidence and intensity of infection; distribution and severity of lesions. Am. J. Trop. Med. Hyg., *19*:982, 1970.
3. Cheever, A.W., Kamel, I.A., Elwi, A.M., et al.: *Schistosoma mansoni* and *Schistosoma haematobium* infections in Egypt: III. Extrahepatic pathology. Am. J. Trop. Med. Hyg., *27*:55, 1978.
4. Wright, W.H.: Geographical distribution of schistosomes and their intermediate hosts. *In* Ansari, N. (Ed.): Epidemiology and Control of Schistosomiasis (Bilharziasis). Basel, S. Karger, 1973, pp. 32–249.

388-D *(Campbell's, pp. 887–888)*

Schistosomal disease results directly from schistosome eggs and from the granulomatous host response to them. The miracidia within eggs produce antigens that "leak" into surrounding interstitial spaces through pores in the egg shell. The host responds to these antigens by forming granulomas around the egg, i.e., an accumulation of macrophages, lymphocytes, and eosinophils. The granulomatous inflammation results in large, bulky, hyperemic, and polypoid masses projecting into the lumen. As oviposition at a site ceases, and trapped eggs are destroyed or calcified, inflammation wanes, being supplanted by fibrous tissue. The polyps and fibrous tissue can lead to obstructive uropathy, which is the most common and dangerous sequela of urinary schistosomiasis. Adult worm pairs and the excretion of schistosome eggs into the urine per se produce no significant disease.

REFERENCES

1. Phillips, S.M., and Colley, D.G.: Immunologic aspects of host responses to schistosomiasis: Resistance, immunopathology and eosinophil involvement. Prog. Allergy, *24*:49, 1978.
2. Warren, K.S.: Schistosomiasis: Host-pathogen biology. Rev. Infect. Dis., *4*:771, 1982.
3. von Lichtenberg, F., Erickson, D.G., and Sadun, E.H.: Comparative histopathology of schistosome granulomas in the hamster. Am. J. Pathol., *72*:149, 1973.

389-A *(Campbell's, pp. 892–894)*

The stage in which eggs are deposited in the tissues, traverse the bladder or rectosigmoid mucosa, and are excreted in the urine is referred to as "active" schistosomiasis. The classic clinical presentation of this stage—hematuria and terminal dysuria—has been recognized for more than 3000 years. Hematuria may be sufficient to cause blood loss anemia. In endemic foci, "active" disease usually arises in children or adolescents. Hematuria, pyuria, and proteinuria vary with the intensity of infection and may be used to measure infection intensity. The first two clinical stages of schistosomiasis — swimmer's itch and acute schistosomiasis—are associated with a pruritic rash and serum sickness-like disease respectively. Azotemia secondary to obstructive uropathy is usually detected during the chronic inactive stage of infection.

REFERENCES

1. Browning, M.D., Narooz, S.I., Strickland, G.T., et al.: Clinical characteristics and response to therapy in Egyptian children infected with *Schistosoma haematobium*. J. Infect. Dis., *149*:998, 1984.
2. Wilkins, H.A., Goll, P.H., and Moore, P.J.: *Schistosoma haematobium* infections and haemoglobin concentrations in a Gambian community. Ann. Trop. Med. Parasitol., *79*:159, 1985b.
3. Diaz Rivera, R.S., Ramos Morales, F., Koppisch, E., et al.: Acute Manson's schistosomiasis. Am. J. Med., *21*: 918, 1956.
4. Smith, J.H., and Christie, J.D.: The pathobiology of *Schistosoma haematobium* infection in humans. Hum. Pathol., *17*:333, 1986.

390-E *(Campbell's, pp. 894–895)*

Urinary egg excretion accurately estimates infection intensity during the early active and early chronic active stages, but is imprecise in late chronic active and inactive cases. Thus, in older infections, patients with severe sequelae may not excrete eggs on multiple examinations when there are 10^6 eggs per gram of tissue. Radiographic findings are better indices of severity than urinary egg count in older age groups. Dipstick proteinuria and hematuria are both sensitive means of screening infected young people in endemic areas. Serologic tests performed with egg-derived antigens have shown high sensitivity-specificity for detecting schistosomal infections; however, these tests do not differentiate active and inactive disease because serologic tests remain positive after live eggs and worms have vanished.

REFERENCES

1. Smith, J.H., Torky, H., Mansour, N., and Cheever, A.W.: Studies on egg excretion and tissue egg burden in urinary schistosomiasis. Am. J. Trop. Med. Hyg., *23*:163, 1974b.
2. Lehman, J.S., Jr., Farid, Z., Smith, J.H., et al.: Urinary schistosomiasis in Egypt: Clinical, radiological, bacteriological, and parasitological correlations. Trans. R. Soc. Trop. Med. Hyg., *67*:384, 1973.
3. Coopan, R.M., Schutte, C.H., Dingle, C.E., et al.: Urinalysis reagent strips in the screening of children for urinary schistosomiasis in the RSA. S. Afr. Med. J., *72*: 459, 1987b.
4. Doehring, E., Ehrich, J.H., and Reider, F.: Daily urinary protein loss in *Schistosoma haematobium* infection. Am. J. Trop. Med. Hyg., *35*:954, 1986b.

391-B *(Campbell's, pp. 896–898)*

Metrifonate (Bilharzil) is an organophosphate compound that is the drug of choice for *S. haematobium* infection in its endemic setting. Cure rates have generally been between 70 to 80 per cent, and no major adverse reactions have been observed among the thousands of individuals treated. Relapses are uncommon. Treatment aims to reduce worm burden, even it if does not achieve total parasitologic cure. In endemic areas, there may be rationale for leaving a few persisting worms if concomitant immunity plays a role in resistance to reinfection. Before sequelae of late infection are surgically treated, continued activity must be interdicted by schistosomicidal medication.

REFERENCES

1. Feldmeier, H., Doehring, E., Duffalla, A.A., et al.: Efficacy of metrifonate in urinary schistosomiasis: Comparison of reduction of *Schistosoma haematobium* and *S. mansoni* eggs. Am. J. Trop. Med. Hyg. *31*:1188, 1982.
2. Siongok, T.K., Ouma, J.H., Houser, H.B., and Warren, K.S.: Quantification of infection with *Schistoma haematobium* in relation to epidemiology and selective population chemotherapy: II. Mass treatment with a single oral dose of metrifonate. J. Infect. Dis., *138*:856, 1978.
3. Feldmeier, H., and Doehring, E.: Clinical experience with metrifonate: Review with emphasis on its use in endemic areas. Acta Trop. (Basel), *44*:357, 1987.

392-D *(Campbell's, pp. 902–903)*

Urinary schistosomiasis has been linked to bladder cancer since the turn of the century. The *bilharzial bladder cancer syndrome* presents with an early onset (between 40 and 50 years of age) and a high frequency of squamous cell carcinomas (60 to 90 per cent) and adenocarcinomas (5 to 15 per cent) and has been exhaustively documented from many regions endemic for *S. haematobium*. It is theorized that urinary schistosomiasis acts as a co-carcinogen or promoter of urothelial cancer and alters the histologic differentiation into squamous cell carcinoma by its direct metaplastic effect. In addition, urinary schistosomiasis predisposes to bacterial infections that increase urinary carcinogens.

REFERENCES

1. Ferguson, A.R.: Associated bilharziasis and primary malignant disease of the urinary bladder with observations on a series of 40 cases. J. Pathol. Bacteriol., *16*:76, 1911.
2. Al-Adnani, M.S., and Salah, K.M.: Schistomiasis and bladder cancer in southern Iraq. J. Trop. Med. Hyg., *86*:93, 1983.
3. Christie, J.D., Crouse, D., Kelada, A.S., et al.: Patterns of *Schistosoma haematobium* egg distribution in the human lower urinary tract: I. Non-cancerous lower urinary tracts. Am. J. Trop. Med. Hyg., *35*:759, 1986.
4. Abdel-Tawab, G.A., Aboul-Azm, T., Ebied, S.A., et al.: The correlation between certain tryptophane metabolites and the N-nitrosamine content in the urine of bilharzial bladder cancer patients. J. Urol., *135*:826, 1986.

393-D *(Campbell's, pp. 902–903)*

Several autopsy series from regions endemic for *S. haematobium* have shown no relationship between bladder cancer and lower urinary tract egg burdens. Most tumors occur on the posterior (40 to 50 per cent) and lateral walls (about 30 per cent) of the bladder and are exophytic. Because the majority are well-differentiated exophytic carcinomas that slough superficially necrotic tumor, necroturia is more frequent than in nonschistosomal bladder cancers. Cytologic criteria separating cancers from schistosomiasis-induced atypia have been developed, so that patients may now be screened by urinary cytology.

REFERENCES:

1. Elem, B., and Purohit, R.: Carcinoma of the urinary bladder in Zambia: A quantitative estimation of *Schistosoma haematobium* infection. Br. J. Urol., *55*:275, 1983.
2. Lucas, S.: Squamous cell carcinoma of the bladder and schistosomiasis. East Afr. Med. J., *59*:345, 1982.
3. Smith, J.H., Torky, H., Mansour, N., and Cheever, A.W.: Studies on egg excretion and tissue egg burden in urinary schistosomiasis. Am. J. Trop. Med. Hyg., *23*:163, 1974b.
4. El-Bolkainy, M.N., Chu, E.W., Ghoneim, M.A., and Ibrahim, A.: Cytologic detection of bladder cancer in rural Egyptian population infected with schistosomiasis. Acta Cytol., *26*:303, 1982.

394-B *(Campbell's, pp. 903–906)*

Both autopsy and clinical studies indicate no association between urinary schistosomiasis per se and pyelonephritis, but document a marked increase in pyelonephritis in patients with severe SOU. SOU with pyelonephritis is even more frequent if histologic cystitis, bladder outlet obstruction, or bacterial cystitis is present. Schistosomal ureteral lesions are most common in the interstitial and juxtavesicular portions with less than 1 per cent of obstruction occurring at the ureteral orifice itself. In active disease, the principal problem may be ureteral dysfunction rather than anatomic stenosis. In late chronic active and inactive urinary schistosomiasis, anatomic obstruction is more prominent. Hydroureter usually precedes hydronephrosis; thus, hydronephrosis represents the final stage in the succession of sequelae. "Balloon dilation" has reportedly proved effective with anatomic stenosis; however, mechanical dilation frequently is followed by repeated episodes of stenosis.

REFERENCES

1. Cheever, A.W., Kamel, I.A., Elwi, A.M., et al.: *Schistosoma mansoni* and *Schistosoma haematobium* infections in Egypt: III. Extrahepatic pathology. Am. J. Trop. Med. Hyg., *27*:55, 1978.
2. Hicks, R.M., Ismail, M.M., Walters, C.L., et al.: Associations of bacteriuria and urinary nitrosamine formation with *Schistosoma haematobium* infection in the Qalyub area of Egypt. Trans. R. Soc. Trop. Med. Hyg. *76*:519, 1982.
3. Al-Shukri, S., and Alwan, M.H.: Bilharzial strictures of the lower third of the ureter: A critical review of 560 strictures. Br. J. Urol. *55*:477, 1983.
4. Wishahi, M.M.: The role of dilatation in bilharzial ureters. Br. J. Urol. *59*:405, 1987.

395-E *(Campbell's, pp. 907–918)*

Filarial diseases are classified either as lymphatic or nonlymphatic afflictions. *Wuchereria bancrofti* accounts for 90 per cent of human *lymphatic* filariasis and is widespread throughout the tropics. It is probably an exclusively human parasite without animal reservoirs. *Brugia malayi* and *Brugia timori*, which cause the remainder of human lymphatic filariasis, spontaneously infect primates and domestic animals, and are confined to the Far East. The *nonlymphatic* filarial parasites rarely cause urogenital manifestation, but *Onchocerca volvulus*, the agent of African river blindness, is known to cause massive inguinal lymphadenopathy, "hanging groin," and scrotal elephantiasis. *Strongyloides stercoralis* is a nematode that has been detected in the urine or urogenital organs.

396-A *(Campbell's, pp. 907–912)*

Serial autopsy studies of men show that the tail of the epididymis and the lower spermatic cord are the most constant locations of filarial worms and often the only sites found in mild infections. Correspondingly, funiculoepididymitis is the most frequent direct consequence of filariasis and hydrocele the most frequent indirect one. Filarial worms are also commonly found in the inguinal lymphatic, especially *B. malayi* and B. timori species. Saturation of inguinal lymphatic trunks may initiate encroachment into femoral lymphatics and proximally to renal lymphangioles producing elephantiasis of the lower extremities and chyluria respectively. Thus far, no filariae have been found in the cisterna chyli or thoracic ducts. Filarial orchitis is rare but may simulate a rapidly developing testicular malignant tumor.

REFERENCE

1. Galindo, L., von Lichtenberg, F., and Baldizon, C.: Bancroftian filariasis in Puerto Rico: Infection pattern and tissue lesions. Am. J. Trop. Med. Hyg., *11*:739, 1962.

397-E *(Campbell's, pp. 907–908)*

The lymphatic filariae are elongated, viviparous nematodes. Their cycle proceeds from human to mosquito and back, through a sequence of larval moults. Mosquitos inject larvae with salivary secretions when biting the human host: multiple injections over a prolonged period are necessary to produce disease. Unable to traverse unbroken skin, the larvae can cross the normal conjunctiva or buccal mucosa. Microfilariae are released into the blood stream by adult females and live for several months. Most endemic patients manifest microfilaremia, but pathologic sequelae rarely develop. Yet this scant proportion of endemic patients in whom pathologic sequelae develops account for the bulk of clinical disease.

REFERENCES

1. Ah, H.S., Klei, T.R., McCall, J.W., and Thompson, P.E.: *Brugia puhangi* infections in Mongolian jirds and dogs following the ocular inoculation of infective larvae. J. Parasitol., *60*:643, 1974b.
2. Ottesen, E.A.: Filariasis now. Am. J. Trop. Med. Hyg. *41*(Suppl.):8, 1989.

398-A *(Campbell's, pp. 914–915)*

The only treatment currently available for genital elephantiasis is excision and plastic reconstruction by full thickness skin grafting. Unless associated bacteria is present, surgical healing is usually decent, despite lymphorrhea during and after surgery. Because the physiologic derangement is not corrected by such procedures, recurrence is common, and repeated operations are less successful, posing greater risk of local complications. The oral antimicrofilarial drugs diethylcarbamazine and ivermectin effectively abolish microfilaremia but have little effect on established pathology in advance filariasis. There is no role for either inguinal lymphadenectomy or radiation in genital elephantiasis.

REFERENCE

1. Jantet, G.H., Taylor, G.W., and Kinmouth, J.B.: Operations for primary lymphedema of the lower limbs: Results after 1–9 years. J. Cardiovasc. Surg. (Torino), *2*:27, 1961.

399-B *(Campbell's, pp. 917–918)*

The hydatid is the larval form of *Echinococcus granulosus*, whose definitive host is the dog and whose principal intermediate host is the sheep. The cysts are acquired by humans who accidently eat the eggs excreted in the feces of dogs or alternate feral hosts. No part of the human anatomy is invulnerable to hydatid cysts, but renal hydatids occur in only 2 per cent of cases. In the kidney or other urogenital sites, hydatid cysts evolve by slow, asymptomatic, concentric growth over years and may invoke pressure symptoms or flank pain, depending upon location and size. The cyst is enveloped by a host fibrous shell with scant inflammatory reaction. Water-clear cyst fluid of high protein and antigen content bathes the germinal structures within the cyst, which can reach 20 cm in diameter but usually rupture earlier. The most frequent urologic presentation is chronic dull flank or lower back discomfort resulting from cystic pressure. Microscopic hematuria is rare. When the x-ray appearance is not diagnostic, the Casoni skin test with hydatid fluid antigen for complement fixation and hemagglutination inhibition serology have proved useful. In most cases, diagnosis, once suspected, presents little difficulty.

Treatment, if warranted, is by surgical excision, an elective procedure unless the cyst becomes superinfected by bacteria and constitutes a nidus of chronic, difficult to eradicate, urinary infection.

REFERENCE

1. Musacchio, F., and Mitchell, N.: Primary renal echinococcosis; A case report. Am. J. Trop. Med. Hyg., *15*:168, 1966.

400-B *(Campbell's, p. 928)*

Fungi belong to the kingdom Eumycetes. Fungi are eukaryotic organisms that contain mitochondria, and have cell membranes composed of ergosterol. They can be dimorphic, and thus unicellular, and reproduce asexually, or they may develop cytoplasmatic filaments known as hyphae or mycelia and reproduce by sexual means.

401-E *(Campbell's, pp. 929–930)*

Blastomycosis, which is caused by the fungus *Blastomyces dermatitidis* is endemic to the Ohio and Mississippi basin area. The fungi inhabit moist soils with high organic content. The primary infection is usually pulmonary; however, dissemination via hematogenous or lymphatic routes may occur. Genitourinary involvement occurs in only 15 to 30 per cent of patients with systemic disease. It involves the epididymis and prostate most commonly; however, involvement of the kidney, testis, penis, and adrenal gland with manifestation of Addison's disease have been reported. The treatment of choice is systemic amphotericin B with or without oral ketoconazole.

402-A *(Campbell's, pp. 930–931)*

The patient in this case illustrates coccidioidomycosis. The responsible fungus is *Coccidioides immitis*, which is a dimorphic fungus indigenous to the semiarid regions of the Western United States, Mexico, and Central and South America. It inhibits warm soil with high salinity. Genitourinary coccidioidomycosis can involve the kidney, adrenal gland, prostate, bladder, and scrotum. Renal coccidioidomycosis can mimic renal tuberculosis with radiographic findings demonstrating moth-eaten calyces, infundibular stenosis, and renal calcification. Prostatic infection is one of the more common manifestations of genitourinary coccidioidal infection, with symptoms indicative of bladder outflow obstruction. The prostate may be boggy or even indurated on examination. The treatment of choice is systemic amphotericin B. Chronic therapy with ketoconazole has been used for up to 1 year. Surgical debridement or excision of isolated lesions is also recommended in cases of epididymal infection.

403-B *(Campbell's, pp. 931–932)*

Histoplasma capsulatum is the fungus responsible for histoplasmosis. This fungus is indigenous to the midwest and southern United States and inhabits nitrogen-rich soil, especially those enriched by bird guano. The genitourinary tract is often involved in disseminated infection and involves the adrenal gland, kidney, prostate, penis, epididymis, and testis. When the adrenal gland is infected, symptoms compatible with Addison's disease have been reported.

404-C *(Campbell's, pp. 932–933)*

The treatment of choice for disseminated histoplasmosis is systemic amphotericin B. The imidazoles, IV miconazole, and oral ketoconazole are not recommended as primary therapy in disseminated disease, but they may have a role in chronic therapy.

405-E *(Campbell's, pp. 935–936)*

Aspergillosis is usually a pulmonary illness in humans; however, genitourinary involvement can occur. Aspergilli are ubiquitous in the environment and can be found throughout the world in soil, decomposed vegetation, paint, and bird excreta. Aspergillus is an opportunistic fungus that afflicts those patients debilitated by malignancy, diabetes mellitus, and immunosuppression. The kidney is the most common site of GU involvement and may demonstrate multiple small abscesses, vascular occlusion, and multiple renal infarcts. Obstructive uropathy may also develop secondary to aspergillar casts or bezoars. Other sites of genitourinary involvement include the prostate, testes, and adrenal gland. The treatment of choice for systemic aspergillosis is IV amphotericin B. In cases of renal aspergillar bezoars, regional irrigation with amphotericin B in conjunction with surgical debulking procedures is recommended.

406-E *(Campbell's, pp. 936–937)*

The patient in this case illustrates prostatic cryptococcal infection in addition to central nervous system involvement. The responsible fungus is *Cryptococcus neoformans*, which can be found in any environment inhabited by birds, particularly pigeons. The primary infection is usually pulmonary and the primary target of hematogenous spread is the central nervous system, with resulting meningitis, meningoencephalitis, or cryptococcoma. Genitourinary tract involvement includes the kidney, prostate, and adrenal. The diagnosis can be made by direct examination of infected fluid with India ink stain which reveals budding yeast with capsules. Since genitourinary cryptococcosis is generally a manifestation of systemic disease, systemic antifungal therapy with amphotericin B with or without oral flucytosine is the treatment of choice.

407-D *(Campbell's, pp. 940–941)*

Urinary candidal colony counts have been helpful in differentiating colonization from infection. Urine specimens obtained by clean catch or single catheterization from patients with histologically proven renal candidiasis show colony counts of 10,000 to 15,000 per milliliters.

408A *(Campbell's, p. 942)*

Candidura is not an uncommon problem encountered in debilitated patients. If candiuria does not resolve following the removal of a chronic indwelling catheter or discontination of broad spectrum antibiotics, regional treatment with intravesical amphotericin B irrigation can be initiated. Studies indicating success rates of 90 per cent have been reported with the use of intravesical amphotericin B irrigation (50 mg/l per day for a minimum of 5 days).

409-C *(Campbell's, pp. 943–944)*

Amphotericin B is a polyene antifungal agent that binds to the orgesterol component of the fungal cell wall and results in the disruption of internal cellular components to cause electrolytic flux. Amphotericin B is poorly absorbed from the gastrointestinal tract and must be administered intravenously to exert systemic antifungal effects. Penetration into cerebrospinal fluid is poor, and minimal amounts are found in amniotic fluid despite crossing the placenta. Biliary excretion is the primary route of elimination. Hemodialysis does not affect plasma levels of the drug. Amphotericin B can also be used in regional therapy as an intravesical irrigation or irrigation of the renal pelvis.

410-C *(Campbell's, pp. 944–945)*

Systemic reactions, such as rigors, chills, and fever, have occurred in 50 per cent of patients in association with intravenous amphotericin B. Other adverse reactions ascribed to IV amphotericin B include generalized pain, headache, convulsions, localized phlebitis, anemia, and thrombocytopenia. The most significant adverse effect of amphotericin B is renal toxicity with its resultant electrolyte imbalance. Amphotericin B-related nephrotoxicity is characterized by hematuria, pyuria, cylindruria, and proteinuria. The nephrotoxicity may be caused by drug impairment of the proximal tubal or ascending loop of Henle that, in turn, activates tubuloglomeruli feedback, which results in vasoconstriction and reduction in GFR. Clinical studies suggest that sodium supplementation and hydration reduced the risk of nephrotoxicity. Electrolytes disturbances include potassium and magnesium depletion. The potassium wasting that accompanies amphotericin B can be corrected by potassium supplementation.

411-A *(Campbell's, pp. 945–946)*

Flucytosine is a fluorinated pyrimidine that requires enzymatic conversion to active metabolites. It is first converted to 5-fluorouracil by cytosine deaminase and then is converted to 5-fluorodoxyuridine monophosphate which adversely affects fungal protein and DNA synthesis. It is readily absorbed by the GI tract, binds poorly to plasma proteins, and primarily excreted by glomerular filtration. Furthermore, it has good penetration into cerebrospinal fluid. The recommended dose is 100 to 150 mg/kg. Adverse effects of 5-fluorouracil include nausea, vomiting, diarrhea, and enterocolitis, abnormalities in liver function tests, and bone marrow depression with the development of anemia, leukopenia, and thrombocytopenia.

412-E *(Campbell's, pp. 946–947)*

Ketoconazole is an imidazole antifungal agent. The primary mechanism of action is interference with fungal ergosterol metabolism that alters cell membrane integrity, thereby disrupting cellular metabolism. It is readily absorbed from the GI tract, primarily metabolized by the liver, and has minimal renal excretion. Adverse effects of ketoconazole may include headaches and skin rashes, but its most significant impact is on liver metabolism through elevation of serum triglycerides and abnormal liver enzymes. It should be given cautiously to those patients requiring cyclosporin, since ketoconazole increases serum cyclosporin levels.

413-D *(Campbell's, p. 940)*

The development of renal candidal infection in infants has been associated with indwelling intravascular catheters, treatment with broad spectrum antibiotics, prematurity, and low birth weight. Oliguria followed by anuria develops secondary to obstruction by fungal accretions. Renal sonography is critical to a diagnosis; it often demonstrates hydronephrosis and fungal excretion within the collecting system. Percutaneous nephrostomy and the use of regional and/or systemic amphotericin B have increased survival dramatically.

414-B *(Campbell's, pp. 953–954)*

In developed countries, reliable evidence exists that (1) the tuberculous incidence has been falling since the turn of the century; (2) under present conditions, irrespective of any treatment, it is diminishing at the rate of 5 per cent per annum; and (3) this decrease in infection rate is exponential. In developed countries the annual decline is about 12 per cent, whereas in developing countries the decline hardly has been noticed. In the Western world only between 8 and 10 per cent of patients with pulmonary tuberculosis develop renal tuberculosis. Vaccination with BCG does not protect the older population from the disease. In addition to having a higher overall incidence of tuberculosis, in developing countries the disease continues to affect adolescents and young adults.

REFERENCES

1. Sutherland, I.: Recent studies in the epidemiology of tuberculosis based on the risk of being infected by the tubercle bacillus. Adv. Tuberc. Res., *19*:1, 1976
2. World Health Organization: Magnitude of the tuberculosis problem of the world. Wkly. Epidemiol. Rec., *50*:393, 1981

415-E *(Campbell's, pp. 954–955)*

M. tuberculosis is the most virulent and infective of all mycobacteria, although the precise nature of this high virulence remains unknown. The cytoplasm of the mycobacterium does not differ essentially from that of other bacteria. Mycobacteria differ from other organisms in that (1) they are extremely slow growing; (2) once phagocytized they are quite resistant to the various intracellular killing mechanisms; (3) they are able to become dormant and remain in tissues for many years without dividing; and (4) they are much more prone than most bacteria to developing resistance, especially when antibiotics are given singly.

REFERENCE

1. Barksdale, L., and Ken, K.S.: Mycobacterium. Bacteriol. Rev., *41*:217, 1977

416-C *(Campbell's, pp. 956–961)*

The primary focus of tuberculosis infection is in the lungs. It is contracted by inhaling droplets of exhaled infected bronchial secretions. Metastatic spread of the organisms occurs by way of the blood stream throughout the body. The sites of metastatic spread within the genitourinary tract include the kidney, epididymis, and prostate. Tuberculosis of the ureter and bladder are without exception secondary to renal tuberculosis. Tuberculosis of the testis is nearly always secondary to infection of the epididymis. Tuberculous orchitis with no epididymal involvement is a very rare presentation. Tuberculosis of the urethra is very rare and is felt to be caused by spread from another focus in the genital tract.

REFERENCE

1. Macmillan, E.W.: Blood supply of the epididymis in man. Br. J. Urol., *26*:60, 1954

417-D *(Campbell's, pp. 956–957)*

Renal calcification is becoming a growing hazard in renal tuberculosis. The incidence of calcification is slowly increasing, and its presence is constantly assuming more importance in the management of renal tuberculosis. Larger areas of calcification should be excised and nonfunctioning kidneys with extensive calcification removed. Most small calcified lesions remain unchanged for more than 20 years; therefore, small lesions can be kept under review on an annual basis and can continue to be managed conservatively, provided that there is no increase in size.

Renal tuberculosis is a secondary manifestation and is caused by a bloodborne metastatic organism. When the organisms reach the kidney, they settle in the blood vessels, usually those close to the glomeruli. Most of these metastatic lesions heal because the bacteremia is not intense. Polymorphonuclear leukocytes disappear early from the lesions. Granulomas consist of a central Langhans' giant cell surrounded by lymphocytes and fibroblasts. There have been many studies linking severe renal tuberculosis with hypertension and it is apparent that two thirds of patients with extensive unilateral tuberculous nephropathy achieve a substantial fall in blood pressure following nephrectomy.

REFERENCES

1. Antonio, D., and Gow, J.G.: Renal calcification in genitourinary tuberculosis—A clinical study. Int. Urol. Nephrol., *7*:289, 1975.
2. Flechner, S.M., and Gow, J.G.: Role of nephrectomy in the treatment of non-functioning or very poorly functioning unilateral tuberculous kidney. J. Urol., *123*:822, 1980.
3. Marks, L.S., and Pontasse, E.F.: Hypertension from renal tuberculosis. Operative cure predicted by renal vein renin. J. Urol., *109*:149, 1973.

418-D *(Campbell's, p. 960)*

Tuberculosis of the prostate is rare, and in many cases the diagnosis is made by the pathologist or is found incidently after a transurethral resection. Severe symptoms and high fever are uncommon and cavitation leading to perineal sinus is very rare. The route of infection is through the hematogenous spread of organisms in the same way as in the kidney. There is no evidence that infection is caused by continuous contact with urine from a kidney with active disease.

On palpation, the tuberculous prostate can be confused with carcinoma as the gland is nodular and usually nontender. Soft areas are extremely uncommon. Once the diagnosis is confirmed, the patient should receive a full course of chemotherapy.

REFERENCE

1. Sporer, A., and Auerback, M.D.: Tuberculosis of the prostate. Urology, *11*:362, 1978.

419-B *(Campbell's, pp. 961–962)*

The patient with genitourinary tuberculosis usually presents with rather vague urinary tract symptoms, and a careful history is important. The most common complaint is that of increasing painless frequency of micturition, at first only at night but later during both day and night. Urgency is uncommon, unless there is extensive bladder involvement. Gross hematuria, which is almost without exception total and intermittent, is present in only 10 per cent of patients, but microscopic hematuria should not be ignored because it is present in up to 50 per cent of patients. Renal and suprapubic pain are rare presenting symptoms and usually mean extensive involvement of the kidney and bladder, respectively. Ureteric colic is uncommon and occurs only when either a small flake of calcification or a clot passes down the ureter.

In a few patients the only first presenting symptom is a painful testicular swelling. The classic triad of lassitude, loss of weight, and anorexia is never seen in the early stages of the disease.

420-B *(Campbell's, pp. 962–963)*

A positive tuberculin skin test is considered an indication that the person has been infected, provided that he or she has not been vaccinated with BCG, but cannot be regarded as an indication of active tuberculous disease. *M. tuberculosis* infection is far more common than tuberculous disease. Nevertheless, an area of induration of 5 mm or less suggests little or no mycobacterial activity because of the high degree of acquired immunity, whereas reactions greater than 15 mm in diameter indicate a high degree of hypersensitivity, which probably reflects active disease. A positive test is of more help when it is known that a previous test was negative; in that case, the infection may be recent and it is likely to produce a lesion that requires treatment.

REFERENCE

1. Youmans, G.P., Paterson, P.Y., and Sommers, H.M.: The Biological and Clinical Basis of Infectious Diseases. Philadelphia, W.B. Saunders Co., 1975, p. 347.

421-E *(Campbell's, p. 958)*

Because bladder lesions are without exception secondary to renal tuberculosis, the earliest forms of infections start around one or another ureteric orifice. When isolated lesions are visible away from the ureteric orifices, which appear normal on inspection and give a clear efflux, it must be assumed that they are not caused by *M. tuberculosis* and are likely to be malignant; biopsy is essential in these patients.

Occasionally, the whole of the bladder is covered by angry, inflamed, velvety granulations with ulcerations. If the disease reaches this stage, it is unlikely that, even with modern chemotherapy, there will be sufficient recovery of the bladder to ensure an adequate capacity with reasonable function.

422-C *(Campbell's, pp. 968–972)*

For the last few years, short courses of chemotherapy have constituted the normal method of treatment because the evidence obtained from treating many thousands of cases showed irrefutably that to treat patients for longer than 9 months was wasteful in time, money, and resources. Certain aspects of genitourinary tuberculosis make it likely to respond equally well, if not better, to short-course chemotherapy. First, fewer organisms are involved in the renal form of the disease than in the pulmonary form. Second, there are high concentrations of isoniazid, rifampicin, pyrazinamide, and streptomycin in the urine. Third, isoniazid and rifampicin pass freely into renal cavities in high concentration. Finally, all of these drugs reach adequate concentrations in the kidney, ureters, bladder, and prostate. The recommended regimen for treatment includes 2 months of treatment with isoniazid, rifampicin, pyrazinamide, followed by 2 months of treatment with isoniazid and rifampicin for a total treatment course of 4 months. Streptomycin adds nothing to the other three drugs in the initial phase; however, it should be given in cases of extensive disease with severe bladder symptoms because it has such a high concentration in the urine.

423-E *(Campbell's, pp. 972–973)*

Toxicity leading to termination of one or more antituberculous drugs occurs in less than 5 per cent of patients. When toxicity does occur, it is usually during the first few weeks of treatment. The two main reactions are hypersensitivity and jaundice. In the event of a severe hypersensitivity reaction, the responsible drug should be identified as quickly as possible. Desensitization can be carried out rapidly and adequate chemotherapy can be resumed, if necessary under steroid cover. When jaundice and associated symptoms occur, all drugs should be stopped. If the jaundice is caused by the drugs, recovery is usually rapid. When the patient is completely recovered, treatment with the same regimen usually can be resumed. Neurologic disturbances, which can occur with isoniazid, can be controlled using pyridoxine.

REFERENCE

1. Hong Kong Chest Service, Tuberculosis Research Centre, Madras, and British Medical Research Council: A controlled trial of 3-month, 4-month, and 6-month regimens of chemotherapy for sputum-smear-negative pulmonary tuberculosis. Am. Rev. Respir. Dis., *139*: 871–876, 1989

424-A *(Campbell's, pp. 974–975)*

The indications for nephrectomy are (1) a nonfunctioning kidney with or without calcification, (2) extensive disease involving the whole kidney, together with hypertension and pelviureteric obstruction, and (3) coexisting renal carcinoma. A localized polar lesion that is increasing in size and threatening to destroy the whole kidney is an indication for *partial* nephrectomy.

425-D *(Campbell's, pp. 976–977)*

The most common site for tuberculous stricture is the ureterovesical junction; stricture may also occur at the pelviureteric junction and, rarely, in the middle third of the ureter. A number of these strictures result from edema, and they will respond to chemotherapy. If there is no improvement after 3 weeks, corticosteroids (prednisone 20 mg three times daily) should be given in addition to the other chemotherapy. The patient can be monitored with weekly intravenous urogram; if there is deterioration or no improvement after a 6-week period, surgical reimplantation is carried out if an initial attempt at dilation has failed.

Endoscopic dilation, even when performed multiple times, is associated with high failure rates. Using the Boari's flap procedure, strictures as long as 14 to 15 cm can be excised and the remaining ureter reimplanted.

REFERENCE

1. Gow, J.G: The results of the reimplantation of the ureter by Boari technique. Proc. R. Soc. Med., *61*:128, 1968.

426-B *(Campbell's, pp. 978–979)*

The main symptoms that warrant consideration of an augmentation cystoplasty are an intolerable frequency both day and night, together with pain, urgency, and hematuria. The appearance on cystoscopy is a diffuse velvet inflammation with a capacity of less than 100 ml. The procedure is not a cystectomy, but a method of increasing the bladder capacity while retaining as much of the bladder as possible. Inflammation of the bladder is no contraindication to surgery, but a two-layer closure and the routine use of the omentum wrapped around the anastomosis reduce the complications.

Renal insufficiency is not a contraindication to augmentation cystoplasty. Enuresis, incontinence, and psychiatric disturbances are contraindications to this procedure. If surgery is necessary in these cases, a urinary diversion is the only treatment. The choice of the segment of bowel used to augment the bladder does not appear to influence the long-term result. The gastrocystoplasty is a more recent technique that requires further evaluation and a prolonged follow-up before it can be considered as an alternative to the use of either colon or cecum.

REFERENCES

1. Kuss, R., Bilker, M., Camey, M., et al.: Indications: and early and late results of intestinocytoplasty. A review of 185 cases. J. Urol., *103*:53, 1970.
2. Smith, R.B., Van Cangh, P., Skinner, D.G., et al.: Augmentation enterocystoplasty—A critical review. J. Urol., *118*:35, 1977

427-A *(Campbell's, pp. 982–989)*

Despite continued attempts at histologic description, the diagnosis of interstitial cystitis is still based primarily on clinical and cystoscopic criteria. Although many histologic abnormalities have been described in patients with interstitial cystitis, there is no histologic finding that is pathognomic for this syndrome. The syndrome is defined by chronic irritative voiding symptoms, sterile and cytologically negative urine, and characteristic cystoscopic findings. Documentation of all three, along with failure to find a more objective cause for this clinical picture must be present before a diagnosis of interstitial cystitis can be established. The characteristic cystoscopic finding is that of pinpoint petechial hemorrhages that develop throughout the bladder after hydrodistention. Because the diagnosis of interstitial cystitis cannot be made in the face of urine infection or cancer, urine cultures and cytology must be negative. The classic symptoms of interstitial cystitis include intense frequency, urgency, nocturia, and superpubic or pelvic pain that is somewhat diminished by voiding.

REFERENCES

1. Messing, E.M., and Stamey, T.A.: Interstitial cystitis: Early diagnosis, pathology, and treatment. Urology, *13*:389, 1978.
2. Walsh, A.: Interstitial cystitis. *In* Harrison, J.H., Gittes, R.F., Perlmutter, A.D., Stamey, T.A., and Walsh, P.C. (Eds): Campbell's Urology, 4th ed. Philadelphia, W.B. Saunders Co., 1978, pp. 693–707.
3. Hand, J.R.: Interstitial cystitis. J. Urol., *61*:291, 1949.

428-C *(Campbell's, pp. 982–983)*

Held and collaborators, using a series of questionnaires, found that household size, marital status, number of male sexual partners, and educational status did not seem to significantly differ in those patients diagnosed as having interstitial cystitis in comparision with the general adult female population. It has also been demonstrated by Oravisto, and supported by others, that symptoms rarely progress after the first few years. In fact, at least 10 per cent of patients experience lasting spontaneous remission.

REFERENCES

1. Held, P., Hanno, P., Wein, A., and Pauly, M.: Epidemiology of interstitial cystitis: Incidence of interstitial cystitis from a national sample of urologists. Presented at the NIH-NIDDK Workshop on Interstitial Cystitis, Bethesda, August 1987.
2. Held, P.J., Hanno, P.M., Wein, A.J., et al.: Epidemiology of interstitial cystitis. *In* Hanno, P., Staskin, D.R., Krane, R.J., and Wein, A.J. (Eds.): Interstitial Cystitis. New York, Springer-Verlag, 1990, pp. 29–48.
3. Oravisto, K.J.: Epidemiology of interstitial cystitis. Ann. Chir. Gynaecol. Fenn., *64*:75, 1975.

429-A *(Campbell's, pp. 983–985)*

It has long been recognized that particular personality traits are common in many patients with interstitial cystitis. However, there is no evidence that such personality traits play a causative role in interstitial cystitis, but, conversely, most evidence points to the fact that the neurotic traits are primarily a response to this chronic debilitating condition rather than its cause.

The etiology of interstitial cystitis remains unknown. It is, however, likely that a variety of factors are responsible and all of the other factors listed have some experimental and/or clinical evidence supporting their role.

REFERENCES

1. Hunner, G.L.: Neurosis of the bladder. J. Urol., *24*:567, 1930.
2. Held, P., Hanno, P., Wein, A., and Pauly, M.: Epidemiology of interstitial cystitis: Incidence of interstitial cystitis from a national sample of urologists. Presented at the NIH-NIDDK Workshop on Interstitial Cystitis, Bethesda, August 1987.
3. Keltikangas-Jorvinan, J., Arvinen, L., Lehtonent, T.: Psychological failure related to interstitial cystitis. Eur. Urol., *15*:69, 1988.

430-C *(Campbell's, p. 987)*

The characteristic cystoscopic finding in patients with interstitial cystitis is the development of pinpoint petechial hemorrhages ("glomerulations") throughout the bladder after hydrodistention at 70 cm of water pressure. These glomerulations are not seen in normal bladders examined similarily, although they may occur in various states of vesical pathology and certainly in those individuals who for any reason do not habitually distend their bladders. The two cystoscopic findings often classically associated with interstitial cystitis—reduced bladder capacity and a Hunner's ulcer—are frequently not found.

REFERENCES

1. Walsh, A.: Interstitial cystitis. *In* Harrison, J.H., Gittes, R.F., Perlmutter, A.D., Stamey, T.A., and Walsh, P.C. (Eds): Campbell's Urology, 4th ed. Philadelphia, W.B. Saunders Co., 1978, pp. 693–707.
2. Hanno, P., Levin, R.M., Monson, R.M., et al.: Diagnosis of interstitial cystitis. J. Urol., *143*:278, 1990.

3. Messing, E.M.: The diagnosis of interstitial cystitis. Urology, *29*(Suppl.):4, 1987a.
4. Messing, E.M., and Stamey, T.A.: Interstitial cystitis: Early diagnosis, pathology, and treatment. Urology, *12*:381, 1978.

431-B *(Campbell's, pp. 988–989)*

Despite continued attempts at histologic description, the diagnosis of interstitial cystitis is still based primarily on clinical and cystoscopic critera. The classically described histopathologic picture consists of a chronic, transmural pancystitis with marked involvement of deeper layers with inflammation and fibrosis. The work by Johansson, however, indicates that the primary abnormalities, even in those with small capacity bladders and ulcers, remain confined to the epithelium and lamina propria. Submucosal edema and vasodilatation (without notable inflammatory infiltrate) compose the major histologic abnormalities. Excessive mast cells in the muscularis, intraepithelial deposition of Tamm-Horsfall protein, and a patchy submucosal vasculitis have all been reported, but are absent in a significant percentage of patients. Perineural inflammation has also been reported, but the diagnostic utility of this finding is not clear.

REFERENCES

1. Johanson, S.L.: Light microscopic findings in bladders of patients with interstitial cystitis. *In* Hanno, P., Staskin, D.R., Krane, R.J., and Wein, A.J. (Eds.): Interstitial Cystitis. New York, Springer-Verlag, 1990, pp. 189–192.
2. Hanno, P., Levin, R.M., Monson, R.M., et al.: Diagnosis of interstitial cystitis. J. Urol., *143*:278, 1990.
3. Fowler, J.E., Lynes, W.L., Lau, J.L.T., et al.: Interstitial cystitis is associated with intraurothelial Tamm-Horsfall protein. J. Urol., *140*:1385, 1988.
4. Matilla, J.: Pathology of interstitial cystitis. *In* Hanno, P., Staskin, D.R., Krane, R.J., and Wein, A.J. (Eds.): Interstitial Cystitis. New York, Springer-Verlag, 1990, pp. 91–94.

432-B *(Campbell's, p. 989)*

Most unanesthetized interstitial cystitis patients have such reduced bladder capacities and pelvic discomfort upon bladder filling that little useful information is usually obtained with urodynamic evaluation. Indeed, misdiagnoses may result, confusing patients, and, at times, delaying the institution of potentially effective therapy.

If the unanesthetized patient has a large bladder capacity and no symptoms (e.g., pain, urgency) with bladder filling, it is difficult to ascribe her problems to interstitial cystitis. Patients with urgency and/or incontinence as their primary symptom(s), may have a neuropathic condition with uninhibited detrusor contractions on cystometry. Urodynamic studies are needed if open surgical procedures (e.g., cystolysis) are contemplated. Baseline urodynamic studies may also be valuable in patients who are to undergo scheduled toleration of increasing volumetric increments ("bladder training").

REFERENCES

1. Steinkohl, W.B., and Leach, G.E.: Urodynamic findings in interstitial cystitis. Urology, *34*:399, 1989.
2. Leach, G.E., and Raz, S.: Interstitial cystitis. *In* Raz, S. (Ed.): Female Urology. Philadelphia, W.B. Saunders Co., 1983, pp. 351–356.
3. McGuire, E.: Neurologic evaluation in interstitial cystitis. *In* Hanno, P., Staskin, D.R., Krane, R.J., and Wein, A.J. (Eds.): Interstitial Cystitis. New York, Springer-Verlag, 1990, pp. 91–94.
4. Parsons, C.L., and Koprowski, P.F.: Interstitial cystitis: Successful management by a pattern of increasing voiding intervals. Urology, *37*:207, 1991

433-B *(Campbell's, p. 992)*

Hanno and associates, using amitriptyline in increasing dosage from 25 to 75 mg nightly, noted improvement in nearly 70 per cent of patients who had been refractory to other treatments. The rationale for its use is that amitriptyline has analgesic properties as well as anticholenergic effects. The use of steroidal and nonsteroidal anti-inflammatory agents, immunosuppressants, and antihistamines has fallen out of favor, in large part because of lack of consistent efficacy. The results of treatment with systemic heparin have been equivocal. Sodium pentosanpolysulfate (Elmiron) has also been shown to be effective by some workers, however, other investigators have not found an advantage over placebo.

REFERENCES

1. Hanno, P., Buehler, J., and Wein, A.J.: Use of amitriptyline in the treatment of interstitial cystitis. J. Urol., 141:846, 1989.
2. Messing, E.M.: The diagnosis of interstitial cystitis. Urology, *29*(Suppl.):4, 1987a.
3. Lose, G., Jespersen, J., Fransden, B., et al.: Subcutaneous heparin in the treatment of interstitial cystitis. Scand. J. Urol. Nephrol., *19*:27, 1985.
4. Holm-Bentzen, M.: Treatment with subcutaneous heparin for interstitial cystitis. Presented at the NIH-NIDDK Workshop on Interstitial Cystitis. Bethesda, August 1987.

434-E *(Campbell's, pp. 992–993)*

Although complete or satisfactory improvement has been demonstrated in 50 to 80 per cent of interstitial cystitis patients treated with DMSO, endoscopic improvement has not been found in those patients with symptomatic relief. Continuous treatment is usually required for long term symptom relief. Its mechanism of action remains unclear, although DMSO has been reported to have analgesic and anti-inflammatory actions and may reduce collagen deposition.

REFERENCES

1. Ek, A., Engberg, A., Frodin, L., and Jonsson, G.: The use of dimethyl-sulfate (DMSO) in the treatment of interstitial cystitis. Scand. J. Urol. Nephrol., *12*:129, 1978.

2. Fowler, J.E.: Prospective study of intravesical dimethyl sulfoxide in treatment of suspected early interstitial cystitis. Urology, *18*:21, 1981.
3. Perez-Mararo, R., Emerson, L.E., and Juma, S.: Urodynamic studies on interstitial cystitis. Urology, *29*(Suppl.):27, 1987.

435-D *(Campbell's, pp. 993–994)*

Surgical therapy should be reserved for patients with severe symptoms who fail to respond to conservative management with several established modalities. Total urinary diversion can be expected to provide immediate and permanant cure. Cystectomy is not necessary to effect relief; however, it is recommended to prevent the development of infection or carcinoma in the defunctionalized bladder. The other procedures listed, although less drastic, are associated with failure rates of at least 25 per cent in the most optimistic series.

REFERENCES

1. Freiha, F.S., and Stamey, T.A.: Cystolysis: A procedure for the selective denervation of the bladder. J. Urol., *123*:360, 1980.
2. Messing, E.M., and Stamey, T.A.: Interstitial cystitis: Early diagnosis, pathology, and treatment. Urology, *12*:381, 1978.
3. Messing, E.M., and Freiha, F.S.: Complication of Clorpactin WCS-90 therapy for interstitial cystitis. Urology, *13*:389, 1979.

436-E *(Campbell's, pp. 986–995)*

It has been shown that the severity and quality of symptoms rarely correlate with the degree of endoscopic pathology. Fewer than half the patients experience burning upon urination, which is more typical of infection or neoplasm. Carcinoma in situ can present with identical symptoms and cystoscopic findings, and thus urinary or bladder lavage specimens must not contain atypical cells on cytologic and/or cytometric examination. Extensive gynecologic evaluation and trials of hormonal therapy are not needed unless physical examination or history indicates the presence of pelvic masses, endometriosis, or other conditions that may symptomatically resemble interstitial cystitis. Cystoscopy and hydrodistention without full anesthesia is not performed, since it is usually unsatisfactory for diagnosing interstitial cystitis.

REFERENCES

1. Hand, J.R.: Interstitial cystitis. J. Urol., *61*:291, 1949.
2. Messing, E.M., and Stamey, T.A.: Interstitial cystitis: Early diagnosis, pathology, and treatment. Urology, *12*:381, 1978.
3. Held, P., Hanno, P., Wein, A., and Pauly, M.: Epidemiology of interstitial cystitis: Incidence of interstitial cystitis from a national sample of urologists. Presented at the NIH-NIDDK Workshop on Interstitial Cystitis, Bethesda, August, 1987.
4. Lamm, D.L., and Gittes, R.F.: Inflammatory carcinoma of the bladder and interstitial cystitis. J. Urol., *117*:49, 1977.

437-D *(Campbell's, p. 996)*

About 90 per cent of patients with interstitial cystitis eventually obtain relief with nonsurgical means. Indeed, the combination of a single hydraulic distention and one chlorpactin WCS–90 instillation, approximately 25 per cent of patients receive the only treatment necessary. It has also been estimated that at least 10 per cent of patients experience lasting spontaneous remission. There is no known serious risk to health or life with interstitial cystitis, and, as mentioned previously, most patients do not experience further progression or deterioration after the diagnosis is established. Patients usually find this information, as well as the confirmation that an organic disease is responsible for their symptoms, reassuring.

REFERENCES

1. Leary, F.J., and Regan, J.B.: Prognosis of interstitial cystitis in women. Presented at Annual Meeting, North Central Section, American Urological Association, West Palm Beach, Fla., November 1985.
2. Messing, E.M., and Stamey, T.A.: Interstitial cystitis: Early diagnosis, pathology, and treatment. Urology, *12*:381, 1978.
3. Rohner, T.J. Jr.: Effectiveness of oxychlorosene (Clorpactin) in interstitial cystitis. J. Urol., *141*:269a; 1989.
4. Oravisto, K.J.: Epidemiology of interstitial cystitis. Ann. Chir. Gynaecol. Fenn., *64*:75, 1975.

438-E *(Campbell's, pp. 997–999)*

The urethral syndrome is an entity in which patients suffer from frequency, urgency, dysuria, and, at times, suprapubic and back pain and urinary hesitancy in the absence of objective urologic findings. The etiology remains unknown, and there is no compelling evidence to support either an anatomically obstructive cause or a link to *Chlamydia* infections. Conversely, there is some evidence supporting a role for external sphincter spasm of possible psychogenic origin. The purpose of cystoscopy is to rule out other diseases causing similar symptoms, as there are no findings that are diagnostic for the urethral syndrome. Urethral biopsies are of negligible value in the absence of objective endoscopic or cytologic findings.

REFERENCES

1. Stamm, W.E.: Relationship of interstitial cystitis to the "urethral syndrome." Presented at the NIH-NIDDK Workshop on Interstitial Cystitis, Bethesda, August 1987.
2. Carson, C.C., Segura, J.W., and Osborne, D.M.: Evaluation and treatment of the female urethral syndrome. J. Urol., *124*:609, 1980.
3. Kaplan, W.E., Firlit, C.F., and Schoenberg, H.W.: The female urethral syndrome: External sphincter spasm as etiology. J. Urol., *124*:48, 1980.

4. Schmidt, R.A., and Tanagho, E.A.: Urethral syndrome or urinary tract infection? Urology, *18*:424, 1981.
5. Splatt, A.J., and Weedon, D.: The urethral syndrome: Experience with the Richardson urethroplasty. Br. J. Urol., *49*:173, 1977.

439-B *(Campbell's, p. 1000)*

Patients with recurrent bacteriuria occasionally experience irritable voiding symptoms when the urine is uninfected, and documented bacteriuria then develops within several months. These patients may benefit from a course of long-term, low-dose antimicrobial prophylaxis. If no improvement is noted with antibiotic therapy, a variety of other approaches can be tried. It should be noted, however, that in some studies the best results occurred in patients managed by observation only.

REFERENCES

1. Kraft, J.K. and Stamey, T.A.: The natural history of symptomatic recurrent bacteriuria in women. Medicine, *56*:55, 1977.
2. Gallagher, D.J., Montgomerie, J.Z., and North, J.D.: Acute infections of the urinary tract and the urethral syndrome in general practice. Br. Med. J., *1*:622, 1965.
3. Carson, C.C., Segura, J.W., and Osborne, D.M.: Evaluation and treatment of the female urethral syndrome. J. Urol., *124*:609, 1980.
4. Zufall, R.: Ineffectiveness of treatment of urethral syndrome in women. Urology, *12*:337,1978.

PART VIII

BENIGN PROSTATIC HYPERPLASIA

CHAPTER 25

DIRECTIONS: Each question below contains suggested responses. Select the ONE BEST response to each question.

440. Prostatic growth is most rapid during which time period?

A. During puberty
B. From birth to puberty
C. During fetal development
D. From puberty to middle age
E. Beyond middle age

441. The exclusive site of origin of BPH within the prostate is the:

A. Anterior fibromuscular stroma
B. Peripheral zone
C. Preprostatic zone
D. Central zone
E. Posterior zone

442. Which of the following statements regarding the histopathology of BPH is *true*?

A. Mitotic figures are common.
B. The most common histologic pattern is fibromyoadenomatous.
C. The most common histologic pattern is muscular.
D. The increase in size of the nodules is mainly stromal.
E. The epithelium is pseudostratified columnar.

443. Which of the following statements regarding experimental studies of BPH in the canine model is *false*?

A. Estrogen has a synergistic effect in the induction of BPH.
B. Prostatic epithelial growth is mediated by the stroma.
C. With aging, the prostate becomes more sensitive to a given level of testosterone.
D. With BPH there is a decrease in the rate of cell death.
E. Aromatase inhibition decreases prostate size.

444. Which of the following statements regarding the etiology of BPH is *false*?

A. There is an increase in androgen receptor content in the nucleus of BPH tissue.
B. The level of dihydrotestosterone (DHT) is higher in BPH tissue than in the unaffected prostate tissue.
C. BPH volume correlates positively with serum levels of free testosterone.
D. BPH volume correlates positively with serum levels of estradiol and estriol.
E. Reversible regression of BPH can be achieved with LHRH agonists.

445. Which of the following statements regarding the natural history of BPH is *true*?

A. Most men with significant amounts of residual urine after voiding develop urinary tract infections.
B. The symptom most strongly predictive of a subsequent prostatectomy is nocturia.
C. Recovery of upper urinary tract function in patients with azotemia is usually good following catheter drainage.
D. Bladder instability rarely resolves with prostatectomy.
E. Once obstructive symptoms develop, spontaneous improvement is rare.

446. Which of the following statements regarding the symptoms associated with BPH is *true*?

A. It is not possible to use symptom scores pre-operatively to predict response to therapy.
B. Hematuria is more common in carcinoma of the prostate than in BPH.
C. Detrusor instability is uncommon in men with clinical prostatism.
D. The symptom of nocturia correlates well with urodynamic findings of obstruction.
E. The symptom of hesitancy does not correlate with the urodynamic findings of obstruction.

447. Which of the following agents has been shown to yield the largest decrease in prostate size?

A. Nafarelin acetate
B. Cyproterone acetate
C. Flutamide
D. Finasteride
E. Prazosin

448. A 62-year-old man presents with moderately severe obstructive voiding symptoms and cystoscopy reveals bladder outlet obstruction secondary to a small prostate. The most effective treatment is:

A. Balloon dilation of the prostate

B. Transurethral incision of the prostate
C. A trial of oral finasteride
D. Transurethral resection of the prostate
E. Placement of self retaining intraurethral stent

449. Which of the following statements regarding the evaluation of patients with BPH is *false*:

A. Maximum flow is the most useful measurement with uroflowmetry.
B. Intravenous urography is indicated only in patients who have associated hematuria.
C. Urinary tract infection should be ruled out in all patients at the time of initial evaluation.
D. The size of the prostate on rectal examination cannot be used to predict the degree of bladder outlet obstruction.
E. Cystoscopy should be performed in the office on most patients suspected of having vesical neck obstruction.

PART VIII

BENIGN PROSTATIC HYPERPLASIA

ANSWERS

440-A *(Campbell's, p. 1009, Figure 25–1)*

From the time of birth until puberty, there is little change in the size of the prostate. At puberty, a rapid increase in size occurs and continues until after the third decade is reached. Prostate growth at this time increases at the rate of 1.6 g per year. Thereafter, prostate growth markedly decreases to 0.4 g per year in men aged 31 to 90.

REFERENCE

1. Berry, S.J., Coffey, D.S., and Walsh, P.C.: The development of human benign prostatic hyperplasia with age. J. Urol., *132*:474–479., 1984.

441-C *(Campbell's, p. 1010)*

The origin and development of BPH (benign prostatic hyperplasia) have been carefully characterized by McNeal. He has noted four distinct zones within the prostate that have morphologic, functional, and pathologic significance: (1) the anterior fibromuscular stroma; (2) the peripheral zone; (3) the central zone; and (4) preprostatic tissue. The last zone is the exclusive site of origin of BPH. Within the preprostatic zone are a cylindrical smooth muscle sphincter and the tiny periurethral glands. A portion of these periurethral glands form the transition zone. The nodules arising within the transition zone enlarge to form the main mass of BPH tissue.

REFERENCE

1. McNeal, J.: Pathology of benign prostatic hyperplasia: Insight into etiology. Urol. Clin. North Am., *17*:477, 1990.

442-B *(Campbell's, pp. 1010–1011)*

On microscopic examination, benign prostatic hyperplasia is characteristically nodular and both epithelial and stromal elements are involved in varying degrees. Several different histologic patterns have been recognized. The fibromyoadenomatous pattern, which is most common, is made up of a stromal component of interlacing strands of smooth muscle and collagen arranged in much the same way as in the normal prostate and glandular elements of differing types.

The marked increase in the size of the nodules that occurs in older men is mainly glandular and is limited to the transition zone. The epithelium is generally made up of tall columnar cells and is not pseudostratified. Few mitotic figures are seen, suggesting that the mitotic cycle is very slow.

REFERENCE

1. Franks, L.M.: Benign prostatic hypertrophy: Gross and microscopic anatomy. Department of Health, Education and Welfare. NIH Publication No. 76-1113: 64, 1976.

443-E *(Campbell's, pp. 1012–1015)*

Estrogen has been shown to have a synergistic effect in the induction of BPH. Decreasing serum estrogen level by aromatase inhibition, however, does not decrease prostate size in the canine model. The release of estrogen feedback on the pituitary gonadal axis induces high levels of serum-luteinizing hormone and markedly stimulates the testis to overproduce testosterone. Because of this confounding variable, it is impossible to know whether or not inhibition of estrogen will reverse the disease in dogs with prostatic hyperplasia and normal testosterone levels.

REFERENCES

1. deKlerk, D.P., Coffey, D.S., Ewing, L.L., et al.: A comparison of spontaneous and experimentally induced canine prostatic hyperplasia. J. Clin. Invest. *64*:842–849, 1979.
2. Walsh, P.C., and Wilson, J.D.: The induction of prostatic hypertrophy in the dog with androstanediol. J. Clin. Invest. *57*:1093–1097, 1976.
3. Oesterling, J.E., Juniewicz, P.E., Walters, J.R., et al.: Aromatase inhibition in the dog. II. Effect of growth, function and pathology of the prostate. J. Urol., *139*: 832–839, 1988.

444-B *(Campbell's, pp. 1015–1017)*

In the 1970s, several studies demonstrated that the content of dihydrotestosterone (DHT) was greater in hyperplastic tissue than in normal prostate tissue. However, these studies used surgically removed specimens as a source for BPH tissue and autopsy specimens for normal tissue. Subsequently, it was demonstrated that the DHT content of prostatic tissue obtained at autopsy is factitiously low. When BPH and normal prostate tissues are obtained in the same manner, no significant difference in the DHT contents is noted. Thus, human BPH occurs in the presence of "normal" levels of dihydrotestosterone. It has, however, been shown both in dogs and in humans, that there is a significant increase in androgen receptor content in the nucleus of BPH tissue. This may be a factor that sensitizes the tissue and facilitates accelerated growth. When the serum hormone levels are corrected for age, BPH volume correlates positively with free testosterone, estradiol, and estriol. Lastly, reversible regression of BPH has been demonstrated with LHRH agonists. All of these findings confirm the concept that BPH is under endocrine control.

REFERENCES

1. Siiteri, P.K., and Wilson, J.D.: Dihydrotestosterone in prostatic hypertrophy. I. The formation and content of dihydrotestosterone in the hypertrophic prostate of man. J. Clin. Invest., *49*:1737, 1970.
2. Walsh, P.C., Hutchins, G.M., and Ewing, L.L.: Tissue content of dihydrotestosterone in human prostatic hyperplasia is not supranormal. J. Clin. Invest., *72*:1772, 1983.
3. Barrack, E.R., Bujnovszky, P., and Walsh, P.C.: Subcellular distribution of androgen receptors in human normal, benign hyperplastic and malignant prostatic tissue: Characterization of nuclear salt-resistant receptors. Cancer Res., *43*:1107, 1983.
4. Partin, A.W., Oesterling, J.E., Epstein, J.I., et al.: The influence of age and endocrine factors on the volume of benign prostatic hyperplasia. J. Urol., *145*:405, 1991.
5. Peters, C.A., and Walsh, P.C.: The effect of nafarelin acetate, a luteinizing hormone-releasing hormone agonist, on benign prostatic hyperplasia. N. Engl. J. Med., *317*:599, 1987.

445-C *(Campbell's, pp. 1020–1021)*

The absolute indications for treatment of BPH include azotemia, hydronephrosis, and bladder decompensation with overflow incontinence. Fortunately, recovery of upper urinary tract function in this group of patients is usually quite good following initial catheter drainage. The recovery of lower urinary tract function is largely dependent upon the severity and duration of bladder decompensation; however, bladder instability will resolve in most patients following treatment.

In most men with significant amounts of residual urine after voiding, urinary tract infections do not develop. Once the urine becomes infected, however, it is difficult to clear the infection without the relief of outlet obstruction. In studies where men with BPH are observed without treatment, approximately one third to two thirds improved spontaneously and 10 to 45 percent required surgery. Arrighi and colleagues demonstrated that the symptom most strongly predictive of subsequent operation was a change in the size and force of the urinary stream.

REFERENCES

1. Bishop, M.C.: Diuresis and renal functional recovery in chronic retention. Br. J. Urol., *57*:1, 1985.
2. McGuire, E.: Detrusor response to obstruction. Department of Health and Human Services, NIH Publication No. 87-2881:227, 1987.
3. Arrighi, H.M., Guess, H.A., Metter, E.J., and Fozard, J.L.: Symptoms and signs of prostatism as risk factors for prostatectomy. Prostate, *16*:253, 1990.

446-A *(Campbell's, p. 1018)*

Symptom scores are valuable for following progression of BPH and quantitating response to therapy. However, it is not possible to use these scores preoperatively to predict response to therapy in individual patients because some patients with low scores do as well after transurethral resection of the prostate as patients with higher scores. Only the symptoms of hesitancy and slow stream have been consistently correlated with urodynamic findings of obstruction. Nocturia is a difficult symptom to evaluate because many elderly men experience increased diuresis at night associated with an alteration in their diurnal secretion of antidiuretic hormone. It is estimated that 50 to 80 per cent of men with clinical prostatism have some degree of detrusor instability. Hematuria is more common in BPH than in carcinoma of the prostate.

REFERENCES

1. Christensen, M.M., and Bruskewitz, R.C.: Clinical manifestations of benign prostatic hyperplasia and indications for therapeutic intervention. Urol. Clin. North Am., *17*:509, 1990.
2. Asplund, R., and Aberg, R.: Diurnal variation in the levels of antidiuretic hormone in the elderly. J. Intern. Med., *229*:131, 1991.

447-C *(Campbell's, pp. 1023–1024)*

In a multicenter randomized double-blind study, a 41 per cent decrease in prostate volume and a 46 per cent increase in urinary flow rate was seen with the pure antiandrogen flutamide. Prazosin, a selective alpha$_1$-adrenergic blocker, decreases the tone of the prostate smooth muscle and does not reduce the size of the prostate. The other agents listed have been shown to decrease prostate size by a range of 25 to 30 per cent. Unlike flutamide and nafarelin, which are associated with a high incidence of breast pain and impotence respectively, finasteride (Proscar), a 5α-reductase inhibitor, offers the possibility of achieving androgen deprivation with few side effects.

REFERENCES

1. Stone, N.N.: Flutamide in treatment of benign prostatic hypertrophy. Urology, *39*:64, 1989.
2. Stoner, E.: The clinical development of a 5 α-reductable inhibitor, finasteride. J. Steroid Biochem., *37*:375, 1990.

448-D *(Campbell's, p. 1022)*

Transurethral incision of the prostate (TUIP) is indicated for the management of bladder outlet obstruction secondary to a small prostate, especially in younger men. The advantage of this procedure is that antegrade ejaculation is preserved in most patients. Bruskewitz and Christensen provided a comparison of TURP and TUIP. In patients who underwent TURP of less than 20 g of tissue, there was a higher incidence of postoperative bladder neck contractures. Conversely, the peak maximum urinary flow rate postoperatively and the percentage of patients who felt improved was higher with patients undergoing TURP (17.2 ml/second, 98 per cent) versus patients undergoing TUIP (12.7 ml/second, 83 per cent). The marginal improvement of patients undergoing TURP and the ability to obtain histologic tissue for evaluation must be balanced against the ability to perform TUIP on an outpatient basis and the reduced frequency of retrograde ejaculation.

REFERENCE

1. Bruskewitz, R.C., and Christensen, M.M.: Critical evaluation of transurethral resection and incision of the prostate. Prostate (Suppl.), *3*:27, 1990.

449-E *(Campbell's, pp. 1018–1020)*

To properly evaluate vesicle neck obstruction, there is no adequate substitution for cystourethroscopy. Therefore, when the diagnosis is uncertain or a urethral stricture is likely, cystoscopy may be performed in the office. In the patient who is markedly symptomatic, however, this examination is best performed immediately prior to prostatectomy to guide the surgeon in choosing an operative approach. The examination should include a complete evaluation of the interior of the bladder, with special reference to trabeculation, cellules, and diverticula. The vesicle neck is examined for the presence of a contracture, bar formation, or intravesical intrusion of the prostate. The length of the posterior urethra is measured from the bladder neck to the verumontanum to aid in estimating the size of the prostate.

PART IX

TUMORS OF THE GENITOURINARY TRACT IN THE ADULT

CHAPTERS 26 THROUGH 31

DIRECTIONS: Each question below contains suggested responses. Select the ONE BEST response to each question.

450. Tumor stem cells in renal cell carcinoma arise from the:
   A. Proximal convoluted tubule
   B. Loop of Henle
   C. Distal convoluted tubule
   D. Collecting duct
   E. Glomerulus

451. Cell theories of tumorigenesis include which of the following?
   A. Primitive cells dedifferentiate from transformed differentiated cells.
   C. Transformation results in blocked terminal differentiation.
   D. Transformation occurs in the stem cell.
   E. All of the above.

452. Based on animal studies, which of the following statements regarding tumors and stem cells is *true*?
   A. Every cell in a solid tumor should be viewed as a stem cell.
   B. Recurrent tumors have the lowest percentage of stem cells.
   C. The lowest stem cell ratio is observed at the time of maximal tumor regression.
   D. One must kill every tumor cell to eradicate a tumor.
   E. Hormone-resistant cells remain hormone resistant throughout their entire life.

453. The mitotic index:
   A. Is an indirect measure
   B. Is the number of mitoses as a percentage of the cells counted
   C. Is unreliable and not very useful
   D. Is inversely proportional to the proliferation rate
   E. Has no relationship to the histologic pattern

454. Which of the following statements regarding tumor growth is *true*?
   A. As tumor size increases, it is more likely that a higher percentage of the cells will respond to therapy.
   B. Every cell division leads to an increase in tumor size.
   C. Most tumors have similar growth rates.
   D. The genome of the transformed cell is unstable and progressive cell division increases heterogenicity.
   E. The maximum tumor burden compatible with life is 10^9 cells.

455. *ras* oncogenes:
   A. Were first isolated from colon cancers
   B. Are the most common oncogenes associated with human cancer
   C. Are identified in a large percentage of urologic malignancies
   D. Are activated by chromosomal rearrangement
   E. Produce proteins that bind to the outside of plasma membranes

456. Growth factors are important in neoplastic disease for the following reasons EXCEPT:
   A. They allow tumors to grow under conditions of reduced serum supplementation.
   B. They have no role in malignant degeneration and are used in treatment.
   C. Mutation of their receptors can result in oncogenic transformation.
   D. They are involved in autocrine growth.

457. The location of the gene felt to be involved in the development of Wilms' tumor is on chromosome:
   A. 2
   B. 3
   C. 7
   D. 10
   E. 11

458. All of the following malignancies have been theorized as having the loss of a tumor suppressor gene as the initiating event in its genesis EXCEPT:
   A. Renal cell carcinoma
   B. Bladder carcinoma
   C. Wilms' tumor
   D. Testicular carcinoma
   E. Retinoblastoma

459. Which of the following regarding metastasis is *true*?

A. Not all cells making up a tumor possess the ability to metastasize.
B. Fibronectin predisposes to invasive potential.
C. Laminin inhibits invasion.
D. Most tumors have equivalent metastatic potential.
E. Chemotherapy can induce differentiation de novo in tumors that lack an inherent capacity for differentiation.

460. All of the following are potent angiogenic factors EXCEPT:

A. Fibroblast growth factor (FGF)
B. Transforming growth factor (TGF)
C. Angiogenin
D. Autocrine motility factor (AMF)
E. Copper

461. Theoretical advantages of primary chemotherapy include all the following EXCEPT:

A. Has the ability to assess effectiveness of therapy by having a "marker lesion."
B. It is well tolerated and not associated with any increased toxicity or death.
C. Potential exists for tumor "downstaging" before definitive surgical therapy.
D. Increased likelihood of fewer resistant cells being present because of earlier initiation of chemotherapy.
E. It is an in vivo chemosensitivity test to guide dosages and number of cycles.

462. Combination chemotherapy is preferred over single-agent therapy because:

A. Tumors tend to be made up of heterogeneous cell populations with differing chemosensitivities.
B. Drugs that are ineffective as single agents are often effective when used in combination.
C. Using several drugs from the same class can increase tumor kill with minimal increased toxicity.
D. Single-agent therapy requires longer cycles with longer intervals between cycles necessary for recovery of bone marrow.
E. Combination chemotherapy has been associated with fewer side effects than single-agent therapy.

463. All of the following factors have been used clinically in the management and/or treatment of neoplastic disease EXCEPT:

A. Life-style changes
B. Granulocyte colony stimulating factor
C. Monoclonal antibody linked to chemical toxins
D. Interleukin-2
E. Pentoxifylline

464. Renal cortical adenomas

A. Arise from distal convoluted tubular cells
B. Can easily be distinguished from renal cell carcinomas by clinical means, so observation is the usual treatment
C. Are caused by a point mutation
D. Are usually asymptomatic and therefore discovered incidentally
E. Are associated with paraneoplastic syndromes

465. A 65-year-old white man is referred after a CT scan of the abdomen performed for abdominal pain revealed bilateral solid renal masses—each approximately 6–7 cm in diameter. A renal arteriogram revealed bilateral "spoke-wheel" patterns, and CT-guided needle biopsy of the masses revealed eosinophilic renal tubular cells with granular cytoplasms packed with mitochondria. The most likely diagnosis is:

A. Renal cortical adenoma
B. Oncocytoma
C. Renal cell carcinoma
D. Angiomyolipoma
E. Leiomyosarcoma

466. The best treatment for an otherwise healthy patient with a right lower pole renal mass, a needle biopsy consistent with oncocytoma, and a normal contralateral kidney is:

A. Observation
B. Chemotherapy
C. Radiation therapy
D. Radical nephrectomy
E. Partial nephrectomy

467. A 60-year-old female complains of left flank pain. Intravenous urography reveals a solid mass in the left kidney. CT scan of the abdomen reveals a 3 cm mass that has the Hounsfield density of 68. The most likely diagnosis is:

A. Renal cell carcinoma
B. Oncocytoma
C. Cortical adenoma
D. Angiomyolipoma
E. Wilms' tumor

468. Which of the following benign renal tumors is most commonly associated with hypertension?

A. Fibroma
B. Lipoma
C. Juxtaglomerular tumors
D. Simple cyst
E. Hemangioma

469. Renal cell carcinoma

A. Is more common in rural populations
B. Is more likely to occur in females than males
C. Has no known etiologic factors
D. Arises from the cells of the distal convoluted tubule
E. Has been associated with the phakomatoses

470. All of the following chromosomal changes have been associated with renal cell carcinoma EXCEPT:

A. Deletion of a small segment of the short arm of chromosome 3
B. Activation of the multidrug resistance gene
C. Deletion of a small segment of the short arm of chromosome 11
D. Overexpression of the genes for transforming growth factor-α (alpha)
E. Translocations involving chromosome 3

471. Which of the following is not one of the classic histologic patterns described for renal cell carcinoma?

A. Clear cell
B. Granular
C. Tubulopapillary

D. Endometroid
E. Sarcomatoid

472. The classic triad of flank pain, flank mass, and hematuria is seen in what percentage of patients with renal cell carcinoma?

A. 5–10
B. 20–30
C. 40–50
D. 60–70
E. 80–90

473. An asymptomatic 58-year-old white male is noted to have microscopic hematuria on routine urinalysis during his annual check-up. Intravenous urogram reveals a large right lower pole renal mass distorting the calyceal system. The mass has an irregular shape with heterogeneous echogenicity and no through transmission on ultrasound. The next step should be:

A. Arteriogram
B. DMSA renal scan
C. CT scan, chest
D. CT scan, abdomen
E. Lower pole partial nephrectomy

474. After undergoing a left radical nephrectomy for a solid mass, a patient has routine postoperative course. The pathology report reveals clear cell carcinoma in the upper pole invading the ipsilateral adrenal gland and a small focus of thrombus extending into the distal aspect of the left renal vein. Lymph nodes are without evidence of metastasis, and the patient has no evidence of metastatic disease. The stage of this tumor is:

A. T3b
B. T4
C. II
D. T3a
E. IV

475. Which of the following is associated with the poorest prognosis in a patient with renal cell carcinoma?

A. Nondiploid tumor
B. Size greater than 3 cm diameter
C. Inferior vena caval involvement completely resected
D. Contralateral renal involvement
E. Lymph node metastasis

476. The advantages of radical nephrectomy in the treatment of renal cell carcinoma include all of the following EXCEPT:

A. The adrenal gland, which is not infrequently involved, is excised.
B. It unequivocally offers improved survival rates over simple nephrectomy alone.
C. Regional lymphatic metastasis may be removed.
D. More adequate margins away from tumor can be achieved.
E. More adequate renal vein division can be achieved.

477. All of the following statements regarding regional lymphadenectomy in renal cell carcinoma are true EXCEPT:

A. Interpretation of the literature in this area is difficult, since the number and location of involved nodes is often not stated.
B. Most patients with positive lymph nodes eventually have bloodborne metastasis.
C. It provides little staging information.
D. Its therapeutic value is still uncertain.
E. Many patients without lymph node metastasis develop disseminated metastasis.

478. As an adjunct to radical nephrectomy, preoperative angiographic occlusion of the renal artery:

A. Has not been associated with reduced bleeding
B. Allows early ligation of the renal vein, which cannot be done without preoperative infarction
C. Has not been associated with significant complications
D. Can be performed without regard to the presence of arteriovenous fistulas
E. Has not been shown to improve survival

479. A 56-year-old obese white female involved in a motor vehicle accident underwent a CT scan of the abdomen to evaluate abdominal pain after blunt trauma. Her CT scan and hospital course were unremarkable except that she was found to have a solitary right kidney with a 4-cm upper pole mass consistent with renal cell carcinoma. An arteriogram was also suggestive of an upper pole renal cell carcinoma. The most appropriate management would be:

A. Autotransplantation following ex vivo surgery
B. In vivo partial nephrectomy combined with regional hypothermia
C. Radical nephrectomy and postoperative dialysis
D. Chemotherapy
E. Immunotherapy

480. Which of the following statements regarding vena caval involvement by renal cell carcinoma is *true*?

A. It is a dire prognostic sign.
B. Thrombus extension into right atrium precludes attempts at surgical removal.
C. If the caval wall is invaded, resection of this part of the cava is contraindicated.
D. Patients with regional or distant metastasis are rarely helped by radical excision.
E. Cardiac surgical techniques have improved exposure but have not decreased operative blood loss.

481. Which of the following currently offers the best response rates in the management of metastatic renal cell carcinoma?

A. Chemotherapy
B. Immunotherapy
C. Hormonal therapy
D. Adjunctive nephrectomy
E. Cryotherapy

482. All of the following statements concerning renal sarcomas are true EXCEPT:

A. They constitute approximately 2 to 3 per cent of malignant renal tumors.
B. They are very chemosensitive.
C. The most common histologic variety is leiomyosarcoma.
D. The treatment of choice is radical nephrectomy.
E. Angiography typically reveals hypovascular lesions without arteriovenous fistulas.

483. Hematologic malignancies involving the kidney:

A. Are best diagnosed by intravenous urogram
B. Require nephrectomy to remove renal involvement and improve survival
C. Are best managed with systemic chemotherapy
D. Can be differentiated from renal cell carcinoma by MRI
E. Initially develop and grow within the renal tubules

484. Metastatic disease involving the kidney is most commonly discovered by:

A. Ultrasound
B. CT scan
C. MRI
D. Autopsy
E. Intravenous urogram

485. Which of the following statements about bladder cancer is *true*?

A. It is more common in blacks than whites.
B. It is more common in Southern states than Northern states.
C. It is more common in females than males.
D. It is the most common cause of cancer death in males.
E. It is associated with a more favorable prognosis in children.

486. Which of the following is *least* important in the development of bladder cancer?

A. Tobacco smoking
B. Ornithine metabolites
C. Exposure to aromatic amines
D. Pelvic irradiation
E. Cyclophosphamide therapy

487. Which of the following is *not* associated with normal bladder urothelium?

A. A transitional layer 3 to 7 cells thick
B. A superficial cell layer composed of flat umbrella cells
C. Cells with the long axis of their nuclei oriented parallel to the basement membrane
D. A lamina propria basement membrane
E. Irregularly arranged muscle fibers in the muscularis mucosa

488. All of the following have been classified as forms of urothelial hyperplasia EXCEPT:

A. Nephrogenic adenoma
B. Cystitis follicularis
C. Cystitis cystica
D. Von Brunn's nests
E. Inverted papilloma

489. Which of the following statements about carcinoma in situ of the urinary bladder is *true*?

A. It should be treated with radical cystectomy.
B. It rarely progresses to invasive cancer.
C. It has a better prognosis if associated with irritative symptoms.
D. It is very sensitive to systemic chemotherapy.
E. It is uncommon in patients with well-differentiated superficial bladder tumors.

490. The most significant pathologic features of transitional cell carcinoma include all of the following EXCEPT:

A. Prominent nucleoli
B. A decreased nuclear-cytoplasmic ratio
C. Clumping of chromatin
D. Increased cell layers
E. Loss of cell polarity

491. Which of the following statements regarding transitional cell carcinoma of the bladder is *true*?

A. It arises most commonly on the anterior wall and dome.
B. The presence of metaplastic elements in a transitional cell carcinoma changes the principal classification of the tumor.
C. It is very unusual to find different tumor types coexisting in the same bladder tumor.
D. Tumor grade is more important in predicting prognosis than tumor stage.
E. There is a high correlation between tumor grade and survival.

492. Squamous cell carcinoma of the bladder:

A. Is associated with chronic inflammation or infection
B. Is the most common type of bladder cancer in England
C. Is not associated with cigarette smoking
D. Is more common in females than males
E. Has a worse prognosis than transitional cell carcinoma—stage for stage and grade for grade

493. The most common type of cancer in exstrophic bladder is:

A. Small cell carcinoma
B. Adenocarcinoma
C. Transitional cell carcinoma
D. Squamous cell carcinoma
E. Melanoma

494. The most common site of hematogenous metastasis from bladder cancer is:

A. Lung
B. Liver
C. Bone
D. Adrenal
E. Intestines

495. Which of the following factors is the *least* important predictor of tumor progression or recurrence in superficial transitional cell carcinoma of the bladder?

A. Tumor stage
B. Tumor grade
C. Tumor size
D. Presence of carcinoma in situ

496. The most common presenting symptom of bladder cancer is:

A. Irritative voiding
B. Flank pain
C. Lower extremity edema
D. Painless hematuria
E. A pelvic mass

497. Which of the following statements regarding urine cytology is *true*?

A. First-voided morning specimens should be used for cytology, since this urine has the greatest concentration of tumor cells.
B. Saline bladder washings are no more accurate than voided urine samples.
C. Urinary tract infection does not produce artifactual changes in urine cytology.
D. Urinary tract instrumentation can shear off sheets of transitional cells which can be misdiagnosed as papillary fragments of tumor.
E. Contrast media usually do not affect cytologic interpretation.

498. When performing transurethral resection of bladder tumors, all of the following are true EXCEPT:

A. It is not invariably necessary to perform formal resection of superficial low-grade papillary tumors.
B. It is not necessarily preferable to completely resect extensive tumors that are obviously muscle-invasive.
C. Tumors arising in a diverticulum should be resected, then treated with intravesical chemotherapy.
D. When resecting large lateral wall tumors, it may be helpful to perform the operation under general anesthesia with the patient profoundly paralyzed with pancuronium.
E. After resection of tumors encroaching on the ureteral orifices, a ureteral stent may help prevent obstruction of the orifice.

499. Which of the following is the most accurate means of staging bladder cancer patients for regional lymph node involvement?

A. CT scan
B. MRI
C. Ultrasound
D. Lymphangiogram
E. Pelvic lymphadenectomy

500. A 74-year-old white male with a 40 pack per year smoking history complained of gross hematuria. IVP revealed urinary tracts without filling defects but left-sided hydronephrosis and a large filling defect on the left wall of the bladder. Transurethral resection of bladder tumor revealed deep muscle invasion of grade III transitional cell bladder cancer. Metastatic work-up was without evidence of extravesical disease. After radical cystectomy and urinary diversion, the final pathology report reveals a deeply muscle-invasive transitional cell carcinoma without metastasis to regional lymph nodes. The stage of the patient's tumor is:

A. T2N0M0
B. T3AN0M0
C. T3*b*N0Mx
D. B*1*
E. C

501. All of the following are candidates for intravesical therapy after transurethral resection EXCEPT:

A. Solitary T1 disease
B. Small grade I T_A bladder tumor
C. Focal CIS
D. Multiple, large T_A tumors
E. Grade III superficial tumor

502. Of the following chemotherapeutic agents used in adjuvant intravesical therapy, which is most often associated with myelosuppression?

A. Etoglucid
B. Mitomycin C
C. Doxorubicin
D. Triethylenethiophosphoramide
E. Epirubicin

503. A 65-year-old white male diagnosed with carcinoma in situ of the bladder is treated with a 6-week course of BCG. Four weeks later, a follow-up cystoscopy and biopsy reveals persistent CIS without evidence of progression. The treatment to recommend next is:

A. Radiation therapy
B. Vitamin therapy
C. Cystectomy
D. Additional BCG therapy
E. Thiotepa

504. The standard treatment for muscle invasive bladder cancer is:

A. Radiation therapy
B. Radical cystectomy
C. Systemic chemotherapy
D. Aggressive transurethral resection
E. Partial cystectomy

505. All of the following statements regarding systemic chemotherapy in stage D2 transitional cell carcinoma of the bladder are true EXCEPT:

A. MVAC appears to be the most effective regimen currently available.
B. Randomized controlled studies have failed to reveal a survival benefit for combination chemotherapy over single agent chemotherapy.
C. Intra-arterial chemotherapy does not appear to be effective in treating lymph node metastases.
D. Granulocyte colony stimulating factor allows the use of higher doses of chemotherapeutic agents.
E. Adjunctive chemotherapy after cystectomy has been unequivocally demonstrated to be effective in increasing survival.

506. The most common malignant nonurothelial tumor of the bladder in adults is:

A. Leiomyosarcoma
B. Pheochromocytoma
C. Primary lymphoma
D. Carcinosarcoma
E. Rhabdomyosarcoma

507. The following statements regarding upper tract urothelial tumors are true EXCEPT:

A. As many as 50 per cent of patients will develop a subsequent bladder tumor.
B. They share the same risk factors as bladder carcinoma.
C. Ureteral tumors are more commonly located in the upper ureter and renal pelvis.
D. Transitional cell carcinoma accounts for the majority of these tumors.

E. Gross hematuria is the most common presenting symptom, occurring in approximately 75 per cent of patients.

508. A patient with muscle-invasive distal left ureteral transitional cell carcinoma undergoes nephroureterectomy with excision of bladder cuff. The subsequent pathology report reveals tumor invading pelviureteral soft tissue without evidence of lymph node or other organ metastases. The stage of this tumor is:

A. T2N0M0
B. II
C. T4N0M0
D. IV
E. T3N0M0

509. A 65-year-old white male with history of asymptomatic microhematuria underwent work-up with a normal intravenous urogram and a normal cystoscopic examination. His bladder washings revealed cells suspicious for transitional cell carcinoma. Follow-up cystoscopy with random biopsies and ureteral washings after retrograde pyelograms were normal except for positive cytologies for transitional cell carcinoma from the left ureter. Ureteroscopy failed to reveal any suspicious lesions. The next step in management should be:

A. Nephroureterectomy
B. Intraureteral instillation of BCG
C. Close follow up with repeat intravenous urogram
D. Radiation therapy
E. Intraureteral instillation of thiotepa

510. The following statements concerning the treatment of upper tract urothelial tumors are true EXCEPT:

A. Low-grade, low-stage tumors do well with either conservative or radical surgery.
B. Recurrent tumors significantly compromise patient survival. Therefore, in patients found to have upper tract urothelial tumors, radical surgery should be recommended initially.
C. Patients with high-grade, high-stage tumors do equally poorly with either conservative or radical surgery.
D. With conservative surgery, tumor recurrences in the retained ipsilateral collecting system vary from 7 to 60 per cent.
E. Patients with unilateral renal pelvic tumors and a normal contralateral kidney are best managed with a total nephroureterectomy.

511. All of the following regarding adenocarcinoma of the prostate are true EXCEPT:

A. No reliably consistent evidence exists for substantial environmental risk factors.
B. Blacks have a mortality two to three times higher than whites.
C. There is a role for genetic factors in prostate cancer.
D. It is the second most common cause of cancer deaths in males in the United States.
E. It is more common in Japan than in the United States.

512. After adenocarcinoma, the next most common type of prostate cancer is:

A. Squamous cell carcinoma
B. Transitional cell carcinoma
C. Leiomyosarcoma
D. Rhabdomyosarcoma
E. Small cell carcinoma

513. The following statements regarding the basal cell layer of the prostatic ducts and acini are true EXCEPT:

A. Invasive adenocarcinomas most frequently arise from this layer.
B. Its cells do not stain for PSA or PAP.
C. It does not function as a myoepithelial cell layer.
D. It may possess the stem cell population for the secretory epithelial cells.
E. Its cells stain keratin-positive.

514. The area of the prostate from which most cancers arise is the:

A. Transitional zone
B. Central zone
C. Peripheral zone
D. Periurethral stroma
E. Preprostatic sphincter

515. All of the following statements regarding prostatic intraepithelial neoplasia (PIN) are true EXCEPT:

A. It is found in approximately 40 per cent of prostates from men older than 50.
B. It is found in approximately 80 per cent of prostates from men with adenocarcinoma.
C. It is associated with alterations in both nuclear characteristics and cell-cell relationships.
D. The basal cell layer is almost always present in the lining of ducts and acini of dysplastic foci.
E. Identification of severe PIN as an isolated lesion on needle biopsy suggests the need for further biopsy.

516. Which of the following statements regarding the Gleason grading system is *true*?

A. The three largest representative areas of the tumor are evaluated.
B. The higher the Gleason score, the more well-differentiated the tumor.
C. The biopsy grade of the tumor usually does not correspond with volume of tumor.
D. Grade is based purely on architectural criteria.
E. The grade of the tumor and knowledge of cancer volume do not accurately predict lymph node metastases.

517. Which of the following statements regarding prostate cancer is *false*?

A. Most clinical stage A cancers arise in the transitional zone.
B. Capsular penetration is more common in transitional zone than in peripheral zone cancers.
C. Most capsular penetration in prostate cancer is along conduits provided by the perineural spaces.
D. Complete capsular penetration correlates strongly with clinical prognosis.

E. Seminal vesical invasion almost always results from direct spread of tumor into the ejaculatory duct wall inside the prostate and near the prostate cancer.

518. A 65-year-old white male was referred after a routine yearly evaluation by his primary physician revealed a normal digital rectal examination (DRE) but a PSA of 14. Transrectal ultrasound was free of hypoechoic areas, but needle biopsy revealed moderately well-differentiated adenocarcinoma from the left lobe only. Bone scan was without evidence of metastatic disease. The patient's clinical stage is:

A. A1
B. A2
C. Ax
D. B1
E. B2

519. Prostate acid phosphatase is:

A. Most accurately measured using an enzymatic assay
B. Just as sensitive as PSA levels at any clinical stage of prostate cancer
C. Not elevated in patients with BPH less than 60 grams
D. Very stable and requires no special treatment before sampling
E. The first tumor marker discovered

520. Which of the following statements regarding prostatic specific antigen (PSA) is *true*?

A. It is a glycoprotein that causes coagulation of the ejaculate.
B. The PSA level is proportional to the volume of prostate cancer.
C. PSA is not organ-specific.
D. The preoperative PSA level is very helpful as a predictor of pathologic stage.
E. The PSA level rises at an average rate of .35 ng/ml/gram of intracapsular cancer.

521. All of the following regarding PSA levels after treatment of prostate cancer are true EXCEPT:

A. Any patient with a Hybritech PSA level >.5 ng/ml 3 weeks or more after radical prostatectomy probably has residual cancer.
B. Stamey has concluded that definitive radiation therapy results in a high local failure rate, which cannot be appreciated by DRE or a PSA level that is in the normal or low-normal range.
C. Serum PSA should be obtained in the early morning since PSA levels display a circadian-type pattern.
D. After beginning hormonal therapy, a fall to an undetectable or near-undetectable level of PSA that is maintained for at least 6 months is predictive of a long-term response.
E. A fall in PSA levels can occur independent of cell inhibition or death.

522. All of the following can cause temporary elevations of PSA levels EXCEPT:

A. Acute urinary retention
B. Nonbacterial prostatitis
C. Rectal examination
D. Cystoscopy
E. Needle biopsy of the prostate

523. A healthy, asymptomatic 61-year-old white male was referred for a PSA level of 25 ng/ml despite a normal DRE. Transrectal ultrasound failed to reveal any suspicious lesions in a small gland and ultrasound guided biopsies revealed benign hyperplasia. The next appropriate step in management is:

A. Follow-up of the patient with a repeat PSA and DRE in 1 year
B. Transurethral resection of the prostate
C. A repeat PSA level 2 weeks after the biopsy to rule out spurious results
D. A bone scan
E. A repeat needle biopsy with sampling of the transition zone

524. With regard to ultrasound guided needle biopsy of the prostate:

A. Hypoechoric lesions are specific for cancer.
B. No isochoic prostate cancers have been reported in studies using TRUS guided biopsies.
C. Well-differentiated tumors tend to be more hypoechoric.
D. Six systemic biopsy specimens taken under TRUS guidance are recommended as the best way to diagnose prostate cancer.
E. Ultrasound guided biopsy of hypoechoric lesions will detect fewer insignificant, microscopic cancers than random systemic biopsies.

525. A healthy 65-year-old white male, who was found to have a left-sided B1 nodule on routine yearly physical examination and a PSA of 3.8, underwent transrectal needle biopsy of the prostate, which revealed moderately well-differentiated adenocarcinoma from the left lobe only. Serum electrolytes, liver function tests, urinalysis, and chest radiography are all within normal limits. The most appropriate next step in management is:

A. A discussion of treatment options with the patient
B. An intravenous urogram
C. A CT scan of abdomen and pelvis
D. An MRI of abdomen and pelvis
E. A bone scan

526. All of the following statements regarding treatment of prostate cancer are true EXCEPT:

A. Treatment is largely determined by the volume and grade of tumor at the time of therapy.
B. Assessing the patient's life expectancy prior to treatment is more important than for any other genitourinary malignancy.
C. Patients should be treated as aggressively as possible due to the rapidly progressive natural history of this cancer.
D. Even a single microscopic metastatic focus in one pelvic lymph node is a hallmark of prostate cancer that is incurable by currently available modalities.
E. CT and MRI are particularly insensitive for pretreatment staging until the spread is gross and more readily discernible by other methods.

527. Patients with clinically localized adenocarcinoma of the prostate who are offered radiation therapy should be told that:

A. External beam radiation therapy has a high failure rate when attempting to sterilize the local cancer.
B. Brachytherapy allows homogeneous distribution of the interstitial seed implants resulting in better survival rates than with external beam therapy.
C. In case of radiation failure, local control of the cancer can subsequently be handled by transurethral resection without significant sequelae.
D. Positive posttreatment biopsies do not correlate with biologically active disease.
E. The combination of gold seed implantation and external beam radiation yields markedly better survival rates than external beam radiotherapy alone.

528. The number of patients with clinical stage B adenocarcinoma of the prostate on DRE that actually have disease confined to the prostate is:

A. 10 per cent
B. 20 per cent
C. 40 per cent
D. 80 per cent
E. 100 per cent

529. A sexually active 65-year-old white male is diagnosed with clinical stage B1 adenocarcinoma of the prostate, a PSA of 8 (Hybritech) and a negative bone scan. He has no significant past medical history. The next step in management is:

A. CT scan
B. MRI of the pelvis
C. External beam radiation therapy
D. Pelvic lymph node dissection, followed by a nerve-sparing radical prostatectomy (if no evidence of lymph node metastases is present)
E. Hormonal therapy

530. A 65-year-old impotent black male with clinical stage B2 adenocarcinoma of the prostate, outlet obstructive symptoms, a PSA of 31 (Hybritech), and a negative CT and bone scan undergoes pelvic lymph node dissection, which reveals no grossly suspicious nodes, but frozen-section shows a microscopic focus of lymph node metastases. The treatment option to recommend is:

A. Radical prostatectomy
B. Early endocrine therapy
C. Radiation therapy
D. Close the incision and follow patient with frequent DRE and serum PSA levels
E. Delayed endocrine therapy

531. After a formal radical prostatectomy, the percentage of patients that can be expected to remain potent is:

A. 10
B. 30
C. 50
D. 70
E. 90

532. Regarding hormonal therapy of prostate cancer, which of the following statements is *true*?

A. LHRH agonists are not equivalent to bilateral orchiectomy in suppressing testosterone or improving survival but are an acceptable alternative in patients who refuse orchiectomy.
B. Early hormonal therapy offers a survival advantage compared to delayed hormonal therapy.
C. Ablation of adrenal androgen effect with flutamide does not appear to offer any advantage in patient survival.
D. Diethylstilbestrol (DES), 3 to 5 mg per day, is an acceptable and cost-effective alternative for most patient who refuse orchiectomy.
E. LHRH agonists can be used safely in patients with significant spinal metastases.

533. Chemotherapeutic agents used in prostate cancer:

A. Should rely on DNA replication for cell killing
B. Have generally been ineffective
C. When effective are associated with long-term responses
D. May decrease the indications for radical prostatectomy
E. Have not been associated with significant toxicity

534. Which of the following statements regarding testicular cancer is *false*?

A. It is the most common malignancy in young adult men.
B. It is one of the most curable of all solid neoplasms.
C. Advances in diagnosis and treatment have led to a decrease in patient mortality to less than 10 per cent.
D. Primary extragonadal germ cell tumors have a better prognosis than testicular germ cell tumors.
E. The majority of primary testicular neoplasms arise from germ cell elements.

535. Which of the following statements regarding testicular neoplasms is *true*?

A. They arise more commonly in the left testis than in the right one.
B. They are bilateral in approximately 6 per cent of the cases.
C. They are more common in blacks than in whites.
D. They are believed to commonly occur in patients with a history of testicular trauma.
E. Their incidence is higher in the United States than in Europe or Scandinavia.

536. The most common pure histologic type of testis cancer is:

A. Embryonal cell
B. Teratoma
C. Yolk sac tumor
D. Choriocarcinoma
E. Seminoma

537. The most common presenting symptom of a testicular neoplasm is:

A. Pain or ache in the scrotum
B. Epididymitis
C. Gynecomastia

D. Painless nodule of the testis
E. Gastrointestinal disturbance (i.e., nausea, vomiting)

538. A 25-year-old white male presents complaining of a 1-month history of pain and swelling in his right hemiscrotum. He denies irritative or obstructive voiding symptoms and has no history of cryptorchidism or recent trauma. Physical examination reveals normal left testis and a tense right hydrocele that precludes palpation of the right testicle. The next step in management should be:

A. Treat empirically for epididymitis and follow up in 3 months
B. Needle aspiration of the hydrocele to allow testis palpation
C. Scrotal ultrasound
D. Obtain serum HCG and alpha-fetoprotein levels
E. Perform right hydrocele repair

539. The primary lymphatic drainage of the left testis is via:

A. Preaortic nodes above the left renal vein
B. Interaortocaval nodes at the level of the left renal vein
C. Precaval nodes at the level of the left renal vein
D. Left common iliac nodes
E. Para-aortic nodes below the left renal vein

540. The most common site for distant, extralymphatic metastasis of testicular tumors is:

A. Bone
B. Liver
C. Brain
D. Lung
E. Viscera

541. A 27-year-old white male undergoes right radical orchiectomy for a solid intratesticular mass. Pathology reveals a teratocarcinoma invading the epididymis. The patient's T stage is:

A. T1
B. T2
C. T3
D. T4a
E. T4b

542. All of the following are important for staging of testicular neoplasms EXCEPT:

A. Pathologic evaluation of the surgical specimen
B. Chest radiograph
C. Chest CT
D. Abdominal CT
E. Serum levels of tumor markers

543. Elevated alpha-fetoprotein levels can be found in all of the following EXCEPT:

A. Embryonal cell tumors
B. Most neonates
C. Yolk sac tumors
D. Pure seminoma
E. Teratocarcinoma

544. Which of the following pituitary hormones can give false positive results in the beta-HCG radioimmunoassay?

A. Adrenocorticotropic hormone
B. Follicle-stimulating hormone
C. Melanocyte-stimulating hormone
D. Luteinizing hormone
E. Thyroid-stimulating hormone

545. What percentage of patients with pure seminoma have elevated levels of HCG?

A. 0 per cent
B. 5–10 per cent
C. 20 per cent
D. 50 per cent
E. 80 per cent

546. Which of the following precludes the diagnosis of pure seminoma?

A. Elevated beta-HCG
B. Elevated alpha-fetoprotein level
C. Elevated lactate dehydrogenase (LDH)
D. Elevated gamma-glutamyl transpeptidase (GGT)
E. Elevated placental alkaline phosphatase (PLAP)

547. All of the following generalizations regarding germ cell tumors are true EXCEPT:

A. Surgical excision of the scrotum is recommended in cases of iatrogenic or neoplastic scrotal violation.
B. Low-volume metastatic seminoma should be treated with radiotherapy after orchiectomy.
C. Patients with large retroperitoneal metastatic deposits are best managed initially with surgical debulking.
D. Most patients with seminomas have disease confined to the testis at diagnosis.
E. Most patients with nonseminomatous germ cell tumors have metastatic disease at diagnosis.

548. Which of the following statements regarding patients with seminomatous germ cell tumor is *true*?

A. One third of patients with histologically pure seminoma who die of the disease have nonseminomatous metastatic deposits.
B. Most present with metastatic disease.
C. After orchiectomy for low stage disease, adjuvant chemotherapy is suggested.
D. High bulk metastatic disease is best treated with radiation therapy.
E. Nonlymphatic metastases are most commonly seen in bone.

549. Compared to other histologic types of seminoma, all the following statements regarding anaplastic seminoma are true EXCEPT:

A. It has more mitotic activity than other histologic types of seminoma.
B. Stage for stage, it has a poorer prognosis for survival.
C. It has a higher rate of local invasion.
D. It has a higher rate of metastases.
E. It has a higher rate of tumor marker production (B-HCG).

550. A 37-year-old white male with history of right orchiopexy as a child undergoes right radical orchiectomy for T2 classical seminoma. Postoperative metastatic work-up reveals no evidence of metastatic disease. The recommended treatment of choice is:

A. Observation and serial tumor markers
B. Platinum-based chemotherapy

C. Irradiation to the para-aortic, ipsilateral pelvic, and bilateral inguinal nodes with shieldings
D. Modified retroperitoneal lymph node dissection
E. Full retroperitoneal lymph node dissection

551. In patients with high bulk retroperitoneal metastases from pure seminomatous germ cell tumors, after radical orchiectomy for local control and diagnosis, the treatment of choice is:

A. Radiation therapy
B. Radiation therapy followed by platinum-based chemotherapy
C. Full retroperitoneal lymph node dissection
D. Platinum-based chemotherapy
E. Modified retroperitoneal lymph node dissection

552. All of the following statements regarding nonseminomatous germ cell tumors are true EXCEPT:

A. The first echelon of spread is most commonly the retroperitoneal lymph nodes.
B. The most common nonlymphatic spread is to the lung.
C. Only 20 per cent of patients have metastatic disease at diagnosis.
D. They have a less favorable natural history than pure seminomas.
E. Combinations of seminomatous and nonseminomatous tumors should be treated as nonseminomatous tumors.

553. Which of the following cells are necessary to diagnose choriocarcinoma of the testis?

A. Syncytiotrophoblasts
B. Cytotrophoblasts
C. Both syncytiotrophoblasts and cytotrophoblasts
D. Yolk sac cells
E. Cells from all three germ cell layers

554. The most common testis tumor of infants and children is:

A. Yolk sac tumor
B. Choriocarcinoma
C. Teratocarcinoma
D. Embryonal cell carcinoma
E. Seminoma

555. In patients with T3 embryonal cell carcinoma with vascular invasion on pathologic section but no evidence of metastatic disease on abdominal CT scan or postoperative tumor marker levels, the treatment of choice is:

A. Observation
B. Radiation therapy
C. Platinum-based chemotherapy
D. Retroperitoneal lymph node dissection
E. Radiation therapy followed by chemotherapy

556. Following various types of modified retroperitoneal lymph node dissection, preservation of ejaculatory function can be expected in approximately:

A. 0–5 per cent
B. 10–15 per cent
C. 20–35 per cent
D. 40–60 per cent
E. 75–95 per cent

557. The treatment of choice following radical inguinal orchiectomy for nonseminomatous germ cell tumor in patients diagnosed with high bulk (>75 cm) retroperitoneal lymph node metastatic disease is:

A. Observation
B. Radiation therapy
C. Platinum-based combination chemotherapy
D. Retroperitoneal lymph node dissection
E. Radiation therapy followed by platinum-based combination chemotherapy

558. The current standard chemotherapeutic regimen for patients with disseminated germ cell tumor is:

A. M-VAC (methotrexate, vinblastine, Adriamycin, cisplatin)
B. CISCA (cisplatin, cytoxan, Adriamycin)
C. VAB (vinblastine, actinomycin, bleomycin)
D. BEP (bleomycin, etoposide, cisplatin)
E. PVB (cisplatin, vinblastine, bleomycin)

559. After primary chemotherapy for a high bulk nonseminomatous testis cancer, a patient has a 4-cm retroperitoneal mass. The next step in management should be:

A. Observation with repeat tumor markers
B. Radiation therapy
C. Further chemotherapy
D. Retroperitoneal lymph node dissection
E. Radiation therapy followed by chemotherapy

560. Primary extragonadal germ cell tumors:

A. Account for 15–20 per cent of all germ cell tumors
B. Are more common in females than in males
C. Present most commonly in patients above the age of 40 years (in contrast to gonadal germ cell tumors)
D. Are generally adequately treated by local excision
E. Most commonly arise in the mediastinum

561. Which of the following statements regarding Leydig cell tumors of the testis is *false*?

A. Radical inguinal orchiectomy is the initial procedure of choice.
B. They are usually malignant.
C. In prepubertal patients, they usually cause precocious puberty.
D. In postpubertal patients, feminizing symptoms tend to occur.
E. They tend to be radioresistant.

562. The most common germ cell element found in gonadoblastomas is similar to:

A. Yolk sac tumor
B. Embryonal cell carcinoma
C. Seminoma
D. Choriocarcinoma
E. Teratocarcinoma

563. The most common nonhematologic primary source of metastases to the testis is:

A. Prostate
B. Lung
C. Gastrointestinal tract
D. Melanoma
E. Kidney

564. The most common epididymal tumor is:

A. Leiomyoma
B. Papillary cystadenoma
C. Lipoma
D. Adenomatoid tumor
E. Fibroma

565. A paratesticular malignant tumor found in an adolescent is most likely to be a(n):

A. Leiomyosarcoma
B. Malignant fibrous histiocytoma
C. Rhabdomyosarcoma
D. Liposarcoma
E. Undifferentiated sarcoma

566. Which of the following penile lesions has been associated with malignant degeneration:

A. Epithelial inclusion cyst
B. Balanitis xerotica obliterans
C. Hirsute papilloma
D. Pseudotumor
E. Angioma

567. All of the following have been associated with a viral etiology EXCEPT:

A. Condyloma acuminata
B. Bowenoid papulosis
C. Kaposi's sarcoma
D. Leukoplakia
E. Verrucous carcinoma of the penis

568. The best treatment for Buschke-Löwenstein tumor is:

A. Topical 5-fluorouracil
B. Radiation therapy
C. Topical podophyllin
D. Local examination
E. Local excision followed by inguinal lymph node dissection

569. All of the following regarding carcinoma in situ (CIS) of the penis are true EXCEPT:

A. It is associated with an increased incidence of subsequent internal malignancy.
B. Human papilloma virus (HPV) has been identified in CIS.
C. Its epidemiology and natural history parallel that of early carcinoma of the penis.
D. In lesions involving the prepuces, circumcision is adequate treatment.
E. Fulguration of the lesion is often associated with recurrence.

570. Which of the following has *not* been associated with increased risk of penile carcinoma:

A. Phimosis
B. Chronic irritation
C. HPV infection
D. Poor hygiene
E. Trauma

571. All of the following regarding circumcision are true EXCEPT:

A. Circumcision in the neonatal period may reduce the incidence of urinary tract infections in male infants.
B. Circumcision at any age is protective against penile carcinoma.
C. Circumcision may not be as important in preventing penile carcinoma in countries where good hygiene is practiced.
D. Carcinoma of the penis is almost unknown in areas where neonatal circumcision is practiced.
E. The current recommendation of the American Academy of Pediatrics is that newborn circumcision has potential medical advantages and disadvantages which must be discussed with the parents.

572. The earliest route of dissemination from penile carcinoma is:

A. Local spread to urethral and bladder.
B. Hematogenous spread to the lung.
C. Lymphatic spread to regional femoral and iliac nodes.
D. Hematogenous spread to liver.
E. Lymphatic spread to para-aortic nodes at level of L_2.

573. Clinically detectable hematogenous metastatic spread occurs in what percentage of patients with penile carcinoma:

A. 0–10
B. 15–20
C. 30–40
D. 50–60
E. 70–80

574. The most common presenting symptom in patients with penile carcinoma is:

A. Pain
B. Hematuria
C. Penile lesion
D. Constitutional symptoms (i.e. fatigue, weight loss, malaise)
E. Nodal lesions

575. A 65-year-old white male diabetic presented with several month history of an erythematous, pruritic lesion in his glans. He was felt to have fungal balanitis and was treated with daily cleansing and Neosporin cream. After 1 month of treatment, his lesion is found to persist without change. The next appropriate step should be:

A. Topical chemotherapy with 5-fluorouracil
B. Radiation therapy
C. Fulguration
D. Penile biopsy
E. Partial penectomy

576. The most common histology found in penile carcinoma is:

A. Basal cell carcinoma
B. Squamous cell carcinoma
C. Transitional cell carcinoma
D. Sarcoma
E. Adenocarcinoma

577. The strongest prognostic indicator for survival in penile carcinoma is:

A. Stage
B. Grade
C. DNA ploidy
D. Size
E. Site on penis

578. A 63-year-old black male with a history of phimosis was referred after biopsy of a glanular penile lesion revealed grade II squamous cell carcinoma. Partial penectomy is performed and pathologic analysis reveals tumor invading the left corpus cavernosum. The patient's T stage is:

A. T_{is}
B. T_1
C. T_2
D. T_3
E. T_4

579. A 72-year-old white male is referred for further management of a superficial appearing 2-cm ulcerative lesion involving the entire right glans. Biopsy revealed grade II squamous cell carcinoma. The recommended treatment for the primary neoplasm should be:

A. 5-Fluorouracil topical chemotherapy
B. Radiation therapy
C. Local wedge resection
D. Partial penectomy with a 2 cm margin proximal to the tumor
E. Neodymium: YAG laser fulguration

580. All of the following regarding performance of lymphadenectomy for penile carcinoma are true EXCEPT:

A. Inguinal lymph node dissection should be performed for persistent clinically palpable nodes after treatment of the primary lesion and a cause of antibodies.
B. Early lymph node dissection yields better survival results than delayed lymph node dissection.
C. Unilateral palpable adenopathy at presentation that persists after treatment of the primary lesion and a cause of antibiotic should be managed with bilateral inguinal lymphadenectomy.
D. Pelvic lymphadenectomy is reasonable for young, healthy males with metastatic disease in inguinal lymph nodes.
E. The development of unilateral palpable adenopathy sometime after the initial presentation and treatment of the primary tumor should be managed with bilateral inguinal lymphadenectomy.

581. The sentinel lymph node is located near which vessel:

A. Inferior epigastric artery
B. Superficial circumflex vein
C. Superficial epigastric vein
D. External iliac vein
E. Obturator vein

582. A 56-year-old white male undergoes partial penectomy for a T_1 grade I squamous cell penile carcinoma. He has no evidence of palpable inguinal adenopathy. Metastatic work up is without evidence of residual disease. The next step in management should be:

A. Observation
B. Ipsilateral sentinel node biopsy
C. Ipsilateral inguinal lymphadenectomy
D. Adjuvant systemic chemotherapy
E. Radiation therapy

583. In patients with stage IV penile carcinoma:

A. Radiation therapy has been found to be very effective with 5 year survivals of approximately 50 per cent.
B. Bleomycin chemotherapy has been shown to be more effective than cisplatin and methotrexate.
C. Inguinal areas tolerate radiation therapy relatively well.
D. Information regarding newer chemotherapy agents comes from trials in the US.
E. Overall a poor prognosis is expected despite chemotherapy and/or radiation therapy.

584. All of the following regarding inguinal lymphadenectomy are true EXCEPT:

A. Transposition of the sartorius muscle over the vessels has minimized the incidence of vascular erosion and thrombosis.
B. The majority of wound problems are secondary to skin loss.
C. In most instances of skin loss, only a small amount of superficial skin is lost.
D. In patients with large, deep skin loss, split thickness skin graft will be necessary.
E. A number of local flaps are available in this area for transposition into areas of tissue defects.

585. The most common malignant sarcoma reported to arise primarily in the penis is:

A. Leiomyosarcoma
B. Hemangioendothelioma
C. Rhabdomyosarcoma
D. Fibrosarcoma
E. Malignant fibrous histiocytoma

586. The most frequent sign of metastatic spread involving the penis is:

A. Pain
B. Penile swelling
C. Priapism
D. Modularity
E. Ulceration

PART IX

TUMORS OF THE GENITOURINARY TRACT IN THE ADULT

CHAPTERS 26 THROUGH 31

ANSWERS

450-A *(Campbell's, pp. 1031–1032)*

A stem cell is defined as a cell that has the characteristics of the extended capacity for self-renewal and the capacity to mature into one or more differentiated forms. Tumor stem cells are the subset of tumor cells responsible for repopulating the tumor following therapy. Tumor stem cells can be considered to be developmentally based on the tissue cell of origin in which they arose. Therefore, kidney tumor stem cells are derived from the proximal tubular cells, bladder carcinomas from the basil cells, and testicular carcinoma from the germinal epithelium.

REFERENCE

1. Steel, G.G.: Growth Kinetics of Tumors. London, Oxford University Press, 1977, p. 217.

451-E *(Campbell's, p. 1032)*

Three theories regarding the origin of tumors from differentiating tissue exist. First of all, homogeneous, primitive cells "dedifferentiate" from transformed differentiated cells. Second, there is homogeneous blocked terminal differentiation through the transformation of transition cells, not stem cell. Finally, the transforming event (initiation) occurs in the stem cell.

452-C *(Campbell's, pp. 1033–1034)*

In most solid tumors, true stem cells constitute a small percentage of the total tumor cell population. A unique feature of tumor cells is that if they are transplanted into a suitable host, they will grow, whereas normal cells will not grow. One technique used to determine stem cell number is to implant different numbers of tumor cells and calculate the number of tumor cells required to achieve tumor growth in 50 per cent of the implanted animals. This technique is referred to as the limiting diluting assay. Using this assay in various animal studies, it was determined that:

1. Not every tumor cell is a stem cell.
2. Hormone-resistant cells surviving after castration still show differential growth when exposed to androgens or estrogens, indicating that hormone resistance is relative.
3. Tumor occurring after treatment appears to be more aggressive with the highest percentage of stem cells noted.
4. The lowest stem cell ratio is observed at the time of maximum tumor regression.

Therefore, if the stem cell is responsible for tumor regrowth and if only the stem cell represents the true reproductive component of the tumor, one does not have to kill every tumor cell to eradicate the tumor, just eliminate the tumor stem cell.

REFERENCE

1. Bruchovsky, N., Rennie, P.S., Coldman, A.J., et al.: Effects of androgen withdrawal on the stem cell composition of the Shionogi carcinoma. Cancer Res., *50*: 2275–2287, 1990.

453-B *(Campbell's, p. 1035)*

The mitotic index is the number of mitoses as a percentage of the cells counted. It is a direct measure and a reliable direct proportional indication of proliferation rate. Higher grades are usually associated with higher mitotic indexes.

REFERENCE

1. Alision, M.R., and Wright, N.A.: Growth Kinetics. Recent Results Cancer Res., *78*:29–43, 1981.

454-D *(Campbell's, pp. 1036–1037)*

The genome of the transformed cell is unstable, and increasing changes occur with each cell division, the cells becoming increasingly heterogeneous. It becomes more likely that cells resistant to therapy will be found with greater frequency as the tumor size increases. Since most tumors have a large fraction of cells dying or leaving the reproductive pool of cells, not every cell division leads to an increase in tumor size. A wide variation in growth rate has been noted even among tumors of the same histologic type. The maximum tumor burden compatible with life is approximately 10^{12} cells.

REFERENCES

1. Goldie, J.H. and Coldman, A.J.: The genetic origin of drug resistance in neoplasms: complications for systemic therapy. Cancer Res., *44*:3543–3563, 1984.
2. Steel, G.G.: Growth Kinetics of Tumors. London, Oxford University Press, 1977, p. 217.

455-B *(Campbell's, pp. 1037–1039)*

The *ras* oncogenes have been reported in approximately 50 per cent of colon and 100 per cent of pancreatic cancers. Although it is the most common oncogene associated with human cancer and was originally isolated from bladder cancer cell lines, *ras* oncogenes are identified in only a small percentage of urologic malignancies. The expressing of *ras* represents a somatic activation of the cellular oncogene by a point mutation. Current research focused on the *ras* protein has shown it to bind to the inner cytoplasmic side of the plasma membrane.

REFERENCES

1. Carter, B.S., Epstein, J.I., and Isaacs, W.B.: *ras* gene mutations in human prostate cancer. Cancer Res., *50*: 6830–6832, 1990.
2. Yao, M., Shuin, T., Misaki, H., and Kubata, Y.: Enhanced expression of C-*myc* and epididymal growth factor receptor (c-*erb* B–1) genes in primary human renal cancer. Cancer Res., *48*:6753–6757, 1988.
3. Carroll, P.R., and Chiganti, R.S.V.: Cytogenetics: Chromosomal abnormalities in urologic tumors. *In* Chisholm, G.D., and Fair, W.R. (Eds): Scientific Foundations of Urology. Oxford, Heinemann Medical Books, 1990, pp. 481–489.

456-B *(Campbell's, p. 1039)*

Characteristic of a number of cancer cells is their ability to grow in tissue culture under conditions of reduced serum supplementation. This suggests the possibility that cancer cells may produce their own growth factors. The growth factors are released by the tumor cell and bind to a cell surface receptor, which leads to growth of the tumor cell. This form of uncontrolled self-stimulation is referred to as autocrine growth. Several growth factors that have been identified include transforming growth factor-alpha (TGF-α), transforming growth factor-beta (TGF-β), and fibroblast growth factor (FGF). In some cases, overproduction of a growth factor is responsible for transformation. In others, mutation of the growth factor receptor can result in oncogenic transformation.

REFERENCE

1. Sporn, M.B., and Roberts, A.B.: Autocrine growth factors and cancer. Nature, *313*:747–751, 1985.

457-E *(Campbell's, p. 1041)*

Depletional analysis of individuals with WAGR syndrome (Wilms' tumor, aniridia, genitourinary abnormalities, mental retardation) revealed that a Wilms' tumor gene is located on chromosome 11p13. This is probably not the only gene implicated in Wilms' tumor, as other genetic and restriction fragment length polymorphism data suggest that multiple loci may be involved.

REFERENCE

1. Call, K.M., Glaser, T., Ito, C.Y., et al.: Isolation and characterization of a zinc finger polypeptide gene at the human chromosome 11 Wilms' tumor locus. Cell, *60*:509–520, 1990.

458-D *(Campbell's, pp. 1040–1041)*

In addition to genes that code for positive regulators of growth, there are genes that code for inhibition of growth. These genes have been called antioncogenes, recessive oncogenes, or tumor suppression genes. Unlike the dominant-acting oncogenes, which require that only one chromosomal allele be affected in order to exhibit the change, in the recessive-acting suppressor gene, both alleles need to be inactivated to cause loss of growth control. Tumor suppressor genes have received widespread attention since the isolation of the retinoblastoma gene in 1985. Wilms' tumor, renal cell carcinoma, and bladder carcinoma have also been associated with antioncogenes. Germ cell testicular cancers, to date, have not been associated with antioncogenes.

REFERENCES

1. Sager, R.: Tumor suppressor genes: the puzzle and the promise. Science, *246*:1406–1412, 1989.
2. Olumni, A.F., Tsai, Y.C., Nichols, P.W., et al.: Allelic loss of chromosome 17p distinguishes high-grade from low-grade transitional cell carcinoma of the bladder. Cancer Res., *50*:7081–7083, 1990.
3. Shimizu, M., Yokota, J., Mori, N., et al.: Introduction of normal chromosome 3p modulates tumorigenicity of a human renal cell carcinoma cell line YCR. Oncogene, *5*:185–194, 1990.

459-A *(Campbell's, pp. 1042–1044)*

The most clinically devastating biologic alteration of malignant tumors is related to their ability to metastasize and colonize different organs. The propensity to metastasize is found in only a minority of the cells in a tumor. The steps involved in the metastatic cascade have been identified.

First, the tumor cells invade and penetrate the vasculature and extracellular matrix. Fibronectin acts as a barrier to this step. Laminim may be chemotactic for some tumor cells. Second, the matrix is dissolved by the release of proteolytic enzymes, such as collagenase. The third step in the invasion process is movement of the cells through the attenuated matrix.

Once the tumor successfully penetrates the endothelial basement membrane, it gains access to the systemic circulation. However, not all cells reaching the circulation survive. The tumor cell then must leave the circulation and evolve into a metastatic deposit. Considering all these steps, it should not be surprising that tumors vary in their metastatic capability.

Chemotherapy does not usually affect tumor differentiation.

REFERENCE

1. Liotta, L.A.: Tumor invasion and metastasis: role of the extracellular matrix. Rhoads Memorial Award Lecture. Cancer Res., *46*:1–7, 1986.

460-D *(Campbell's, pp. 1043–1044)*

A feature common to many malignancies is the formation of new blood vessels, called angiogenesis. Tumor growth requires a vascular supply. FGF, TGF, angiogenion, and copper are all potent angiogenic factors. Autocrine motility factor is a positive-acting factor for tumor motility and metastatic tumor spread, but is not associated with angiogenesis.

REFERENCE

1. Folkman, J., and Klagsburn, M.: Angiogenic factors. Science, *235*:442–447, 1987.

461-B *(Campbell's, p. 1046)*

The theoretical advantages of primary chemotherapy includes the ability to assess the effectiveness of therapy by having a "marker lesion" in place at the time chemotherapy is given. In the absence of a demonstrable effect of the therapy on the local lesion, primary chemotherapy can be discontinued, thus avoiding unnecessary toxicity in some patients who are unresponsive. This "in vivo chemosensitivity test" will guide the clinician to the proper dosage and number of cycles necessary to achieve maximal effect. There is also the potential for tumor "downstaging," making it possible to reduce the extent and severity of subsequent surgery. The likelihood of fewer resistant cells being present as a result of the initiation of treatment before surgery or radiation is another advantage of primary chemotherapy.

Disadvantages of primary chemotherapy exist too. Practically, chemotherapy may delay the timing and impair the effectiveness of subsequent surgery. In addition, it exposes the patients who would be cured by definitive treatment alone to unnecessary toxicity and death.

REFERENCE

1. DeVita, V.T.: Principles of chemotherapy. *In* DeVita, V.T., Hellman, S., and Rosenberg, S.A. (Eds.): Cancer: Principles and Practice of Oncology. Philadelphia, J.B. Lippincott, Co., 1989, pp. 276–290.

462-A *(Campbell's, pp. 1046–1047)*

With few exceptions, such as choriocarcinoma and Burkitt's lymphoma, combination chemotherapy is generally required to cure chemotherapy-sensitive human tumors. Because tumors are heterogeneous, combination therapy may provide broader coverage and decrease the likelihood of resistance. If a drug is ineffective when used as a single agent, it is unlikely to be effective in combination. When several drugs of the same class are available, a drug should be selected to minimize overlapping toxicity with other drugs in combination.

REFERENCE

1. DeVita, R.T.: Principles of chemotherapy. *In* DeVita, V.T., Hellman, S., and Rosenberg, S.A. (Eds.): Cancer: Principles and Practice of Oncology. Philadelphia, J.B. Lippincott, Co., 1989, pp. 276–290.

463-C *(Campbell's, pp. 1047–1048)*

Numerous reports of increased risk for the development of cancer from various environmental and life-style factors are reported. Elimination of tobacco products and alteration in nutritional habits have all been recommended.

The introduction of hematopoietic growth factor (G-CSF) has significantly reduced the toxicity associated with some types of combination chemotherapy. Another approach is using genetically manipulated cells to produce agents that can kill tumor cells, such as tumor necrosis factor (TNF) or interleukin-2 (IL-2), which activates immunotherapeutic responses.

Pentoxifylline has been found to reverse some of the negative aspects of cancer with improvement in appetite, sense of well-being, and performance status.

Although the use of monoclonal antibodies linked to chemical toxins has been theorized for the treatment of human tumors, pharmacologic amounts of toxin and the chemical means for linking the toxin to an antibody are currently not available.

REFERENCES

1. Lerman, C., Rimer, B., and Engstrom, P.F.: Reducing available cancer mortality through prevention and early detection regimens. Cancer Res., *49*:4955–4962, 1989.
2. Rosenberg, S.A., Aebersold, P., Cornetta, K., et al.: Gene transfer into humans: Immunotherapy of patients with advanced melanoma using tumor-infiltrating lymphocytes modified by retroviral gene transduction. N. Engl. J. Med., *323*:570–578, 1990.
3. Dezube, B.J., Fridovich-Keil, J.L., Bouvard, I., et al.: Pentoxifylline and well-being in patients with cancer. Lancet, *335*:662, 1990.

464-D *(Campbell's, p. 1056)*

Renal cortical adenomas, commonly encountered at autopsy, are benign tumors both clinically and histologically. The etiology of renal cortical adenomas is unknown. The renal adenoma is characterized by uniform acidophilic or clear cells, with monotonous nuclear and cellular characteristics, believed to arise from the proximal convoluted tubule. Most renal cortical adenomas are discovered incidentally. Paraneoplastic syndromes are usually not seen in benign renal tumors. Since renal cortical adenomas are clinically indistinguishable from renal cell carcinoma, they are treated as such.

465-B *(Campbell's, pp. 1056–1058)*

Renal oncocytoma accounts for 3 to 7 per cent of solid renocortical tumors. They are more common in men than women and generally have the same age incidence as that of renal cell carcinoma. Oncocytomas vary in size and have a median diameter of 6 cm. Grossly, the tumors have a typical appearance: usually tan or light brown in color, they are round, well circumscribed, encapsulated, and have a central stellate scar. Microscopically, the tumor is characterized by large eosinophilic cells with granular cytoplasm. Electron microscopy demonstrates the abundance of mitochondria that distinguishes this cell type from renal cell carcinoma. The typical cell appearance suggests an origin from the distal renal tubules.

Renal oncocytomas are usually asymptomatic, and the majority of tumors are discovered incidentally. No typical CT scan or MRI appearance has been identified. The typical arterial phase of the angiogram reveals a "spoke-wheel" or stellate pattern seldom associated with venous pooling or arteriovenous fistula. However, the angiogram may be indistinguishable from that of a hypovascular renal cell carcinoma.

REFERENCES

1. Lieber, M.M.: Renal oncocytoma: Prognosis and treatment. Eur. Urol., *18*(Suppl.2):17, 1990.
2. Lieber, M.M., and Tsukamato, T.: Renal oncocytoma. *In* deKernion, J.B., Pavone-Macaluso, M. (Eds.): Tumors of the Kidney. Baltimore, Williams and Wilkins, 1986, p. 257.
3. Noguiera, E., and Bannosch, P.: Cellular origin of rat renal oncocytoma. Lab. Invest., *59*:337, 1988.
4. Landier, J.F., Desligneres, S., Boccon-Gibod, L., and Steg, A.: Renal oncocytomas. Sem. Hop. Paris, *55*: 1275, 1979.

466-E *(Campbell's, p. 1058)*

The management of renal oncocytomas is dictated by two characteristic features: (1) the unreliability and nonspecificity of current radiographic studies, and (2) the possibility of the presence of malignant elements and oncocytoma cells in the same tumor. A reliable preoperative diagnosis of renal oncocytoma merits an attempt at more conservative surgery, i.e., partial nephrectomy. Radical nephrectomy is still the safest method of therapy unless contraindicated by other factors (e.g., solitary kidney, small size, poor renal function). For poor operative risks, "observation treatment" of suspected oncocytomas may be appropriate.

REFERENCE

1. Lieber, M.M.: Renal oncocytoma: Prognosis and treatment. Eur. Urol., *18*(Suppl. 2):17, 1990.

467-D *(Campbell's, pp. 1058–1061)*

Renal hamartomas (angiomyolipomas) are benign tumors that may occur as an isolated phenomenon or as part of the syndrome associated with tuberous sclerosis. Approximately 80 per cent of patients with tuberous sclerosis will be found to have renal hamartomas. This is a disease that is both hereditary and familial and is characterized by mental retardation, epilepsy, and adenoma sebaceum. Patients with tuberous sclerosis require careful screening for the presence of renal tumors.

Renal hamartomas are frequently bilateral. Microscopically, they are found to have three primary components—blood vessels, clusters of adipocytes, and sheets of smooth muscle. These tumors are usually asymptomatic; however, large tumors may cause local discomfort or gastrointestinal symptoms. Patients may also present with sudden pain or hypotension due to hemorrhage.

Ultrasound of these lesions reveals a solid, hyperechoic mass; however, the diagnostic procedure of choice at present is CT scan or MRI, which reveals the high fat content that accurately defines the presence of angiomyolipoma in most cases.

The management of angiomyolipoma is controversial; however, due to the multiplicity of these benign tumors, conservative surgery is recommended. Asymptomatic lesions can be observed with CT scans at regular intervals—any increase in size in these lesions can be managed with exploration. Symptomatic lesions should initially be treated with selective embolization or partial nephrectomy.

REFERENCES

1. McCollough, D.L., Scott, R., Jr., and Seybold, H.M.: Renal angiomyelolipoma (hematoma): Review of the literature and report of 7 cases. J. Urol., *105*:32, 1971.
2. Oesterling, J.E., Fishman, E.K., Goldman, S.M. and Marshall, F.F.: The management of renal angiomyolipoma. J. Urol., *135*:1121, 1986.

468-C *(Campbell's, pp. 1061–1062)*

Juxtaglomerular tumor is a rare, benign renal tumor that secretes renin. Young patients typically present with hypertension, elevated serum renin levels, and hyperaldosteronism. These tumors are typically small ($\leq$2–3 cm in diameter), and are often not detectable radiographically.

Fibromas are rare benign tumors of the renal parenchyma. They may grow to large size, become adherent to the kidney, and often resemble uterine fibroids. Angiographically, they are usually hypovascular. A radical nephrectomy is usually performed because of the uncertainty of the diagnosis.

Lipoma, leiomyoma, angioma, rhabdomyoma, neurofibroma, dermoid, and endometriosis are other rare, benign renal tumors.

REFERENCE

1. Orjauvik, O.S., Aas, M., Fauchald, P., et al.: Renin-secreting renal tumor with severe hypertension. Acta Med. Scand., *197*:329, 1975.

469-E *(Campbell's, p. 1062)*

Renal cell carcinoma is an uncommon tumor, accounting for approximately 3 per cent of adult malignancies and approximately 24,000 new cases per year in the United States. It is more common among urban dwellers and is more common in males by a factor of 2:1. Although it may occur in younger age groups, renal cell carcinoma occurs primarily in the 5th to 7th decades of life. It has been noted to occur with increased frequency in patients with tuberous sclerosis, von Hippel-Lindau disease, and other phakomatoses.

Renal cell carcinomas seem to arise from the proximal convoluted tubule, the same cell of origin as that of renal adenomas. Tobacco smokers have been noted to have an increased incidence of renal cell carcinoma. No definitive relationship between occupational and industrial carcinogens and renal carcinoma has been documented.

REFERENCES

1. Lauritsen, J.G.: Lindau's disease: A study of one family through six generations. Acta Chir. Scand., *139*:482, 1975.
2. Bennington, J.L., and Beckwith, J.B.: Tumors of the kidney, renal pelvis, and ureter. *In* Atlas of Tumor Pathology. Washington, D.C., Armed Forces Institute of Pathology, 1975, Facs. 12.
3. LaVecchia, C., Negri, E., D'Avanzo, B., and Franceschi, S.: Smoking and renal cell carcinoma. Cancer Res., *50*:5231, 1990.

470-C *(Campbell's, pp. 1062–1063)*

The most consistent chromosomal changes observed in renal cell carcinoma are deletions and translocations involving the short arm of chromosome 3 (3p). Transforming growth factors (TGFs) alpha and beta are two tumor-produced regulatory growth factors that may be related to the development of renal cell carcinoma.

Renal cell carcinoma remains relatively resistant to currently available chemotherapeutic agents. The basis for this appears to be related to 170-kilodalton transmembrane glycoprotein (P-glycoprotein, P170) and coded by the multidrug resistance 1 (MDR1) gene that functions as an energy-dependent drug efflux pump.

REFERENCES

1. Kovacs, G., Erlandsson, R., Boldog, F., et al.: Consistent chromosome 3p deletion and loss of heterozygosity in renal cell carcinoma. Proc. Natl. Acad. Sci. USA, *85*:1571, 1988.
2. Linehan, W.M., Robertson, C.N., Anglard, P., et al.: Clinical perspective—renal cell carcinoma: Potential biologic and molecular approaches to diagnosis and therapy. *In* Cancer Cells 7, Molecular Diagnostics of Human Cancer. Cold Spring Harbor Laboratory, 1989, p. 59.
3. Fojo, A.T., Shen, D.W., Mickley, L.A., et al.: Intrinsic drug resistance in kidney cancers is associated with expression of a human multidrug resistance gene. J. Clin. Oncol., *5*:1922, 1987.

471-D *(Campbell's, pp. 1064–1066)*

Although it is unusual to see absolutely pure examples, renal cell carcinomas can be broadly grouped into four histologic types: clear cell, granular cell, tubulopapillary, and sarcomatoid. A number of investigators have related various types of grading systems to prognosis; however, with any given stage, the microscopic grading has little significance as compared to some other tumors. Measurements of DNA ploidy may be the reflection of tumor heterogeneity and an indication of biologic potential; however, the clinical value of this technique remains to be determined for renal cell carcinoma.

REFERENCE

1. Murphy, W.M.: Diseases of the kidney. *In* Urological Pathology. Philadelphia, W.B. Saunders, 1989, p. 409.

472-A *(Campbell's, pp. 1066–1067)*

The classic triad of pain, hematuria, and flank mass occurs in approximately 10 per cent of patients and generally indicates advanced disease. The most frequent findings in patients with renal cell carcinoma are pain (41 per cent), hematuria (38 per cent), weight loss (36 per cent), mass (24 per cent), hypertension (22 per cent), fever (18 per cent), hypercalcemia (6 per cent), and erythropoiesis (<3 per cent). Few tumors are associated with such a diversity of paraneoplastic syndromes. Renal malignancies may elaborate parahormone-like factors, glucagon, insulin, and human chorionic gonadotropin. The most dramatic syndrome is associated with nonmetastatic hepatic dysfunction and is referred to as Staufer syndrome. Patients with this syndrome have abnormal liver function tests without hepatic metastasis. Return of liver function to normal after nephrectomy is a good prognostic sign. Persistence or recurrence of this syndrome is almost invariably associated with recurrence of the tumor.

REFERENCES

1. Sufrin, G., Chasan, S., Golio, A., and Murphy, G.P.: Paraneoplastic and serologic syndromes of renal adenocarcinomas. Semin. Urol., 7:158, 1989.
2. Boxer, R.J., Waisman, J., Leiber, M.M., et al.: Nonmetastatic hepatic dysfunction associated with renal carcinoma. J. Urol., *119*:468, 1978.

473-D *(Campbell's, pp. 1067–1072)*

With the greater use of ultrasound, CT, and MRI, the ability to detect renal tumors in earlier stages has significantly increased. In fact, many more renal masses are now being demonstrated with US and CT than with urography.

Ultrasound evaluation can usually distinguish among cystic, solid, and complex masses. The sonographic criteria for a simple benign cyst include an absence of internal echoes, a smooth, well-defined wall, and good through transmission with posterior acoustic enhancement. Solid lesions have variable echogenecity, no or little through transmission, and irregular shape. Any lesion that on ultrasound is not clearly a simple cyst should be studied further by CT scan. The role of MRI in the diagnosis and staging of renal cell carcinoma is currently under investigation, but MRI may be useful in patients with renal insufficiency or a history of allergy to contrast dyes. The emergence of CT and MRI has resulted in a marked narrowing of indications for angiography in the evaluation of renal masses. Angiography is useful in situations where parenchymal-sparing procedures are anticipated, e.g., solitary kidney or bilateral renal masses. Classic findings of renal cell carcinomas on angiography include neovascularity, arteriovenous fistulas, capsular vessels, and venous poolings.

REFERENCES

1. Lang, E.: Comparison of dynamic and conventional computed tomography, angiography, and ultrasonog-

raphy in the staging of renal cell carcinoma. Cancer, *54*:2205, 1984.
2. Stewart, R.R., and Dunnick, N.R.: Imaging renal neoplasms. Prob. Urol. *4*:175, 1990.

474-A *(Campbell's, pp. 1072–1074)*

The staging system most commonly employed in the United States is Robson's modification of the system of Flocks and Kadesky. In this system, stage I signifies tumor confirmed within the renal capsule; stage II is associated with tumor outside the kidney but confined to Gerota's fascia (which includes ipsilateral adrenal involvement). Stage III lesions involve the renal vein, inferior vena cava, or regional lymph nodes, and stage IV signifies involvement of adjacent organs or distant metastasis.

The tumor, node, metastasis (TNM) system for the staging of renal cell carcinoma is seen below:

Tx	primary tumor cannot be assessed
T0	no evidence of primary tumor
T1	tumor ≤2.5 cm in greatest dimension, limited to the kidney
T2	tumor >2.5 cm in greatest dimension, limited to the kidney
T3a	tumor invades adrenal gland or perinephric tissues but confined to Gerota's fascia
T3b	tumor extends into renal vein or vena cava
T4	tumor beyond Gerota's fascia
N0	no identifiable nodes
N1	metastasis in a single lymph node, ≤2 cm in greatest dimensions
N2	metastasis in lymph nodes >5 cm in greatest dimension
M0	tumor without distant metastasis
M1	tumor with distant metastasis

REFERENCES

1. Robson, C.J., Churchill, B.M., and Anderson, W.: The results of radical nephrectomy for renal cell carcinoma. Trans. Am. Assoc. Genetourin. Surg., *60*:122, 1968.
2. Hermanek, P., and Schrott, K.M.: Evaluation of the new tumor, nodes, and metastasis classification of renal cell carcinoma. J. Urol., *144*:238, 1990.

475-E *(Campbell's, pp. 1073–1074)*

The factors that have been associated with a poor prognosis in renal cell carcinoma are extension to regional lymph nodes, extension through Gerota's fascia, involvement of contiguous organs, distant metastasis, and renal vein involvement (although some studies have failed to show an increased risk of recurrence or decreased survival with renal vein or inferior vena caval involvement).

Involvement of the regional lymph nodes draining the renal parenchyma is a dire prognostic sign, associated with a 5-year survival rate of 0 to 30 per cent. Invasion through Gerota's fascia decreases the 5-year survival rate to approximately 45 per cent. Preliminary DNA flow cytometry data suggest that both prognosis and tumor progression rate may well correlate with nondiploid tumor patterns. In patients with localized bilateral renal tumors, the 5-year survival after bilateral partial nephrectomy is approximately 71 per cent. The size of the renal tumor is only indirectly correlated with survival.

REFERENCES

1. deKernion, J.B., and Berry, D.: The diagnosis and treatment of renal cell carcinoma. Cancer, *45*:1947, 1980.
2. Skinner, D.G., Pfister, R.F., and Colvin, R.: Extension of renal cell carcinoma into the vena cava: The rationale for aggressive surgical management. J. Urol., *107*: 711, 1972.

476-B *(Campbell's, pp. 1074–1076)*

Surgery remains the only effective method of treatment of primary renal cell carcinoma. Radical nephrectomy is the procedure of choice in patients with renal cell carcinoma and a normal contralateral kidney. Simple nephrectomy was practiced for decades but has been supplanted by radical nephrectomy, which is presumed, although not absolutely proved, to increase the surgical cure rate.

Radical nephrectomy accomplishes several objectives: (1) the adrenal gland, which is not infrequently involved, is excised; (2) lymphatic metastases are removed; (3) a more adequate margin away from the tumor is achieved; and (4) more adequate renal vein division is also accomplished.

REFERENCE

1. Patel, N.P., and Lavengood, R.W.: Renal cell carcinoma: Natural history and results of treatment. J. Urol., *119*:722, 1978.

477-C *(Campbell's, pp. 1074–1075)*

Regional lymphadenectomy is often added to radical nephrectomy, and increased survival has been attributed to removal of involved lymph nodes. Interpretation of the literature is difficult because the number and location of involved lymph nodes are often not stated as fully as other factors. On the other hand, several characteristics of renal carcinoma argue against a therapeutic role for lymphadenectomy. First, most patients with positive lymph nodes eventually have bloodborne metastases. Second, the lymphatic drainage of renal carcinoma is variable. Third, many patients without lymph node metastasis develop disseminated metastasis. Although the practical therapeutic value of lymphadenectomy is still uncertain, it can generally be accomplished simply and safely, and provides valuable staging information.

REFERENCES

1. deKernion, J.B.: Lymphadenectomy for renal cell carcinoma: Therapeutic implications. Urol. Clin. North Am., *7*:697, 1980.
2. Golimbu, M., Joshi, P., Sperber, A., et al.: Renal cell carcinoma: Survival and prognostic factors. Urology, *27*:291, 1986.

478-E *(Campbell's, p. 1075)*

Since the advent of sophisticated angiographic methods, preoperative occlusion of the renal artery has been advocated as an adjunct to radical nephrectomy. In patients with arteriovenous fistulas, pulmonary embolization can occur, and must be cautiously avoided. Hemorrhage is reduced, especially in patients with very large tumors supplied by many parasitized vessels. The renal vein can be ligated prior to dissection of the renal artery, and a host-immune stimulation has been attributed to renal infarction. However, a salutary effect on survival has not been demonstrated, and the procedure can be associated with complications that may compromise the ability of the patient to tolerate surgery. Early ligation of the renal vein can be performed safely without preoperative embolization if necessary; however, embolization may be a reasonable adjunct in patients with large vascular tumors, especially in the presence of large caval thrombi.

479-B *(Campbell's, p. 1076)*

In the patient with renal cell carcinoma involving a solitary kidney, partial nephrectomy in vivo, combined with regional hypothermia, is the most common approach. Although autotransplantation following ex vivo excision has been used, most tumors are now excised without the need for the "workbench" approach. In localized tumors, partial nephrectomy has been associated with a 5-year survival approaching 71 per cent. This survival is independent of whether a patient has tumor in the contralateral kidney. Survival is mostly dependent on the stage of the tumor. Total radical nephrectomy with dialysis is seldom necessary, but would depend on the size of the tumor and the amount of residual renal parenchyma.

REFERENCE

1. Marberger, M., Pugh, R.C.B., Auvert, J., et al.: Conservative surgery of renal carcinoma: The EIRSS experience. Br. J. Urol., *53*:528, 1981.

480-D *(Campbell's, pp. 1077–1078)*

The propensity for renal cell carcinoma to invade the renal veins and extend into the main renal vein is well recognized. Continued growth of the thrombus into the vena cava occurs in a small number of cases. Suspected extension of thrombus into the inferior vena cava should be evaluated with inferior venacavogram, CT, or MRI. Vena caval extension was once thought to be a dire prognostic sign; however, it is now recognized that most patients can still be cured surgically. The feasibility of resection of extensive caval thrombi and successful short-term outcome has been improved by collaboration with cardiac surgeons, resulting in decreased intraoperative hemorrhage. The current experience indicates that excision of renal cell carcinoma with caval extension remains the treatment of choice and can be safely performed, even with extension into the right atrium. However, patients with regional and distant metastases are rarely helped by radical excision.

Occasionally, the tumor may invade the wall of the vena cava. Resection of the cava is feasible, with preservation of a sleeve to accommodate venous drainage, or excision of an obstructed segment of the vena cava if necessary.

REFERENCES

1. Shefft, P., Norvick, A.C., Straffin, R.A., and Stewart, B.H.: Surgery for renal cell carcinoma extending into the inferior vena cava. J. Urol., *120*:P28, 1978.
2. Cherrie, R.J., Goldman, D.G., Lindner, A., and deKernion, J.B.: Prognostic implications of vena caval extension of renal cell carcinoma. J. Urol., *128*:910, 1982.
3. Clayman, R.V., Gonzalez, R., and Fraley, E.E.: Renal cell carcinoma invading the inferior vera cava: Clinical review and anatomical approach. J. Urol., *123*:157, 1980.

481-B *(Campbell's, pp. 1079–1084)*

In spite of the remarkable advances realized with the other tumors, renal cell carcinoma has remained refractory to chemotherapy. Vinblastine appears to be the most commonly used single agent; however, to date neither single agent nor combination chemotherapy has been found to be very effective.

Progesterone therapy continues to be a method of management in the absence of more effective agents. However, no proper study has proved the efficacy of these agents in the management of advanced renal cell carcinoma.

The theory underlying immunotherapy for metastatic renal carcinoma is that host immune functions play a role in tumor control, and that these immune functions can be further stimulated. Quesada and co-workers used alpha-interferon to treat patients with metastatic renal cell carcinoma with response rates of up to 26 per cent. Although interferons have unquestionable activity against renal cell carcinoma, most patients who respond are those with limited metastases, especially limited pulmonary metastases. Other agents used in the immunotherapy of metastatic renal cell carcinoma include interleukin-2 (IL-2), lymphokine-activated killer cells (LAK), and tumor-infiltrating lymphocytes (TIL).

Adjunctive nephrectomy (removal of the primary tumor in the patient with metastases for the purpose of either prolonging survival or causing regression of metastatic lesions) has been tried. Following adjunctive nephrectomy, regression of metastasis can be expected in less than 1 per cent of patients. Adjunctive nephrectomy is no longer recommended except for patients in planned treatment protocols, e.g., in conjunction with immunotherapy or other therapies. Palliative nephrectomy is best reserved for the control of severe hemorrhage, pain, or paraneoplastic syndromes. Presently, cryotherapy has no role in the treatment of renal cell carcinoma.

REFERENCES

1. Yagoda, A.: Chemotherapy of renal cell carcinoma: 1983–1989. Semin. Urol., 7:199, 1989.
2. Quesoda, J.R., Evans, L., Saks, S.R., et al.: Recombinant interferon alpha and gamma combination as treatment in metastatic renal cell carcinoma. J. Biol. Response Mod., 7:234, 1988.
3. Montie, J.E., Stewart, B.H., Straffon, R.A., et al.: The role of adjunctive nephrectomy in patients with metastatic renal cell carcinoma. J. Urol., *117*:272–275, 1977.

482-B *(Campbell's, pp. 1084–1085)*

Sarcomas constitute only about 2 to 3 per cent of malignant tumors of the kidney. Differentiation from renal cell carcinoma is usually difficult or impossible, except that angiographically, sarcomas are usually hypovascular without arteriovenous fistulas. Leiomyosarcomas are the most common variety, composing about 60 per cent of sarcomas. Virtually every other variety of sarcoma has been noted to arise from the kidney including osteogenic sarcoma, liposarcoma, fibrosarcoma, carcinosarcoma, angiosarcoma, rhabdomyosarcoma, malignant fibrous histiocytoma, and hemangiopericytomas.

The treatment of choice for renal sarcomas is radical nephrectomy; however, the prognosis is generally poor when patients are treated with surgery alone. Adjuvant chemotherapy may be beneficial, although these tumors are not very chemosensitive.

REFERENCE

1. Farrow, G.M., Harrison, E.G., Utz, D.C., and Remie, W.H.: Sarcomas and sarcomatoid and mixed malignant tumors of the kidney in adults. Cancer, *22*:545, 1968.

483-C *(Campbell's, pp. 1085–1087)*

Renal lymphomas are uncommon and generally occur as only one manifestation of the systemic disease. The lymphoma initially grows between the nephrons and subsequently expands and produces the typical lymphomatous mass. CT scan appears to be the method of choice in diagnosing renal lymphoma. The major diagnostic problem is differentiating a renal lymphoma mass from a renal cell carcinoma. CT-guided needle aspiration may help in arriving at a histologic diagnosis.

The treatment of renal lymphomas is usually the indicated systemic treatment of lymphoma, i.e., chemotherapy and radiotherapy. Nephrectomy is seldom, if ever, indicated, except in the case of a solitary lesion or in the patient with severe symptoms, such as uncontrollable hemorrhage.

REFERENCE

1. Silber, S.J., and Chang, C.Y.: Primary lymphoma of the kidney. J. Urol., *110*:282, 1973.

484-D *(Campbell's, p. 1087)*

Due to its profuse vascularity and high blood flow, the kidney is a frequent site of metastatic deposits from a variety of solid tumors and hematologic malignancies. Metastases to the kidney are seldom clinically identified and are most often discovered at autopsy. The most common solid tumor metastasizing to the kidney is lung carcinoma. Virtually every other solid neoplasm may metastasize to the kidney. The principal method of detection of metastatic lesions within the kidney, in patients who present with symptomatic metastases, is CT scan. With pyelographic or ultrasonographic identification, it is difficult to distinguish metastatic tumors from primary renal neoplasms.

REFERENCES

1. Klinger, M.E.: Secondary tumors of the genitourinary tract. J. Urol., *65*:144, 1951.
2. Barbaric, Z.L.: Genitourinary Radiology. New York, Thieme Medical Publishers, Inc., 1991, p. 171.

485-E *(Campbell's, pp. 1094–1095)*

In 1993, approximately 52,600 new cases of bladder cancer were diagnosed in the United States. Bladder cancer is 2.7 times more common in men than women, and is approximately 2 to 3 times more common in whites than blacks. The incidence of bladder cancer has been reported to be 30 to 50 per cent higher in the northern United States than in the South.

Bladder cancer is the fourth most common cause of cancer death in men (after lung, prostate, and colorectal cancer) accounting for approximately 5 per cent of all cancer deaths in men and about 3 per cent of all cancer deaths in women.

Although bladder cancer can occur at any age, it is generally a disease of the elderly, with the median age at diagnosis of approximately 67 to 70 years. Younger patients appear to have a more favorable prognosis because they present more frequently with superficial, low-grade tumors; however, grade-for-grade, the risk of disease progression is the same in young patients as in older patients.

REFERENCES

1. Silverberg, E., Boring, C.C., and Squires, T.S.: Cancer statistics, 1990. CA, *40*:9, 1990.
2. Morrison, A.S.: Advances in the etiology of urothelial cancer. Urol. Clin. North Am., *11*:557, 1984.
3. Wan, J., and Grosman, H.B.: Bladder carcinoma in patients age 40 years or younger. Cancer, *64*:178, 1989.

486-B *(Campbell's, pp. 1095–1098)*

Many data suggest that many bladder cancer are carcinogen-induced. Carcinogens produce lesions in the genome of the transitional epithelial cells, initiating the process of carcinogenesis.

It is estimated that occupational exposure (i.e., exposure to aromatic amines) accounts for 25 to 30 per cent of bladder cancer cases in the United States.

Cigarette smokers have up to a fourfold higher incidence of bladder cancer than nonsmokers. Other forms of tobacco use are associated with only a slightly increased risk for bladder cancer.

Consumption of large quantities of the analgesic phenacetin is associated with an increased risk for transitional cell carcinoma of the renal pelvis and bladder, with the latency period usually longer for bladder tumors (25 years) than for renal pelvic tumors (10 to 20 years). Other factors associated with an increased risk of bladder cancer include chronic cystitis, pelvic irradiation, and cyclophosphamide.

Metabolites of the amino acid tryptophan have been reported, though not proved, to be potentially carcinogenic.

REFERENCES

1. Morrison, A.S.: Advances in the etiology of urothelial cancer. Urol. Clin. North Am. *11*:557, 1984.

2. Piper, J.M., Tonascia, J., and Metanoshi, G.M.: Heavy phenacetin use and bladder cancer in women aged 20–49 years. N. Engl. J. Med., *313*:292, 1985.

487-C *(Campbell's, p. 1098)*

The urothelium of the normal bladder is a transitional cell epithelium three to seven cell layers thick. There is a basement cell layer upon which rests one or more layers of intermediate cells. The most superficial layer is composed of large flat umbrella cells, and the cells of the urothelium are oriented with the long axis of the oval nuclei being perpendicular to the basement membrane (cellular polarity). The urothelium rests on a lamina propria basement membrane which contains scattered muscle fibers, which are irregularly arranged.

REFERENCES

1. Koss, L.G., Esperanza, M.T. and Robbins, M.A.: Mapping cancerous and precancerous bladder changes: A study of the urothelium in ten surgically removed bladders. JAMA, *227*:281, 1974.
2. Keep, J.C., Pichl, M., and Miller, A., et al.: Invasive carcinomas of the urinary bladder: Evaluation of the tunica musculis mucosae involvement. Am. J. Clin. Pathol., *91*:575, 1989.

488-A *(Campbell's, pp. 1098–1100)*

The term epithelial hyperplasia is used to describe an increase in the number of cell layers without nuclear or architectural abnormalities, and included in this category are epithelial hyperplasia, inverted papilloma, cystitis cystica, and von Brunn's nests. Metaplastic changes include cystitis glandularis, nephrogenic adenoma, and squamous metaplasia.

Nephrogenic adenoma is a rare lesion that histologically resembles primitive renal collecting tubules. It is a metaplastic response of the urothelium to trauma, infection, or radiation therapy with little nuclear atypia or mitotic activity noted. It is more common in men and is often associated with symptoms of dysuria and frequency. Treatment of choice is transurethral resection.

REFERENCE

1. Navarre, R.J., Jr., Loening, S.A., Platz, C., et al.: Nephrogenic adenoma: A report of 9 cases and review of the literature. J. Urol., *127*:775, 1982.

489-E *(Campbell's, pp. 1102–1103)*

Carcinoma in situ (CIS) appears as a velvety patch of erythematous mucosa on cystoscopic examination. Histologically, it consists of poorly differentiated transitional cell carcinoma confined to the urothelium. It occurs more commonly in men, and urine cytopathology study results are positive in 80 to 90 per cent of patients with CIS.

CIS occurs only rarely in patients with well-differentiated, superficial bladder tumors. Its presence portends a poor prognosis with high tumor recurrence rates and a 40 to 83 per cent risk of progression to invasive cancer. Patients with marked urinary symptoms generally have a shorter interval preceding the development of invasive cancer.

In the early 1970s, radical cystectomy was recommended for carcinoma in situ. In recent years, intravesical therapy has become the preferred primary treatment for CIS, and the most effective agent is bacillus Calmette-Guérin (BCG). Radiation therapy and systemic chemotherapy are not effective in the treatment of CIS.

REFERENCES

1. Utz, D.C., and Farrow, G.M.: Carcinoma in situ of the urinary tract. Urol. Clin. North Am., *11*:735, 1984.
2. Soloway, M.S.: Intravesical and systemic chemotherapy in the management of superficial bladder cancer. Urol. Clin. North Am., *11*:623, 1984.
3. Coplen, D.E., Marcus, M.D., Myers, J.A., et al.: Long-term follow up of patients treated with one or two 6-week courses of intravesical bacillus Calmette-Guérin: Analysis of possible predictors of response free of tumor. J. Urol., *144*:652, 1992.

490-B *(Campbell's, p. 1103)*

More than 90 per cent of bladder cancers are transitional cell carcinomas. These tumors differ from normal urothelium by having an increased number of epithelial cell layers with papillary folding of the mucosa, loss of cell polarity, abnormal cell maturation from the basal to superficial layers, giant cells, nuclear crowding, increased nuclear-cytoplasmic ratio, prominent nucleoli, clumping of chromatin, and increased number of mitoses.

REFERENCE

1. Koss, L.G.: Tumors of the urinary bladder. *In* Atlas of Tumor Pathology, Second Series, Fascile 11, Washington, D.C., Armed Forces Institute of Pathology, 1975, p. 1.

491-E *(Campbell's, pp. 1105–1107)*

Transitional cell epithelium has a great metaplastic potential. Therefore, transitional cell carcinomas have been found to contain spindle cell, squamous cell, or adenocarcinomatous elements in up to 30 per cent of cases. Transitional cell carcinomas arise most commonly in the trigone/bladder base area and on the lateral walls; however, they may arise anywhere within the bladder. It is not unusual for different tumor types to coexist in the same bladder, with the most frequent combination being a papillary transitional cell carcinoma with flat carcinoma in situ. The presence of these metaplastic elements in a transitional cell carcinoma does not change the principal classification of the tumor as a transitional cell carcinoma.

A strong correlation exists between tumor grade and prognosis; however, the correlation between tumor stage (Ta to T4) and prognosis is even stronger.

REFERENCES

1. Koss, L.G.: Tumor of the urinary bladder. *In*: Atlas of Tumor Pathology, Second Series, Fascile 11. Washing-

ton, D.C., Armed Forces Institute Pathology, p. 1, 1975.
2. Jewett, H.J., and Strong, G.H.: Infiltrating carcinoma of the bladder: Relation of depth of penetration of the bladder wall to incidence of local extension and metastasis. J. Urol., *55*:366, 1946.

492-A *(Campbell's, pp. 1107–1108)*

Considerable variability is noted in the prevalence of squamous cell carcinoma (SCC) of the bladder in different parts of the world. For example, SCC accounts for only about 1 per cent of bladder cancers in England, 3 to 7 per cent in the United States, but more than 75 per cent in Egypt. SCC can be divided into two categories. First, bilharzial bladder cancers are associated with chronic infection with *S. hematobium* and account for 80 per cent of SCC in Egypt. They occur in patients who are, on the average, 10 to 20 years younger than patients with transitional cell carcinoma, and are usually well differentiated with a relatively low incidence of lymph node and distant metastasis. Second, nonbilharzial SCC are usually associated with chronic irritation. Cigarette smoking has also been reported to be significantly associated with an increased risk of SCC. Male predominance is less striking in SCC (1.3:1) than in transitional cell carcinoma. Treatment of choice in muscle invasion SCC is radical cystectomy. Radiation therapy and chemotherapy are ineffective in SCC of the bladder. While SCC more commonly presents with invasive disease, stage-for-stage, the prognosis of SCC is comparable to that of transitional cell carcinoma.

REFERENCES

1. Ghoneim, M.A., Awad, H.K.: Results of treatment in carcinoma of the bilharzial bladder. J. Urol., *123*:850, 1980.
2. Bejany, E.C., Lockhart, J.L., and Rhamy, R.K.: Malignant vesical tumors following spinal cord injury. J. Urol., *138*:1390, 1987.

493-B *(Campbell's, pp. 1108–1109)*

Adenocarcinoma accounts for less than 2 per cent of primary bladder cancers. They are classified into three groups: (1) primary vesical, (2) urachal, and (3) metastatic.

Primary vesical adenocarcinoma most commonly arises at the base or the dome of the bladder. Adenocarcinoma is the most common type of cancer in exstrophic bladders. These tumors usually develop in response to chronic inflammation and irritation. Most bladder adenocarcinomas are mucin-producing, poorly differentiated, and invasive at diagnosis. Radical cystectomy with pelvic lymphadenectomy offers the best chance for cure.

Urachal carcinomas are extremely rare tumors. Adenocarcinoma is the most common histologic type. Patients with urachal adenocarcinomas have a worse prognosis than those with primary bladder adenocarcinoma. Tumors treated with partial cystectomy have local recurrence rates between 15 and 50 per cent; therefore, radical cystectomy with bilateral pelvic lymphadenectomy and en block excision of the urachus is the treatment of choice for all except the small, well-differentiated urachal carcinomas. As with other adenocarcinomas, radiation therapy and chemotherapy are ineffective in urachal carcinomas.

One of the most common forms of adenocarcinoma of the bladder is metastatic adenocarcinoma. The sites of origin for these tumors include the rectum, stomach, breast, prostate, endometrium, and ovary.

REFERENCES

1. Kantor, A.F., Hartge, P., Hoover, R.N., et al.: Epidemiological characteristics of squamous cell carcinoma and adenocarcinoma of the bladder. Cancer Res., *48*: 3853, 1988.
2. Sheldon, C.A., Clayman, R.V., Gonzolez, R., et al.: Malignant urachal lesions. J. Urol., *131*:1, 1984.
3. Klinger, M.E.: Secondary tumors of the genitourinary tract. J. Urol., *65*:144, 1951.

494-B *(Campbell's, p. 1110)*

The common sites of vascular metastasis from bladder cancer are liver, 38 per cent; lung, 36 per cent; bone, 27 per cent; adrenal gland, 21 per cent; and intestine, 13 per cent. Lymphatic metastasis occur earlier and independent of hematogenous metastasis in some patients. In fact, the most common sites of metastases in bladder cancer are the pelvic lymph nodes, occurring in about 78 per cent of patients. Among these, the obturator nodes are involved in 74 per cent, the external iliac nodes in 65 per cent, the juxtaregional common iliac nodes in 20 per cent, and perivesical nodes in 16 per cent.

REFERENCES

1. Babaian, R.J., Johnson, D.E., Llamos, L., et al.: Metastasis from transitional cell carcinoma of the urinary bladder. Urology, *16*:142, 1980.
2. Smith, J.A. Jr., and Whitmore, W.F. Jr.: Regional lymph node metastasis from bladder cancer. J. Urol., *126*: 591, 1981.

495-C *(Campbell's, pp. 1111–1113)*

The most clinically useful prognostic parameters for tumor recurrence and subsequent cancer progression in the patient with a superficial bladder tumor are tumor grade, tumor stage, and the presence of carcinoma in situ.

Tumor grade and depth of invasion are also the most important factors in predicting the likelihood of lymph node metastasis in patients with invasive bladder cancer.

REFERENCES

1. Fitzpatrick, J.M., West, A.B., Butler, M.R., et al.: Superficial bladder tumors (stage pTa, grades 1 and 2): The importance of recurrence pattern following initial resection. J. Urol., *135*:920, 1986.
2. Kern, W.H.: The grade and pathologic stage of bladder cancer. Cancer, *53*:1185, 1984.

496-D *(Campbell's, p. 1113)*

The most common presenting symptom of bladder cancer is painless hematuria, which occurs in approximately 85 per cent of patients. Irritative voiding symptoms (e.g., frequency, urgency, dysuria) constitute the second most common form of presentation, and are usually associated with diffuse CIS or invasive bladder cancers. Other signs and symptoms of bladder cancer include flank pain from ureteral obstruction, lower extremity edema, pelvic mass, weight loss, or bone pain.

REFERENCE

1. Varkarokic, M.J., Garta, J., Moore, R.H., et al.: Superficial bladder tumor: Aspects of clinical progression. Urology, *4*:414, 1974.

497-D *(Campbell's, pp. 1113–1115)*

Malignant transitional cells can be observed on microscopic examination of the urinary sediment or bladder washings. The limitations of microscopic cytology are due to the fact that cells from well-differentiated tumors are cytologically normal-appearing and are not readily shed into the urine. False-positive cytologic findings may occur in 1 to 12 per cent of patients, and false-negative results can be expected in up to 20 per cent of patients.

Saline bladder washings are more accurate than voided urine samples. In urine that has remained in the bladder for prolonged periods, cellular degeneration occurs; therefore, first-voided morning specimens should not be sampled for cytology. Urinary tract infections, indwelling catheters, calculi, or bladder instrumentation can produce artifactual changes in urinary cytology. If sheets of transitional cells are sheared off by one of these, the cell fragments may be mistaken for tumor fragments. Osmotic changes from contrast media may also cause difficulties in interpreting cytologic preparations.

REFERENCE

1. Gamarra, M.C., and Zein, T: Cytologic spectrum of bladder cancer. Urology, *23*:23, 1984.

498-C *(Campbell's, pp. 1115–1116)*

The ideal method for resecting a bladder tumor is to first resect the superficial portion of the tumor. Then, the deep portion along with some underlying bladder muscle is resected and sent as a separate specimen for histologic examination. After the tumor has been completely resected, the base is fulgurated. It is not always necessary to perform a formal resection of superficial low-grade papillary tumors, especially those that are difficult to reach with the resectoscope. Although it does not provide tumor for histologic study, it is acceptable to treat these tumors with simple fulguration.

If a tumor is very extensive and broad-based (i.e., almost certain to require cystectomy), it is not always necessary to attempt complete resection. In some cases, it may be more prudent to begin resection at the margin of the tumor resecting only enough tissue to establish the presence of muscle invasion, with frozen section documenting the adequacy of the biopsy specimens.

Tumors encroaching on the ureteral orifices should be resected. It is important not to fulgurate the orifice after tumor resection, and a ureteral stent may be left in place for several days to prevent obstruction of the orifice by scar.

Resection of tumors on the lateral bladder wall can be performed with the patient under general anesthesia with intravenous administration of pancuronium to minimize the risk of inadvertent bladder perforation associated with the obturator reflux.

Tumors arising in a bladder diverticulum are best treated with partial or total cystectomy. Transurethral resection carries a the high risk of bladder perforation.

REFERENCE

1. Soloway, M.S.: The management of superficial bladder cancer. *In* Javadpour, N. (Ed.): Principles and Management of Urologic Cancer. Baltimore, Williams & Wilkins, 1983, p. 446.

499-E *(Campbell's, pp. 1116–1118)*

Because tumor stage is important in determining therapy, accurate staging of bladder cancer is desirable. The first treatment decision based on tumor stage is whether the patient has a superficial or invasive tumor. The most important test for judging the depth of penetration of the tumor is the primary transurethral resection of the tumor.

The second treatment decision made on the basis of stage is based on the identification of patients with invasive tumors who may benefit from aggressive, potentially curative therapy. For this purpose, CT scanning, ultrasonography, and magnetic resonance imaging (MRI) have been used but are inaccurate in determining the presence or absence of microscopic muscle invasion or minimal extravesical tumor spread.

Pelvic lymphadenectomy is the most accurate means of staging bladder cancer patients for regional lymph node involvement, and is usually performed in conjunction with cystectomy rather than as an independent procedure. In patients with limited pelvic lymph node metastases, the performance of cystectomy and pelvic lymph node dissection may be associated with cure rates of 10 to 35 per cent.

A metastatic evaluation to rule out distant metastases should be performed before pelvic lymphadenectomy. The recommended metastatic evaluation for patients with invasive bladder cancer includes chest radiography, excretory urogram, abdominopelvic CT scan has also been recommended, though one must be cautious about overinterpretation, and bone scan is recommended in patients with elevated alkaline phosphatase or bone pain and liver function tests.

REFERENCE

1. Skinner, D.G.: Management of invasive bladder cancer: A meticulous pelvic lymph node dissection can make a difference. J. Urol., *128*:34, 1982.

500-B *(Campbell's, pp. 1118–1119)*

Two main staging systems for bladder cancer are currently in use. In the United States, most urologists choose the Jewett-Strong system as modified by Marshall. The other staging system is the tumor, node, metastasis system (TNM) developed jointly by the International Union Against Cancer and the American Joint Committee on Cancer Staging. These staging systems are seen below.

Finding	Jewett-Strong Marshall Stage	1987 TNM Stage
No tumor in specimen	0	T0
CIS	0	Tis
Papillary tumor confined to mucosa	0	Ta
Submucosal invasion	A	T1
Superficial muscle invasion	B_1	T2
Deep muscle invasion	B_2	T3a
Invasion of perivesical fat	C	T3b
Invasion of contiguous organs	D_1	T4
Regional lymph node metastasis	D_1	N1-3
Juxtaregional lymph node metastasis	D_2	N1-3
Distant metastasis	D_2	M1

REFERENCES

1. Marshall, V.F.: The relation of the preoperative estimate to the pathologic demonstration of the extent of vesical neoplasms. J. Urol., *68*:714, 1952.
2. Hermanck, P., and Sobin, L.H. (Eds): UICC — International Union Against Cancer TNM Classification of Malignant Tumors, ed. 4. Heidelberg, Springer-Verlag, 1987, p. 135.

501-B *(Campbell's, pp. 1119–1120)*

Most patients with superficial bladder cancer can be adequately treated with transurethral resection or fulguration of the tumor. The overall survival rate for these patients is approximately 70 per cent at 5 years. The traditional follow up program recommended for patients with superficial bladder cancer includes serial cystoscopies every 3 months for 2 years, then every 6 months for 2 years, and yearly thereafter. Annual excretory urograms have also been recommended. Follow-up cystoscopy can be readily performed as an office procedure with the flexible cystoscope.

Either adjuvant intravesical chemotherapy or intravesical immunotherapy is indicated in patients who are at a high risk for tumor recurrence, including patients with recurrent tumors, multiple tumors, high-grade tumors (II or greater), lamina propria invasion, or carcinoma in situ.

REFERENCE

1. Rubben, H., Lutzeyer, W., Fischer, N., et al.: Natural history and treatment of low and high risk superficial bladder tumors. J. Urol., *139*:283, 1988.

502-D *(Campbell's, pp. 1120–1121)*

Triethylenethiophosphoramide (Thiotepa) is an alkylating agent that acts by cross-linking nuclear acids and proteins. A frequently recommended regimen includes 30 mg in 30 ml of saline for 6 weekly treatments. Thiotepa is less valuable for the treatment of CIS. Because of its low molecular weight, thiotepa is readily absorbed through the urothelium and causes myelosuppression in 15 to 20 per cent of patients. White blood cell and platelet counts should be obtained before each thiotepa treatment.

Etoglucid (Epodyl), available in Europe but not in the United States, is an alkylating agent similar to thiotepa but with a slightly higher molecular weight. It, therefore, causes myelosuppression less frequently than thiotepa; however, it causes a more severe chemical cystitis. It is commonly administered in a 1 per cent solution weekly for 12 weeks, and then monthly thereafter.

Mitomycin C is an antibiotic chemotherapeutic agent that acts by inhibition of DNA synthesis. It has a higher molecular weight than thiotepa or etoglucid, and, therefore, causes fewer problems via transurothelial absorption. It is usually administered in a dose of 20 to 40 mg intravesically weekly for 6 to 8 weeks. Monthly maintenance therapy has been recommended but has not been demonstrated to be superior. Genital skin rashes have been noted with the use of mitomycin C in up to 15 per cent of patients.

Doxorubicin is also an antibiotic chemotherapeutic agent with a high molecular weight. A variety of dose schedules have been proposed. Epirubicin is an agent with characteristics similar to Adriamycin.

All agents for intravesical chemotherapy are about equally effective with the possible exception that etoglucid was reported to be more effective than doxorubicin in preventing tumor recurrences in patients with primary bladder cancers. The complete response rates for these agents range from 33 to 57 per cent for the treatment of residual papillary tumors, 55 to 66 per cent for the treatment of CIS, and approximately 60 per cent when used as prophylaxis against tumor recurrence.

Thiotepa and BCG are the least expensive intravesical agents available. Mitomycin C is the most expensive.

REFERENCES

1. Soloway, M.S.: The management of superficial bladder cancer. *In* Javadpour, N. (Ed.): Principles and Management of Urologic Cancer. Baltimore, Williams and Wilkins, 1983, p. 446.
2. Kurth, K.H., Schroder, F.H., Tunn, U., et al.: Adjuvant chemotherapy of superficial transitional cell bladder carcinoma: Preliminary results of a European Organization for Research on Treatment of Cancer randomized trial comparing doxorubicin, hydrochloride, etoglucid, and transurethral resection alone. J. Urol., *132*:258, 1984.
3. Newling, D.: Intravesical therapy in the management of superficial transitional cell carcinoma of the bladder: Experience of the EORTC group. Br. J. Cancer, *61*:497, 1990.

503-D *(Campbell's, pp. 1122–1124)*

BCG, an attenuated strain of *Mycobacterium bovis* with stimulatory effects on immune responses, has emerged as the most effective intravesical agent for the treatment of superficial bladder cancer.

Prospective randomized trials have shown that BCG is effective for prophylaxis against tumor recurrence. It has also been used to treat residual unresectable tumors, although BCG should not be considered as a substitute for the resection of resectable tumors. BCG has been reported to delay tumor progression. BCG is perhaps most useful in the treatment of CIS, with response rates of up to 89 per cent. Studies suggest that patients who fail to respond to initial induction therapy may respond to a second, more intensive regimen. The alterative therapy for failure to 2 courses of BCG depends on the type of tumor present at the time of failure. Low-grade superficial tumors can be treated with other intravesical agents; however, in patients with high-grade or invasive tumors, cystectomy should be considered.

The main side effect of BCG therapy is bladder irritability, occurring in up to 91 per cent of patients. Other side effects include hematuria (46 per cent), low-grade fever (24 per cent), malaise (18 per cent), chills (8 per cent), arthralgias (2 per cent), and granulomatous prostatitis. Symptoms severe enough to require antitubercular antibiotics occur in up to 6 per cent of patients. Patients having fever persisting for more than 48 hours following intravesical BCG therapy and not responding to antipyretics should be treated with oral isoniazid, 300 mg/day, plus pyridoxine, 50 mg/day. Patients with more prolonged or severe symptoms should be treated with isoniazid, pyridoxine, and rifampicin, 600 mg/day. Corticosteroids (40 mg prednisone daily) have been recommended for severe reactions. No data exist on the necessary duration of treatment for symptomatic disseminated BCG infections. It is possible that a 6-week course of treatment may suffice; however, it is prudent to recommend a 3- to 6-month course. BCG administration is contraindicated in immunocompromised or pregnant patients, in patients with cystitis, or after traumatic catheterization.

REFERENCES

1. Lamm, D.L.: Intravesical therapy of superficial bladder cancer. AUA Update, 2:2, 1983.
2. Lamm, D.L., Stogdill, V.D., Stogdill, B.J., et al.: Complications of bacillus Calmette-Guérin immunotherapy in 1,278 patients with bladder cancer. J. Urol., *135*: 272, 1986.
3. Herr, H.W., Laudone, V.P., Badalament, R.A., et al.: Bacillus Calmette-Guérin therapy alters the progression of superficial bladder cancer. J. Clin. Oncol., 6: 1450, 1988.

504-B *(Campbell's, pp. 1125–1128)*

In recent years, two essentially different approaches to the treatment of muscle-invasive bladder cancer have been adopted: (1) bladder preservation and (2) bladder reconstruction. Radical cystectomy, the most effective local therapy for patients with bladder cancer, is associated with pelvic recurrence rates of only 10 to 20 per cent as compared with recurrence rates of 50 to 70 per cent with radiation therapy alone, chemotherapy alone, or combination of the two. The operative mortality of radical cystectomy is less than 2 per cent.

Transurethral resection should probably be reserved for patients with small, low-grade tumors with only superficial muscle invasion and for patients who are not medically fit for cystectomy.

Partial cystectomy is a legitimate treatment option in selected patients with solitary invasive bladder cancer who cannot be managed safely with transurethral resection and who have no prior history of bladder tumor. Severe atypia or CIS elsewhere in the bladder and inability to achieve adequate margins and still preserve bladder function are contraindications to partial cystectomy. Disturbingly high tumor recurrence rates (70 per cent) have been reported in patients with high-grade tumors treated with partial cystectomy.

REFERENCES

1. Herr, H.W.: Conservative management of muscle-infiltrating bladder cancer: Prospective experience. J. Urol., *138*:1162, 1987.
2. Montie, J.E., Straffon, R.A., and Stewart, B.H.: Radical cystectomy without radiation therapy for carcinoma of the bladder. J. Urol., *131*:477, 1984.
3. Resnick, M.I., and O'Connor, V.J., Jr.: Segmental resection for carcinoma of the bladder: Review of 102 patients. J. Urol., *109*:1007, 1973.

505-E *(Campbell's, pp. 1131–1133)*

Chemotherapeutic agents that have documented activity against transitional cell carcinoma include cisplatin, methotrexate, vinblastine, and doxorubicin. Combination therapy with three or four of these drugs is associated with higher objective response rates than with my single-agent therapy. The four-drug combination, MVAC, is believed to be the most effective regimen currently available, with overall response rates of 57 to 70 per cent.

Intra-arterial chemotherapy does not appear to be effective in treating lymph node metastases; however, some favorable responses have been noted in patients with metastatic disease, suggesting that intra-arterial infusion may increase the therapeutic index of chemotherapy. Granulocyte colony-stimulating factor is another agent that may aid in the chemotherapy of metastatic bladder cancer by allowing the use of higher doses of chemotherapeutic agents and decreasing the interval between cycles. Side effects of the growth factor include skin rash, fever, malaise, hypotension, chest pain, and pleuritis.

Systemic chemotherapy has been employed as an adjunct to both radical cystectomy and radiation therapy; however, these trials have yielded conflicting results. To date, no generally accepted prospective, randomized trials demonstrate the effectiveness of adjuvant chemotherapy.

REFERENCES

1. Sternberg, C.N., Yagoda, A., Scher, H.I., et al.: Preliminary results of MVAC (methotrexate, vinblastine, doxorubicin, and cisplatin) for transitional cell carcinoma of the urothelium. J. Urol., *133*:403, 1985.
2. Troner, M., Brick, R., Omura, G.A., et al.: Phase III comparison of cisplatin alone versus cisplatin, doxorubicin, and cyclophosphamide in the treatment of bladder (urothelial) cancer: A Southeastern Cancer Study Group Trial. J. Urol., *137*:660, 1987.
3. Logothetis, C.J., Dexeus, F.H., Sella, A., et al.: Escalated therapy for refractory urothelial tumors: Methotrexate-vinblastine-doxorubicin-cisplatin plus unglycosylated recombinant human granulocyte-macrophage colony-stimulating factor. JNCI, *82*:667, 1990.
4. Soloway, M.S.: Learning to integrate systemic chemotherapy into a treatment plan for patients with advanced bladder cancer. J. Urol., *133*:440, 1985.

506-A *(Campbell's, pp. 1133–1136)*

Leiomyosarcoma is the most common malignant mesenchymal tumor of the bladder occurring in adults. It is twice as common in men as in women. Grossly, it appears as a submucosal nodular or ulcerating mass. Histologically, spindle cells are arranged in parallel bundles. The treatment of choice is radical cystectomy. Other sarcomas of the bladder include rhabdomyosarcoma (most common in young children), angiosarcoma, liposarcoma, chondrosarcoma, and osteosarcoma. The most effective treatment for these tumors is also total cystectomy; however, the prognosis of patients with bladder sarcoma is generally poor regardless of treatment.

Primary bladder lymphoma is the second most common nonepithelial bladder tumor. The peak age at diagnosis is 40 to 60 years, and women are affected more often than men. The treatment of choice is radiation therapy, with or without chemotherapy, depending on the extent of tumor.

Bladder pheochromocytoma accounts for less than 1 per cent of all bladder tumors and less than 1 per cent of all pheochromocytomas. They arise from paraganglionic cells within the bladder wall. There is no sex predilection, and the peak age of incidence is between 20 and 40 years. Most bladder pheochromocytomas are metabolically active, causing paroxysmal attacks of hypertension on filling and emptying of the bladder in two thirds of patients. Hematuria is noted in approximately 50 per cent of patients. The treatment of choice is partial cystectomy.

Other nonurothelial bladder tumors include small-cell carcinoma and carcinosarcoma, both rare and associated with uniformly poor prognosis. Aggressive management with radical cystoprostatectomy is the treatment of choice for these tumors.

The bladder may be secondarily involved by cancers from any other primary site. The most common primary sites are melanoma, colon, prostate, lung, and breast.

REFERENCES

1. Swartz, D.A., Johnson, D.E., Ayala, A.E., et al.: Bladder leiomyosarcoma: A review of 10 cases with 5-year follow-up. J. Urol., *133*:200, 1985.
2. Koss, L.G.: Tumors of the urinary bladder. *In* Atlas of Tumor Pathology, Second Series, Fascile 11. Washington, D.C., Armed Forces Institute of Pathology, 1975, p. 1.

507-C *(Campbell's, pp. 1137–1140)*

Upper urinary tract epithelial tumors are relatively uncommon, accounting for 5 to 10 per cent of all renal tumors and about 5 per cent of all urothelial tumors. They are twice as common in men as in women with the peak incidence being in the sixth and seventh decades of life. Risk factors for upper tract urothelial tumors are similar to those for bladder cancer and include occupational exposure to aromatic amines, cigarette smoking, analgesic abuse, chronic infection or irritation, and exposure to cyclophosphamide.

Bilateral involvement occurs in 2 to 5 per cent of upper track transitional cell carcinoma, and upper tract tumors occur in 2 to 4 per cent of patients with bladder cancer. Approximately 30 to 75 per cent of patients with upper tract urothelial tumors will develop bladder tumors at some time.

Ureteral tumors are located most commonly in the lower ureter and least commonly in the upper ureter.

Transitional cell carcinoma accounts for more than 90 per cent of upper tract urothelial tumors; squamous cell carcinomas account for up to 7 per cent of upper urinary tract tumors; and adenocarcinoma represents less than 1 per cent of upper urinary tract tumors. Rarely, sarcomas occur in the upper urinary tract. Surgical excision is the preferred treatment.

The most common presenting symptom of upper tract urothelial tumors is gross hematuria, occurring in about 75 per cent of patients. Other symptoms include flank pain (approximately 30 per cent), flank mass, weight loss, anorexia, or bone pain. The natural history of this disease reveals a high correlation between tumor stage and grade and progression.

The diagnosis of upper tract urothelial tumors is made using a combination of modalities including intravenous urography, retrograde urography, cytology, and ureteropyeloscopy with biopsy as needed.

REFERENCES

1. Fraley, E.E.: Cancer of the renal pelvis. *In* Skinner, D.G., and deKernion, J.B. (Eds.): Genitourinary Cancer. Philadelphia, W.B. Saunders Co., 1978, p. 134.
2. Babarian, R.J., and Johnson, D.E.: Primary carcinoma of the ureter. J. Urol., *123*:357, 1980.
3. Gittes, R.F.: Retrograde brushing and nephroscopy in the diagnosis of upper-tract urothelial cancer. Urol. Clin. North Am., *11*:617, 1984.

508-E *(Campbell's, pp. 1143–1144)*

Two staging systems are commonly used for transitional cell carcinoma of the upper urinary tract. These include the staging system described by Grabstald and coworkers and the TNM staging system. These systems are seen below.

Finding	Grabstald–Cummings Stage	1987 UICC Stage
Carcinoma in situ	I	Tis
Noninvasive papillar tumor	I	Ta
Tumor involving submucosa	II	T1
Muscle-invasive tumor	III	T2
Tumor invading renal parenchyma	III	T3
Tumor invading peripelvic or periureteral tissue	III	T3
Invasion of contiguous organs or beyond renal capsule	IV	T4
Lymph node metastases	IV	N (1-3)
Distant metastases	IV	MI

REFERENCES

1. Grabstald, H., Whitmore, W.F., and Melamed, M.R.: Renal pelvic tumors. JAMA, *218*:845, 1971.
2. Spiessl, B., Beahrs, O.H., Hermanek, P., et al.: Renal pelvis and ureter. *In* Spiessl, B., Beahrs, O.H., Hermanek, P., Hutter, R.V., Scheibe, O., Sobin, L.H., and Wagoner, G. (Eds.): UICC-TNM Atlas Illustrated Guide to the TNM/pTNM-Classification of Malignant Tumors. Berlin, Springer-Verlag, 1989, p. 260.

509-C, 510-B *(Campbell's, pp. 1144–1146)*

Current data suggest that the following generalizations are valid concerning the treatment of upper tract urothelial tumors. Patients with low-grade, low-stage tumors do well with either conservative or radical surgery. Patients with intermediate grade tumors do better with radical surgery. Patients with high-grade, high-stage tumors do equally poorly with either conservative or radical surgery.

With conservative surgery, tumor recurrence rates in the retained ipsilateral collecting system vary from 7 to 60 per cent; however, little evidence exists that recurrences compromise patient survival.

Patients with only positive cytologic findings of the upper tracts and normal radiographic findings and ureteroscopic examinations should be followed closely with excretory or retrograde urography and should *not* be treated blindly.

The traditional treatment for upper tract urothelial tumors is total nephroureterectomy with excision of a cuff of bladder due to the high incidence of tumor recurrence in the ureteral stump in patients treated with more conservative operations. Conservative excision of upper tract urothelial tumors can be considered in patients with low-grade, low-stage tumors or in patients in whom renal sparing surgery is needed (i.e., bilateral tumors, or solitary kidneys). In patients with renal pelvic tumors, conservative surgery is only recommended in situations in which it is necessary to avoid renal failure.

Limited data exist on the results of endoscopic management of upper tract urothelial tumors; however, only patients with small, single, low-grade tumors should be considered for this approach. Only anecdotal information is available concerning instillation therapy for upper tract urothelial tumors.

The chemotherapeutic regimens for the treatment of upper tract urothelial tumors are the same as those for the treatment of bladder cancer; however, long-term results have been disappointing.

REFERENCES

1. Murphy, D.M., Zincke, H., and Furlow, W.L.: Management of high grade transitional cell cancer of the upper urinary tract. J. Urol., *135*:25, 1981.
2. Zungri, E., Chechile, G., Algaba, F., et al.: Treatment of transitional cell carcinoma of the ureter: Is the controversy justified? Eur. Urol., *17*:276, 1990.
3. Tannock, I., Gospodarowicz, M., Connolly, J., et al.: MVAC chemotherapy for transitional cell carcinoma: The Princess Margaret Hospital experience. J. Urol., *142*:28, 1989.

511-E *(Campbell's, pp. 1159–1160)*

Adenocarcinoma of the prostate is the most common internal cancer of males in the United States, and the second most common cause of cancer deaths in males. No consistent evidence exists for substantial risk factors associated with diet, occupation, socioeconomic status, infectious disease history, sexual practices, body build, or hormonal factors.

The differences between countries in mortality rate and incidence of clinical prostate cancer are striking, with the United States near the high end of the continuum and Japan near the low end. In the United States, blacks have a mortality rate for prostate cancer that is two to three times the rate for whites; however, in an autopsy study, the frequency of incidental prostate cancer was found to be similar between the two races.

A probable role for genetic factors in prostate cancer has also been uncovered in several studies of familial aggregation in prostate cancer cases. A two- to threefold increase in risk has been reported for men having a father or brother with clinical carcinoma of the prostate, and the relative risk may exceed 5 if two or more first-degree relatives have had clinical prostate cancer.

REFERENCES

1. Carter, B.S., Carter, H.B., and Isaacs, J.T.: Epidemiologic evidence regarding predisposing factors to prostate cancer. Prostate, *16*:187, 1990.
2. Steinberg, G.D., Carter, B.S., Beaty, T.H., et al.: Family history and the risk of prostate cancer. Prostate, *17*: 337, 1990.

512-B *(Campbell's, pp. 1162–1164)*

Acinar adenocarcinoma comprises more than 95 per cent of all prostate cancers, and more than 90 per cent of the remainder are transitional cell carcinomas. These cancers are derived from a common precursor cell type, the embryonic urogenital sinus epithelium. Transitional cell carcinoma in the prostate, in the majority of the cases, is found in patients with a history of bladder or urethral cancer and, in rarer cases, it arises from a primary focus in the prostate. See Table 29–1.

REFERENCE

1. Schellhammer, P.F., Bean, M.A., and Whitmore, W.F., Jr.: Prostatic involvement by transitional cell carcinoma: Pathogenesis, patterns and prognosis. J. Urol., *118*:399, 1977.

513-A *(Campbell's, pp. 1164–1166)*

In the prostate, malignant tumors rarely arise from any cells other than those that are found lining normal ducts and acini. Even among these populations, there is one cell type, the basal cell, which appears to rarely undergo malignant transformation. These basal cells are not myoepithelial cells, and they have been proposed to contain the stem cell population, which renews the secretory epithelium. They are distinguished immunohistochemically by absent PSA and PAP stainings and by expression of keratin intermediate filaments 5 and 14. Invasive adenocarcinomas of the prostate are never seen to form a basal cell layer, even an incomplete one.

514-C *(Campbell's, pp. 1166–1168)*

McNeal has delineated precisely the anatomic landmarks of the prostate. All of the major ducts of the prostate enter the urethra in its distal segment, and the proximal segment is completely sheathed by the preprostatic sphincter, a continuous sleeve of smooth muscle fibers that would preclude the passage of major ducts.

The periurethral stroma contains scattered tiny periurethral glands which branch proximally toward the bladder neck. The periurethral glands and stroma are often involved in BPH (corresponding to median lobe hypertrophy).

The transitional zone is represented by two small lobes of glandular tissue, whose ducts leave the urethra immediately below the distal border of the preprostatic sphincter. This area accounts for the origin of approximately 20 per cent of adenocarcinomas, and these are usually recognized clinically as incidental findings in transurethral resection for BPH.

The central zone comprises a separate set of ducts arising on the convexity of the verumontanum in proximity to the ejaculator duct orifices. The central zone gives rise to only 5 to 10 per cent of all adenocarcinomas.

More than half of all cancers arise in the peripheral zone, which is normally the largest region and the one most accessible to rectal palpation of cancer.

REFERENCE

1. McNeal, J.E., Redwine, E.A., Freiha, F.S., and Stamey, T.A.: Zonal distribution of prostatic adenocarcinoma. Am. J. Surg. Pathol., *12*:897, 1988.

515-D *(Campbell's, pp. 1169–1171)*

Prostatic intraepithelial neoplasia (PIN), also known as intraductal dysplasia, is found in approximately 40 per cent of prostates from men older than 50 years without adenocarcinoma and in 80 per cent of prostates from men with adenocarcinoma.

Nuclear enlargement, cell crowding or pseudostratification, and alterations of cytoplasmic staining are cytologic changes that are usually seen in dysplasia. Dysplasia is most specifically characterized by increased variation in nuclear size. Almost equally significant is some degree of disorder in cell-cell relationships. These histologic features are thought to represent a temporal continuum of deviation from normal toward the emergence of invasive carcinoma.

The basal cell layer, which probably provides the most reliable morphologic distinction between invasive and noninvasive epithelium, is often focally absent in the lining of the ducts and acini of dysplastic foci.

The higher degrees of dysplasia are not often found in prostates without cancer. The identification of severe PIN as on isolated lesion on needle biopsy suggests a need for further biopsy to rule out concurrent invasive cancer.

REFERENCES

1. Quinn, B.D., Cho, K.R., and Epstein, J.I.: Relationship of severe dysplasia to stage B adenocarcinoma of the prostate. Cancer, *65*:2328, 1990.
2. Bostwick, D.G., and Brawer, M.K.: Prostatic intraepithelial neoplasia and early invasion of prostate cancer. Cancer, *59*:788, 1987.

516-D *(Campbell's, pp. 1174–1175)*

The grading system for prostate cancer in most general use is the Gleason system, based purely on architectural criteria. The diversity of histologic patterns in biopsy samples is handled by assigning a "primary" grade to that pattern occupying the greatest area of the specimen and a "secondary" grade to that pattern occupying the second largest area. Primary and secondary grades are added to give a "score" or "sum." Because there are five possible grades, the score or sum comprises nine intervals from 2 to 10.

Grades 1 to 3 share the general architectural pattern of independent glands, each lined by a single row of epithelial cells, which completely encloses a lumen, and, in turn, is completely enclosed by stroma. The malignant glands of grade 1 to 3 cancer show loss of the orderly branching pattern of benign ducts with loss of intervening stroma. The Gleason grade 4 histologic pattern is defined by the absence of "complete" gland formation as defined for the lower grades. Grade 5 carcinoma often has a pattern distinguished by the near absence of any true lumens in the cell cords. Usually, cytoplasm is distinctively scant in this grade.

It has been the general experience that the biopsy grade of a tumor has often not been an accurate predictor of clinical course for the individual patient. In a series of radical prostatectomies for adenocarcinoma, knowledge of quantitated cancer volume and whole tumor Gleason grade together provided an extremely accurate prediction of lymph node metastasis.

REFERENCES

1. Gleason, D.F.: Histologic grading and staging of prostate carcinoma. *In* Tannenbaum, M. (Ed.): Urologic Pathology: The Prostate. Philadelphia, Lea & Febiger, 1977, pp. 171–197.
2. McNeal, J.E., Villers, A.A., Redwine, E.A., et al.: Histologic differentiation, cancer volume, and pelvic lymph node metastasis in adenocarcinoma of the prostate. Cancer, *66*:1225, 1990.

517-B *(Campbell's, pp. 1178–1182)*

The boundary between the peripheral zone and transition zone appears to represent a barrier to invasion for most cancers. This compartmentalization tends to prevent many peripheral zone carcinomas from spreading anteriorly, possibly increasing the likelihood of their detection by rectal examination. Conversely, the restricted local spread of transitional zone cancers tends to confine them to the tissues near to the proximal segment of the prostate urethra, remote from the rectal surface. Hence, transition zone cancers are usually detected incidentally at TUR for BPH.

Clinical stage A carcinomas are nearly equivalent to transition zone cancer. They have a relatively low frequency of capsule penetration compared with stage B tumors, and they seldom show seminal vesical invasion.

The weight of evidence now indicates that only complete penetration through the prostate capsule with perforation of its external surface correlates with prognosis or other measures of aggressive behavior. Most penetration of the capsule by prostate cancer is *facilitated spread* represented by the extension of cancer through the capsule along conduits provided by the perineural spaces. The importance of perineural space invasion through the capsule is evident in the striking regional localization of capsule penetration to the areas of the superior and inferior pedicles, where nerve fibers cluster as they penetrate the capsule. Overall, capsule penetration is only about half as frequent in transition zone carcinomas and tends to be of lesser extent.

Seminal vesical invasion almost always results from direct spread of tumor into the ejaculatory duct wall inside the prostate and near the prostate base.

REFERENCES

1. McNeal, J.E., Price, H.M., Redwine, E.A., et al.: Stage A versus stage B adenocarcinoma of the prostate: Morphological comparison and biological significance. J. Urol., *139*:61, 1988.
2. Villers, A., McNeal, J.E., Redwine, E.A., et al.: The role of perineural space invasion in the local spread of prostatic adenocarcinoma. J. Urol., *142*:763, 1989.
3. Villers, A., McNeal, J.E., Redwine, E.A., et al.: Pathogenesis and biological significance of seminal vesicle invasion in prostatic adenocarcinoma. J. Urol., *143*: 1183, 1990.

518-C *(Campbell's, pp. 1182–1186)*

The staging system devised by the Organ Systems Coordinating Center (OSCC) of the National Cancer Institute was published in 1988 by Whitmore. It is based on the TNM system. See Table 29–2.

Primary Tumor	T Stage	
Digitally unrecognizable cancer	A	
$\leq$5% of total surgical specimen of Gleason grade <8		A1
>5% of specimen, or $\leq$5% with Gleason grade $\geq$8		A2
detectable by ultrasound or PSA, confirmed by biopsy		Ax
Digitally palpable cancer, organ-confined	B	
$\leq$ 1/2 of one lobe	B1	
>1/2 of one lobe but not >1 lobe		B2
>1 lobe or bilaterally palpable	B3	
Palpable cancer extending beyond the prostate capsule	C	
unilateral extension (may include seminal vesicle)	C1	
bilateral extension (may include seminal vesicle)	C2	
extension into bladder, rectum, levators, pelvic side wall	C3	
Lymph node status	N stage	
No regional lymph node metastases		N0
Microscopic regional lymph node metastases		N1
Gross regional lymph node metastases	N2	
Extraregional lymph node metastases	N3	
Distant metastases	M stage	
No evidence of metastases		M0
Elevated acid phosphatase only (3 consecutive samples)	M1	
Visceral (V) or bone (B) metastases	M2	

519-E *(Campbell's, pp. 1186–1187)*

Prostate carcinoma was the first malignancy for which the biochemical evaluation of a tumor marker became possible with tests for serum acid phosphatase.

Serum enzymatic acid phosphatase was initially the standard marker for prostate cancer; however, the radioimmunoassay (RIA-PAP), with its ability to measure precisely minute quantities of prostatic acid phosphatase, have virtually replaced all enzymatic assays in the United States. although RIA-PAP assays are several times more sensitive than enzymatic assays, they are almost never as sensitive as PSA levels at any given clinical stage.

Prostatic acid phosphatase is unstable at room temperature (requiring immediate icing after venepuncture or stabilization with an acid citrate buffer). It has a half-life of 0.5 to 2.5 hours.

BPH causes elevations of RIA-PAP in 14 per cent of patients, primarily in those with greater than 40 grams of benign hyperplasia.

REFERENCES

1. Heller, J.E.: Prostatic acid phosphatase: Its current clinical status. J. Urol., *137*:1091, 1987.
2. Stamey, T.A., Yang, N., Hay, A.R., et al.: Prostate-specific antigen as a serum marker for adenocarcinoma of the prostate. N. Engl. J. Med., *317*:909, 1987.

520-B *(Campbell's, pp. 1187–1190)*

PSA is a serine protease, produced only by prostatic epithelial cells, which hydrolyzes the coagulin of the ejaculate. Several publications from Roswell Park between 1980 and 1986 confirmed that PSA was organ-specific, that serum elevations of PSA occurred in both prostate cancer and BPH, and that PSA was an important marker for monitoring patients with prostatic cancer.

Stamey and colleagues showed that the PSA level rises at in overall rate of 3.5 ng/ml/gram of intracapsular cancer, whereas in prostates without cancer, BPH causes serum levels of PSA to rise by only 0.3 ng/ml/gram of BPH.

Although PSA level is proportional to the volume of prostate cancer present, investigators have not found preoperative serum PSA levels to be very helpful as a predictor of pathologic stage.

REFERENCES

1. Oesterling, J.E.: Prostate-specific antigen: A critical assessment of the most useful tumor marker for adenocarcinoma of the prostate. J. Urol., *145*:907, 1991.
2. Stamey, T.A., Yang, N., Hay, A.R., et al.: Prostate-specific antigen as a serum marker for adenocarcinoma of the prostate. N. Engl. J. Med., *317*:909, 1987.

521-C *(Campbell's, pp. 1190–1192)*

Although the PSA level is most useful in estimating the tumor burden in patients with untreated prostate cancer, it is also helpful in monitoring patients after radical prostatectomy, radiation therapy, and hormonal therapy.

Given a half-life of 3.2 days, any patient with a Hybritech PSA level >0.5 ng/ml (or a Yang PSA level >0.3 ng/ml) three weeks or more after radical prostatectomy has residual cancer. Following serum PSA levels at frequent intervals after radical prostatectomy allows for earlier assessment of therapeutic efficacy and also creates the possibility of initiating adjunctive therapy when tumor burden is extremely small.

Kabalin and coworkers performed systemic, TRUS-guarded biopsies of the prostate in 27 patients after definitive radiation therapy, most of whom had normal digital rectal examination (DRE) and low or undetectable serum PSA levels. A total of 93 per cent had histologically identified prostate cancer. It was concluded that there is an unacceptably high failure rate to radiation therapy, which cannot be appreciable by DRE, or a normal PSA level.

Data suggest that an early fall to near undetectable or undetectable levels of PSA that is maintained for at least 6 months can be predictive of a long-term response to hormonal therapy. Although PSA is undoubtedly androgen-dependent, evidence has been presented that the fall in PSA levels may be independent of cell inhibition or death.

Serum PSA levels can be drawn at any time during the day since there is no evidence for a circadian-type pattern in PSA levels from 8 a.m. to 8 p.m.

REFERENCES

1. Oesterling, J.E.: Prostate-specific antigen: A critical assessment of the most useful tumor marker for adenocarcinoma of the prostate. J. Urol., *145*:907, 1991.
2. Kabalin, J.N., Hodge, K.K., McNeal, J.E., et al.: Identification of residual cancer in the prostate following radiation therapy: Role of transrectal ultrasound guided biopsy and prostate-specific antigen. J. Urol., *142*:326, 1989.
3. Stamey, T.A., Kablin, J.N., Ferrari, M., and Yang, N.: Prostate specific antigen in the diagnosis and treatment of adenocarcinoma of the prostate: IV. Anti-androgen treated patients. J. Urol., *141*:1088, 1989.

522-B *(Campbell's, pp. 1182–1194)*

Acute bacterial prostatitis elevates serum PSA levels dramatically, often requiring several months to return to baseline values. Nonbacterial prostatitis causes neither an elevation in PSA levels or a change in the TRUS appearance of the prostate.

Although there is some controversy over whether DRE elevates serum levels of PSA, some studies have shown nearly a twofold increase in serum PSA levels after rectal examination. Cystoscopy has been associated with a fourfold increase in serum PSA values, and needle biopsy of the prostate has been shown to cause a 57-fold increase in serum PSA with elevated levels persisting for up to 1 month after the procedure. Men who present with acute urinary retention from BPH tend to have higher serum PSA levels than those who present for elective surgery.

REFERENCES

1. Stamey, T.A., Yang, N., Hay, A.R., et al.: Prostate-specific antigen as a serum marker for adenocarcinoma of the prostate. N. Engl. J. Med., *317*:909, 1987.
2. Armitage, T.G., Cooper, E.H., Newling, D.W.W., et al.: The value of the measurement of serum prostate specific antigen in patients with BPH and untreated prostate cancer. Br. J. Urol., *62*:584, 1988.

523-E *(Campbell's, pp. 1194–1196)*

McLeary noted that transrectal ultrasound is not a technique for the detection of anteromedially located prostate cancers (i.e., cancer located in the transition zone). If the PSA level is very elevated and systemic biopsies in the peripheral zone produce negative results, then random sampling of the transition zone may be indicated to disclose cancer.

REFERENCE

1. McLeary, R.D.: Biopsy techniques, strategic and systemic. Presented at the 5th International Symposium on Transrectal Ultrasound in the Diagnosis and Management of Prostate Cancer. Chicago, Ill., September 14, 1990, pp. 7–17.

524-D *(Campbell's, pp. 1194–1198)*

We have relied on DRE and digitally guided biopsies for the diagnosis of prostate cancer for many decades. The advent of PSA and transrectal ultrasound (TRUS), especially TRUS-guided biopsies of hypoechoic areas, has clearly increased the detection rate of prostate cancer. It is important to understand, however, that normal prostate tissue, areas of inflammation, and even BPH can appear hypoechoic on TRUS of the peripheral and central zones. In fact, in one study, 47 per cent of the hypoechoic lesions biopsied revealed "benign" prostate tissue, a number that clearly emphasizes the nonspecificity of hypoechoic findings on TRUS. Because hypoechoic lesions in the peripheral and central zones are not specific for cancer, it is recommended that six systemic biopsies taken under TRUS guidance are the best way to diagnose prostate cancer. In addition, systemic biopsies represent the only technique currently available to detect isoechoic cancers, which represent up to 21 per cent of palpable stage B cancers.

It is well known that the more differentiated cancers (Gleason grades 3 or less) tend to be less hypoechoic to isoechoic.

The only criticism of systemic biopsies is the possibility of detecting microscopic small—and therefore insignificant—foci of cancer. Because 47 per cent of all biopsies directed at hypoechoic areas show histologically normal prostate tissue, a 15-mm-long biopsy is just as easily hit an insignificant cancer as can systemic, spatially oriented biopsies.

REFERENCES

1. McLeary, R.D.: Biopsy techniques, strategic and systemic. Presented at the 5th International Symposium on Transrectal Ultrasound in the Diagnosis and Management of Prostate Cancer. Chicago, IL., September 14, 1990, pp. 7–17.
2. Shinohara, K., Wheeler, T., and Scardino, P.T.: The appearance of prostate cancer on transrectal ultrasonography: Correlation of imaging and pathological examinations. J. Urol., *142*:76, 1989.

525-A *(Campbell's, pp. 1198–1199)*

Unless the patient has microscopic hematuria, there is no need for either a cystoscopy or intravenous urogram in the evaluation of patients with clinical stage A or B prostate cancer. In most cases, CT scan and MRI add little information. If the biopsy cores are loaded with undifferentiated cancer, and the PSA level is greater than 100 ng/ml by the Yang assay (some say >20 ng/ml), there may be some reason to seek the presence of large retroperitoneal lymph nodes, which might be aspirated to save surgical exploration.

Bone scans are useful, but PSA testing has greatly restricted their need. Oesterling has argued convincingly that any radical prostatectomy candidate with a Hybritech serum PSA level ≤ 20 ng/ml has *almost* no chance of demonstrating bone metastases.

REFERENCE

1. Oesterling, J.E.: Prostate-specific antigen: A critical assessment of the most useful tumor marker for adenocarcinoma of the prostate. J. Urol., *145*:907, 1991.

526-C *(Campbell's, pp. 1199–1201)*

The treatment of prostate cancer is largely determined by the volume and grade of tumor at the time of therapy. Because escape of prostate cancer into the periprostatic fat and seminal vesicles and lymph node invasion are usually microscopic, there is no imaging modality capable of signaling early spread into these areas. CT and MRI are insensitive to the spread of cancer until the invasion is gross and more readily discernible by other methods.

A critical issue in the treatment of prostate cancer is the prolonged natural history of this disease in the absence of interventional therapy, especially in the early clinical stages. Stamey and coworkers reported that over two thirds of all clinical stage A and B cancers double at rates exceeding 4 years. It is fair to state, therefore, that assessing the life expectancy of patients with prostate cancer prior to treatment is far more important than for any other genitourinary malignancy. If the patient does not have an estimated 10- to 15-year life expectancy, neither radical prostatectomy nor irradiation therapy should be considered unless there are unusual mitigating circumstances.

The risk of lymph node metastasis is directly proportional to stage in patients with adenocarcinoma of the prostate. Even a single microscopic metastatic focus in only one of multiple pelvic lymph nodes is a hallmark of prostate cancer that is incurable by any currently available modality of treatment; 70 per cent of these patients will die of prostate cancer rather than unrelated causes. However, because of the long natural history of the disease, many of these patients will do well for 10 years.

REFERENCES

1. Stamey, T.A., McNeal, J.E., Freiha, F.S., and Redwine, E.: Morphometric and clinical studies on 68 consecutive radical prostatectomies. J. Urol., *139*:1235, 1988.
2. Stamey, T.A., and Kabalin, J.N.: Prostate-specific antigen in the diagnosis and treatment of adenocarcinoma of the prostate: I. Untreated patients. J. Urol., *141*:1070, 1989.
3. Scardino, P.T.: Early detection of prostate cancer. Urol. Clin. North Am., *16*:635, 1989.

527-A *(Campbell's, pp. 1201–1203)*

Studies have demonstrated an extraordinarily high failure rate of external beam radiation therapy to sterilize local prostate cancer.

Scardino and Wheeler compared the actuarial 5-, 10-, and 15-year survival rates for combined radiotherapy to survival rates for external beam therapy alone. For all clinical stage A2 and B patients, the actuarial survival rates at 5, 10, and 15 years for combined therapy were 86 per cent, 59 per cent, and 28 per cent, compared with 81 per cent, 60 per cent, and 34 per cent for external beam therapy.

One of the limitations of all forms of brachytherapy has been the nonhomogeneous distribution of the interstitial seed implants despite the best of efforts. Survival rates with external beam therapy have generally been better than those with brachytherapy.

One serious problem of irradiation for stage C or D1 cancer is the 33 per cent rate of urinary incontinence after a TURP for progressive urinary obstruction months or years after completion of irradiation. Early hormonal therapy or simple vesical neck incisions instead of TURP may help to decrease the risk of incontinence in this group of patients.

Several studies have clearly documented that the presence of positive biopsy findings 18 months or more after irradiation therapy strongly correlates with biologically active disease and treatment failure. A rising or elevated PSA level 1 year or longer after radiotherapy also indicates irradiation failure.

REFERENCES

1. Kabalin, J.N., Hodge, K.K., McNeal, J.E., et al.: Identification of residual cancer in the prostate following radiation therapy: Role of transrectal ultrasound guided biopsy and prostate specific antigen. J. Urol., *142*:326, 1989.
2. Scardino, P.T., and Wheeler, T.M.: Local control of prostate cancer with radiotherapy: Frequency and prognostic significance of positive results of postirradiation prostate biopsy. NCI Monogr., *4*:95, 1988.

528-C *(Campbell's, pp. 1203–1204)*

The nerve-sparing retropubic radical prostatectomy and the recognition of an unsuspected and extraordinarily high failure rate of external beam radiotherapy to sterilize local prostate cancer have greatly increased the number of radical prostatectomies performed in the United States for clinically localized stage A and B cancer. It should be noted, however, that only 40 per cent of clinical stage B prostate cancers thought to be localized on DRE are actually confined to the prostate. Capsular penetration into the periprostate fat most commonly occurs in the area of the neuromuscular bundle.

REFERENCES

1. Stamey, T.A., McNeal, J.E., Freiha, F.S. and Redwine, E.: Morphometric and clinical studies on 68 consecutive radical prostatectomies. J. Urol., *139*:1235, 1988.
2. Bigg, S.W., Kavonssi, L.R., and Catalona, W.J.: Role of nerve-sparing radical prostatectomy for clinical stage B_2 prostate cancer. J. Urol., *144*:1420, 1990.

529-D *(Campbell's, pp. 1205–1209)*

In general, 80 per cent of B1 nodules will be less than 4 ml in volume, and almost all are curable by radical prostatectomy if positive surgical margins are not created. As repeatedly emphasized in this chapter, MRI and CT scans are not useful for clinical stage A and B cancers. Radiation therapy has been shown to have a high failure rate in attempting to sterilize local cancer. Hormonal therapy is generally reserved for patients with extraprostatic spread of their disease.

REFERENCES

1. Walsh, P.C., Lepor, H., and Eggleston, J.C.: Radical prostatectomy with preservation of sexual function: Anatomical and pathological considerations. Prostate, *4*:473, 1983.
2. Sogani, P.C., and Farri, W.R.: Treatment of advanced prostate cancer. Urol. Clin. North Am., *14*:353, 1987.

530-A *(Campbell's, p. 1209)*

The increase in practice of radical retropubic prostatectomy has created the following dilemmas: (1) what to do when the lymph nodes are found unexpectedly to be positive at surgical staging, and (2) what to do for the 10 per cent of patients in whom the results of surgical examination of the pelvic nodes are initially negative but later, with more extensive and permanent histologic sectioning, are found to be positive. No clear answers can be given in response to these questions. The disadvantages of radiation therapy for large stage B and C cancers have been pointed out. Steinberg and associates reported that there was no difference in local progression in clinical stage D1 disease between these patients expectantly treated (without surgery), and those treated with radiation.

In the 1990s, there is a definite tendency toward removing these prostates for local control, recognizing that the surgery is not curative. Without question, the impotent patient with obstructive urinary symptoms will do better treated with a noncurative radical prostatectomy in the presence of unexpected D1 disease of microscopic volume.

However, all of these options will require a decade of research to learn what is best for the patient.

REFERENCE

1. Steinberg, G.D., Epstein, J.I., Piantodosi, S., and Walsh, P.C.: Management of stage D1 adenocarcinoma of the prostate: The Johns Hopkins Experience 1974 to 1987. J. Urol., *144*:1425, 1990.

531-A *(Campbell's, p. 1210)*

Complications of radical retropubic prostatectomy include death (<1 per cent), pulmonary emboli (2.7 per cent), urinary incontinence (5 per cent), anastomotic stricture (<10 per cent), rectal injury (1–2 per cent), and significant lymphoceles (<1 per cent). Erectile impotency occurs in 90 per cent of patients after radical prostatectomy. The risk of this complication may be decreased with the performance of a nerve-sparing procedure as described by Walsh and colleagues. Fortunately, because orgasmic function is invariably maintained even when all the periprostatic fascia with their enclosed neurovascular bundles are excised, there are numerous ways to provide satisfactory erectile function for the impotent patient. Moreover, the wait for spontaneous return of the erectile function can be much longer than 12 months.

REFERENCE

1. Igel, T.C., Barrett, D.M., Segura, J.W., et al.: Perioperative and postoperative complications from bilateral pelvic lymphadenectomy and radical retropubic prostatectomy. J. Urol., *137*:1189, 1987.

532-B *(Campbell's, pp. 1210–1214)*

Approximately 75 per cent of all new patients who present with prostate cancer will ultimately require some form of therapy other than radical prostatectomy (see Table 29–4). Given the fact that all forms of radiation therapy now appear essentially incapable of sterilizing prostate cancer confined to the pelvis, and recognizing that currently there exists no effective chemotherapeutic agent, hormonal therapy will be required for most patients diagnosed with prostate cancer unless there are significant improvements in early detection.

In the presence of untreated metastatic bone disease confirmed by bone scans, hormonal therapy produces improvement in 60 to 80 per cent of men; however, hormonally resistant progression appears during the first 12 months of therapy in 35 to 40 per cent of these patients. Studies suggest that neuroendocrine cells may be important in the final, progressive androgen-resistant phase of metastatic prostate cancer.

Evidence from current studies suggests that early hormonal therapy may increase the patient survival in comparison to delayed hormonal therapy, even though a definitive randomized study to test this possibility has not been reported.

A 1989 multicenter trial combined leuprolide, an analogue of gonadotropin-releasing hormone, with either placebo or flutamide, a nonsteroidal antiandrogen that competitively inhibits the binding of androgens to the cell nucleus. It found an increased median length of survival of 28.3 months versus 35.6 months for the flutamide combination. Androgen deprivation therapy is clearly superior to leuprolide alone in prolonging life.

Bilateral orchiectomy has been the gold standard for hormonal therapy since the report by Huggins and associates in 1941. LHRH agonist therapy can be considered equivalent to bilateral orchiectomy. The initial "flare" from temporary release of testosterone can cause bone pain in the first week of therapy. A potential for spinal cord injury exists if vertebral metastases are present; therefore, LHRH agonists should be avoided in any patient with metastatic cancer who has the slightest suggestion of neurologic symptoms.

Diethylstilbestrol (DES) is associated with a high cardiovascular risk at dosages of 3 to 5 mg/day. The dosage of 1 mg/day of DES, however, is as effective as 5 mg/day in delaying progression of stage C to D2 disease, without having the associated cardiovascular risk.

REFERENCES

1. Sogani, P.C., and Fair, W.R.: Treatment of advanced prostate cancer. Urol. Clin. North Am., *14*:353, 1987.
2. Cohen, R.J., Glezerson, G., Hoffejee, Z., and Afrika, D.: Prostatic carcinoma: Histological and immunohistological factors affecting prognosis. Br. J. Urol., *66*: 405, 1990.
3. Crawford, E.D., Eisenbeyer, M.A., McLeod, D.G., et al.: A controlled trial of leuprolide with and without

flutamide in prostatic carcinoma. N. Engl. J. Med., *321*:419, 1989.

533-B *(Campbell's, p. 1214)*

Effective chemotherapeutic agents are urgently needed for prostate cancer. Unfortunately, there are no effective chemotherapeutic drugs for prostate cancer. Those that have been tried show short responses without any significant survival advantage. Most chemotherapeutic agents tried have been associated with substantial toxicity.

In view of the 3-year doubling time for most cancers, cell cycle nonspecific agents will be required rather than those that rely on DNA replication for cell killing. Effective chemotherapeutic agents could greatly increase the indications for radical prostatectomy when provided as adjunctive therapy.

REFERENCES

1. Eisenberger, M.A.: Chemotherapy for prostatic carcinoma. NCI Monogr., 7:151–163, 1988.
2. Johnson, D.E., Logothetis, C.J., and von Eschenbach, A.C.: Systemic Therapy for Genitourinary Cancer. Chicago, Year Book Medical Publishers, 1989.

534-D *(Campbell's, pp. 1222–1223)*

Testicular cancer, although relatively rare, represents the most common malignancy in men in the 15- to 35-year old age group. It has become one of the most curable solid neoplasms. This dramatic improvement in survival resulting from the combination of effective diagnostic techniques, improved tumor markers, effective multidrug chemotherapy, and modifications of surgical technique has led to a diminution of patient mortality to less than 10 per cent.

Most primary neoplasms of the testis arise from germinal elements, accounting for 90 to 95 per cent of all testicular neoplasms. The nongerminal elements, accounting for approximately 5 per cent of all primary testicular neoplasms, include neoplasms arising from gonadal stroma, mesenchymal structures, and ducts. Metastatic tumors to the testis are distinctly uncommon.

It is of interest that in patients whose germ cell tumors arise outside the testis (extragonadal germ cell tumors), the prognoses with similar treatment is approximately half that expected in patients whose tumors are of primary germ cell region.

535-B, 536-E *(Campbell's, pp. 1225–1227)*

The average annual rate of testicular cancer is highest in Scandinavia; intermediate in the United States and Great Britain; and low in Africa and Asia.

The highest incidence of testicular cancers is noted in young adults (20 to 40 years). Seminoma is the most common histologic type overall, with a peak incidence between the ages of 35 and 39 years. Embryonal carcinoma and teratocarcinoma occur predominantly between the ages of 25 and 35 years. Choriocarcinoma occurs more often in the 20- to 30-year age group. Yolk sac tumors are the predominant lesions of infancy and childhood, rarely occurring in pure form in the adult. Malignant testicular lymphomas are predominantly tumors of men over the age of 50.

The incidence of testicular tumors in the American black is roughly one third of that in the American white.

Testicular neoplasms appear to be slightly more common in the right testis than in the left, similar to the slightly greater incidence of right-sided cryptorchidism. Approximately 2 to 3 per cent of testicular tumors are bilateral.

Approximately 7 to 10 per cent of patients with testicular tumors have prior histories of cryptorchidism and nearly 50 per cent of these were associated with intra-abdominal testis. Most investigators have concluded that trauma to an enlarged testis is an event that prompts medical evaluation rather than being a causative factor.

REFERENCE

1. Mostofi, F.K.: Testicular tumors: Epidemiologic, etiologic, and pathologic features. Cancer, *32*:1186, 1973.

537-D *(Campbell's, p. 1228)*

The usual presentation of a testicular tumor is a nodule or painless swelling of one gonad. Approximately 30 to 40 per cent of patients may complain of a dull ache or heavy sensation in the lower abdomen or scrotum. Acute scrotal pain will be the presenting symptom in approximately 10 per cent of patients. Although almost 50 per cent of patients will have metastatic disease at the time of diagnosis, only 10 per cent will have manifestations of these metastases (e.g., neck mass, respiratory symptoms, gastrointestinal disturbances, back pain, nervous system manifestations, or lower extremity swelling). Gynecomastia will be seen in approximately 5 per cent of patients.

538-C *(Campbell's, p. 1229)*

A hydrocele may be present in patients with testicular neoplasms, and it may increase the difficulty of appreciating a testicular neoplasm. Ultrasonography of the scrotum is a rapid and reliable technique to exclude epididymitis and should be utilized in patients if there is any suspicion of testicular tumor. Needle aspiration of the hydrocele should be discouraged since it would alter the pattern of metastatic spread in the event of the presence of a testicular tumor.

REFERENCE

1. Richie, J.P., Birnholz, J., and Garnick, M.B.: Ultrasonography as a diagnostic adjunct for the evaluation of masses in the scrotum. Surg. Gynecol. Obstet., *154*: 695, 1982.

539-E *(Campbell's, pp. 1229–1230)*

The majority of testicular cancers spread through the lymphatics in an orderly fashion, although vascular dissemination can occur early in some tumors. The primary lymphatic drainage from the right testicle is to the interaortocaval lymph nodes, and subsequently to precaval, preaortic, and paracaval lymph nodes. Once the interaortocaval nodes are involved, there tends to be spread to the left para-aortic area, more commonly from right to left. The primary drainage of the left testis is to the left para-aortic nodes just below the level of the left renal vein and, subsequently, to the preaortic nodes.

Cross-metastases occur more commonly in patients with right-sided tumors. Iliac lymph nodes may be involved primarily when the tumor has invaded the epididymis or spermatic cord. Inguinal metastases may occur when the tunica albuginea has been involved or when previous surgery, such as inguinal herniorrhaphy or orchiopexy, has altered the normal lymphatic flow. Although the suprahilar area was thought to be involved commonly in patients with more extensive retroperitoneal nodal cases, the lymphatics tend to follow the aorta below the crus of the diaphragm into the retrocrural space.

REFERENCE

1. Donohue, J.P., Zachary, J.M., and Maynard, B.R.: Distribution of nodal metastases in nonseminomatous testis cancer. J. Urol., *128*:315, 1982.

540-D *(Campbell's, p. 1230)*

Distant spread of testicular cancer occurs most commonly to the pulmonary region, with intraparenchymal pulmonary involvement. Subsequent spread may be noted to the liver, viscera, brain, or bone. In general, bony metastases are encountered rather late in the course of disease. Central nervous system metastases may be understaged.

REFERENCE

1. Johnson, D.E., Appelt, G., Samuels, M.C., and Luna, M.: Metastases from testicular carcinoma. Urology, *8*: 234, 1976.

541-C *(Campbell's, pp. 1230–1231)*

A variety of clinical staging systems have been advocated during the past 40 years. The system proposed by Goden and Gibb in 1951 has been the mainstay of clinical staging. This ABC system was refined by Skinner with subclassification of regional nodal involvement into B1, B2, and B3. The American Joint Committee TNM Staging System can also be seen below (see also Tables 30–3 and 30–4).

Boden/Gibb Stage	Skinner Stage	TNM Stage
A (I) Tumor confined to testis	A Tumor confined to testis	TX3 unknown status TO → no evidence of tumor T1 → confined to testis T2 → beyond tunica T3 → invasion of rete testis or epididymis T4a → invasion of cord T4b → invasion of scrotum
B (II) Spread to regional nodes	B1-<6 positive retroperitoneal nodes,no node > 2 cm	N1
	B2->6 positive retroperitoneal nodes, any node > 2 cm	N2
C (III) Spread beyond retroperitoneal nodes B3-massive retroperitoneal disease		N3
	C Metastatic spread	M+

REFERENCES

1. Boden, G., and Gibb, R.: Radiotherapy and testicular neoplasms. Lancet, *2*:1195, 1991.
2. Skinner, D.G.: Nonseminomatous testis tumor: A plan of management based on 96 patients to improve survival in all stages by combined therapeutic modalities. J. Urol., *115*:65, 1976.

542-C *(Campbell's, pp. 1231–1232)*

Radical or inguinal orchiectomy, with early clamping of the spermatic cord at the deep inguinal ring, effectively removes the primary tumor and allows staging in patients with testicular cancer. Posteroanterior and lateral chest radiographs should be the initial radiographic procedure performed for clinical staging. CT scan of the chest is so sensitive that a high false positive rate makes its use questionable. Abdominal CT scans have been recommended as being the most effective means to identify retroperitoneal lymph node involvement. Tumor markers may be capable of detecting small tumor burdens (10^5 cells) that are not distinguishable by currently available imaging techniques.

543-D *(Campbell's, p. 1232)*

Alpha-fetoprotein (AFP) is a single-chain glycoprotein with a molecular weight of approximately 70,000. In the fetus, AFP is produced by the fetal yolk sac, liver, and gastrointestinal tract. The highest concentrations of AFP noted during the 12th to 14th weeks of gestation gradually decline so that 1 year following birth, AFP is detectable only at low levels (<40 ng/ml). The metabolic half-life of AFP in humans is between 5 and 7 days.

After the first 6 weeks of postnatal life, an elevated AFP level may be detected in association with a number of malignancies (testis, liver, pancreas, stomach, lung), normal pregnancy, and benign liver disease. AFP may be produced by pure embryonal carcinomas, teratocarcinoma, yolk sac tumor, or combined tumors but not by pure choriocarcinoma or pure seminoma.

REFERENCE

1. Javadpour, N.: The role of biologic tumor markers in testicular cancer. Cancer, *45*:1755, 1980.

544-D, 545-B *(Campbell's, p. 1232)*

Human chorionic gonadotropin (HCG) is a glycoprotein (molecular weight 38,000) composed of an alpha and a beta polypeptide chain, and is normally produced by trophoblastic tissue. Pituitary hormones (luteinizing hormone, follicle-stimulating hormone, thyroid-stimulating hormone) possess alpha subunits closely resembling that of HCG. The beta subunit of HCG is structurally and antigenically distinct from that of the pituitary hormones; however, some of the RIA techniques for β-HCG variously cross-react with luteinizing hormone (LH).

The serum half-life of HCG is between 24 and 36 hours. Beta-HCG is elevated in all patients with choriocarcinoma, 40 to 60 per cent of patients with embryonal carcinoma, and 5 to 10 per cent of patients with pure seminomas.

REFERENCE

1. Fraley, E.E., Lange, P.H., and Kennedy, B.J.: Germ-cell testicular cancer in adults. N. Engl. J. Med., *301*:1270, 1979.

546-B *(Campbell's, pp. 1233–1234)*

Relative to seminoma, the detection of an elevated AFP level strongly suggests the presence of a nonseminomatous element. Step sections of the primary tumor may further defuse the source of the marker abnormality. Approximately 30 to 45 per cent of patients dying with seminoma are found to have elements of nonseminomatous histology at autopsy. It is generally accepted that between 5 and 10 per cent of patients with "pure" seminoma will have mild elevation of β-HCG level because of the presence of syncytiotrophoblastic giant cell forms.

Lactic acid dehydrogenase (LDH) is a nonspecific tumor marker in patients with germ cell testicular neoplasms, and may be helpful as a marker substance in the surveillance of patients with advanced seminoma. Gamma-glutamyl transferase (GGT) and placental alkaline phosphatase (PLAP) are also nonspecific markers that may be elevated in patients with seminoma as well as those with nonseminomatous testis tumors.

REFERENCE

1. Javadpour, N.: Multiple biochemical tumor markers in testicular cancer. Cancer, *52*:887, 1983.

547-C *(Campbell's, p. 1234)*

Principal treatment strategies for patients with germ cell tumor of the testis have evolved from conceptions of tumor natural history, clinical staging, and effectiveness of treatment. Each of the major treatment alternatives, surgery, irradiation, and chemotherapy, has a particular but imperfectly defined role in the management of testicular tumors. As a means of establishing local control, inguinal or "radical" orchiectomy is clearly preferred. Surgical excision of retained spermatic cord remnant or of the "contaminated" scrotum is recommended following scrotal violation or tumor spillage. Because more than 50 per cent of patients with testicular tumors present with metastatic disease, further treatment following orchiectomy is usual. It is generally accepted that the majority of patients with large retroperitoneal metastatic deposits are best managed initially by chemotherapy.

Between 65 and 85 per cent of all seminomas are clinically confined to the testis, whereas 60 to 70 per cent of nonseminomas appear with recognizable metastatic disease.

548-A *(Campbell's, pp. 1235–1236)*

Seminoma is the most common histologic testis tumor in adults and accounts for approximately 60 to 65 per cent of all pure testicular germ cell tumors. Approximately 75 per cent of patients with seminomas will present with stage I disease, and in this group, greater than 90 per cent survival should be anticipated. Postorchiectomy external beam radiation therapy to the retroperitoneal lymph nodes achieves very high cure rates for these patients.

The optimum treatment of patients who present with distant metastases or bulk retroperitoneal disease is initially chemotherapy.

Autopsy studies in patients dying with seminoma reveal that liver and lung involvement is common and is seen in approximately 75 per cent of patients. Bone and brain metastases are observed in 50 and 25 per cent of patients, respectively. Of major import is the fact that approximately 30 per cent of patients with histologically pure seminoma of the testis who ultimately die of the disease are found to harbor nonseminomatous elements in metastatic sites.

REFERENCES

1. Oliver, R.T., Lore, S., and Ong, J.: Alternatives to radiotherapy in the management of seminoma. Br. J. Urol., *65*:61, 1990.
2. Whitmore, W.F., Jr.: The treatment of germinal tumors of the testis. *In* Proceeding of the Sixth National Cancer Conference. Philadelphia, J.B. Lippincott Co., 1968, pp. 347–355.

549-B *(Campbell's, pp. 1236–1237)*

Three subtypes of pure seminoma have been described: classic, anaplastic, and spermatocytic. Classic or typical seminoma accounts for 82 to 85 per cent of all seminomas. Histologically, it is composed of islands or sheets of relatively large cells with clear cytoplasm and densely staining nuclei.

Anaplastic seminoma accounts for between 5 and 10 per cent of all seminomas. Histologically, anaplastic seminoma is typed by increased mitotic activity (three or more mitoses per high-power field), nuclear pleomorphism, and cellular anaplasia. The less favorable results of treatment for patients with anaplastic seminoma may merely reflect a greater metastatic potential; however, there is no difference from classic seminoma when patients are treated appropriately and compared stage for stage.

Spermatocytic seminoma accounts for 2 to 12 per cent of all seminomas, and nearly half occur in men over the age of 50 years. Its metastatic potential is extremely low, and prognosis is accordingly favorable.

REFERENCES

1. Percarpio, B., Clements, J.C., McLeod, D.G., et al.: Anaplastic seminoma: An analysis of 77 patients. Cancer, *43*:2510, 1979.
2. Shulman, Y., Ware, S., Al-Askari, S., and Morales, P.: Anaplastic seminoma. Urology, *21*:379, 1983.

3. Weitzner, S.: Spermatocytic seminomas. Urology, *6*:74, 1979.

550-C *(Campbell's, p. 1237)*

The natural history and radiosensitivity of seminoma favor megavoltage irradiation in relatively modest amounts as the treatment of choice in the majority of patients following inguinal orchiectomy with 5-year survival rates of 90 to 95 per cent in stage I disease and roughly 80 per cent in stage II disease.

In stage I and low-volume stage II seminoma, irradiation of para-aortic and inguinopelvic lymphatics is delivered through anterior and posterior parallel opposing fields. In patients with a retained spermatic cord remnant or contaminated scrotum, the field may be widened considerably (see Fig. 30–1).

In patients with histories of herniorrhaphy or prior orchiopexy, the inferior portion of the field should include the contralateral inguinal region as well. The contralateral testis should be shielded. Prophylactic treatment of the mediastinum or supraclavicular area is not indicated.

REFERENCE

1. Thomas, G.M., Rider, W.D., Dembo, A.J., et al: Seminoma of the testis: Results of treatment and patterns of failure after radiation therapy. Int. J. Radiat. Oncol. Biol. Phys., *8*:165, 1982.

551-D *(Campbell's, pp. 1238–1239)*

The overall disease-free survival in patients with high bulk (>5 cm) retroperitoneal or advanced disease treated with abdominal irradiation is only approximately 50 per cent. In patients with bulk or advanced disease, the initial treatment should be platinum-based chemotherapy with surgery or radiation therapy reserved for those patients in whom treatment fails.

Patients with advanced seminomas seem to have chemosensitive tumors, and more than 85 per cent of these patients have achieved continuous disease-free status with cisplatin combination chemotherapy.

REFERENCES

1. Oliver, R.T., Lore, S., and Ong, J.: Alternatives to radiotherapy in the management of seminomas. Br. J. Urol., *65*:61, 1990.
2. Fossa, S., Borge, L., Aass, N., et al.: The treatment of advanced metastatic seminoma: Experience in 55 cases. J. Clin. Oncol., *5*:1071, 1987.

552-C *(Campbell's, p. 1239)*

Tumors designated as "nonseminoma" include those that are histologically composed of embryonal carcinomas, teratoma, choriocarcinoma, and yolk sac elements, alone or in various combinations. Tumors containing both seminomatous and nonseminomatous elements are generally regarded as nonseminomas, and treated as such.

Clinical evidence is strong that nonseminomas have a potentially less favorable natural history than do pure seminomas. Approximately 50 to 70 per cent of patients with nonseminomas, but only 20 to 30 per cent of patients with seminomas, will present with metastatic disease at the time of diagnosis. The first echelon of spread for all germ cell tumors is most commonly the retroperitoneal lymph nodes. After retroperitoneal lymph nodes, lung is the next most common site of metastatic spread, followed by liver, brain, bone, and kidney.

553-C, 554-A *(Campbell's, pp. 1239–1240)*

Embryonal carcinoma is generally discovered as a small round but irregular mass invading the tunica vaginalis. Its cut surface reveals a variegated, grayish, fleshy tumor, often with areas of necrosis or hemorrhage. Pleomorphism, mitotic figures, and giant cells are common.

Pure choriocarcinoma may present with evidence of advanced distant metastasis and what seems to be a paradoxically small intratesticular lesion. Grossly, it is noted to have a grayish-white color with central hemorrhage. Microscopically, two distinct cell types must be demonstrated to satisfy the histologic diagnosis of choriocarcinoma: syncytiotrophoblasts and cytotrophoblasts.

Teratoma contains more than one germ cell layer in various stages of maturation. "Mature" elements resemble benign structures from normal endoderm, ectoderm, and mesoderm. "Immature" teratomas consist of undifferentiated primitive tissues from each of the three germ cell layers.

Yolk sac tumor is the most common testis tumor of infants and children. In adults, it occurs most frequently in combination with other histologic types. In its pure form, the lesion has a homogeneous yellowish, mucinous appearance.

In approximately 40 per cent of testis tumors, more than one histologic pattern is identified. The most common mixed testicular tumor is teratocarcinoma, the combination of teratomas and embryonal carcinoma, occurring in approximately 24 per cent of testis tumors.

REFERENCE

1. Mostofi, F.K.: Testicular tumors: Epidemiologic, etiologic, and pathologic features. Cancer, *32*:1186, 1973.

555-D *(Campbell's, pp. 1240–1244)*

In patients with nonseminomatous germ cell tumors, following inguinal orchiectomy, the accuracy of clinical staging is critical as a determinant for further treatment selection. Because of the inaccuracy of clinical staging, retroperitoneal lymphadenectomy (RPLND) remains the mainstay of surgical therapy in patients with nonseminomatous germ cell tumors. The cure rate for patients with pathologically confirmed stage I disease is roughly 95 per cent with surgery alone. The 5 to 10 per cent of patients who experience relapse following a negative RPLND for stage I disease have 100 per cent survival with salvage chemotherapy.

Several series have evaluated prognostic factors associated with relapse. Factors associated with an increased risk of relapse include embryonal cell elements in the primary tumor, high T stage (T2 or greater), and the presence of vascular or lymphatic invasion. The presence of one or more of these factors precludes surveillance therapy.

The main objections to retroperitoneal lymph node irradiation have been the inaccuracy of clinical staging of the retroperitoneal lymph nodes; the resultant lack of survival data that could be reasonably compared with surgical data; and the concern that, in the event of postirradiation relapse, the prior irradiation might preclude adequate chemotherapy or surgical excision.

REFERENCES

1. Fraley, E.E., Lang, P.H., and Kennedy, B.J.: Germ-cell testicular cancer in adults. N. Engl. J. Med., *301*:1370, 1979.
2. Fung, C.Y., Kalish, L.A., Brodsky, G.L., et al.: Stage I nonseminomatous germ cell testicular tumor: Prediction of metastatic potential by primary histopathology. J. Clin. Oncol., 6:1467, 1988.

556-E *(Campbell's, pp. 1242–1243)*

Richie reported a prospective study of modified lymph node dissection in 85 patients with clinical stage I nonseminomatous germ cell testis tumor. The dissection is bilateral above the level of the inferior mesenteric artery (IMA) but unilateral below the IMA. With respect to preservation of ejaculatory function, up to 94 per cent of patients have recovered antegrade ejaculation. Several other studies have confirmed these results with anywhere from 66 to 98 per cent rates of preservation of ejaculation in low stage disease. Thus far, recurrence rates with these modified techniques are no different from those with standard techniques.

REFERENCES

1. Richie, J.P.: Modified retroperitoneal lymphadenectomy for clinical stage I testicular cancer. J. Urol., *144*: 1160, 1990.
2. Donohue, J.P., Foster, R.S., Rowland, R.G., et al.: Nerve-sparing retroperitoneal lymphadenectomy with preservation of ejaculation. J. Urol., *144* (2 Pt. 1):287, discussion 291, 1990.

557-C *(Campbell's, pp. 1245–1246)*

The high relapse and unresectability rates in patients with bulky retroperitoneal disease, coupled with the demonstrated effectiveness of multidrug regimens in treating disseminated cancer, makes platinum-based combination chemotherapy the treatment of choice for the initial management for those with advanced nodal or pulmonary nonseminomatous metastases (see Fig. 30–4). The efficacy of lymph node irradiation still remains in question. The main drawback to radiation therapy is that, if relapse occurs following radiation therapy, the effectiveness of chemotherapy may be undermined by cumulative myelosuppression. Furthermore, surgical treatment of locally persistent disease may be complicated by prior irradiation.

558-D *(Campbell's, pp. 1247–1248)*

One of the major contributors to the development of combination chemotherapy for patients with disseminated testicular cancer has been the group at Indiana University. Beginning in 1974, cisplatin (the single most active agent in testis cancer) was added to the standard two-day regimen of vinblastine and bleomycin. Five year disease-free survival rates in stage III disease were improved from the 74 per cent to 83 per cent when VP–16 (etoposide) was substituted for vinblastine. Thus bleomycin, etoposide, platinum (BEP) is superior combination chemotherapy to PVB and has become the standard treatment for patients with disseminated germ cell tumor. The response rates for three cycles of BEP are equivalent to four cycles; therefore, three cycles of BEP chemotherapy should suffice in most cases.

REFERENCES

1. Einhorn, L.H., and Williams, S.D.: Chemotherapy of disseminated testicular cancer. Cancer, *46*:1339, 1980.
2. Williams, S.D., Birch, R., Einham, L.H., et al: Treatment of disseminated germ cell tumors with cisplatin, bleomycin, and either vinblastine or etoposide. N. Engl. J. Med., *316*:1435, 1987.

559-D *(Campbell's, p. 1248)*

Cisplatin combination chemotherapy will effect cure rates in approximately 70 to 80 per cent of patients with disseminated germ cell tumors. In patients in whom serum markers have normalized after four cycles of chemotherapy, residual masses >3 cm should be resected surgically. Surgeons should be aware of potential bleomycin-related complications, especially with pulmonary fibrosis. Bleomycin toxicity can be minimized by restriction of crystalloid and free water intraoperatively and by reducing the forced inspiratory oxygen (less than 0.25).

REFERENCE

1. Barneveld, P.W., Sleijfer, D.T., VanderMark, T.W., et al.: Natural cause of bleomycin-induced pneumonitis. Am. Rev. Respir. Dis., *135*:43, 1987.

560-E *(Campbell's, pp. 1249–1250)*

Primary tumors of extragonadal origin are rare, accounting for 3 to 5 per cent of all germ cell tumors. The most common sites of origin, in decreasing frequency, are the mediastinum, retroperitoneum, sacrococcygeal region and pineal gland. Males are predominantly affected, and these tumors are seen most commonly in young adults, with the exception of sacrococcygeal tumors, which are most often diagnosed in the neonate. Histologically, all germ cell types are represented, with pure seminoma accounting for roughly half the tumors in the mediastinum and retroperitoneum.

Complete local excision of mediastinal or retroperitoneal tumors is rarely feasible because of frequent local extension and high rates of metastatic disease at diagnosis. Response rates with radiation and/or chemotherapy (depending on histology and stage of the tumor) are not as good as for gonadal germ cell tumors. The rarer sacrococcygeal tumors, which are usually benign, may be treated with wide local excision alone.

REFERENCE

1. Recondo, J., and Libshitz, H.I.: Mediastinal extragonadal germ cell tumors. Urology, *11*:369, 1978.

561-B *(Campbell's, pp. 1250–1251)*

Sex cord-mesenchyme tumors make up between 5 and 10 per cent of all testis tumors. These include Leydig cell tumors, Sertoli cell tumors, granulosa cell, and theca cell tumors. Leydig cell tumors are the most common of these lesions, making up between 1 and 3 per cent of all testis tumors. The majority of these tumors occur between the ages of 20 and 60 years, although 25 per cent have been reported before puberty. The etiology of Leydig cell tumors is unknown, and there appears to be no association with cryptorchidism.

Approximately 10 per cent of Leydig cell tumors are malignant; however, no malignant cases have ever been reported in the prepubertal age group. In the prepubertal cases (average age 5 years), presenting symptoms are usually those of isosexual precocity, whereas in adults, the most common presenting feature is a testicular mass. Adults may also present with symptoms of a feminizing nature, such as impotence, decreased libido, and gynecomastia.

Radical inguinal orchiectomy is the treatment of choice. In the event of pathologic suspicion of malignancy, CT scan or ultrasound of the retroperitoneum is indicated to search for retroperitoneal adenopathy. RPLND has been recommended as routine in patients with malignant appearing lesions; however, total experience with any form of therapy is limited by the small number of patients who have been treated. These tumors are relatively radioresistant, and chemotherapy regimens have not demonstrated a convincing benefit in patients with metastatic spread.

The prognosis for Leydig cell tumors is good because of their generally benign nature. Average survival time from surgery, in patients with metastatic disease, is approximately 3 years.

REFERENCE

1. Gabrilove, J.L., Nicolis, G.L., Mitty, H.A., and Sohval, A.R.: Feminizing interstitial cell tumor of the testis: Personal observation and a review of the literature. Cancer, *35*:1184, 1975.

562-C *(Campbell's, pp. 1252–1253)*

Gonadoblastomas are rare tumors occuring almost exclusively in patients with some form of gonadal dysgenesis, with the majority of patients under 30 years of age at diagnosis. The tumors consist of three elements, Sertoli cells, interstitial tissue, and germ cells, the proportions of which show considerable variation. The germ cells of gonadoblastoma are similar to those of seminoma.

Approximately four fifths of patients with gonablastomas are phenotypic female and the remainder are phenotypic males, almost always presenting with cryptorchidism, hypospadias and some female internal genitalia. In general, 90 per cent of patients with gonadal dysgenesis and gonadoblastoma have chromatin-negative findings and more than half have an XY karyotype, with the remainder demonstrating mosaicism.

Radical orchiectomy is the first stage in therapy, and the high incidence of bilaterality (50 per cent) argues for contralateral gonodectomy when gonodal dysgenesis is present. As with germ cell tumors of the adult testis, further therapy may logically be based on the histology of the germ cell element and the results of clinical staging.

REFERENCES

1. Scully, R.E.: Gonodoblastoma: A gondal tumor related to dysgerminoma (seminoma) and capable of sex-hormone production. Cancer, *6*:455, 1953.
2. Taterman, A.: A distinctive gondal neoplasm related to gonodoblastoma. Cancer, *30*:1219, 1972.

563-A *(Campbell's, p. 1255)*

Approximately 200 cases of metastatic carcinoma to the testis have been reported. In the majority, it is discovered incidentally at autopsy in cases of widespread disease. The common primary sources in decreasing order of frequency are prostate, lung, gastrointestinal tract, melanoma, and kidney.

The testicle appears to be a prime initial site of relapse in male children with acute lymphocytic leukemia. Biopsy is essential to the diagnosis; however, orchiectomy is probably unwarranted. Appropriate treatment in patients with testicular involvement of leukemia is testicular irradiation with 2000 cGy in 10 fractions plus reinstitution of adjunctive chemotherapy.

564-D *(Campbell's, p. 1256)*

Adenomatoid tumors are the most common tumors of the paratesticular tissues, accounting for 30 per cent of all paratesticular tumors. In men they arise most commonly in or adjacent to the lower pole of the epididymis. The majority of these tumors occur in the third or fourth decade of life, but cases have been seen in patients ranging from 20 to 80 years of age. These tumors are usually small, solid, and asymptomatic.

These tumors behave in a benign fashion, and there has never been a documented case of metastasis. The long history of these tumors and the absence of distant metastases suggest a benign nature. Treatment, therefore, is only surgical excision.

REFERENCES

1. Soderstrom, J., and Leidberg, C.F.: Malignant "adenomatoid" tumor of the epididymis. Acta Pathol. Microbiol. Scand., *67*:165, 1966.
2. Mostofi, F.K., and Price, E.B.: Tumors of the male genital system. *In* Atlas of Tumor Pathology, Second Series, Fascicle 8. Washington, D.C., Armed Forces Institute of Pathology, 1973.

565-C *(Campbell's, pp. 1257–1258)*

Most investigators agree that rhabdomyosarcoma, in its juvenile form, accounts for approximately 40 per cent of all paratesticular tumors, benign and malignant. Leiomyosarcoma appears to be the second most common lesion in this area, followed by fibrosarcoma, liposarcoma, and undifferentiated mesenchymal tumors.

Paratesticular rhabdomyosarcoma occurs predominantly in children and adolescents and is most commonly seen during the first 2 decades of life. Clinically, the tumor usually appears as a large intrascrotal mass that compresses the testis and epididymis.

The primary paratesticular tumor should be removed by inguinal orchiectomy with high ligation of the cord. Adjuvant therapy for all paratesticular malignancies depends on histology and grade, with most being treated with radiation therapy and combination chemotherapy (e.g., CAV: Cytoxan, actinomycin D, vincristine). Since the risk of retroperitoneal lymph node metastases in patients with rhabdomyosarcoma is between 25 and 40 per cent, routine RPLND has been recommended in patients with paratesticular rhabdomyosarcoma as well.

REFERENCES

1. Johnson, D.E.: Trends in surgery for childhood rhabdomyosarcoma. Cancer, *35*:916, 1975.
2. Kingston, J.E., McElwain, T.J., and Malpas, J.S.: Childhood rhabdomyosarcoma: Experience of the Children's Solid Tumor Group. Br. J. Cancer, *48*:195, 1983.
3. Gowing, N.F., and Morgan, A.D.: Paratesticular tumors of connective tissue and muscle. Br. J. Urol., *36* (suppl):78, 1964.

566-B *(Campbell's, pp. 1264–1266)*

Congenital inclusion cysts have been reported to occur in the penoscrotal raphe, but acquired inclusion cysts subsequent to trauma are more common. Other benign tumors of the penis include angiomas, fibrosis, neuromas, lipomas, pseudotumors from self-administered infections or foreign bodies, and hirsutoid papillomas. Hirsutoid papillomas are pearly penile papules located on the glans near the coronal sulcus or frenulum. Treatment is rarely necessary, and no association with infection or malignancy has been reported. When a diagnosis is in question, all benign lesions are best treated with local excision and careful histologic examination to rule out malignancy.

The most frequent manifestation of balanitis xerotica obliterous (BXO) is a white patch on the prepuce or glans that extends to and around the urethral meatus. Glandular erosions, fissures, and meatal stenosis may occur. Histologically, it is similar to lichen sclerosus et atrophicus. Diagnosis requires a biopsy of the lesion. Treatment is directed at relief of meatal stenosis by meatotomy, urethral dilation, or local application of topical steroids. Because of reports of malignant degeneration, the lesions require periodic examination, with follow up biopsies if a change in clinical appearance occurs.

Other premalignant cutaneous lesions of the penis include leukoplakia and cutaneous horns.

REFERENCES

1. Bainbridge, D.R., Whitaker, R.H., and Shepheard, B.G.F.: Balanitis xerotica obliterous and urinary obstruction. Br. J. Urol., *43*:487, 1971.
2. Rheinschild, G.W., and Olsen, B.S.: Balanitis xerotica obliterous. J. Urol., *104*:860, 1970.

567-D *(Campbell's, pp. 1266–1268)*

A number of penile lesions have been associated with viral infection. Condyloma acuminata are typically soft, pliable, reddish, papillary lesions, also called "veneral" or "genital" warts. In the male, condylomata occur most commonly on the prepuce, penile shaft, or glans, with only approximately 5 per cent of patients demonstrating intraurethral involvement. This disease is believed to be sexually transmitted and caused by HPV. A 5 per cent acetic acid soak of the penis may help identify subclinical disease in patients at risk, and urethroscopy is indicated for any patient with condyloma at the urethral meatus. A variety of different options exist for the treatment and even alpha-interferon. Intra urethral lesions are best managed by neodymium:YAG laser or intraurethral 5-fluorouracil cream.

Bowenoid papulosis occurs as multiple papules on the penile skin, with a peak incidence during the 2nd and 3rd decades of life. It appears similar to carcinoma in situ but has a benign clinical cause. DVA studies of biopsy specimens have found DNA-sequences closely related to HPV 16. Treatment of the lesion includes electrofulgation, cryotherapy, laser, and 5-fluorouracil cream.

Kaposi's sarcoma is a disease of the reticuloendothelial system which can manifest itself as an elevated, painful, bleeding papule or ulcer on the penis. Kaposi's sarcoma has been closely associated with patients with AIDS, and in these patients, it is a much more virulent malignancy. Kaposi's sarcoma restricted to penile involvement should be treated aggressively with local excision or radiation therapy. In patients with AIDS, Kaposi's sarcoma of the penis is rarely the first area of involvement, therefore, treatment is radiation therapy or chemotherapy. Verrucous carcinoma of the penis has also been shown to have a viral etiology (see next question).

Leukoplakia is a premalignant whitish plaque believed to be caused by chronic irritation. A viral etiology has not been found.

REFERENCES

1. Carpiniello, V.L., Schoenberg, M., and Malloy, T.R.: Long-term follow up subclinical human papillomavirus infected patients, treated with the CO_2 laser and intraurethral 5-fluorouracil: A treatment protocol. J. Urol., *143*:726, 1990.
2. Gross, G., Hagedorn, M., Ikenberg, H., et al.: Bowenard papulosis: Presence of human papillomavirus (HVP) structural antigens and of HPV 16-related DNA sequences. Arch. Dermatol., *121*:858, 1985.
3. Bayne, D., and Wise, G.J.: Kaposi's sarcoma of the penis and extended genitalia: A disease of our times. Urology, *31*:22, 1988.

568-D *(Campbell's, pp. 1268–1269)*

Buschke-Lowenstein tumor, also known as verrucous carcinoma or giant condyloma acuminata, is a peculiar low grade variant of squamous cell carcinoma of the penis. As in the case of condyloma acuminata, the etiology may be viral (HPV 6 and 11). Verrucous carcinoma displaces, penetrates, and destroys adjacent structures by compression; however, on histologic examination, it shows no signs of malignancy.

Excisional biopsy or multiple deep biopsies are necessary to distinguish this lesion from true penile carcinoma. Once the diagnosis is established, treatment consists of local excision, sparing as much of the penis as possible. Treatment with podophyllin has proved unsuccessful, as has treatment with topical 5-fluorouracil cream. Since lymph node metastases are extremely rare with verrucous carcinoma, inguinal lymph node dissection is not indicated. Radiation therapy is not advised since it has been associated with rapid malignant changes when directed at verrucous carcinoma in other locations.

REFERENCES

1. Bruns, T.N.C., Lavvetz, R.J., Kerr, E.S., and Ross, G.: Buschke-Lowenstein giant condylomas: Pitfalls in management. Urology, *5*:773, 1975.
2. Dawson, D.F., Duckworth, J.K., Bernhardt, H., and Young, J.M.: Giant condyloma and verrucous carcinoma of the genital area. Arch. Pathol., *79*:225, 1965.

569-A *(Campbell's, pp. 1269–1270)*

Carcinoma in situ of the penis (also known as erythroplasia of Queyrat or Bowen's disease) has a natural history that parallels that of early carcinoma of the penis. It is characterized by noninvasive replacement of normal mucosa with atypical hyperplastic cells with vacuolation, multiple, hyperchromatic nuclei, and mutatic figures at all levels. HPV has also been identified in carcinoma in situ. Although, traditionally, Bowen's disease was believed to be a marker for internal malignancy, case-controlled studies have not confirmed this association. Therefore, penile carcinoma in situ does not warrant a specific search for internal malignancy.

Since treatment requires proper identification of malignancy, biopsies should be multiple and of adequate depth to detect invasion. If a lesion is small and noninvasive, local excision that spares penile structure and function (e.g., Mohs technique) is adequate. Preputial lesions are best managed with circumcisions. Fulguration is occasionally successful, but is often associated with recurrences. Other treatment options for patients with carcinoma in situ of the penis include radiation therapy, topical 5-fluorouracil, liquid nitrogen cryosurgery, and laser therapy (CO_2 or Nd:YAG).

REFERENCES

1. Grabstold, H., and Kelley, C.D.: Radiation therapy of penile cancer. Urology, *15*:575, 1980.
2. Graham, J.H., and Helwig, E.B.: Erythroplasia of Queyrat. Cancer, *32*:1396, 1973.

570-E *(Campbell's, pp. 1270–1271)*

Penile carcinoma constitutes less than 1 per cent to fall malignancies in the United States' male population, an increase of 1 to 2 cases per 100,000 per year. It is most commonly diagnosed during the 6th and 7th decade of life. Some series have found that blacks have a higher incidence than whites.

The incidence of carcinoma of the penis varies markedly with the hygienic standards and the cultural and religious practices of different countries. Circumcision in neonates and children has been well established as a prophylactic measure that virtually eliminates the occurrence of penile carcinoma. Adults circumcision, however, offers little or no protection against the future appearance of penile carcinoma.

Chronic irritation from retained smegma has been postulated to increase the risk of the development of penile carcinoma. Phimosis, which is present in 25 to 75 per cent of patients presenting with penile cancer, is another risk factor. Penile carcinoma has also been associated with sexually transmitted HPV. Of note, there is a threefold to eightfold increase in the incidence of cervical cancer among the sexual partners of patients with penile carcinoma.

Although a history of trauma often predates the appearance of carcinoma of the penis, it is thought that this finding is coincidental rather than causal. No consistent etiologic relationship of penile carcinoma to veneral disease (syphilis, granuloma inguinale, and choroid) has been found, and any association of these diseases with penile carcinoma is probably coincidental.

REFERENCES

1. Gursel, E.D., Georgountzos, C., Uson, A.C., et al.: Penile cancer. Urology, *1*:569, 1973.
2. Hanash, K.A., Furlow, W.L., Utz, D.C., and Harrison, E.G.: Carcinoma of the penis: A clinicopathologic study. J. Urol., *104*:291, 1970.

571-B *(Campbell's, p. 1271)*

Carcinoma of the penis is almost unknown among the Jewish population, among whom neonatal circumcision is customary. In the United States, where neonatal circumcision is frequent, penile carcinoma comprises less than 1 per cent of malignancies in males. Adult circumcision offers little or no protection against the future appearance of penile carcinoma. It is reasonable to consider that circumcision may not be as important in countries in which good hygiene is practiced and soap and water is readily available.

New evidence has suggested possible medical benefits from newborn circumcision, such as a reduction in the incidence of urinary tract infections. As a result, the American Academy of Pediatrics Task Force on Circumcisions has revised its assessment as follows: "Newborn circumcision has potential advantages as well as disadvantages. When circumcision is being considered, the benefits and risks should be explained to the parents and informed consent obtained."

REFERENCE

1. Schoen, E.J., Anderson, G., Bohon, C., et al.: Task force on circumcision, report of the task force on circumcision. Pediatrics, *84*:388, 1989.

572-C, 573-A *(Campbell's, pp. 1271–1272)*

Carcinoma of the penis usually begins with a small lesion, which gradually extends to involve the entire glans, shaft, and corpora. Buck's fascia acts as a temporary natural barrier.

Metastases to the regional femoral and iliac nodes represents the earliest route of dissemination from penile carcinoma. Multiple cross-communications exist throughout all levels of drainage, as that penile lymphatic drainage is bilateral to both inguinal areas.

Metastatic enlargement of regional lymph nodes eventually leads to skin necrosis, chronic infection, and death (from inanition, sepsis, or hemorrhage) in the majority of untreated patients within 2 years of diagnosis. Clinically detectable distant metastatic lesions to the lung, liver, bone, or brain are uncommon, and are reported as occurring in 1 to 10 per cent of large series. Urethral and bladder involvement is also rare.

REFERENCES

1. Cabanas, R.: An approach to the treatment of penile carcinoma. Cancer, *39*:456, 1977.
2. Skinner, D.G., Leadbetter, W.F., and Kelley, S.B.: The surgical management of squamous cell carcinoma of the penis. J. Urol., *107*:273, 1972.
3. Riveros, M., and Gorostiaga, R.: Cancer of the penis. Arch. Surg., *85*:377, 1962.

574-C *(Campbell's, pp. 1272–1273)*

Almost without exception, the penile lesion itself calls attention to the possibility of carcinoma. Phimosis may obscure a lesion and thus result in a prolonged period of neglect. Penile carcinoma is most frequent in the glans, the coronal sulcus, and the prepuce. Occasionally, a mass on ulceration, a necrosis or hemorrhage in the inguinal area resulting from nodal metastases present before the lesion concealed in the phimotic preputial sac. Urinary retention and urinary fistula are rare presenting symptoms.

Pain does not develop in proportion to the extent of the local destructive process. Presenting symptoms referable to distant metastases are also rare because local and regional nodal disease are usually far advanced before distant metastases are detectable.

The time from the initiation of signs and symptoms to the time of the patient's presentation to a physician averages approximately 1 year. At presentation, the majority of lesions are confined to the penis. Examination should include characterization of the penile lesion, inspection of the base of the penis and scrotum, rectal and bimanual examination, and palpation of both inguinal areas to attempt to fully assess the extent of disease

REFERENCES

1. Gursel, E.D., Georgountzos, C., Usm, A.C., et al.: Penile cancer. Urology, *1*:569, 1973.
2. Johnson, D.E., Fuerst, D.E., and Ayala, A.G.: Carcinoma of the penis: Experience in 153 cases. Urology, *1*:404, 1973.

575-D *(Campbell's, p. 1274)*

Identifying carcinoma of the penis and the depth of invasion by microscopic study of a biopsy specimen is mandatory before initiation of therapy. No harmful effects regarding tumor dissemination secondary to biopsy are recognized. Biopsy with confirmation of tumor by frozen section while the patient is still anesthetized, and immediate surgical excision (with full prior informed consent of the patient) constitutes an alternative means of diagnosis and simultaneous treatment.

576-B *(Campbell's, p. 1274)*

The majority of tumors of the penis are squamous cell carcinomas demonstrating keratinization, epithelial pearl formation, and various degrees of mitotic activity. The normal rete pegs are disrupted, and invasive lesions penetrate the basement membrane and surrounding structures.

577-A *(Campbell's, pp. 1274–1276)*

Most malignancies of the penis are low grade. Several series have noted reduced survival rates among patients with high-grade neoplasms. The loss of cell surface blood group antigens has also been associated with invasion and metastases. Aneuploidy may also predict disease of greater biologic potential for growth and metastases. However, the strongest prognostic indicator for survival is the presence or absence of nodal metastases (see Tables 31–1 and 31–2).

REFERENCE

1. Fraley, E.E., Zhang, G., Manivel, C., and Niehans, G.A.: The role of ilioinguinal lymphadenectomy and significance of histological differentiation in treatment of carcinoma of the penis. J. Urol., *142*:1478–1482, 1989.

578-C *(Campbell's, pp. 1276–1277)*

No universally accepted staging system for penile carcinoma exists. The most commonly employed classification was suggested by Jackson; however, it fails to specifically characterize both the initial primary lesion and any nodal metastases. The tumor, node, and metastasis (TNM) staging system most precisely described the depth of invasion of the primary lesion, and it also more accurately describes the status of the regional lymph nodes.

JACKSON CLASSIFICATION FOR PENILE CARCINOMA

Stage I (A)	Tumor confined to glans, prepuce or both
Stage II (B)	Tumor involves penile shaft
Stage III (C)	Tumor with operable inguinal metastases present
Stage IV (D)	Tumor involving adjacent structures; tumor associated with inoperable inguinal metastases or distant metastases

TNM CLASSIFICATION OF PENILE CARCINOMA

Primary Tumor (T)

Tx	Primary tumor cannot be assessed
T0	No evidence of primary tumor
Tis	Carcinoma in situ
TA	Verrucous carcinoma of the penis
T1	Tumor invades subepithelial connective tissue
T2	Tumor invades corpus spongiosum or cavernosum
T3	Tumor invades urethra or prostate
T4	Tumor invades other adjacent structures

Regional Lymph Nodes (N)

NX	Regional lymph nodes cannot be assessed
N0	No regional lymph node metastases
N1	Metastases in a single, superficial inguinal lymph node
N2	Metastases in multiple, superficial inguinal lymph nodes (unilateral or bilateral)
N3	Metastases in deep inguinal or pelvic lymph nodes

Distant Metastases (M)

MX	Presence of distant metastases cannot be assessed
M0	No distant metastases
M1	Distant metastases

REFERENCES

1. Jackson, S.M.: The treatment of carcinoma of the penis. Br. J. Surg., *53*:33, 1966.
2. Union Internatinale Contre le Cancer (UICC): TNM Atlas: Illustrated Guide to the TNM/pTNM—Classi-

fication of Malignant Tumors, 3rd ed. New York, Springer-Verlag, 1989, pp. 237–244.

579-D *(Campbell's, pp. 1276–1282)*

Amputation by partial or total penectomy is the gold standard of therapy for penile carcinoma. For lesions involving the glans and distal shaft, even when they are apparently superficial, partial amputation with a 2-cm margin proximal to the tumor is necessary to minimize local recurrence. In contrast, local wedge resection has been associated with recurrence rates of approximately 50 per cent. Adequate partial amputation in the absence of inguinal metastases can produce 5-year survival rates of 70 to 80 per cent.

If the proximal penile shaft is involved by malignancy to the extent that resection will leave a close margin and a stump that prohibits upright voiding, total penectomy, and perineal urethrostomy, should be performed.

In an attempt to preserve as much normal tissue as possible, the Mohs micrographic surgery technique (MMS) has been suggested for the management of small penile lesions with cure rates at least equal to the results of partial penectomy in select patients.

Laser therapy has been employed to treat stage Tis, Ta, T1, and some T2 penile cancer. It is imperative to adequately stage the tumor with deep biopsies before applying laser therapy. Treatment of T1 and T2 tumors has not been as successful as with Tis (recurrence rates of up to 15 per cent have been rated).

When radiation therapy is employed as the initial treatment for penile carcinoma, control of the primary lesions occurs with much less frequency than when surgery is primarily employed.

Topical chemotherapy has no role in the initial management of invasive carcinoma of the penis.

REFERENCES

1. deKernion, J.B., Tynbery, P., Persky, L., and Fegen, J.P.: Carcinoma of the penis. Cancer, *32*:1256, 1973.
2. McDougal, W.S., Kirchner, F.K., Jr., Edwards, R.H., and Killion, L.T.: Treatment of carcinoma of the penis: The case of primary lymphadenectomy. J. Urol., *136*: 38, 1986.
3. Bandieramonte, G., Santoro, O., Borocchi, P., et al.: Total resection of glans penis surface by CO_2 laser microsurgery. Acta Oncol., *27*:575, 1988.
4. Kelly, C.D., Arthur, K., Rogoff, E., and Grabstald, H.: Radiation therapy of penile cancer. Urology, *4*:571, 1974.

580-E *(Campbell's, pp. 1282–1287)*

Inguinal lymph node dissection should be performed in the presence of clinically palpable nodes after appropriate treatment of the primary lesion and subsidence of inflammation. Up to 50 per cent of patients with inguinal metastasis who are treated with inguinal lymphadenectomy achieve a 5-year disease-free survival, as opposed to almost certain death within 2 years for those patients who do not undergo treatment. Palpable adenopathy at initial presentation does not inevitably indicate the presence of tumor. A false-positive rate of up to 50 per cent related to inflammation has been reported. A 6-week course of antibiotics can be used to help differentiate inflammation from metastatic disease. Due to the anatomic crossover of lymphatic of the penis, contralateral metastases have been noted in up to 50 per cent of patients treated with bilateral inguinal node dissection at diagnosis, even if the contralateral nodal region appears negative to palpation. Therefore, in patients presenting with unilateral adenopathy at initial presentation in the treatment of the primary tumor, the absence of clinical adenopathy on one side dictates a higher probability of freedom from disease on that side. Therefore, in this case, it is recommended to perform only unilateral lymph node dissection.

Immediate adjunctive lymph node dissection yields better survival results that delayed lymph node dissection. This finding has led to controversy regarding how to treat patients with clinically negative groin examination findings at the time of presentation of the primary lesion since inguinal lymph node dissection is associated with significant morbidity. In these cases, it is important to identify indicators that predict for increased risk of nodal involvement (e.g., stage T2 or higher, or high grade tumors) so as to be able to select patients who are most likely to harbor subclinical metastases.

The therapeutic gain of extending nodal dissection to include the iliac nodes is undetermined. However, because involvement of pelvic nodes on microscopic examination may occur with some frequency, because survival with positive pelvic nodes has been documented, and because duration of survival has been lengthened after iliac node dissection, the procedure is reasonable for the young males, who are a good surgical risk.

REFERENCES

1. Fraley, E.E., Zhang, G., Manivel, C., and Nichans, G.A.: The role of ilioinguinal lymphadenectomy and significance of histological differentiation in the treatment of carcinoma of the penis. J. Urol., *142*:1478, 1989.
2. McDongol, W.S., Kirchner, F.K., Jr., Edwards, R.H., and Killion, L.T.: Treatment of carcinoma of the penis: The case of primary lymph adenectomy. J. Urol., *136*: 38, 1986.
3. Puras, A., Foruno, R., Gonzales-Flores, B., and Sottongo, A.: Staging lymphadenectomy in the treatment of carcinoma of the penis. Proc. Kimbrough Urol. Semin., *14*:15, 1980.

581-C *(Campbell's, p. 1285)*

Sentinel node biopsy as described by Cabanas is predicated on detailed penile lymphangiographic studies that have demonstrated consistent drainage of the penile lymphatics into a "sentinel" node or group of nodes located superomedial to the junction of the saphenous and femoral veins in the area of the superficial epigastric vein. Metastases to this node indicate the need for a complete inguinal lymph node dissection.

The accuracy of sentinel node biopsy to identify inguinal metastases has been questioned with false negative rates of 6 to 50 per cent (average 10 per cent) in various series.

REFERENCES

1. Cobanas, R.: An approach to the treatment of penile carcinoma. Cancer, *39*:456, 1977.

2. McDougal, W.S., Kirchner, F.K., Jr., Edwards, R.H., and Killion, L.T.: Treatment of carcinoma of the penis: The case of primary lymphadenectomy. J. Urol., *136*: 38, 1986.

582-A *(Campbell's, pp. 1287–1288)*

Patients with stages Tis, Ta, or T1 have lesions that involve only the glans mucosa or shaft skin and that are totally exophytic and superficial. These penile lesions, in the absence of palpable adenopathy, are found to have nodal metastases in less than 10 per cent of the cases, and therefore, may be followed with periodic examination of the inguinal area after treatment of the primary tumor. The subsequent appearance of unilateral adenopathy provides indications for unilateral inguinal node dissection.

Patients with stages T2 or T3 have lesions that invade Buck's fascia, tunica albuginea, and the corporal bodies. The incidence of nodal metastases increases significantly in the presence of T2 disease or greater (approximately 66 per cent). Therefore, immediate bilateral adjunctive node dissection is indicated.

Patients with penile carcinoma and palpable adenopathy require control of the primary tumor, followed by a reevaluation of the inguinal nodes after 2 to 6 weeks of antibiotic therapy in an attempt to control infection and allows time for inflammatory adenopathy to resolve. If adenopathy persists, bilateral inguinal node dissections are recommended. If adenopathy resolves with antibiotic therapy, then the decision for adjunctive lymphadenectomy is based on primary tumor stage.

REFERENCE

1. McDougal, W.S., Kirchner, F.K. Jr., Edwards, R.H., and Killion, L.T.: Treatment of carcinoma of the penis: The case of primary lymphadenectomy. J. Urol., *136*: 38, 1986.

583-E *(Campbell's, pp. 1288–1290)*

Given the overall poor prognosis, the treatment of patients with distant metastases, inoperable inguinal metastases, or extensive adjuvant organ invasion is often limited to palliative chemotherapy or radiation therapy, but in young patients, aggressive confined modality therapy with surgical and chemotherapy is warranted.

Objections to radiation therapy of inguinal node metastases are that inguinal areas tolerate radiation poorly and are subject to skin maceration and ulceration. Radiation therapy for inguinal metastases documented by histologic examination has been compared with surgery for the node-positive groin. A 50 per cent 5-year survival rate was observed among the surgically treated group, and a 25 per cent 5-year survival rate was observed among the irradiated group. Other series have also reported that radiation to the inguinal areas has not proved therapeutically effective.

The route of penile carcinoma in the United States will make it difficult to accumulate sufficient numbers of patients to adequately test chemotherapeutic agents in Phase II or III trials. This information will need to come from trials in South America or Asia. Several studies have shown that cis-platinum and methotrexate have greater activity than bleomycin. Response rates using both chemotherapy and radiation therapy have been disappointing as well.

REFERENCES

1. Jensen, M.S.: Cancer of the penis in Denmark 1942–1962 (511 cases). Dan. Med. Bull., *24*:66, 1977.
2. Ahmed, T., Sklaroff, R., and Yagoda, A.: Sequential trials of methotrexate, cis-platin, and bleomycin for penile cancer. J. Urol., *132*:465, 1984.
3. Sklaroff, R.B., and Yagoda, A.: Penile cancer: Natural history and therapy. *In* Chemotherapy and Urological Malignancy. New York, Springer-Verlag, 1982, pp. 98–105.

584-D *(Campbell's, p. 1291)*

Changes in the technique and the incisions employed have limited the complications seen previously with lymph node dissection. The transposition of the sartorius muscle over the femoral vessels has minimized the incidence of vascular erosion and thrombosis.

The majority of wound problems are secondary to the loss of skin at the edge of the wound. In most instances, however, only a small amount of superficial skin is lost. These small areas of skin loss can be simply covered with split-thickness skin grafting. However, with deeper skin loss or with the excision of a larger cuticular area with the specimen, more substantial tissue transfer is required. A number of local flaps are available for transposition into these tissue defects including gracilis, tensor fascia lata, and rectus abdominis flaps.

REFERENCE

1. Trier, W.C.: Local skin flaps, Chap. 321. *In* Strauch, B., Vasconex, L.O., and Hall-Findlay, E.J. (Eds): Grabb's Encyclopedia of Flaps, Vol III. Boston, Little, Brown, and Co., 1990, pp. 1393–1395.

585-B *(Campbell's, pp. 1291–1292)*

Nonsquamous malignancies of the penis are extremely rare. Primary mesenchymal tumors of the penis can present at any age with signs and symptoms of subcutaneous mass, penile pain, priapism, or urinary obstruction. Malignant lesions are found more frequently on the proximal shaft; benign lesions are more often located distally. The most common malignant lesions are those of vascular origin (hemangioendothelioma), followed in frequency by those of neural, myogenic, and fibrous origin. To avoid local recurrences, total penile amputation, even for superficial malignancies of any cell type, should be considered. Regional metastases are rare; therefore, unless adenopathy is palpable, node dissections are not recommended. Distant metastases are also unusual. Radiation therapy and chemotherapy have not been used extensively enough to comment upon their efficacy.

REFERENCE

1. Dehner, L.P., and Smith, B.H.: Soft tissue tumors of the penis. Cancer, *25*:1431, 1970.

586-C *(Campbell's, p. 1293)*

Metastatic lesions to the penis are unusual. The most common sites of origin of metastatic lesions to the penis are the bladder, the prostate, and the rectum. Renal and respiratory neoplasms have also metastasized to the penis.

Penile metastases represent an advanced form of virulent disease and usually appear rather rapidly after recognition and treatment of the primary lesion. Because of the association of a penile metastatic lesion with advanced disease, survival after its presentation is limited, and the majority of patients die within 1 year.

Penectomy is occasionally indicated after failure of other modalities to palliate intractable pain. Treatment with radiation therapy has been generally unsuccessful, and chemotherapy has not been employed in a sufficient number of cases to warrant definitive recommendations.

REFERENCES

1. Abeshouse, B.S., and Abeshouse, G.A.: Metastatic tumors of the penis: A review of the literature and a report of two cases. J. Urol., *86*:99, 1961.
2. Mukamel, E., Farrer, J., Smith, R.B., and deKernion, J.B.: metastatic carcinoma of the penis: When is total penectomy indicated? Urology, *24*:15, 1987.

PART X

EMBRYOLOGY AND ANOMALIES OF THE GENITOURINARY TRACT

CHAPTERS 32 THROUGH 43

DIRECTIONS: Each question below contains suggested responses. Select the ONE BEST response to each question.

587. The mesoderm originates from the:
A. Yolk sac
B. Amnion
C. Cell migration between ectoderm and endoderm
D. Allantois
E. Germ cells

588. The period of the embryo, during which the germ layers form the organs of the body, is completed by the end of:
A. 4 weeks
B. 8 weeks
C. 12 weeks
D. 16 weeks
E. 20 weeks

589. The urinary system arises from the:
A. Endoderm
B. Mesoderm
C. Ectoderm
D. Ectoderm and mesoderm
E. Mesoderm and endoderm

590. The mesonephric (wolffian) duct arises from the:
A. Pronephric duct
B. Paramesonephric duct
C. Müllerian duct
D. Ectoderm
E. Endoderm

591. The ureteral bud arises from the:
A. Pronephric duct
B. Mesonephric duct
C. Metanephric duct
D. Ectoderm
E. Endoderm

592. The ureter and kidney arise from the:
A. Endoderm
B. Mesoderm
C. Ectoderm
D. Mesoderm and ectoderm
E. Mesoderm and endoderm

593. Based on current theories of renal development, the most likely explanation for renal dysplasia is:
A. Abnormal interaction between defective metanephrogenic mesenchyme and ureteral bud ampullae
B. Toxic damage to normal renal blastema
C. Obstruction of developing ureter
D. Failure during nephron vascularization
E. Failure of nephron segmentation

594. The bladder arises from the:
A. Ectoderm
B. Mesoderm
C. Endoderm
D. Mesoderm and endoderm
E. Mesoderm and ectoderm

595. The Weigert-Meyer rule states that in a patient with complete ureteral duplication, the ureter draining the upper pole of the kidney is:
A. Cranial and medial to the lower pole ureter
B. Cranial and lateral to the lower pole ureter
C. Caudal and medial to the lower pole ureter
D. Caudal and lateral to the lower pole ureter
E. Lateral to the lower pole ureter

596. During human embryologic and early fetal development, the genitalia are structurally the same in males and females until the:
A. 4th week
B. 8th week
C. 10th week
D. 16th week
E. 20th week

597. The penile urethra arises from the:
A. Genital swelling
B. Vesicoallantoic canal
C. Tourneux's fold
D. Paramesonephric duct
E. Urogenital sinus

598. The embryologic origin of the prostate is the:
A. Vesicoallantoic canal
B. Urogenital sinus

C. Müller's tubercle
D. Mesonephric duct
E. Yolk sac

599. Dihydrotestosterone mediates the development of the:

A. Seminal vesicle
B. Epididymis
C. Vas deferens
D. Prostate
E. Genital swelling

600. The paraurethral glands of Skene in the female are homologues of the male:

A. Prostate
B. Cowper's gland
C. Utricle
D. Seminal vesicle
E. Urethral glands

601. Bartholin's glands in the female are homologues of the male:

A. Prostate
B. Cowper's glands
C. Utricle
D. Seminal vesicles
E. Seminal colliculus

602. The appendix of the epididymis orignates from the:

A. Müllerian duct
B. Paramesonephric duct
C. Mesonephric tubules
D. Wolffian duct
E. Paragenitalis

603. The organ of Giraldés derives from the:

A. Müllerian duct
B. Pronephros
C. Metanephros
D. Müller's tubercle
E. Mesonephric tubules

604. The origin of the seminal vesicle is the:

A. Müllerian duct
B. Paramesonephric duct
C. Mesonephric duct
D. Urogenital sinus
E. Prostatic urethra

605. Müllerian inhibiting substance is produced by:

A. Leydig cells
B. Sertoli cells
C. Genital ridge
D. Paragenitalis
E. Germ cells

606. The prostatic utricle is a remnant of the:

A. Müllerian duct
B. Mesonephric duct
C. Urogenital sinus
D. Wolffian duct
E. Gartner's duct

607. The appendix of the testis is a remnant of the:

A. Mesonephric duct
B. Mesonephric tubules
C. Gubernaculum
D. Müllerian duct
E. Organ of Giraldés

608. Gartner's duct is a remnant of the:

A. Müllerian duct
B. Gubernaculum
C. Urethral groove
D. Uterovaginal primordium
E. Mesonephric duct

609. Which of the following statements about the anatomic development of the fetal kidney is *true*?

A. The pronephros is the first stage of renal development and is important because its ductal system gives rise to the ureteric bud.
B. The mesonephros degenerates by 12 weeks gestation and has little impact on the definitive kidney.
C. The mesonephros is felt to transiently function but then quickly degenerates.
D. The metanephros gives rise to the definitive kidney independent of the pronephros and mesonephros.
E. The metanephric kidney develops centrifugally with the medullary nephrons being the last to complete development.

610. The following statements about functional fetal renal development are true EXCEPT:

A. The human kidney first produces urine around 10 to 12 weeks.
B. Throughout gestation, salt and water homeostasis is handled by the placenta.
C. Fetal renal blood flow is approximately 10 times less that of the newborn.
D. GFR progressively increases with gestational age.
E. Potassium excretion decreases with gestation in response to fetal plasma aldosterone concentration.

611. Neonatal renal fuction is characterized by all of the following EXCEPT:

A. The GFR slowly rises.
B. A blunted response to sodium loading persists.
C. Concentrating ability remains fairly limited.
D. Bicarbonate reabsorption increases.
E. Calcium handling reverses to active reabsorption.

612. When evaluating glomerular function in the postnatal period, which of the following is *true*?

A. Checking the serum creatinine in the first 24–48 hours of life provides an accurate baseline of glomerular function.
B. A preterm infant may have a serum creatinine as high as 1.5 mg/dl for the first few weeks of life.
C. Due to rapid changes in postnatal renal function, serum creatinine values are of little use.
D. The creatinine clearance can be accurately derived from the serum creatinine concentration and a newborn's height.
E. While a ^{99m}TC-diethylenetriminepentaacetic acid (T_c-DTPA) renal scan provides information about the relative function of each kidney, it provides a poor measurement of the GFR.

613. A healthy-appearing infant is found to have the following laboratory values: serum sodium of 136 mg/dl, serum chloride of 104 mg/dl, serum potassium of 5.8 mg/dl, serum total CO_2 of 19, and a urine pH of 5.0. Which of the following best describes the status of this child?

A. No abnormality is present.
B. Type I RTA is present.
C. Type II RTA is present.
D. Type III RTA is present.
E. Type IV RTA is present.

614. In reference to the patient in the previous question, after the diagnosis has been made all of the following would be an appropriate next evaluation or treatment EXCEPT:

A. Initiate alkali therapy with Shohl's solution or Bicitra.
B. Sonographic examination of the urinary tract.
C. 24-hour urine collection for creatinine clearance, protein and calcium excretion, and phosphorus reabsorption.
D. Initiate therapy with furosemide to manage the concomitant volume overload.
E. Urinalysis to screen for glucosuria.

615. Which of the following conditions is *not* felt to cause a disorder of urinary concentration in infants and children?

A. Unilateral renal agenesis
B. Obstructive nephropathy
C. Pyelonephritis
D. Renal tubular acidosis
E. Sickle cell nephropathy

616. Which of the following statements concerning the hormonal control of renal function during fetal development is *true*?

A. The renin-angiotensin system develops very early in the fetus and as in the adult, fetal renin is localized to the juxtaglomerular apparatus.
B. A marked increase in plasma renin activity occurs in the perinatal period.
C. Atrial natriuretic peptide (ANP) levels decrease in response to intrauterine blood transfusion.
D. In contrast to maternal ANP plasma levels, fetal levels are low due to increased numbers of "clearance" receptors in the fetus.
E. The fetal collecting duct is considerably more sensitive to arginine vasopressin (AVP) than its adult counterpart.

617. Which of the following statements regarding the response of the developing kidney to ureteral obstruction is *false*?

A. The earlier in development urinary obstruction develops, the more severe the resulting renal impairment.
B. Chronic partial ureteral obstruction results in a marked increase in vascular resistance of the affected kidney.
C. Presence of a normal contralateral kidney affects the degree of maturation occurring in the congenitally obstructed kidney.
D. Congenital ureteral obstruction decreases the renin content of the obstructed kidney.
E. Unilateral ureteral obstruction alters the postnatal renin distribution of the contralateral kidney.

618. All the following are accurate descriptions of the typical Potter's facial appearance EXCEPT:

A. Prominent fold and skin crease beneath each eye
B. Blunted nose
C. Depression between lower lip and chin
D. Low-set ears
E. Dry, loose skin

619. A 14-year-old girl is being evaluated for abdominal pain and a pelvic mass. A KUB is normal except for medial displacement of the splenic flexure. Pelvic ultrasonography reveals uterus didelphys with left hematocolpos. Which of the following is the best embryologic explanation for these findings?

A. Unilateral renal agenesis resulting from an insult occurring before the 4th week of gestation
B. Unilateral renal agenesis resulting from a defect occurring early in the 4th week of gestation
C. Unilateral renal agenesis resulting from a defect occurring after the 4th week of gestation
D. Ectopic left pelvic kidney due to incomplete ascent during the 5th week of gestation
E. Left-to-right crossed, fused ectopia due to abnormal rotation of the caudal end of the fetus late in the 5th week of gestation

620. A 40-year-old man being evaluated for an abdominal mass is found on excretory urogram to have an accessory left kidney. Which of the statements regarding this condition is *false*?

A. A supernumerary kidney generally will have its own blood supply and collecting system.
B. It is a very rare condition with a higher predilection for the left side.
C. The nonaccessory kidney is generally ectopic due to displacement by the accessory kidney.
D. When two completely independent ureters are present, the Weigert-Meyer principle is generally obeyed.
E. The vascular supply to the accessory kidney is very anomalous.

621. An excretory urogram of an 8-year-old girl who was born with an omphalocele is likely to show which of the following anomalies?

A. Right unilateral kidney
B. Horseshoe kidney
C. Right-to-left renal ectopia
D. Lump kidney
E. Bilateral cephalad renal ectopia

622. A 6-year-old boy is found to have a right sigmoid kidney. Which of the following statements about this anomaly is true?

A. Fusion of the two kidneys occurred relatively late in renal development.
B. Fusion of the two kidneys occurred relatively early in renal development.
C. The crossed kidney will be found superior to the uncrossed kidney.
D. Generally, a normal kidney will be found in the left renal fossa.
E. On cystoscopy, the left hemitrigone will be absent.

623. All of the following findings on excretory urogram are suggestive of a horseshoe kidney EXCEPT:

A. Low insertion of the ureter into the pelvis
B. Anteriorly displaced upper ureter which appears to drape over a midline mass
C. Kidneys that are low lying and close to the vertebral bodies
D. Vertical or outward axis with the upper poles pointing laterally
E. Continuation of the outer border of the lower pole of each kidney toward the midline

624. A patient is found to have a malrotated kidney with the renal pelvis facing laterally. Which of the following findings would confirm that the anomaly occurred due to hyperrotation of the developing kidney?

A. Presence of a flattened and elongated renal pelvis
B. Lateral displacement of the upper third of the ureter
C. Stretching of the superior calyx
D. Renal vessels that course ventral to the kidney
E. Renal vessels that course dorsal to the kidney

625. In a hypertensive patient with a renal artery aneurysm, which of the following conditions is *not* an indication for surgical excision of the aneurysm?

A. Hypertension is uncontrollable.
B. An incomplete ringlike calcification is present.
C. The aneurysm is 1.5 cm in diameter.
D. The aneurysm increased in size on serial angiograms.
E. An arteriovenous fistula is present.

626. All of the following are felt to be possible etiologic factors in the formation of a calyceal diverticulum EXCEPT:

A. Localized cortical abscess draining into a calyx
B. Achalasia of a calyx
C. Dysfunction of the sphincter surrounding a minor calyx
D. Early degeneration of a fourth generation ureteral branch
E. Obstruction of a calyx due to infection

627. Which of the following findings is seen in a kidney with megacalycosis?

A. Dilated, thick-walled renal pelvis
B. Underdeveloped, crescent appearing medulla
C. Cortical thinning in the area of the affected calyx
D. Impaired acid excretion
E. Dilated collecting tubules

628. During a work-up for recurrent urinary tract infections, a 1-year-old boy is found to have a left ureteropelvic junction obstruction (see Fig. 34–1). Before any surgical intervention, which of the following should be performed?

A. Renal ultrasound to evaluate the degree of cortical thinning
B. Cystoscopy with retrograde pyelogram to delineate the area of obstruction
C. Voiding cystourethrogram to rule out obstruction secondary to vesicoureteral reflux
D. Furosemide renal scan to confirm the presence of obstruction
E. Placement of a percutaneous nephrostomy tube and performance of a Whittaker test to quantitate the degree of obstruction

629. If the patient in the question above was 25 years old rather than 1 year old, which of the following would be the most likely cause of the ureteropelvic junction obstruction?

A. Atrophic, widely separated smooth muscle cells within the wall of the distal renal pelvis
B. Persistent fetal convolution of the upper ureter
C. Upper ureteral polyps
D. Kinking of the upper ureter by an aberrant renal vessel passing *anteriorly* to the ureteropelvic junction
E. Secondary obstruction due to severe vesicoureteral reflux

630. A 4-year-old boy is found to have double ureters of the left kidney. Which of the following statements regarding this condition is *false*?

A. The second ureter is felt to result from an additional ureteral bud arising from the mesonephric duct.
B. The ureteral bud closest to the urogenital sinus becomes the lower pole ureter.
C. Medial and caudal rotation of the mesonephric duct places the upper pole orifice distal to the lower pole orifice.
D. Immediate fission of a single ureteral bud is felt to produce double ureters that do not follow the Weigert-Meyer rule.
E. Due to its ectopic orifice, the upper pole ureter will more commonly reflux.

631. A 6-year-old girl is being evaluated for incontinence. An excretory urogram reveals an ectopic right ureter that empties into the vagina. All of the following statements regarding this condition are true EXCEPT:

A. A low (caudal) origin of the ureteral bud results in an ectopic orifice.
B. Due to its abnormal origin, the ureteral bud has little time for migration and ascent away from the mesonephric duct.
C. Failure of the ureter to separate from the mesonephric duct results in drainage via the genital tract.
D. The placement of the orifice within the vagina is explained by the close association of mesonephric and paramesonephric ducts during ureteral development.
E. In a male patient, a similar anomaly would result in an ectopic ureter emptying into the seminal vesical or ejaculatory duct.

632. Which of the following statements regarding ureteral duplications is *true*?

A. They are rare anomalies most commonly seen in males.
B. An increased incidence of duplications is seen in children with urinary infections.
C. The terms bifid ureter and double ureter may be used interchangeably.
D. Duplication is felt to be genetically determined by an autosomal recessive trait.
E. An extravesical Y junction of a bifid ureter prevents ureteroureteral reflux of urine.

633. Which of the following findings is commonly seen in a primary obstructed megaureter?

A. Calyceal blunting
B. Increased collagen between muscle cells
C. Poor renal function
D. Female predominance
E. Normal smooth muscle cell density

634. A 20-year-old man is found to have a single, ectopic right ureter. The left side is normal. Which of the following symptoms was this patient *least* likely to have had?

A. Painful defecation
B. Urinary frequency
C. Urinary incontinence
D. Scrotal swelling
E. Painful ejaculation

635. In a female with a single ectopic ureter, which of the following is the most common presenting symptom?

A. Painful defecation
B. Urinary frequency
C. Urinary incontinence
D. Labial swelling
E. Flank pain

636. Which of the following statements regarding ureteroceles is *false*?

A. Ectopic ureteroceles most commonly involve the upper pole of a double ureter.
B. A stenotic ureterocele has a narrowed orifice located on its dome.
C. A sphincteric ureterocele empties only during voiding when the bladder neck opens.
D. Contralateral ureteral obstruction may be produced by a large ectopic ureterocele.
E. Histologically, a stenotic ureterocele is recognized by the absence of muscle within its wall.

637. A preureteral cava (circumcaval ureter) results from which of the following developmental events?

A. Persistence of the lumbar portion of the right subcardinal vein to become the dominant vein
B. Atrophy of the left supracardinal veins and the lumbar portion of the right posterior cardinal vein
C. Persistence of the ventral and dorsal right subcardinal veins
D. Fusion of the lumber portion of the left and right posterior cardinal veins
E. Abnormal migration of the ureteral bud dorsal to the right posterior cardinal vein

638. Which of the following statements about dysplastic kidneys is *false*?

A. The kidney may be of normal size.
B. Only a portion of the kidney may be affected.
C. The diagnosis may be confirmed radiographically.
D. The anomaly results from abnormal metanephric differentiation.
E. Histologically, focal, diffuse or segmentally arranged primitive ducts are seen.

639. Which of the following histologic findings confirms the diagnosis of dysplastic kidney?

A. Presence of primitive glomeruli
B. Presence of ductules surrounded by connective tissue devoid of smooth muscle cells
C. Presence of multiple cysts
D. Presence of loose, disorganized mesenchyme
E. Presence of primitive ducts surrounded by connective tissue devoid of elastin

640. In a patient with renal hypoplasia, which of the following findings help to distinguish segmental hypoplasia (Ask-Upmark kidney) from oligomeganephronia?

A. Small renal size
B. Severe hypertension
C. Proteinuria
D. Decreased creatinine clearance
E. Autosomal recessive inheritance

641. A boy is found to have posterior urethral valves and a severely hypodysplastic left kidney. Cystourethroscopy with ablation of the valves is performed. Which of the following cystoscopic findings was most likely present?

A. Normal position of left ureteral orifice
B. Slight lateral displacement of left ureteral orifice
C. Marked lateral displacement of left ureteral orifice
D. Absence of left ureteral orifice
E. Normal position of left ureteral orifice but caudal ectopia of the right

642. Which of the following disorders is *not* classified as a genetically determined form of renal cystic disease?

A. Medullary sponge kidney
B. Infantile polycystic kidney
C. Adult polycystic kidney
D. Juvenile nephronophthisis
E. Medullary cystic disease

643. All patients with autosomal recessive polycystic kidney disease have been found to have which of the following lesions?

A. Degeneration of the retina
B. Cerebellar hemangioblastomas
C. Cysts within the small bowel mesentery
D. Periportal lesions of the liver
E. Hyperpigmentation of the lips

644. The gene for the autosomal dominant form of polycystic kidney disease (adult polycystic kidney) has been localized to which chromosome?

A. Long arm of chromosome 3
B. Long arm of chromosome 5
C. Short arm of chromosome 11
D. Short arm of chromosome 16
E. Short arm of chromosome 22

645. Which of the following anomalies is *not* associated with autosomal dominant polycystic kidney disease?

A. Retinal angiomas
B. Colonic diverticula
C. Mitral valve prolapse
D. Aneurysms of the circle of Willis
E. Pancreatic cysts

646. Juvenile nephronophthisis and medullary cystic disease share all of the following characteristics EXCEPT:

A. Development of polyuria and polydipsia
B. A renal tubular defect resulting in an inability to conserve sodium
C. Polyuria resistant to correction with vasopressin
D. Absence of proteinuria and hematuria
E. Autosomal recessive inheritance

647. Which of the following is *not* a characteristic of tuberous sclerosis?

A. Autosomal dominant inheritance
B. Cerebellar hemangioblastomas
C. Epilepsy
D. Mental retardation
E. Adenoma sebaceum

648. The kidneys of patients with tuberous sclerosis are often involved with multiple cysts and/or angiomyolipomas. Which of the following characteristics are typical of the renal cysts associated with tuberous sclerosis?

A. They are commonly in excess of 4 cm in diameter.
B. They are lined with a single layer of cells with small pale nuclei.
C. The cells lining the cysts do not appear to be associated with the development of renal cell carcinoma.
D. The cells lining the cysts often aggregate into masses of tumorlets.
E. They are not associated with the development of renal failure.

649. All of the following are manifestations of Von Hippel-Lindau disease EXCEPT:

A. Autosomal dominant inheritance
B. Retinal angiomas
C. Hepatic cysts
D. Pheochromocytoma
E. Renal cell carcinoma

650. The contralateral kidney in a patient with a multicystic dysplastic kidney often displays each of the following EXCEPT:

A. Ureteropelvic junction obstruction
B. Obstructive megaureter
C. Vesicoureteral reflux
D. Persistence of fetal folds of the ureter
E. Complete ureteral duplication

651. A newborn is being evaluated for a large left abdominal mass. Which of the following sonographic findings would help to identify the mass as being due to a multicystic dysplastic kidney rather than due to severe hydronephrosis?

A. Presence of a large central cyst surrounded by smaller peripheral cysts
B. Absence of an identifiable renal sinus
C. Absence of interfaces between cysts
D. Presence of marked hydroureter
E. Presence of cortical thickening

652. A patient who has had a multicystic dysplastic kidney left in place is most likely to develop which of the following?

A. Flank pain
B. Hypertension
C. Renal cell carcinoma
D. Transitional cell carcinoma
E. Wilms' tumor

653. A 3-year-old boy is found to have a large multilocular cyst of the left kidney and a normal right kidney. The decision to perform a left nephrectomy is best supported by which of the following?

A. Multilocular cysts are believed to be a part of a spectrum of neoplasia related to Wilms' tumor.
B. Hematuria, commonly associated with multilocular cysts in this age group, could cause severe anemia.
C. Nephrectomy would best relieve the flank pain commonly seen in these patients.
D. Further bouts of pyelonephritis are best prevented with nephrectomy.

654. All of the following findings may be associated with simple renal cysts EXCEPT:

A. Abdominal mass
B. Hematuria
C. Hypertension
D. Destruction of adjacent calyces
E. Calyceal or renal pelvis obstruction

655. Which of the following sonographic findings is *not* consistent with the diagnosis of a simple renal cysts?

A. Sharply defined, thin walls with a distinct margin
B. Well-defined internal echoes
C. Acoustic enhancement behind the lesions
D. Spherical or ovoid shape
E. Absence of internal echoes

656. Magnetic resonance imaging (MRI) can help to identify a cyst as being hemorrhagic rather than simple, based on which of the following findings?

A. Demonstration of wall thickening on birth T1- and T2-weighted images
B. Low signal intensity on T1-weighted images
C. Extremely bright image intensity on T2-weighted images
D. Contrast enhancement on T1- but not T2-weighted images
E. Enhancement of fine intralesional calcifications

657. A child is found to have a Bosniak Type IV right renal cyst. The most appropriate management of this lesion is:

A. Do nothing
B. Cyst puncture and sclerosis
C. Repeat ultrasonography in 3 months
D. Right partial nephrectomy
E. Right radical nephrectomy

658. The characteristic histologic feature of medullary sponge kidney is:

A. Cystic dilatation of the intrapapillary collecting ducts
B. Cystic dilatation of the ascending loop of Henle
C. Cystic dilatation of the distal convoluted tubule
D. Cystic dilatation of the proximal convoluted tubule
E. Cystic dilatation of the Bowman's space

659. The renal calculi most commonly formed by uninfected patients with medullary sponge kidney are composed of:

A. Magnesium ammonium phosphate
B. Calcium oxalate
C. Uric acid
D. Cystine
E. Lysine

660. Acquired renal cystic disease has been noted to occur and progress in all of the following patients EXCEPT:

A. Those being managed by hemodialysis
B. Those being managed by peritoneal dialysis
C. Those being managed medically
D. Those being managed after successful renal transplantation
E. Those returning to hemodialysis after failed renal transplantation

661. Calyceal diverticula most commonly arise from which of the following sites?

A. Upper pole papilla
B. Lower pole papilla
C. Fornix of upper pole calyx
D. Fornix of lower pole calyx
E. Renal sinus

662. After what week of development do the human male and female fetus normally begin to become phenotypically distinct?

A. 4th
B. 8th
C. 12th
D. 16th
E. 20th

663. The gene thought to encode for human testis-determining factor (TDF) has been localized to the:

A. Short arm of the Y chromosome, between the centromere and pseudoautosomal region
B. Short arm of the Y chromosome, distal to the pseudoautosomal region
C. Long arm of the Y chromosome, between the centromere and pseudoautosomal region
D. Long arm of the Y chromosome, distal to the pseudoautosomal region
E. Y chromosome, but the exact region has not been identified

664. All of the following are true statements regarding normal human gonadal differentiation EXCEPT:

A. The gonadal ridges are formed during the 4th week of development.
B. Prior to the 2nd month of gestation, the gonadal ridges are devoid of germ cells.
C. Germ cells are initially located in the endoderm of the yolk sac.
D. Germ cell division is delayed until migration is complete.
E. Late in the 5th week of gestation, the male and female gonad are indistinguishable.

665. Which of the following statements regarding the sexual differentiation of the human gonad is *true*?

A. Around the 7th week of gestation primitive granular cells organize around the dividing oocyte to form primordial follicle.
B. The first morphologic sign of sexual dimorphism in the gonads is development of primordial Leydig cells in the fetal testis.
C. Müllerian-inhibiting substance is the primordial hormone of the fetal testis.
D. Onset of estrogen synthesis by the fetal ovary lags behind the onset of testosterone synthesis by the fetal testis.
E. Endocrine differentiation of the fetal ovary and testis involves the differential expression of numerous enzymes.

666. All of the following genital organs are derived from cells of the mesonephric kidney EXCEPT:

A. Epididymis
B. Seminal vesicle
C. Vas deferens
D. Uterus
E. Fallopian tubes

667. The initial event in the virilization of the male urogenital tract is the:

A. Production of testosterone by the fetal testis
B. Development of luteinizing hormone receptors in the fetal testis
C. Onset of paramesonephric duct regression
D. Posterior migration of the genital swellings
E. Fusion of the genital folds

668. Which of the following is *not* a derivative of the wolffian ducts?

A. Epididymis
B. Prostatic utricle
C. Vas deferens
D. Appendix epididymis
E. Ejaculatory ducts

669. All of the following statements regarding testicular descent are true EXCEPT:

A. Initially, the testis and mesonephros are attached to the posterior abdominal wall by a peritoneal fold.
B. Herniation of the processus vaginalis through the ventral abdominal wall results in formation of the inguinal canal.
C. Contraction of the gubernaculum pulls the testis down the inguinal canal and into the scrotum.
D. The process of testicular descent is thought to be androgen-dependent.
E. After testicular descent, further development of the abdominal musculature closes the deep and superficial inguinal rings.

670. Which of the following female genital structures is thought to be derived from the wolffian duct?

A. Gartner's ducts
B. The fallopian tubes
C. The body of the uterus
D. The upper vagina
E. The uterine cervix

671. The gene that codes for müllerian-inhibiting substance has been localized to the:

A. Short arm of the Y chromosome
B. Long arm of the Y chromosome
C. Short arm of the X chromosome
D. Long arm of the X chromosome
E. Short arm of chromosome 19

672. Müllerian-inhibiting substance is thought to have all of the following actions EXCEPT:

A. Dissolution of the basement membrane
B. Condensation of mesenchymal cells
C. Blocking phosphorylation of tyrosine residues on membrane proteins
D. Induction of intracellular lysosomal enzymes
E. Antagonism of epidermal growth factor

673. All of the following steps are involved in the action of androgens within target cells EXCEPT:

A. Testosterone enters the target cell by passive diffusion.
B. Within the cells, testosterone binds to a specific receptor protein to form a hormone-receptor complex.
C. The hormone-receptor complex binds with high affinity to receptor sites on the chromatin.
D. The hormone-receptor complex induces a second messenger to increase levels of cyclic-AMP.
E. An increase in transcription of specific messenger RNAs occurs, and new proteins are synthesized.

674. A deficiency of 5α-reductase will result in abnormal development of which of the following structures?

A. Testes
B. Scrotum
C. Epididymis
D. Vas deferens
E. Seminal vesicles

675. All of the following are classified as disorders of chromosomal sexual differentiation EXCEPT:

A. Klinefelter's syndrome
B. Turner's syndrome
C. Mixed gonadal dysgenesis
D. True hermaphroditism
E. Gonadal agenesis

676. Which of the following findings is *not* found in patients with the classic form of Klinefelter's syndrome?

A. Increased incidence of hypospadias
B. Increased average body height
C. Decreased testicular length
D. Elevated plasma levels of FSH
E. Gynecomastia

677. In Turner's syndrome, all of the following features are seen EXCEPT:

A. Primary amenorrhea
B. Sexual infantilism
C. Ambiguous genitalia
D. Bilateral streak gonads
E. Elevated plasma levels of FSH

678. The final adult height of patients with Turner's syndrome has been most successfully increased by treating with:

A. Recombinant human growth hormone alone
B. Ethinyl estradiol alone
C. Oxandrolone alone
D. Recombinant human growth hormone with oxandrolone
E. Ethinyl estradiol with medroxy progesterone acetate

679. The most common malignant germ cell tumor occurring in patients with mixed gonadal dysgenesis is:

A. Gonadoblastoma
B. Seminoma
C. Embryonal cell
D. Teratoma
E. Choriocarcinoma

680. In a true hermaphrodite with a male phenotype, menstruation usually presents:

A. As cyclic hematuria
B. As cyclic testicular pain
C. As cyclic pelvic pain
D. As perineal bleeding
E. Without any signs of menstruation

681. Patients with pure gonadal dysgenesis have the same clinical features as those with gonadal dysgenesis (Turner's syndrome) EXCEPT:

A. Presence of streak gonads
B. Sexual infantilism
C. Short stature
D. Primary amenorrhea
E. Failure of breast development

682. Which of the following enzymes is *not* involved in the synthesis of androgens?

A. 20,22-Desmolase
B. 17α-Hydroxylase
C. 17β-Hydroxysteroid dehydrogenase
D. 17,20-Desmolase
E. 11-Hydroxylase

683. All of the following may be seen in a female newborn with 21-hydroxylase deficiency EXCEPT:

A. Clitoral hypertrophy and chordee
B. Absent uterus
C. Salt loss
D. Fusion of labioscrotal folds
E. A prostate gland

684. In which of the following characteristics do patients with 11β-hydroxylase deficiency significantly differ from those with 21-hydroxylase deficiency?

A. Mode of genetic inheritance
B. Effect on plasma ACTH levels
C. Effect on development of external genitalia
D. Degree of salt loss
E. Effect on internal genitalia

685. All of the following are true statements regarding vaginal agenesis EXCEPT:

A. It is one of the more common causes of primary amenorrhea.
B. The uterus may be rudimentary or normal.
C. One third of patients will have associated renal abnormalities.
D. Successful pregnancies have been reported after corrective vaginal surgery.
E. This condition is inherited as an autosomal recessive trait.

686. A defect or deficiency of which of the following hormones results in male pseudohermaphroditism without congenital adrenal hyperplasia?

A. 17,20-Desmolase
B. 20,22-Desmolase

C. 3β-Hydroxysteroid dehydrogenase
D. 17α-Hydroxylase
E. 11-Hydroxylase

687. A 14-year-old girl is found to have primary amenorrhea, clitoral enlargement, mild breast enlargement, and development of facial and body hair. Pelvic examination reveals a blind-ending vagina. The plasma androstenedione concentration is elevated and the karyotype is 46,XY. The best diagnosis is:

A. 17α-Hydroxylase deficiency
B. 17β-Hydroxysteroid dehydrogenase deficiency
C. 17,20-Desmolase deficiency
D. 20,22-Desmolase deficiency
E. 3β-Hydroxysteroid dehydrogenase deficiency

688. An adolescent suffering from 5α-reductase deficiency exhibits all of the following EXCEPT:

A. Involution müllerian duct derivatives
B. Blind vaginal pouch
C. Involution of wolffian duct derivatives
D. Female body habitus
E. Normal male plasma testosterone level

689. All of the following disorders are felt to result from an androgen receptor defect EXCEPT:

A. Complete testicular feminization
B. Incomplete testicular feminization
C. Reifenstein syndrome
D. Pure gonadal dysgenesis
E. Infertile male syndrome

690. A phenotypically normal, asymptomatic girl is found to have complete testicular feminization. Castration:

A. Is not necessary
B. Should be performed at the time of diagnosis
C. Should be performed before puberty
D. Should be performed at menarche
E. Should be performed after puberty

691. The most appropriate surgical intervention for a patient with persistent müllerian duct syndrome is:

A. No surgical intervention
B. Bilateral orchiectomy
C. Removal of uterus and upper vagina
D. Primary or staged orchiopexy
E. Creation of an artificial vagina

692. All of the following are true statements regarding microphallus EXCEPT:

A. In the newborn, stretched penile length less than 1.9 cm is consistent with microphallus.
B. Microphallus is frequently associated with testicular maldescent.
C. Microphallus is considered the consequence of defective androgen secretion during the first trimester.
D. Initial management of patients younger than age 3 years is low-dose, short-term, systemic testosterone.
E. Postpubertal treatment of previously undiagnosed hypogonadotropic hypogonadism with systemic testosterone may improve penile size.

693. When evaluating a newborn with sexual ambiguity, the most important finding on physical examination is:

A. Hyperpigmentation of the areola
B. Palpation of a gonad
C. Palpation of a midline uterus
D. Size of the phallus
E. Location of the urethral meatus

694. Which of the following findings is most significant when establishing the sex of rearing of a child with ambiguous genitalia?

A. Degree of phallic development
B. Chromosomal sex
C. Presence of palpable gonads
D. Results of gonadal biopsy
E. Response to hCG administration

695. Psychosexual identity is usually well-differentiated after what age?

A. 6–8 months
B. 9–13 months
C. 18–24 months
D. 2 1/2–3 years
E. After 4 years

696. Which of the statements concerning the embryology of the male genitourinary system is *false*?

A. The indifferent gonad differentiates into the fetal testis by gestational week 7 under the influence of a protein secreted by the XY primordial germ cell.
B. The wolffian duct differentiates into the male ductal system under the influence of testosterone during the eighth week of gestation.
C. Fetal Leydig cells secrete müllerian-inhibiting factor, which causes complete degeneration of the müllerian ductal system.
D. The male external genitalia develop under the influence of dihydrotestosterone between the 8th and 16th weeks of gestation.
E. The process of testicular descent is essentially dormant between the 12th week and 7th month of gestation but rapidly resumes its course by the end of the 8th month of gestation.

697. ____ of full-term infants and ____ of premature infants have cryptorchidism at birth.

A. 1 per cent, 10 per cent
B. 1 per cent, 30 per cent
C. 3 per cent, 10 per cent
D. 3 per cent, 30 per cent
E. 10 per cent, 30 per cent

698. The incidence of cryptorchidism in adults is:

A. 0.1 per cent
B. 0.5 per cent
C. 0.8 per cent
D. 2 per cent
E. 5 per cent

699. By one year of age, ____ of cryptorchid testes in premature infants and ____ of cryptorchid testes in full-term infants spontaneously descend.

A. 33 per cent, 66 per cent
B. 50 per cent, 75 per cent
C. 75 per cent, 95 per cent
D. 66 per cent, 33 per cent
E. 95 per cent, 75 per cent

700. Unilateral or bilateral anorchia is found in ____ of cases at the time of inguinal exploration for cryptorchidism.

A. 1 per cent
B. 3 per cent
C. 10 per cent
D. 15 per cent
E. 20 per cent

701. Which mechanism is generally accepted as playing the major role in promoting testicular descent?

A. Hormonal
B. Epididymal maturation
C. Traction theory
D. Differential growth
E. Intra-abdominal pressure

702. Cryptorchidism is associated with all of the following EXCEPT:

A. Kallman's syndrome
B. Cystic fibrosis
C. Klinefelter's syndrome
D. Noonan's syndrome
E. Von Hippel-Lindau disease

703. The most common location for an ectopic testis is in the:

A. Superficial inguinal pouch
B. Suprapubic region
C. Contralateral scrotum
D. Femoral canal
E. Perineum

704. A 2-year-old male undergoes exploratory laparoscopy for an impalpable right testis. Intraoperatively, he is noted to have blind-ending testicular vessels on the right. What should the next step be?

A. Inguinal exploration
B. Do nothing and close
C. Hormonal treatment
D. Abdominal ultrasound
E. Scrotal exploration

705. Which statement concerning the histologic and ultrastructural changes associated with cryptorchid testes is *false*?

A. Chronologically, histologic alterations appear by 1 1/2 years of age and include smaller seminiferous tubules, fewer spermatogonia, and more peritubular tissue.
B. Histologic changes do not occur in the contralateral testis of the unilateral cryptorchid male.
C. Ultrastructural changes in the seminiferous tubule include degeneration of mitochondria, loss of ribosomes in cytoplasm and smooth endoplasmic reticulum, and increase in collagen fibers in the spermatogonia and Sertoli cells.
D. Histologic abnormalities are more pronounced if the testis resides further away from the bottom of the scrotum.
E. Ultrastructural changes in the seminiferous tubules occur as early as the second year of life.

706. Which of the following statements regarding the association between testicular neoplasia and cryptorchidism is *true*?

A. Choriocarcinoma is the most frequent neoplasm encountered in cryptorchid testes.
B. The undescended testis is 100 times more likely to undergo malignant degeneration than the normal testis.
C. Orchiopexy is recommended between 1 and 1 1/2 years of age since histologic and ultrastructural changes begin to occur at an early age.
D. About 30 per cent of testicular tumors arise from an undescended testis.
E. Abdominal testes and inguinal testis have similar potential to undergo malignant degeneration.

707. Which of the following statements concerning complications associated with undescended testes is *true*?

A. Despite successful unilateral orchiopexy during childhood, sperm counts are lower in adulthood in comparison to normal adults.
B. The incidence of testicular torsion in the undescended testis is greater in the prepubertal period.
C. Hernia sacs are found in approximately 50 per cent of patients with cryptorchidism.
D. Cryptorchidism strictly affects the spermatogenic compartment of the testis and leaves the interstitial testicular compartment free of defects.
E. Vasal and epididymal abnormalities are not associated with the cryptorchid state.

708. Which statement regarding hormonal therapy for undescended testes is *false*?

A. HCG stimulates Leydig cell production of testosterone, which in turn promotes testicular descent.
B. Both hCG and Gn-RH can be administered intranasally to treat testicular maldescent.
C. Gn-RH stimulates production of LH by the hypothalamus and induces testicular descent.
D. Doses of hCG above 15,000 I.U. cause significant side effects such as changes in testicular histology, increase in penile size, and bone age alteration.
E. About 10 per cent of patients treated with Gn-RH relapse 6 months after therapy.

709. The incidence of hydroceles in full-term males is:

A. 0 per cent
B. 2 per cent
C. 6 per cent
D. 10 per cent
E. 15 per cent

710. Extravaginal testicular torsion is most common in:

A. Utero
B. Puberty
C. Adulthood
D. The newborn period
E. The geriatric period

711. Which statement is true concerning testicular torsion?

A. Testicular torsion is most common during the neonatal period.
B. Intravaginal torsion rarely occurs in adolescence.
C. The torsed testicle is viable if operated upon within 48 hours.

D. Torsion of the appendix testis mimics true testicular torsion.
E. Contralateral orchiopexy is not recommended at the time of scrotal exploration.

712. Each of the following is felt to be a specific indication for ultrasonographic genitourinary evaluation in utero EXCEPT:

A. A finding of persistent breech presentation
B. A lower than expected fundal height
C. A higher than expected fundal height
D. A history of urinary developmental abnormalities in a sibling
E. A low maternal serum alpha-fetoprotein level

713. The fetal kidney can be reliably detected with ultrasound after what gestational age?

A. 10 weeks
B. 12 weeks
C. 15 weeks
D. 20 weeks
E. 24 weeks

714. The most common genitourinary defect detected in utero has been reported to be:

A. Hydronephrosis
B. Multicystic dysplastic kidney
C. Renal agenesis
D. Adrenal hyperplasia
E. Neuroblastoma

715. Which of the following sonographic findings is *not* consistent with a prenatal diagnosis of posterior urethral valves?

A. Bilateral hydroureteronephrosis
B. Thin-walled, dilated bladder
C. Incomplete bladder emptying
D. Suggestion of a dilated posterior urethra
E. Male sex identification

716. During a routine maternal fetal sonogram, intraluminal intestinal calcifications are noted in the fetus. This finding suggests the presence of:

A. Anorectal malformation
B. Congenital adrenal hyperplasia
C. Neuroblastoma
D. Teratoma
E. Mesoblastic nephroma

717. In a fetus noted to have genitourinary anomalies on prenatal ultrasonography, the strongest indicators of a poor prognosis include all of the following EXCEPT:

A. Early onset of severe renal parenchymal changes
B. Bladder outlet obstruction
C. Severe nonrenal congenital anomalies
D. Hydronephrosis
E. Oligohydramnios

718. When evaluating a fetus for possible prenatal intervention, which of the following has *not* been recommended as a means of assessing potential fetal renal function?

A. Aspiration of the fetal bladder to determine fetal urine electrolytes
B. Ultrasound-guided biopsy of the fetal kidney
C. Evaluation of the degree of renal sonographic echogenicity
D. Sonographic documentation of bladder refilling and emptying
E. Estimation of the volume of amniotic fluid

719. In a neonate diagnosed with hydronephrosis on prenatal ultrasound examination, the clearest indication for immediate postpartum ultrasonography is:

A. Preterm delivery
B. Suspicion of ureteropelvic junction obstruction
C. Suspicion of primary obstructive megaureter
D. Evidence of autosomal recessive polycystic kidney disease
E. Suspicion of bladder outlet obstruction

720. The mouse model for autosomal recessive polycystic kidney suggests that cystogenesis may be related to all of the following EXCEPT:

A. A sodium-potassium ion pump in the tubular cells
B. Tubular basement membrane changes
C. Disordered cell migration in the developing medullary pyramids
D. Disordered regulation of epidermal growth factor gene expression
E. Induction of the c-*myc* proto-oncogene

721. The prenatal and postnatal kidney differ in all of the following ways EXCEPT:

A. The fetal kidney performs little of the dialysis of the fetal circulation.
B. The renal blood flow of the prenatal kidney is dramatically less.
C. Oxygen tension is markedly reduced in the fetal kidney.
D. The fetal kidney is much more sensitive to the natriuretic effects of atrial natriuretic peptide.
E. The principal activity of the fetal kidney is growth and development rather than function.

722. The principal advantage to working with opossum pups to study congenital renal obstruction is:

A. A naturally high incidence of congenital ureteral obstruction
B. Glomerulogenesis continues until age 2 weeks postnatally
C. A long gestation similar to that of humans
D. "Birth" into the marsupium of the mother allowing surgical manipulation without inducing preterm labor
E. Tolerance of multiple procedures on a given pup to explore the dynamics of renal response to obstruction

723. The response of the fetal kidney to obstruction is determined by all of the following EXCEPT:

A. Time of onset of obstruction during gestation
B. Duration of the obstruction
C. Severity of the obstruction
D. Status of the contralateral kidney
E. Dialysis of the fetal circulation by the placenta

724. Postnatally, all of the following changes in renal physiology are noted in an individual with prenatal obstructive uropathy EXCEPT:

A. Increased sodium reabsorption
B. Reduced glomerular filtration
C. Impaired acid excretion
D. Reduced water reabsorption
E. Reduced renal blood flow

725. Which of the following statements regarding the results of animal studies on the effect of prenatal obstruction on renal growth and development is *false*?

A. In the fetal rabbit, impaired nephrogenesis is reversed with early postnatal decompression.
B. Kidney obstruction in the opossum has produced histologic dysplasia.
C. Experimental production of in utero compensatory renal hypertrophy has not been documented.
D. In the avian kidney, obstruction alone will not produce dysplasia.
E. Hydrostatic pressure is felt to be involved in the development of dysplasia.

726. Which of the following changes is seen in prenatally obstructed bladders?

A. Smooth muscle cell hypertrophy
B. Retarded development of myosin heavy chain isoforms
C. Increased density of muscarinic cholinergic receptors
D. Bladder wall thinning on ultrasonography
E. Connective tissue elements increased to a greater degree than smooth muscle mass

727. Which of the following statements regarding the relationship of renal and pulmonary development in the fetus is *true*?

A. No significant relationship between pulmonary and renal development appears to exist.
B. Renal agenesis results in pulmonary hypoplasia with diminished airway branching.
C. Bladder outlet obstruction occurring during the last one third of gestation does not appear to effect pulmonary development.
D. In models where oligohydramnios is induced without bladder outlet obstruction, lung development proceeds normally.
E. In utero decompression of bladder outlet obstruction will not prevent pulmonary hypoplasia.

728. Which of the following statements regarding the neonatal period are *true*?

A. It encompasses the first 3 months of life.
B. Most infant deaths occur during the neonatal period.
C. Approximately 50 per cent of neonatal deaths are attributed to gross congenital malformations.
D. One third of all infant deaths occur during the first year of life.
E. Approximately 40 per cent of neonatal deaths are associated with urologic abnormalities.

729. Clues to the presence of genitourinary disorders during pregnancy include all of the following EXCEPT:

A. Family history of fetal wastage or chromosomal abnormalities.
B. Oligohydramnios or polyhydramnios on prenatal ultrasound.
C. First trimester bleeding.
D. Diabetes mellitus in the mother.
E. Maternal age greater than 30 years.

730. The incidence of single umbilical artery, which is associated with a 4-fold increase in infant mortality, in the neonate is approximately:

A. 1 per cent
B. 5 per cent
C. 10 per cent
D. 15 per cent
E. 30 per cent

731. Abnormalities commonly associated with renal abnormalities include all of the following EXCEPT:

A. Widely spaced eyes
B. Low set ears
C. External ear abnormality
D. Flattened nose
E. Widely spaced nipples

732. All of the following statements regarding fetal intervention are true EXCEPT:

A. In utero therapy for urinary tract decompression is still under clinical investigation.
B. The most important prognostic feature in the fetus with bilateral hydronephrosis and distended bladder is the volume of amniotic fluid.
C. Fetal intervention is usually effective since early obstructive uropathy tends to be reversible.
D. The rate of diagnostic error in prenatal evaluation can be as high as 30 to 40 per cent.
E. Early delivery should not be performed in the fetus with unilateral hydronephrosis.

733. Regarding abdominal masses in neonates:

A. Most are detected by abdominal ultrasound
B. The majority are caused by gastrointestinal pathology
C. Approximately 50 per cent arise in the kidney
D. The most common cause is multicystic dysplastic kidney
E. The recommended initial diagnostic procedure is an intravenous urogram

734. A urology consult is requested for a term newborn male with a right upper quadrant abdominal mass on physical examination. Ultrasound reveals a normal left kidney but on the right side, there is a cystic mass with interfaces between the cysts, the largest of which are located laterally, and no identifiable renal sinus. The most likely diagnosis is:

A. Congenital mesoblastic nephroma
B. Neuroblastoma
C. Ureteropelvic junction obstruction
D. Multicystic dysplastic kidney
E. Vesicoureteral reflux

735. Umbilical artery catheters have increased the incidence of which of the following conditions?

A. Renal artery thrombosis
B. Renal vein thrombosis
C. Adrenal hemorrhage
D. Renal cortical necrosis
E. Renal calculus formation

736. The most common cause of hypertension in the neonate is:

A. Renal artery stenosis
B. Renal artery thrombosis
C. Renal vein thrombosis
D. Polycystic kidney disease
E. Coarctation of the aorta

737. A urology consult is obtained for a 6-hour-old term male who has not voided yet. The pregnancy was complicated by preeclampsia requiring the administration of magnesium sulfate to the patient's mother. Physical examination reveals a normal-appearing neonate with a palpable bladder and normal external genitalia. The next step in management should be:

A. Intravenous urogram
B. Renal ultrasound
C. Voiding cystometrogram
D. Urethral catheterization and later reevaluation
E. Cystoscopy

738. All of the following statements regarding neonatal ascites are true EXCEPT:

A. The most common fluid found is urine.
B. Urinary ascites occurs more commonly in the female.
C. The most common cause of urinary ascites is posterior urethral valves.
D. The diagnostic method of choice when ascites is suspected is abdominal ultrasound.
E. In approximately 15 per cent of cases, the etiology remains unknown.

739. The most common cause of a neonatal abdominal mass is:

A. Adrenal hemorrhage
B. Hydronephrosis
C. Wilms' tumor
D. Congenital mesoblastic nephroma
E. Neuroblastoma

740. All of the following are indications for early pyeloplasty EXCEPT:

A. Solitary kidney
B. Bilateral ureteropelvic junction obstruction
C. Asymptomatic unilateral ureteropelvic junction destruction
D. An obstructed kidney contributing less than 40 per cent of overall function by DTPA scan
E. Unilateral ureteropelvic junction obstruction with contralateral multicystic dysplastic kidney

741. In the majority of cases, multicystic dysplastic kidneys are now being diagnosed by:

A. Prenatal ultrasound
B. Postnatal ultrasound
C. CT scan
D. MRI
E. Intravenous urogram

742. All of the following are features of renal vein thrombosis EXCEPT:

A. Hematuria
B. Thrombocytopenia
C. Proteinuria
D. Delayed excretion or nonfunction intravenous pyelogram
E. Polycythemia

743. All of the following are recommended as part of the initial management of renal vein thrombosis EXCEPT:

A. Hydration
B. Correction of electrolyte imbalance
C. Antibiotics
D. Heparin
E. Nephrectomy

744. Which of the following is *not* a risk factor for adrenal hemorrhage?

A. Prolonged labor
B. Traumatic delivery
C. Perinatal anoxia
D. Low birth weight
E. Hypoprothrombinemia

745. A term newborn male is found to have an abdominal mass, anemia, and jaundice. The most valuable radiologic tool to confirm the diagnosis is:

A. Intravenous urogram
B. CT scan
C. MRI
D. Ultrasound
E. Bone scan

746. The optimal initial management of uncomplicated adrenal hemorrhage includes:

A. Percutaneous drainage
B. Adrenalectomy
C. Surveillance with serial ultrasounds, hematocrit, and bilirubin determinations
D. Percutaneous embolization of adrenal artery
E. Epsilon amino caproic acid (Amikar) administration

747. The most common renal tumor in neonates is:

A. Congenital mesoblastic nephroma
B. Wilms' tumor
C. Polycystic kidney disease
D. Angiomyolipoma
E. Oncocytoma

748. All of the following statements regarding hydrometrocolpos are true EXCEPT:

A. It is less common than hematocolpos that occurs at menarche.
B. It is usually caused by vaginal atresia.
C. It may result in ureteral obstruction.
D. Management should consist of observation since spontaneous resolution is common.
E. It is likely to occur to female infants with imperforate anus or cloacal anomalies.

749. After what age is nocturnal enuresis generally considered a cause for concern?

A. 2 years
B. 4 years
C. 5 years
D. 8 years
E. 12 years

750. Which of the following statements regarding the early development of urinary control is *false*?

A. In infants, micturition occurs spontaneously as a spinal cord reflex.
B. The striated (external) urinary sphincter of an infant does not play a role in preventing incontinence.
C. After the first year of life, the frequency of urinations per day decreases while the mean voided volume increases.

D. Control of the external urinary sphincter is usually complete by the age of 3 years.
E. Direct volitional control of the spinal micturition reflex is required to prevent incontinence.

751. In the normal sequence of development of bowel and bladder control, which of the following events generally occurs first?

A. Control of bowel function at night
B. Control of bowel function by day
C. Control of bladder function by day
D. Control of bladder function by night
E. No sequence of development has been noted

752. Which of the following urodynamic findings is usually *not* seen in children with enuresis?

A. Reduced bladder capacity while awake
B. Normal bladder capacity while under anesthesia
C. Frequent, high amplitude, spontaneous bladder contractions during sleep
D. Presence of uninhibited bladder contractions
E. Pelvic floor muscle activity during spontaneous bladder contractions

753. All of the following statements support the belief that enuresis is a result of developmental delay or lag EXCEPT:

A. Increased prevalence of bed wetting in lower socioeconimic groups
B. Increased prevalence of enuresis in children from broken homes
C. Increased incidence of bed wetting in children who are delayed in talking
D. Increased incidence of bed wetting in deep sleepers
E. Association of primary enuresis and retardation in skeletal maturation

754. A 7-year-old boy is being evaluated for diurnal enuresis. Work-up with history and physical examination, neurologic examination, urinalysis, and urine culture are normal. The next appropriate step in management is:

A. Ultrasound evaluation of kidneys, ureters, and bladder
B. Voiding cystourethrography
C. Intravenous pyelography
D. Retrograde urethrography
E. Cystourethroscopy

755. When using anticholinergics to treat enuresis, it has been found to be most effective in patients with:

A. Normal cystometrograms
B. Pure nocturnal enuresis
C. Proven uninhibited bladder contractions
D. Symptoms of day and night incontinence, frequency, and urgency
E. Decreased functional bladder capacity

756. Which of the following statements regarding the use of desmopressin (DDAVP) in the treatment of enuresis is *true*?

A. It works well for day and night wetting.
B. Better results occur in younger children.
C. Despite widespread use, no controlled studies have proved its effectiveness over placebo.
D. Upon discontinuation of treatment, most children resume wetting.
E. Given intranasally, the drug's effect lasts only 3 to 4 hours.

757. The effectiveness of imipramine in the treatment of enuresis is felt to be due to all of the following actions EXCEPT:

A. Alteration of sleep patterns
B. Antidepressant activity
C. Anticholinergic activity
D. Antispasmodic activity on bladder smooth muscle
E. Effect on sympathetic input to the bladder

758. Which of the following treatments for bed wetting has been shown to be the most effective?

A. Bladder training
B. Conditioning therapy
C. Responsibility reinforcement
D. Imipramine
E. Desmopressin (DDAVP)

759. Withdrawal of which of the following substances has been shown to significantly reduce bed wetting in adult enuretics?

A. Caffeine
B. Nicotine
C. Red-dye
D. Dairy products
E. Chocolate

760. External urethral sphincter electromyography (EMG) recorded using a needle electrode measures which of the following?

A. Sphincter muscle tone
B. Sympathetic nerve impulses
C. Somatic nerve impulses
D. Parasympathetic nerve impulses
E. Motor unit action potentials

761. In an 8-year-old boy, the predicted average bladder capacity is:

A. 50 ml
B. 80 ml
C. 150 ml
D. 200 ml
E. 300 ml

762. The most accurate term to describe the condition in which the meninges and neural tissue extend beyond the confines of the vertebral canal is:

A. Myelodysplasia
B. Spina bifida
C. Meningocele
D. Myelomeningocele
E. Lipomyelomeningocele

763. The Arnold-Chiari malformation consists of:

A. Cysts of the jaw, vertebral abnormalities, and intracranial calcifications
B. Herniation of the cerebellar tonsils down through the foramen magnum and obstruction of the fourth ventricle
C. Microcephaly, polydactyly, and posterior encephalocele

D. Hypotonia, a high forehead, and hepatosplenomegaly
E. Cerebellar hemangioblastomas, retinal angiomas, and cysts of the pancreas, kidney, and epididymis

764. The use of the Credé maneuver in a newborn who has recently undergone closure of an open lumbar myelomeningocele:

A. Is required in the majority of patients
B. Is strongly discouraged due to the high risk of bladder rupture
C. Is performed instead of clean intermittent catheterization if it adequately empties the bladder
D. Is associated with higher rates of pyelonephritis
E. Should be delayed until a formal urodynamic evaluation has been completed

765. In a newborn with myelodysplasia, which of the following patterns of urodynamic findings is associated with the highest risk of urinary tract deterioration?

A. Detrusor-sphincter dyssynergia without detrusor hypertonicity
B. Detrusor-sphincter synergia with detrusor hypertonicity
C. Detrusor-sphincter synergia without detrusor hypertonicity
D. Denervated sphincter with detrusor hypertonicity
E. Denervated sphincter without detrusor hypertonicity

766. In an adolescent with myelodysplasia noted to have a significant change on urodynamic assessment, radiologic investigation of the central nervous system is *least* likely to reveal:

A. Recurrent evagination of meninges and nerve roots
B. Tethering of the spinal cord
C. A syrinx of the cord
D. Increased intracranial pressure due to a shunt malfunction
E. Partial herniation of the brain stem and cerebellum

767. Which of the following is *not* considered to be an indication for performing antireflux surgery in a child with myelodysplasia and vesicoureteral reflux?

A. Recurrent symptomatic urinary tract infection while on adequate antibiotic therapy and appropriate catheterization techniques
B. Persistent hydroureteronephrosis despite effective bladder emptying and lowering of intravesical pressure
C. Severe reflux with an anatomic abnormality at the ureterovesical junction
D. Reflux persisting beyond the age of 8 years
E. Implantation of an artificial urinary sphincter

768. A 6-year-old boy with myelodysplasia is being managed with oxybutynin and CIC. Urodynamic testing is done to evaluate persistent incontinence and reveals a drop in urethral resistance with bladder filling. The most appropriate initial therapeutic intervention would be:

A. Maximize dose and frequency of oxybutynin
B. Discontinue oxybutynin and begin hyoscyamine
C. Continue oxybutynin and begin phenylpropanolamine
D. Perform a Young-Dees bladder neck reconstruction
E. Implant an artificial urinary sphincter

769. Which of the following statements regarding sexual development and sexuality in myelodysplastic individuals is *true*?

A. Few myelodysplastic women have an uneventful pregnancy.
B. Myelodysplastic males reach puberty at an age similar to that for normal males.
C. Male erectile function is generally normal.
D. Breast development and menarche tend to be delayed.
E. Reproductive function in the female is greatly impaired.

770. A newborn is found to have a small dimple overlying the lower spine and is suspected of having an occult spinal dysraphism. Examination will most likely reveal which of the following?

A. Perineal sensation will be absent.
B. The lower extremities will be hyperreflexic.
C. The lower extremities will be areflexic.
D. Urodynamic testing will reveal detrusor hyperreflexia.
E. Neurologic examination will be normal.

771. In addition to magnetic resonance imaging (MRI) of the spine, which of the following tests should also be performed on an infant with questionable skin or bony abnormality of the lower spine?

A. Excisional biopsy of the superficial skin lesion
B. Myelogram with a water-based contrast material
C. Renal ultrasonography
D. Urodynamic testing
E. Voiding cystourethrography

772. Which of the following maternal conditions has been implicated in the etiology of sacral agenesis?

A. Age over 40 years
B. Gestational, insulin-dependent diabetes
C. Rheumatoid arthritis
D. Ethanol abuse
E. Cocaine abuse

773. Which of the following structures is *not* generally affected in the Vacterl syndrome?

A. Vertebral
B. Anal
C. Cranial
D. Renal
E. Limb

774. Which of the following is a true statement regarding cerebral palsy?

A. Early neurosurgical intervention is required due to the progressive nature of this disease.
B. The incidence is decreasing because smaller and younger premature infants are surviving in intensive care units.
C. Most affected children will develop total urinary control.

D. Urodynamic evaluation of all affected children should be performed within the first few months of life.
E. The majority of patients undergoing urodynamic evaluation will have evidence of a mixed upper and lower motor neuron lesion.

775. A newborn delivered via a high forceps delivery is subsequently noted to have loss of sensation and paralysis of the lower limbs. Evaluation of this patient is most likely to show which of the following?

A. A lack of bony abnormalities on plain radiography of the spine
B. Swelling of the cord above the lesion on computed tomography (CT)
C. Early restoration of bladder and rectal function followed by delayed return of sensation and motor function
D. Detrusor hyperreflexia and detrusor-sphincter dyssynergia on immediate postinjury urodynamic evaluation
E. In the case of permanent injury, delayed urodynamic evaluation reveals detrusor areflexia

776. When evaluating a child for enuresis, which of the following is *not* considered an indication for performing urodynamic studies?

A. A girl who voids normally but is constantly damp both day and night
B. A pubertal child with nocturnal enuresis resistant to conventional therapy
C. A boy with bladder trabeculation on voiding cystography
D. A boy with diurnal incontinence with no associated pathology
E. A girl with recurrent urinary tract infections despite continuous antibiotics

777. In a girl with recurrent urinary tract infections, periodic tightening and relaxation of the external sphincter during voiding (stop-and-start voiding), when unrecognized or untreated, is thought to be the forerunner of which of the following conditions?

A. Stress urinary incontinence
B. Interstitial cystitis
C. Vesicoureteral reflux
D. Urethral diverticulum
E. Bladder diverticulum

778. Incontinence in a patient with profound constipation is felt to be due to which of the following?

A. Overflow incontinence due to bladder neck obstruction by the fecal mass
B. Stress incontinence due to loss of the normal vesicourethral angle
C. Development of a rectovesical fistula
D. Development of uninhibited contractions of the bladder
E. Marked reduction in bladder capacity

779. The term "Vincent's curtsy" refers to which of the following?

A. Frequent dips in the flow rate curve occurring during staccato voiding
B. The abnormal gait assumed by some patients with myelomeningocele
C. The sudden drop in sphincter EMG activity noted in children with periodic relaxation of the sphincter
D. The abnormal posture produced by lower extremity contractures noted in patients with cervical cord lesions
E. A characteristic posturing assumed by some children in an attempt to prevent voiding due to detrusor hyperreflexia

780. Which of the following findings is *not* likely to be seen in a child with an infrequent voiding pattern?

A. Bladder capacity larger-than-normal for age
B. High residual volume on catheterization
C. Cystogram with vesicoureteral reflux
D. Urinary flow rate with intermittent flow and sudden peaks
E. Incomplete bladder emptying

781. Radiologic evaluation of a child with Hinman syndrome is most likely to reveal which of the following?

A. Hydroureteronephrosis
B. Smooth bladder wall
C. Small-capacity, contracted bladder
D. Little or no post-void residual urine volume
E. Lesions of the sacral spine

782. The most reliable way to collect a urine sample for urinalysis and urine culture in infants and small children is by:

A. Bagged specimen
B. Midstream specimen
C. Urethral catheterization
D. Suprapubic aspiration
E. Retrograde ureteral catheterization

783. All of the following are reasons for a UTI to persist EXCEPT:

A. Inadequate therapy
B. Periurethral colonization
C. Bacterial resistance
D. Inadequate urinary concentration of drug
E. Multiple organism infection

784. In which of the following age groups are urinary tract infections more common in boys than girls?

A. 0–3 months
B. 3 months to 1 year
C. 1 year to 5 years
D. 5–10 years
E. Around puberty

785. Host factors contributing to bacteriuria include all of the following EXCEPT:

A. P-fimbriae
B. Periurethral colonization
C. P_1 blood group phenotype
D. Reflux
E. Immune status

786. The best clinical sign/symptom to differentiate pyelonephritis from cystitis in children is:

A. Flank pain
B. Nausea and vomiting
C. Fever >38°C
D. Incontinence
E. Dysuria

787. Papillary impressions are first lost in which grade of reflux?

A. I
B. II
C. III
D. IV
E. V

788. What percentage of grade II reflux will resolve after 3 years of conservative therapy?

A. 15 per cent
B. 25 per cent
C. 50 per cent
D. 65 per cent
E. 90 per cent

789. All of the following are true regarding renal scarring EXCEPT:

A. 17 per cent of children with bacteriuria have renal scarring.
B. Most renal scars are found on the first evaluation.
C. 30 per cent of children with renal scarring have reflux.
D. Renal scarring rarely occurs after age 10.
E. Renal scarring can be lessened with early antibiotic therapy.

790. All of the following factors affect renal scar development after infection EXCEPT:

A. Intrarenal reflux
B. Pressure effect of reflux
C. Host immune response
D. Age
E. Sex

791. The risk of hypertension with reflux nephropathy is:

A. No greater than in controls
B. 3–5 per cent
C. 10–20 per cent
D. 50 per cent
E. 80 per cent

792. Which of the following is predictive of progressive renal deterioration?

A. Recurrent infections
B. Renal scarring
C. Hypertension
D. Proteinuria
E. Persistent reflux

793. Untreated bacteriuria during pregnancy will result in pyelonephritis in what percentage of patients?

A. There is no increased incidence of pyelonephritis
B. 2 per cent
C. 7 per cent
D. 40 per cent
E. 75 per cent

794. The most common urine culture result in children presenting with hemorrhagic cystitis is:

A. No growth
B. Enterococcus
C. *E. coli*
D. Adenovirus 11
E. Adenovirus 21

795. All of the following antibiotics are good choices for prophylaxis of UTI in children EXCEPT:

A. Nitrofurantoin
B. Cephalexin
C. Bactrim
D. Trimethoprim
E. Nalidixic acid

796. All of the following are indications for surgical management of reflux EXCEPT:

A. Multiple breakthrough infections while on prophylaxis
B. Renal scarring 3 months after the last infection
C. Poor compliance with medical therapy
D. Reflux that fails to resolve after many years of medical therapy
E. Open bladder surgery required to correct another problem

PART X

EMBRYOLOGY AND ANOMALIES OF THE GENITOURINARY TRACT

CHAPTERS 32 THROUGH 43

ANSWERS

587-C *(Campbell's, pp. 1301–1303; Fig. 32–1)*

Development begins after a sperm fertilizes an ovum. The zygote begins its development by division into about 30 smaller cells, blastomeres. The blastomeres form a hollow sphere, or blastula. An inner cell mass then develops which gives rise to tissues of the embryo. During the second week, the inner cell mass flattens. A separate sheet of cells, the endoderm, appears on the underside of the inner cell mass. The ectoderm is composed of cells that appose the endoderm. A cleft appears above the ectoderm and enlarges as the yolk sac. During the third week, cell migration between the endoderm and ectoderm forms the primitive streak noted on the surface of the blastoderm. These cells develop into mesoderm.

REFERENCES

1. Austin, C.R., and Short, R.V.: Reproduction in Mammals, Book 2. Embryonic and Fetal Development, 2nd ed. Cambridge, Cambridge University Press, 1973.
2. Avey, L.B.: Developmental Anatomy. Philadelphia, W.B. Saunders Co., 1974.

588-B *(Campbell's, pp. 1302–1303; Table 32–2)*

As stated above, the first few weeks of development involve primitive cellular arrangements and conversion form the zygote to laminar embryo. Between the third and sixth weeks, mesenchyme condenses as blocklike structures, the somites, to form the somite embryo. Next, the period of the embryo (8 weeks of gestation) ensues, and the germ layers form the organs of the body. From week 9 to term, the period of the fetus, development involves maturation of the formed organs.

589-E *(Campbell's, pp. 1303–1304)*

The definitive urinary system results from complex interactions of embryonic mesoderm with itself and with endoderm. The pronephros is the first urinary tissue to appear, followed by the mesonephros, and finally, the metanephros. The pronephros appears in the cervical region of the ten-somite embryo between the second and sixth somites. Pronephric tubules develop from intermediate mesoderm, but the tubules do not function. The pronephros then quickly degenerates. Next, the mesonephric (wolffian) duct descends from the level of the cervical somites to reach the caudal region of the embryo. The mesonephric duct apposes intermediate mesoderm and mesonephric tubules develop. These tubules differentiate into glomerulus, proximal tubule, distal tubule, and collecting duct. By 28 days, the mesonephric duct contacts the urogenital sinus and later drains into the sinus. A brief period of function is believed to exist, but after 10 weeks of development the caudal mesonephric tubules degenerate. The cranial nephrons will persist and be incorporated into the genital duct system. The metanephros will develop next and ultimately become the definitive kidney.

REFERENCES

1. Hamilton, W.J., and Mossman, H.W. (Eds.): The urogenital system. *In* Human Embryology Prenatal Development of Form and Function. New York, Macmillan Press Ltd., 1976, p. 377.
2. Felix, W.: The development of the urinogenital organs. *In* Keibel, F., and Mall, F.P. (Eds.): Manual of Human Embryology. Philadelphia, J.B. Lippincott Co., 1912. (Vol. II, Chapt. XIX., p. 866).

590-A *(Campbell's, pp. 1303–1305; Fig. 32–4)*

As stated above, the pronephros is the first urinary tissue to appear, and it forms pronephric tubules from intermediate mesoderm. It is believed that the duct of the pronephric tubule continues caudally as the mesonephric (wolffian) duct. This duct plays a critical role in the development of male genital organs and gives rise to the transiently functioning mesonephros.

591-B *(Campbell's, pp. 1304–1307; Fig. 32–6)*

After the mesonephric duct drains into the urogenital sinus, the ureteral bud appears. The bud originates as a diverticulum from the posteromedial aspect of the mesonephric duct at the point where the terminus of the duct bends to enter the cloaca. The ureteral bud appears to develop further over four periods. During these periods, the ureteral bud makes contact with metanephric mesenchyme and undergoes symmetric and asymmetric branchings to form the renal collecting system and induce renal tubules and nephrons.

REFERENCE

1. Potter, E.L.: Normal and Abnormal Development of the Kidney. Chicago, Year Book Medical Publishers, 1972.

592-B *(Campbell's, pp. 1306–1308; Fig. 32–6)*

It is the ureteral bud that induces nephrogenesis. The mesonephric duct, derived from the mesoderm, gives rise to the ureteral bud. This bud extends into and is surrounded by metanephric mesenchyme, which is also of mesodermal origin. Nephrogenesis involves the interaction of the metanephric mesenchyme and the ureteral bud. The ureteral bud develops further over four periods. In period 1 (from the 5th to the 14th week of gestation), four to six symmetrical branchings occur to mold the renal pelvis. The subsequent three to five generations of branching contribute to the calyces. These branches also induce nephron development within the metanephric mesenchyme. During periods 2 (15th to 22nd week) and 3 (22nd to 32nd week) the ureteral bud branches less frequently, but it continues to induce formation of nephrons. As each ureteral ampulla extends toward the cortex, a family of about four nephrons is laid down as arcades or tiers of nephrons. The medullary nephrons develop first, followed by cortical nephrons. During period four (32nd to 36th week to adulthood), no new nephrons are induced, but the previously formed collecting ducts elongate, the proximal tubules convolute, and the loops of Henle penetrate deeper into the medulla.

REFERENCE

1. Potter, E.L.: Normal and Abnormal Development of the Kidney. Chicago, Year Book Medical Publishers, 1972.

593-A *(Campbell's, pp. 1311–1313)*

Clinical observations led to inferences that obstruction of urine drainage may cause renal dysplasia, but this has not been supported by experimental or clinical data. Obstruction of the ureters of normal renal blastemas leads to hydronephrosis, not to dysplasia. Abnormal ureteral bud and metanephrogenic mesenchyme interactions, however, are felt to lead to the formation of a dysplastic kidney. For example, when the ureters of a duplex kidney drain onto the trigone, their associated renal units are normally formed. When the ureters drain outside the trigone, however, their associated renal units are poorly formed or dysplastic. The ureters, which drain outside the trigone, are presumed to have originated from defective ureteral buds. These malpositioned buds may interact poorly with the metanephrogenic mesenchyme. The mesenchyme does not become specialized enough to elaborate tubules and thus differentiates abnormally. Furthermore, the development of dysplasia may be accentuated by coexisting renal obstruction.

REFERENCES

1. Bernstein, J.: The morphogenesis of renal parenchymal maldevelopment (renal dysplasia). Pediatr. Clin. North Am., *18*:395, 1971.
2. Stephens, F.D.: Embryopathy of malformations. J. Urol. (Guest editorial), *127*:13, 1982.

594-D *(Campbell's, pp. 1323–1327)*

The bladder arises from the endoderm of the urogenital sinus and mesoderm of the mesonephric duct caudal to the ureteral bud origin. After the mesonephric ducts drain into the urogenital sinus, the epithelium of the urogenital sinus fuses with that of the mesonephric duct. By 33 days of gestation, the segment of the mesonephric duct beyond the ureteral bud dilates as the common excretory duct—the precursor of the hemitrigone. Continued growth of the epithelium and mesoderm of the common excretory duct separates the ureteral orifices laterally and establishes the framework of the primitive trigone. As development continues, the bladder becomes a cylindric tube lined by connective tissue. Later, mesenchyme surrounding the bladder develops into circular, interlacing, and longitudinal strands of smooth muscle. These muscle fibers continue to organize and develop. The mechanics of bladder distention may stimulate further muscularization. Continence of bladder urine may be possible at about 16 weeks, when the urethral sphincter muscle encircles the urethra.

REFERENCES

1. Alcaraz, A., Vinaixa, F., Tejedo-Mateu, A., et al.: Congenital obstructive disease of the ureter. Acta Urol. Esp., *13*:318, 1989.
2. Lowsley, O.S.: The development of the human prostate gland with reference to the development of other structures at the neck of the urinary bladder. Am. J. Anat., *13*:299, 1912.

595-C *(Campbell's, pp. 1323–1324; Fig. 32–29)*

As stated previously, after the mesonephric ducts drain into the urogenital sinus, the epithelium of the urogenital sinus fuses with that of the mesonephric duct. As the caudal segments of mesonephric ducts dilate to form the common excretory ducts, their mesenchyme migrates toward the midline. The epithelia of the ducts fuse toward the midline as a triangular area—the primitive trigone. If a duplex kidney has developed, both ureters drain into a single common excretory duct. As the common excretory duct is absorbed into the urogenital sinus, the ureters become incorporated into the primitive hemitrigone. Initially the lower pole orifice is caudal and medial to the upper pole orifice. (See Fig. 32–29,B). As viewed from outside the bladder, the ureteral orifice draining the upper pole of the kidney rotates clockwise so that the orifice lies caudal and medial to the orifice of the lower pole ureter. Weigert, and later Meyer, recognized the regularity of this relationship, which has come to be known as the Weigert-Meyer rule.

596-C *(Campbell's, pp. 1327–1328)*

Development of the genitalia is covered in detail in Chapter 36. It is important to note, however, that the development of the external genitalia is closely related to the development of the urethra. The urethra forms from the urogenital sinus, and this initially proceeds through a phenotypically indifferent stage. During the fifth week, a plate of endodermal cells thickens the inner portion of the urogenital membrane. By 6 weeks of development, the urogenital sinus is apparent. Over the next 4 weeks, the urethral plate and grooves develop and mesenchyme proliferates to form laterally positioned urethral folds. At 10 weeks of gestation, the genital tubercle is prominent and is flanked laterally by labioscrotal swellings. The ventral side of the genital tubercle shows the superficial and deep urethral grooves. At this point, the indifferent stage ends and the external genitalia of the male and female develop differently.

REFERENCE

1. Waterman, R.E.: Human embryo and fetus. *In* Hafez, E.S.E., and Kenemans, P. (Eds.): Atlas of Human Reproduction. Hinghom, MA, Kluwer, Boston, Inc., 1982.

597-E *(Campbell's, pp. 1328–1329)*

By the 10th week, the external genitalia of a boy masculinize. The genital tubercle elongates into a cylindric phallus. Mesenchyme in the tubercle condenses as the primitive cavernous tissue. The phallic portion of the urogenital sinus forms the bulbar and penile urethra. The endodermal edges of the secondary urethral groove fuse to tubularize the penile urethra. The ectodermal edges of the groove fuse as the median raphe. The scrotal swellings round, migrate caudally, and fuse to form the scrotum at the base of the penis. By term, the urethra shows an outer circular and an inner longitudinal layer, both of which are contiguous with their respective layers of the bladder.

REFERENCE

1. Rowsell, A.K., and Morgan, B.D.G.: Hypospadias and the embryogenesis of the penile urethra. Br. J. Plast. Surg., *40*:201, 1987.

598-B *(Campbell's, p. 1330; Fig. 32–34)*

The pelvic portion of the urogenital sinus develops into the lower portion of the prostatic urethra and the membranous urethra. Prostatic differentiation begins in the mesenchyme of the prostatic part of the urethra. Mesenchymal cells under the basal lamina develop into fibroblasts by the eighth week of development. By the 10th week, epithelial outgrowths from the prostatic segment of the urethra grow and branch out into the surrounding mesenchyme. By 12 weeks, five groups of tubules form the lobes of the prostate.

REFERENCES

1. Hamilton, W.J., and Mossman, H.W. (Eds.): The urogenital system. *In* Human Embryology Prenatal Development of Form and Function. New York, Macmillan Press Ltd., 1976, p. 201.
2. Lowsley, O.S.: The development of the human prostate gland with reference to the development for other structures of the neck of the urinary bladder. Am. J. Anat., *13*:299, 1912.

599-D *(Campbell's, pp. 1330–1332)*

Development of the external genitalia is under hormonal control. Male differentiation is dependent on testosterone and dihydrotesterone, the more potent, 5α reduced form of testosterone. The urogenital sinus epithelium and genital tubercle can convert the testosterone produced by the fetal testis to dihydrotesterone due to the presence of 5α-reductase. Dihydrotesterone mediates the differentiation of the derivatives of the urogenital sinus, namely, the prostate, from the pelvic portion of the urogenital sinus, and the external genitalia, from the phallic portion of the urogenital sinus. Testosterone mediates the differentiation of the derivatives of the wolffian duct, namely, the seminal vesicle, epididymis, and vas deferens.

REFERENCES

1. George, F.W., Peterson, K.G., Frankel, P.A., and Wilson, J.D.: The androgen receptor in the fetal epididymis is similar to that in the mature rabbit. Proc. Soc. Exp. Biol. Med., *188*:500, 1988.
2. Cunha, G.R.: Epithelio-mesenchymal interactions in primordial gland structures which become responsive to androgen stimulation. Anat. Rec., *172*:179, 1972.
3. Kellokumpu-Lehtinen, P., and Pelliniemi, L.J.: Hormonal regulation of differentiation of human fetal prostate and Leydig cells in utero. Folia Histachem. Cytobiol., *26*:113, 1988.
4. Siiteri, P.K., and Wilson, J.D.: Testosterone formation and metabolism during male sexual differentiation of the human embryo. J. Clin. Endocrin. Metab., *38*:113, 1974.

600-A *(Campbell's, p. 1332)*

The pelvic portion of the urogenital sinus in the female develops into the lower portion of the definitive urethra and vagina. Epithelial tubules originate from the primitive urethra after about 11 weeks to become the paraurethral glands of Skene. These glands are the female homologues of the prostate. As expected, mesenchymal differentiation in the female is less prominent than in the analogous segment in the male.

REFERENCES

1. Hamilton, W.J., and Mossman, H.W. (Eds.): The urogenital system. *In* Human Embryology Prenatal Development of Form and Function. New York, Macmillan Press Ltd., 1976, p. 201.
2. Stephen, F.D.: Congenital Malformations of the Urinary Tract. New York, Praeger Publishers, 1983.
3. Kellokumpu-Lehtinen, P., and Pelliniemi, L.J.: Hormonal regulation of differentiation of human fetal prostate and Leydig cells in utero. Folia Histochem. Cytobiol., *26*:113, 1988.

601-B *(Campbell's, p. 1333)*

In the female, the phallic portion of the urogenital sinus remains a vestibule because the ureteral plate does not extend as far to the genital tubercle as in the male. The urethra and vagina open into the vestibule. The labial swellings grow posterior to the vestibule and meet to form the posterior commissure. The swellings also grow lateral to the vestibule to form the labia majora. Urethral folds that flank the urogenital sinus develop into the labia minora. After the ninth week of development, Bartholin's glands begin as evaginations of the vestibule endoderm and then grow into the labia majora. These glands are the homologues of Cowper's glands in the male.

REFERENCES

1. Hamilton, W.J., and Mossman, H.W. (Eds.): The urogenital system. *In* Human Embryology Prenatal Development of Form and Function. New York, Macmillan, 1976, p. 201.
2. Stephens, F.D.: Congenital Malformation of the Urinary Tract. New York, Praeger Publishers, 1983.

602-C *(Campbell's, pp. 1334–1335; Fig. 32–39)*

After 12 weeks of gestation, urogenital union, the fusion of testicular and mesonephric ducts, begins. The rete tubules in the testis connect to the epigenitalis of the mesonephros. These epigenital ducts now become the efferent ducts, and the mesonephric duct becomes the vas deferens. During the fourth month, the efferent ducts adjacent to the testis remain straight, whereas those adjacent to the vas deferens coil. The upper portion of the vas deferens also coils and becomes the epididymis, whereas the lower portion near the müllerian tubercle dilates fourfold to become an ampulla. The remaining mesonephric tubules become vestigial. Epigenital tubules that do not participate in urogenital union remain as the appendix of the epididymis.

REFERENCES

1. Wood-Jones, F.: The musculature of the bladder and urethra. Anatomical Society, Great Britain and Ireland. J. Anat. Physiol., *36*:51(2), 1901–2.
2. Felix, W.: The development of the urinogenital organs. *In* Keibel, F. and Mall, F.P. (Eds.): Manual of Human Embryology, Vol. 2. Philadelphia, J.B. Lippincott Co., 1912, Chap. 19.

603-E *(Campbell's, pp. 1334–1335; Fig. 32–39)*

As stated above, during urogenital union, some mesonephric tubules join the rete tubules of the testis to become the efferent ducts, while the upper tubules become the appendix of the epididymis. The epididymis is comprised of the lower group of the lumbar mesonephric tubules (paragenitalis). The paragenitalis degenerates, but tubules between the head of the epididymis and the testis may remain as the organ of Giraldés.

604-C *(Campbell's, p. 1334)*

During urogenital union, the wolffian or mesonephric duct becomes the vas deferens. The upper portion of the vas deferens coils and becomes the epididymis. The lower portion of the vas deferens near the müllerian tubercle dilates fourfold to become an ampulla. This segment of the vas deferens develops concentric layers of mesenchyme by 12 weeks, but muscle fibers are not seen until 28 weeks. After 12 weeks, a septum divides the ampulla of the distal portion of the vas deferens into the ejaculatory duct and the seminal vesicle.

REFERENCE

1. Felix, W.: The development of the urinogenital organs. *In* Keibel, F. and Mall, F.P. (Eds.): Manual of Human Embryology, Vol. 2. Philadelphia, J.B. Lippincott Co., 1912, Chap. 19.

605-B *(Campbell's, p. 1337)*

After 8 weeks of development in the male, the müllerian ducts begin to degenerate. This occurs due to exposure to müllerian inhibiting substance (MIS). MIS is a polypeptide produced by fetal Sertoli cells. In the laboratory, the cranial portion of the duct is more sensitive to the effect of MIS than the caudal portion of the duct. Clinically, however, regression extends both caudally and cranially. The gene for MIS has been localized to the short arm of chromosome 19. The exact mechanism of action is MIS is not known, but after local adsorption of the substance, the mesenchyme may then alter the extracellular matrix by increased hyaluronidase activity or fibronectin lysis. These alterations may facilitate breakdown of the müllerian duct basement membrane.

REFERENCES

1. Donohoe, P.K., Ito, Y., and Hendren, W.H., III: A graded organ culture assay for detecting of müllerian inhibiting substance. J. Surg. Res., *23*:141, 1977.
2. Jirasek, J.E.: Morphogenesis of the genital system in the human. Birth Defects. The National Foundation, Original Article Series, *15*:13, 1977.
3. Cohen-Haguenaur, O., Picard, J.V., Mattei, M.G., et al.: Mapping of the gene for anti-müllerian hormone to the short arm of human chromosome 19. Cytogenet. Cell Genet., *44*:2, 1987.
4. Ikawa, H., Hutson, J.M., Budzik, G.P., et al.: Steroid enhancement of müllerian duct regression. J. Pediatr. Surg., *17*:453, 1982.

606-A *(Campbell's, p. 1337)*

Under the influence of müllerian inhibiting substance, the müllerian ducts degenerate as male sexual development proceeds. By 16 weeks, the caudal end of the müllerian duct is degenerated to the level of the ejaculatory ducts. The müllerian vagina does not form, and testosterone inhibits formation of the sinus vagina. At this level, the müllerian ducts are fused as the enterovaginal primordium. This primordium persists in the male as the prostatic utricle. The utricle becomes quite large and a dense layer of stroma surrounds it. The utricle opens into the urogenital sinus in the midline, adjacent to the orifices of the ejaculatory ducts.

REFERENCE

1. Deibert, G.A.: The separation of the prepuce in the human penis. Anat. Rec., *57*:387, 1933.

607-D *(Campbell's, p. 1337)*

As stated above, as male sexual differentiation proceeds, the müllerian ducts degenerate due to the effects of müllerian inhibiting substance. As with the regressing mesonephric tubules, portions of the degenerating müllerian duct may persist as vestigial structures. The cranial end of the degenerating müllerian duct may persist as the appendix of the testis. This structure has no functional importance, but it must be kept in mind when evaluating a patient for acute scrotal pain. Torsion of the appendix testis can present with acute scrotal pain and lead to an erroneous diagnosis of epididymitis or testicular torsion.

608-E *(Campbell's, pp. 1338–1339)*

After about 9 weeks gestation, the septum between the fused müllerian ducts is absent. The mesonephric ducts degenerate around the 10th week. By the 11th week, the vaginal plate lined by squamous epithelium is seen. The uterovaginal primordium remains Y-shaped until the 12th week. The cranial unfused portion of the müllerian ducts becomes the oviducts; the caudal fused portion becomes the uterus and cervix. The bicornuate uterus becomes a single chamber by upward expansion of the fused müllerian ducts as the fundus.

The müllerian ducts develop in the feminine manner spontaneously unless they are inhibited by MIS. The mesonephric duct degenerates, but remnants may remain as Gartner's duct. The duct lies along the margin of the oviduct and uterus and opens adjacent to the cervix.

REFERENCE

1. Fitzgerald, M.J.T. (Ed.): Abdominal and pelvic organs. *In* Human Embryology. New York, Harper and Row, 1978, p. 106.

609-C *(Campbell's, p. 1344; Fig. 33–1)*

The kidney develops in three major stages. The pronephros is the first to appear (at 3 weeks) but never progresses beyond a rudimentary stage and completely involutes by 5 weeks. The mesonephros develops at 5 weeks and has some excretory function. It, too, quickly degenerates by 11 to 12 weeks, but is critical to the development of the definitive kidney in that it gives rise to the ureteric bud. This ultimately gives rise to the collecting system and induces nephrogenesis. The metanephros develops into the kidney proper. It develops and matures with a centrifugal pattern, with the outer cortical nephrons being the last to complete development.

REFERENCE

1. Potter, E.L.: Normal and Abnormal Development of the Kidney. Chicago, Year Book, 1972.

610-E *(Campbell's, pp. 1344–1345)*

Urine production begins around 10–12 weeks, but the placenta is responsible for salt and water homeostasis throughout gestation.

Fetal renal blood flow is low in the fetus with a ratio of renal blood flow to cardiac output at 20 weeks of 0.03 compared to the postnatal ratio of 0.2–0.3. This is related to a number of factors including a low number of vascular channels with high arteriolar resistance seen in early gestation and may also be related to the renin-angiotensin system.

Glomerular filtration rate (GFR) increases with gestational age and parallels renal mass because nephrogenesis continues from 10 to 12 weeks gestation until 34 weeks.

Fetal handling of sodium and potassium are related to plasma aldosterone levels. The aldosterone concentration increases with gestational age, resulting in increasing sodium retention (and a negative fractional excretion of sodium [FE_{Na}]) and increasing potassium excretion.

REFERENCES

1. Rudolph, A.M., and Heyman, M.: Circulatory changes during growth in the fetal lamb. Circ. Res., *26*:289, 1976.
2. Ichikawa, I., Maddox, D.A., and Brenner, B.M.: Maturational development of glomerular ultrafiltration in the rat. Am. J. Physiol., *236*:F465, 1979.
3. Robillard, J.E., Gomez, R.A., Meernik, J.G., et al.: Role of angiotensin II on the adrenal and vascular responses to hemorrhage during development of fetal lambs. Circ. Res., *50*:645, 1982.
4. Smith, F.G., and Robillard, J.E.: Pathophysiology of fetal renal disease. Semin. Perinatol., *13*:305, 1989.

611-A *(Campbell's, pp. 1345–1346)*

At birth, a number of dramatic events occur that alter renal function. Renal blood flow increases 5- to 18-fold with a redistribution of flow from inner to outer cortex and decreased intravascular resistance. The GFR doubles during the first week of life. For infants born prematurely (before 34 weeks), GFR rises slowly until a postconceptual age of 34 weeks, when a rapid rise is then observed. This increase is due to decreased vascular resistance and increased perfusion pressure, glomerular permeability, and filtration surface. This rise in GFR is also associated with increases in bicarbonate reabsorption and glucose transport.

A blunted response to sodium loading persists due to the inability of the distal tubule to appropriately decrease its fractional excretion of sodium. This is related to high circulating renin and aldosterone levels and a poor renal response to atrial natriuretic peptide.

Concentrating ability is also altered in that the neonatal kidney can dilute well (to 25–35 mOsm), but poorly concentrates (to 600–700 mOsm) due to immaturity of the renal medulla, decreased medullary concentrations of sodium chloride and urea, and poor responsiveness of the collecting ducts to antidiuretic hormone.

Calcium-phosphate metabolism also changes after birth. Parathyroid hormone (PTH) is suppressed at birth, and serum calcium concentration falls. This then causes an increase in PTH release, calcium reabsorption, and phosphate excretion.

REFERENCES

1. Gruskin, A.B., Edelmann, C.A. Jr., and Yuan, S.: Maturational changes in renal blood flow in piglets. Pediatr. Res., *4*:7, 1970.

2. Guignard, J.P., Torrado, A., DaCunha, O., et al.: Glomerular filtration rate in the first three weeks of life. J. Pediatr. 87:268, 1975.
3. Arant, B.S., Jr.: Developmental patterns of renal functional maturation compared in the human neonate. J. Pediatr, 92:705, 1978.
4. Kim, M.S., and Mandell, J.: Renal Function in the Fetus and Neonate. *In* King, L.R., Jr. (Ed.) Urologic Surgery in Neonates and Young Infants. Philadelphia, W.B. Saunders Co., 1988, p 41.

612-B *(Campbell's pp. 1346–1347)*

Determining the GFR in an infant is difficult for a number of reasons. These include technical difficulties in collecting timed urine and blood samples, inaccuracies in measuring serum creatinine and the rapid change of GFR with normal growth. During the first 48 hours of life, serum creatinine reflects maternal creatinine. By one week the creatinine of a term infant is normally less than 1 mg/dl but in a preterm infant it may be as high as 1.5 mg/dl for the first month of life. Serial creatinine determinations are very helpful because a progressive increase suggests renal insufficiency regardless of gestational age.

Using the serum creatinine and the patient's height, one can calculate an estimate of creatinine clearance only. As in adults, a 24-hour urine collection can be used to accurately calculate creatinine clearance. It is important to correct for adult body surface area to reduce confusion when comparing results to expected normal ranges.

A Tc-DTPA renal scan allows for precise measurement of GFR and differential renal function because it is cleared solely by glomerular filtration. Difficulty with venous access and patient cooperation during imaging may limit its usefulness.

REFERENCES

1. Trompeter, R.A., Al-Dahhan, J., Haycock, G.B., et al.: Normal values for plasma creatinine concentration related to maturity in normal term and preterm infants. Int. J. Pediatr. Nephrol., *4*:145, 1983.
2. Schwartz, G.J., Brion, L.P., and Spitzer, A.: The use of plasma creatinine concentration for estimating glomerular filtration rate in infants, children, and adolescents. Pediatr. Clin. North Am., *34*:571, 1987.

613-E *(Campbell's, pp. 1347–1348; Fig. 33–4)*

The condition present is most likely a type IV renal tubular acidosis (RTA), where the kidney has normal distal tubular acidification but impaired potassium secretion. In this case, the diagnosis is made from the presence of a metabolic acidosis reflected in a low total CO_2, a normal anion gap of 13 (Gap = $[Na^+] - [C1^-] + [CO_2]$), appropriate acidification of the urine below a pH of 5.5, and an elevated serum potassium.

In type I RTA, defective distal tubular acidification is present resulting in metabolic acidosis, a normal anion gap, and an inappropriately high urine (pH >5.5). In type II RTA, a decreased threshold for proximal tabular bicarbonate reabsorption results in a low serum total CO_2, normal anion gap, and appropriate acidification of the urine (pH <5.5). Type III RTA is a combined proximal and distal tubular abnormality.

Prior to evaluating any patient for RTA, it is important to be sure that diarrhea or some other source of gastrointestinal bicarbonate loss is not causing or adding to the metabolic acidosis.

614-D *(Campbell's, pp. 1347–1349)*

The simplest way to manage all types of RTA is to initiate therapy with sodium bicarbonate or sodium citrate (Shohl's solution or Bicitra) at a dosage of 3 mEq/kg/day divided into four daily doses. Ultimately, one should try to raise the total CO_2 to the normal range (>20 mEq/L) and the urine pH above 7.8.

A number of causes of RTA in children are known. Thus congenital obstructive nephropathy and Fanconi's syndrome should always be ruled out. As a result, evaluation with ultrasonography and tests for serum electrolytes, calcium, phosphorus, parathyroid hormone, and thyroid function should be obtained, along with a urinalysis to screen for glucosuria and aminoaciduria. A 24-hour urine collection for calculation of creatinine clearance, protein excretion, and tubular reabsorption of phosphorus should also be performed.

Most infants with RTA will respond well to alkali therapy, but some patients with type IV may have persistent hyperkalemia despite correction of acidosis. This is best managed using chlorothiazide 10 to 20 mg/kg/day or Kayexalate 1 g/kg/day. When using diuretics, it is important to watch for development of volume contraction that may reduce potassium excretion. Kayexalate may cause sodium retention and volume expansion of bowel obstruction from inspissated resin in the intestinal tract. Furosemide, 1 mg/kg in infusion, may be used to differentiate type IV from type I RTA as it will result in acidification of the urine of patients with type IV but not type I RTA. No volume overload is associated the RTAs.

REFERENCES

1. Chan, C.M.: Renal tubular acidosis. J. Pediatr., *102*: 327, 1983.
2. Hutcheon, R.A., Shibuya, M., Leumann, E., et al.: Distal renal tubular acidosis in children with chronic hydronephrosis. J. Pediatr., *89*:372, 1976.
3. Rodriguez-Soriano, J., Vallo, A., and Oliveros, R.: Transient pseudohypoaldosteronism secondary to obstruction uropathy in infancy. J. Pediatr., *103*:375, 1983.

615-A *(Campbell's, p. 1349)*

Renal maldevelopment causes most disorders of urinary concentration in infants and children. Renal dysplasia, obstructive nephropathy, and pyelonephritis all effect the concentrating ability of the kidney. Renal tubular acidosis, sickle cell nephropathy, and medullary cystic disease may also result in impaired concentrating ability. In all of these, a mild impairment is seen such that the urine specific gravity is greater than 1.005. A urine specific gravity greater than 1.020 generally rules out a serious abnormality of concentrating ability. In unilateral renal agenesis, however, the remaining kidney is generally functionally and anatomically normal.

Infants with diabetes insipidus usually have a urine specific gravity less than 1.005. Also, any infant with unexplained dehydration or hypernatremia should be screened for a urine concentrating defect. Evaluation should include serum electrolytes, BUN and creatinine, urinalysis and urine culture, renal ultrasonography and possibly voiding cystourethrogram.

Further work-up with a formal water deprivation test or testing for renal response to DDAVP may be necessary.

616-B *(Campbell's, pp. 1349–1351)*

Fetal and neonatal renal function is controlled by a number of circulating hormones. The renin-angiotensin system (RAS) develops quite early. Renin is present in the mesonephros and has been detected as early as the eighth week of gestation. Until early in the postnatal period, renin is distributed along arcuate and interlobular arteries. Postnatally, it localizes to the juxtaglomerular apparatus. Plasma renin activity (PRA) is low during fetal life until the perinatal period when a marked increase occurs in response to vaginal delivery and other perinatal events.

Atrial natriuretic peptide (ANP) is secreted by cardiac myocytes. It causes an increase in GFR, natriuresis, diuresis, and vascular permeability, inhibits renin and aldosterone release, and stimulates vasorelaxation. ANP acts via specific receptors and is removed from plasma by "clearance" receptors. Overall, ANP plays a role in the physiologic adaption of the fetus and neonate to its changing environment and, more specifically, it aids in regulation of fetal blood volume. Fetal plasma levels of ANP are significantly higher than maternal levels and are altered by a number of stimuli. For example, intrauterine blood transfusions, which increase fetal blood volume, have been shown to increase fetal plasma ANP levels.

As in the adult, arginine vasopressin (AVP) is released by the fetus in response to osmolar and nonosmolar stimuli. In contrast to the adult, however, the fetal collecting duct is less sensitive to AVP. Normal responsiveness to AVP develops in the postnatal period. Inappropriate AVP secretion or unresponsiveness to AVP can have life threatening consequences for the newborn.

REFERENCES

1. Pernollet, M.G., Devynek, M.A., MacDonald, G.J., et al.: Plasma renin activity and adrenal angiotensin II receptors in fetal, newborn, adult and pregnant rabbits. Biol. Neonate., *36*:119, 1979.
2. Fiselier, T., Monnens, L., and van Munster, P., et al.: The renin angiotensin aldosterone system in infancy and childhood in basal conditions and after stimulation. Eur. J. Pediatr., *143*:18, 1984.
3. Goetz, K.L.: Physiology and pathophysiology of atrial peptides. Am. J. Physiol., *254*:E1, 1988.
4. Robillard, J.E., and Weiner, C.: Atrial natriuretic factor in the human fetus: Effect of volume expansion. J. Pediatr., *113*:552, 1988.
5. Leake, R.D., Weitzman, R.E., Weinberg, J.A., et al.: Control of vasopressin secretion in the newborn lamb. Pediatr. Res., *13*:257, 1979.

617-D *(Campbell's, pp. 1352–1353)*

The developing kidney differs from the adult in its response to ureteral obstruction, and the timing of the obstruction is critical to determining the degree of resulting abnormalities. Early in gestation, ureteral atresia results in irreversible multicystic dysplasia of the affected kidney. If obstruction occurs later in development, the effects are less severe and may be minimized by early intervention. Due to impairment of glomerular recruitment, chronic partial unilateral ureteral obstruction results in a marked increase in vascular resistance of the affected kidney. This impairment in recruitment is felt to be due to alterations in levels of growth factors regulated by the obstructed and nonobstructed renal tissue.

The renin angiotensin system is also affected by unilateral ureteral obstruction. The renal renin content is increased in the obstructed kidney. Furthermore, the distribution of renin is altered in both the obstructed and unobstructed kidney, resulting in persistence of the early neonatal distribution of renin along the afferent arteriole.

REFERENCES

1. King, L.R., Coughlin, P.W.F., Bloch, E.C., et al.: The case for immediate pyeloplasty in the neonate with ureteropelvic junction obstruction. J. Urol., *132*:725, 1984.
2. Chevalier, R.L.: Glomerular number and perfusion during normal and compensatory renal growth in guinea pig. Pediatr. Res., *16*:436, 1982.
3. Chevalier, R.L., and Gomez, R.A.: Response of the renin-angiotensin system to relief of neonatal ureteral obstruction. Am. J. Physiol., *255*:F1070, 1989.
4. El Dahr, S., Gomez, R.A., Gray, M.S., et al.: In situ localization of renin and its mRNA in neonatal ureteral obstruction. Am. J. Physiol., *285*:F854, 1990.

618-D *(Campbell's, pp. 1358–1359; Fig. 34–2)*

Potter's facies is one of many anomalies associated with bilateral renal agenesis. Potter described the characteristic facial appearance, which consists of a prominent fold and skin crease beneath each eye, a blunt nose, and a prominent depression between the lower lip and chin. The ears appear to be low set because the lobes are broad and drawn forward, but the ear canals are placed normally. Other characteristics include dry, loose-appearing skin, large clawlike hands, and clubbing of the feet. These facial and limb abnormalities appear to be due to compression of the fetus by the uterine walls secondary to oligohydramnios.

REFERENCES

1. Potter, E.L.: Bilateral renal agenesis. J. Pediatr., *29*:68, 1946; Potter, E.L.: Facial characteristics in infants with bilateral renal agenesis. Am. J. Obstet. Gynecol., *51*: 885, 1946.
2. Bain, A.D., and Scott, J.S.: Renal agenesis and severe urinary tract dysplasia: A review of 50 cases, with particular reference to associated anomalies. Br. Med. J., *1*:841, 1960.
3. Thomas, I.T., and Smith, D.W.: Oligohydramnios, cause of the nonrenal features of Potter's syndrome, including pulmonary hypoplasia. J. Pediatr., *84*:811, 1974.

619-B *(Campbell's, pp. 1360–1364; Figs. 34–3, 34–5)*

This patient has unilateral renal agenesis with uterus didelphys and obstruction of the ipsilateral uterine horn and vagina resulting in hematocolpus. These abnormalities develop due to a defect occurring early in the fourth week of gestation. It affects both the mesonephric and ureteral buds. As a result, not only does failure of induction of the metanephric blastema occur, but the maldeveloped mesonephric duct prevents crossover of the müllerian duct and subsequent fusion, thereby producing didelphic uterus with obstruction of the ipsilateral uterine horn and vagina. Magee and colleagues would classify this as a type II genital and renal anomaly.

In this particular case, the KUB revealing medial displacement of the splenic flexure suggests either left renal agenesis or ectopia because the colon now occupies the area normally occupied by the left kidney. This characteristic gas pattern, Lebowitz' sign, is felt to be a very reliable sign of renal agenesis.

REFERENCES

1. Magee, M.C., Lucey, D.T., and Fried, F.A.: A new embryologic classification for uro-gynecologic malformations: the syndromes of mesonephric duct induced mullarian deformities. J. Urol., *121*:265, 1979.
2. Muscatello, V., and Lebowitz, R.L.: Malposition of the colon in left renal agenesis and ectopia. Radiology, *120*:371, 1976.

620-C *(Campbell's, pp. 1364–1365)*

Supernumerary kidney is a very rare condition with only 75 reported cases. It effects males and females equally and has a higher predilection for the left side. The accessory kidney will have its own blood supply and collecting system, and is a distinct parenchymatous mass that may be separate or attached to the normal kidney by loose areolar tissue. Generally, the normal kidney will be in correct position in the renal fossa and the accessory kidney will be located caudally. The ureter draining the supernumerary kidney will converge with the normal ureter in 50 per cent of cases and will be completely independent in the other 50 per cent. When a complete ureter is present, it will enter the trigone following the Weigert-Meyer principle in 90 per cent of cases. In almost half of the reported cases, however, the ureter is obstructed, resulting in severe dilatation of the collecting system. The vascular supply is very anomalous.

REFERENCES

1. McPherson, R.I.: Supernumerary kidney: Typical and atypical features. Can. Assoc. Radiol. J., *38*:116, 1987.
2. Geisinger, J.F.: Supernumerary kidney. J. Urol., *38*:331, 1937.
3. N'Guessan, G., and Stephens, F.O.: Supernumerary kidney. J. Urol., *130*:649, 1983.
4. Tada, Y., Kokado, Y. Hashinaka, Y., et al.: Free supernumerary kidney: A case report and review. J. Urol., *126*:231, 1981.

621-E *(Campbell's, pp. 1365–1371; Fig. 34–13)*

In a patient with an omphalocele, the liver may herniate into the omphalocele sac with the intestines. As a result, cephalad ectopia develops, as the kidneys will ascend until they are stopped by the diaphragm. Normally, after acquiring a cap of metanephric blastema during the fifth week of gestation, the developing kidney migrates on its own, is extruded from the pelvis, or appears to migrate as the embryonic tail uncurls and differential growth between the body and tail occurs. It normally reaches its adult location by the end of the eighth week of gestation and its accent is limited by organs occupying a more cephalad position, i.e., the liver and spleen. If the more cephalad organs are displaced due to an omphalocele, the kidneys continue to migrate until stopped by the diaphragm. Other than having excessively long ureters and a more cephalad origin of the renal arteries, the kidneys are structurally and functionally normal.

REFERENCE

1. Pinckney, L.E., Moskowitz, P.S., Lebowitz, R.L., and Fritzsche, P.: Renal malposition associated with omphalocele. Radiology, *129*:677, 1978.

622-A *(Campbell's, pp. 1371–1376; Fig. 34–16)*

A sigmoid kidney is an anomaly of crossed ectopia with fusion where one kidney is located opposite from the side on which its ureter enters the bladder, is normally rotated, and is fused to the inferior pole of the normally positioned kidney. Each renal pelvis is oriented correctly and faces in opposite directions from one another. As each kidney has already completed rotation on the vertical axis, fusion must occur relatively late in renal development. Classification of fusion anomalies was refined and expanded to include crossed ectopia by McDonald and McClellan in 1957. Generally the kidneys function normally and patients are asymptomatic. The trigone is usually normal as ureters enter from both sides of the bladder. Finally, these patients have an excellent prognosis but may be at increased risk for developing urinary tract infections or renal calculi due to partial obstruction of the collecting system.

REFERENCES

1. McDonald, J.H., and McClellan, D.S.: Crossed renal ectopia. Am. J. Surg., *93*:995, 1957.
2. Kron, S.D., and Meranze, D.R.: Completely fused pelvic kidney. J. Urol., *62*:278, 1949.

623-A *(Campbell's, pp. 1376–1381; Figs. 34–28, 34–29)*

Horseshoe kidney is the most common of all renal fusion anomalies. The anomaly consists of two distinct renal masses lying vertically in either side of the midline connected at their lower poles by a parenchymatous or fibrous isthmus that crosses the midline. The abnormality occurs between the fourth and sixth weeks of gestation, after the ureteral bud has entered the renal blastema. Some disturbance causes joining of the inferior poles of the developing metanephric masses. The classic radiographic features consist of kidneys that are low lying and close to the vertebral column; vertical or outward axis; continuation of the outer border of the lower pole of each kidney toward and across the midline; high insertion of the ureter into the pelvis; and an anteriorly displaced upper ureter that appears to drape over a midline mass.

REFERENCE

1. Boyden, E.A.: Description of a horseshoe kidney associated with left inferior vena cava and disc-shaped suprarenal glands, together with a note on the occurrence of horseshoe kidneys in human embryos. Anat. Rec., *51*:187, 1931.

624-E *(Campbell's, pp. 1381–1383; Fig. 34–30)*

As the adult kidney assumes its final location in the renal fossa, it rotates such that the calyces point laterally and the pelvis faces medially. When this orientation is not achieved, it is termed malrotation. The kidney starts with the pelvis facing ventrally and as it migrates caudally, it normally rotates 90 degrees toward the midline. Malrotation can occur due to failure of rotation, incomplete rotation, hyperrotation, or reverse rotation. The abnormal phases of rotation have been labeled based on the position of the renal pelvis. Many characteristic features are present in the malrotated kidney including distortion of the renal pelvis, calyces, or ureter, but only the relationship of the renal blood supply to the renal parenchyma provides a clue to the actual direction of rotation. Vessels coursing ventral to the kidney suggest reverse rotation while dorsally coursing vessels suggest hyperrotation.

REFERENCE

1. Weyrauch, H.M. Jr.: Anomalies of renal rotation. Surg. Gynecol. Obstet., *69*:183, 1939.

625-C *(Campbell's, pp. 1386–1387)*

Renal artery aneurysms occur with an overall incidence of 0.1–0.3 per cent. They are classified as saccular, fusiform, dissecting, and arteriovenous. Fusiform aneurysms are felt to be congenital and occur at the bifurcation of the main renal artery and one of its divisions or at the bifurcation of a more distal branching. Saccular aneurysms are the most common type and are localized outpouchings which communicate with the arterial lumen.

Most renal artery aneurysms are asymptomatic but may produce symptoms over time due to their tendency to enlarge. Pain, hematuria, and hypertension may develop. The diagnosis may be suspected when a pulsatile mass is palpated in the area of the renal hilum or an abdominal bruit is heard. Excision is recommended if: (a) hypertension cannot be controlled easily; (b) an incomplete ringlike calcification is found; (c) the aneurysm is larger than 2.5 cm; (d) the patient is female and may become pregnant; (e) an increase in aneurysm size is noted on serial angiogram or (f) an arteriovenous fistula is present. The risk of spontaneous rupture is about 10 per cent.

REFERENCES

1. Abeshouse, B.S.: Renal aneurysm: Report of two cases and review of the literature. Urol. Cutan. Rev., *55*:451, 1951.
2. Puutasse, E.F.: Renal artery aneurysm: Report of 12 cases, two treated by excision of the renal aneurysm and repair of renal artery. J. Urol., *77*:697, 1957.
3. Zinman, L., and Libertino, J.A.: Uncommon disorders of the renal circulation: renal artery aneurysm. *In* Breslin, D.J., Swinton, N.W., Libertino, J.A., and Zinman, L. (Eds.): Renovascular Hypertension. Baltimore, Williams & Wilkins, 1982, pp. 110–114.
4. Poutasse, E.F.: Renal artery aneurysms. J. Urol., *96*: 593, 1966.

626-D *(Campbell's, p. 1388)*

A calyceal diverticulum is a cystic cavity lined by transitional epithelium within the renal parenchyma and located peripherally to a minor calyx to which it is connected by a small infundibulum. The upper calyx is most frequently affected. They are felt to develop via congenital and acquired factors. Third and fourth generation ureteral branches, which usually degenerate, may persist as isolated branches forming the diverticulum. Acquired factors include a localized cortical abscess draining into a calyx, obstruction due to infection or stone within the calyx, renal injury, achalasia, and spasm of the sphincter which is felt to surround a minor calyx.

Calyceal diverticula are generally asymptomatic and found incidentally, but may cause problems due to incomplete drainage. This may result in distention and pain during diuresis, infection, or stone formation.

REFERENCES

1. Lister, J., and Singh, H.: Pelvicalyceal cysts in children. J. Pediatr. Surg., *8*:901, 1973.
2. Siegel, M.J., and McAlister, W.H.: Calyceal diverticula in children: unusual features and complications. Radiology, *131*:79, 1979.

627-B *(Campbell's, pp. 1389–1390; Figs. 34–38, 34–39)*

Megacalycosis is an enlargement of calyces due to malformation of the renal papillae. It is not due to any obstructive processes. An increased number of malformed, dilated calyces is seen. The renal pelvis is not dilated and is of normal thickness. The ureteropelvic junction is nonobstructed and is normally funneled. The renal cortex shows no signs of scarring or chronic inflammation; it is of normal thickness. The abnormality is in the medulla which is underdeveloped and crescent shaped rather than its normal pyramidal shape. The collecting tubules are shorter than normal and oriented transversely rather than vertically from the corticomedullary junction, but they are not dilated. Acid excretion after an acid load is normal, but a mild disorder of maximum concentrating ability has been reported.

Megacalycosis is felt to be congenital in origin. A transient delay in recanalization of the upper ureter after the branches of the ureteral bud hook up with the metanephric blastema occurs resulting in a brief period of obstruction as the embryonic glomeruli begin producing urine. As a result, fetal calyces dilate and then retain an obstructed appearance in postnatal life. No obstruction persists in these kidneys. Diuretic venogram and Whitaker testing fail to demonstrate evidence of obstruction in these kidneys and long-term follow-up has failed to show further anatomic changes or functional deterioration.

REFERENCES

1. Puigvert, A.: Megacaliosis: diagnostio diferencial con la hidrocaliectasia. Med. Clin., *41*:294, 1963.
2. Vela Navarrete, R., and Garcia Robledo, J.: Polycystic disease of the renal sinus: structural characteristics. J. Urol., *129*:700, 1983.
3. Gittes, R.F., and Talner, L.B.: Congenital megacolyces vs. obstructive hydronephrosis. J. Urol., *108*:833, 1972.
4. Johnston, J.H., and Sandomirsky, S.K.: Intrarenal vascular obstruction of the superior infundibulum in children. J. Pediatr. Surg., *7*:318, 1972.
5. Gittes, R.F.: Congenital megacalices. Monogr. Urol., *5*:(1):1, 1984.

628-C *(Campbell's, pp. 1393–1401)*

Upper urinary tract obstruction due to ureteropelvic junction (UPJ) obstruction is a common anomaly of childhood. It is defined as an impediment to urinary flow from the renal pelvis into the ureter. Most cases are found perinatally due to the increased use of prenatal ultrasonography. Its etiology is not clear but appears to be due to a developmental arrest occurring at the ureteropelvic junction. This may be due to fetal vessels compressing the ureter or failure of complete canalization of the upper ureter. UPJ obstruction may be further classified as intrinsic, extrinsic, or secondary depending on the anatomic abnormality causing obstruction.

Diagnosis is often made by prenatal ultrasound revealing hydronephrosis. In this setting, the diagnosis must be confirmed with a postnatal examination. In older children, the diagnosis is often made via excretory urogram which reveals a distended renal pelvis and calyces, with a sharp cutoff at the UPJ. Delayed films are needed to evaluate for presence of a hydroureter. If the diagnosis is equivocal, a diuretic renogram is helpful in that the rate of isotope uptake will access renal function while the diuretic induced washout curve will access the degree of obstruction. Similarly, a Whitaker test, which involves measuring renal pelvis pressure during constant infusion of saline or contrast via a percutaneous nephrostomy tube, will also help identify UPJ obstruction if less invasive studies remain inconclusive. A retrograde pyelogram performed at the time of surgical correction can delineate the limits of the narrowed area, but is not needed in most cases and may be technically difficult to perform, especially in young males. Finally, a voiding cystourethrogram is mandatory on every patient with UPJ obstruction to rule out the possibility of secondary obstruction due to severe vesicoureteral reflux. Vesicoureteral reflux will coexist in 10 per cent of patients with UPJ obstruction.

REFERENCES

1. Allen, T.D.: Congenital ureteral strictures. *In* Lutzeyer, W., and Melchior, H. (Eds.): Urodynamic Upper and Lower Urinary Tract. Berlin, Springer-Verlag, 1973, pp. 137–147.
2. Ruano-Gil, D., Coca-Payeras, A., and Tejedo-Maten, A.: Obstruction and normal re-canalization of the ureter in the human embryo: Its relation to congenital ureteric obstruction. Eur. Urol., *1*:287, 1975.
3. Krueger, R.P., Ash, J.M., Silver, M.M., et al.: Primary hydronephrosis: Assessment of diuretic renography, pelvis perfusion pressure, operative findings and renal and ureteral histology. Urol. Clin. North Am., *7*:231, 1980.
4. Whitaker, R.H.: Methods of assessing obstruction in dilated ureters. Br. J. Urol., *45*:15, 1973.
5. Lebowitz, R.L., and Blickman, J.G.: The coexistence of ureteropelvic junction obstruction and reflux. Am. J. Roentgenol., *140*:231, 1983.

629-D *(Campbell's, pp. 1393–1401; Fig. 34-48)*

Most cases of ureteropelvic junction (UPJ) obstruction are found before puberty. In adults, the vast majority of cases are due to an aberrant vessel to the lower pole of the kidney crossing anteriorly to the UPJ or upper ureter. The ureter will course behind the vessel and may angulate at two places—the UPJ and the point at which it drapes over the vessel. As the pelvis distends and bulges anteriorly, the ureter is compressed and kinks resulting in a two-point obstruction. This extrinsic UPJ obstruction may be seen in children and may be due to exacerbation of a preexisting intrinsic lesion. As opposed to infants and young children who often present after incidental discovery on prenatal ultrasound or due to urinary tract infection, older patients often present with intermittent flank pain, especially during diuresis, or renin-mediated hypertension.

REFERENCES

1. Lowe, F.C., and Marshall, S.F.: Ureteropelvic junction obstruction in adults. Urology, *23*:331, 1984.
2. Stephens, F.D.: Ureterovascular hydronephrosis and the "aberrant" renal vessels. J. Urol., *128*:984, 1982.
3. Snyder, H.M., III, Lebowitz, R.L., Colodny, A.H., et al.: Ureteropelvic junction obstruction in children. Urol. Clin. North Am., *7*:273, 1980.
4. Williams, D.I., and Kenawi, M.M.: The prognosis of pelviureteric obstruction in childhood: A review of 190 cases. Eur. Urol., *2*:57, 1976.
5. Belman, A.B., Kropp, K.F., and Simon, N.M.: Renal pressor hypertension secondary to unilateral hydronephrosis. N. Engl. J. Med., *278*:1133, 1968.

630-E *(Campbell's, pp. 1402–1405; Figs. 34–57, 34–58)*

Double ureters (or complete ureteral duplication) is felt to result from an additional ureteral bud arising from the mesonephric duct. The bud normally develops from the mesonephric duct at its "elbow" where it bends ventrally and medially to join the urogenital sinus. When a second bud develops, the bud closest to the urogenital sinus becomes the lower pole ureter and is absorbed into the developing bladder first. The second bud arises from higher on the mesonephric duct, migrates with it, and then rotates medially and caudally before it is attached and absorbed into the bladder. This ureter becomes the upper pole ureter and its orifice is found medial and distal to the upper pole orifice, obeying the Weigert-Meyer law. If the double ureter forms as the result of immediate fission of a single (or junctional) ureteral bud, the common base of the junctional bud is absorbed into the developing bladder and is not effected by rotation of the mesonephric duct. As a result, the upper pole ureter is positioned cephalad to the lower pole orifice providing a rare exception to the Weigert-Meyer law. The lower pole ureter most commonly will reflux into the lower pelvis. The first ureteral bud originates too close to the urogenital sinus but the second bud arises more normally at the bend of the mesonephric duct. The lower pole orifice is placed high and lateral on the trigone with decreased muscularization. As a result, it tends to reflux. The upper pole ureter is generally ectopically located, but terminates more normally on the trigone and does not reflux.

REFERENCES

1. Stephens, F.D.: Anatomical vagaries of double ureters. Aust. N.Z. J. Surg., *28*:27, 1958.
2. Tanagho, E.A.: Embryologic basis for lower ureteral anomalies: A hypothesis. Urology, *7*:451, 1976.

631-A *(Campbell's, pp. 1405–1406; Figs. 34–59, 34–60)*

An ectopic ureter in a single or duplex system may be explained by a high or cranial origin of the involved ureteral bud from the mesonephric duct. Because the bud is further away from the urogenital sinus, it is incorporated into the bladder later and migrates with the mesonephric duct for a longer period and a greater distance. Upon absorption into the developing bladder, the ureteral orifice and mesonephric duct separate, with the orifice migrating cephalad and laterally as the bladder continues to develop. Due to its late absorption into the bladder, there is little time for ascent and migration of the ureteral orifice. In extreme cases, the ureter may not separate and empties into a derivative of the mesonephric duct resulting in drainage via the genital tract. In a male, the ureter may empty into the seminal vesical or ejaculatory duct, but continence is maintained as these structures are proximal to the external sphincter. In a female, the mesonephric duct degenerates but remains in its medial and distal portion as Gartner's duct. Gartner's duct lies within the muscular wall of the genital tract from the internal cervical or along the lateral vaginal wall to the hymen. Distention of Gartner's duct with urine results in its rupture and drainage into the genital tract. Incontinence results because the external sphincter is bypassed by the ectopic ureteral orifice.

REFERENCES

1. Tanagho, E.A.: Embryologic basis for lower ureteral anomalies: A hypothesis. Urology, *7*:451, 1976.
2. Arey, L.B.: Developmental Anatomy: A Textbook and Laboratory Manual of Embryology, 7th ed. Philadelphia, W.B. Saunders Co., 1974.
3. Ellerker, A.G.: The extravesical ectopic ureter. Br. J. Surg., *45*:344, 1958.
4. Grey, S.W., and Skandalakis, J.E.: Embryology for Surgeons. The Embryological Basis for the Treatment of Congenital Defects. Phildelphia, W.B. Saunders Co., 1972.
5. Meyer, R.: Normal and abnormal development of the ureter in the human embryo-a mechanistic consideration. Anat. Rec., *96*:355, 1946.

632-B *(Campbell's, pp. 1406–1409)*

Ureteral duplication is the most common ureteral anomaly with an incidence of about 0.8 per cent. It is twice as common in females. Duplications are classified as bifid ureter, a partial duplication of the ureter with one ureteral orifice, or double ureters, a complete duplication with two orifices. Generally, ureteral duplication is asymptomatic; however, there is an increased incidence of duplications in children being evaluated for urinary tract infections and when the Y junction is extravesical, stasis and infection can occur due to reflux of urine from one system into the other. If the Y junction is intravesical, however, ureteroureteral reflux is much less pronounced. Genetic studies of patients with ureteral duplications reveal an autosomal dominant pattern with incomplete penetrance.

REFERENCES

1. Campbell, M.F.: Anomalies of the Ureter. *In* Campbell, M.F., and Harrison, J.H. (Eds.): Urology, 3rd ed. Philadelphia, W.B. Saunders Co., 1970.
2. Nation, E.F.: Duplication of the kidney and ureter: A stastistical study of 230 new cases. J. Urol., *51*:456, 1944.
3. Cohen, N., and Berant, M.: Duplications of the renal collecting system in the hereditary osteo-onychodysplasia syndrome. J. Pediatr., *89*:261, 1976.

633-B *(Campbell's, pp. 1412–1415; Tables 34–4, 34–5)*

Megaureter means large ureter. It includes both primary and secondary lesions which result in dilatation of the ureter from near the ureterovesical junction to the renal pelvis but without significant dilatation of the renal pelvis or calyces. The International Pediatric Urologic Seminar in 1976 produced a classification system for megaureters. This system includes three main types of megaureter: reflux, obstructed, and nonreflux–nonobstructed. Each of the three main types is further subclassified as primary or secondary. A primary obstructed megaureter generally is seen as a nontortuous dilatation of the upper ureter that progressively widens distally to a fusiform or bulbous dilation before abruptly narrowing to a short undilated ureteral segment entering the bladder. The calyces and pelvis are generally normal and renal function is only mildly impaired. The dilatation of the ureter results from a distal adynamic segment or rarely, may be due to distal ureteral stenosis. The adynamic segment will usually show abnormal muscular development with maloriented and deficient muscle fibers. A excess of collagen is noted in the ureteral wall and adventitia. There is also an increased amount of collagen between muscle cells and muscle bundles. The disruption of the normal helical pattern of smooth muscle halts the normal persistaltic wave and may cause regurgitation of the urine bolus back up into the dilated ureter. Primary obstructed megaureter occurs up to five times more often in males.

REFERENCES

1. Smith, D.E.: Report of Working Party to Establish an International Nomenclature for the Large Ureter. *In* Bergsma, D., and Duckett, J.W., Jr. (Eds.): Urinary System Malformations in Children. Birth Defects: Original Article Series, Vol. 13, No. 5, New York, Alan R. Liss, p.3, 1977.

2. MacKinnon, K.J., Foote, J.W., Wiglesworth, F.W., et al.: The pathology of the adynamic distal ureteral segment. J. Urol., *103*:134, 1970.
3. Hanna, M.K., Jeffs, R.D., Sturgess, J.M., et al.: Ureteral structure and ultrastructure. Part II. Congenital uroteropelvic junction obstruction and primary obstructive megaureter. J. Urol., *116*:725, 1976.
4. Notley, R.G.: The structural basis for normal and abnormal ureteric motility. The innervation and musculature of the human ureter. Ann. R. Coll. Surg. Engl., *49*:250, 1971.
5. Pfister, R.C., McLaughlin, A.P., III, and Leadbetter, W.F.: Radiological evaluation of primary megaureter. Radiology, *99*:503, 1971.

634-C *(Campbell's, pp. 1419–1422; Fig. 34–60)*

An ectopic ureter is one that does not have its orifice at the normal position on the trigone. It results from delay in, or lack of, separation of the ureteral bud from the mesonephric duct. Approximately 20 per cent of ectopic ureters are associated with a single ureter and most of these occur in males. The ectopic orifice may be found in the urinary or genital tract along the course of the mesonephric duct. In males, the ectopic orifice may be found from the trigone to the verumontanum or in the genital tract via the seminal vesicle, vas deferens, or ejaculatory duct. Because all of these structures empty proximal to the external sphincter, incontinence is not a symptom. Urinary frequency and urgency may result from the trickle of urine in the posterior urethra. Other symptoms may result from inflammation or infection of genital organs and may include painful defecation or constipation from seminal vesiculitis, scrotal swelling and pain from epididymitis, and painful ejaculation or hematospermia from prostatitis. In the rare case of bilateral single ectopic ureters, incontinence may be seen.

REFERENCES

1. Schulman, C.C.: The single ectopic ureter. Eur. Urol., *2*:64, 1976.
2. Stephens, F.O.: Anatomical vagaries of double ureters. Aust. N.Z. J. Surg., *28*:27, 1958.
3. Stephens, F.D.: Congenital Malformations of the Rectum, Anus, and Genitourinary Tracts. London, E & S Livingstone Ltd., 1963.
4. Ellerker, A.G.: The extravesical ectopic ureter. Br. J. Surg., *45*:344, 1958.
5. Brannan, W., and Henry, H.H., II: Ureteral ectopia: Report of 39 cases. J. Urol., *109*:192, 1973.
6. Schnitzer, B.: Ectopic ureteral opening into seminal vesicle: A report of four cases. J. Urol., *93*:567, 1965.

635-C *(Campbell's, pp. 1419–1422; Fig. 34–60)*

As in males, the ectopic ureteral orifice tends to follow an ectopic pathway which extends from the urinary to the genital tracts. More than 80 per cent of ectopic ureters in females, however, are duplicated. The orifice is most frequently located in the urethra, vestibule, and vagina. As a result, about 50 per cent of females present with urinary incontinence. A normal voiding pattern is usually maintained with constant wetness. Urinary frequency, flank pain, and recurrent urinary tract infections may also be seen but are less frequent. Painful defecation and labial swelling generally are not seen.

REFERENCES

1. Stephens, F.D.: Anatomical vagaries of double ureters. Aust. N.Z. J. Surg., *28*:27, 1958.
2. Stephens, F.D.: Congenital Malformations of the Rectum, Anus, and Genitourinary Tracts. London, E & S Livingstone Ltd., 1963.
3. Schulman, C.C.: The single ectopic ureter. Eur. Urol., *2*:64, 1976.

636-E *(Campbell's, pp. 1422–1424)*

A ureterocele is a cystic dilation of the submucosal ureter. Ericson classified ureteroceles as simple or intravesical and ectopic. Intravesical ureteroceles are completely contained within the bladder and end in a fairly normal location. Ectopic ureteroceles extend into the bladder neck or urethra and the orifice is ectopically located. Ectopic ureteroceles differ from intravesical ureteroceles in that they tend to involve the upper pole of a double ureter and tend to be larger. A second classification system also exists and includes stenotic, sphincteric, and sphincterostenotic ureteroceles. A stenotic ureterocele is intravesical, tends to be normally located, and has a narrowed orifice located on the dome of the spherical mass. A sphincteric ureterocele is ectopic and has its orifice within the internal sphincter. As a result, it will empty only during voiding when the bladder neck opens. As the name implies, a sphincterostenotic ureterocele is ectopically located and has a tiny orifice. They tend to be large and can fill the bladder or prolapse through the urethra. Large ectopic ureteroceles may also cause obstruction of the lower ureter of an ipisilateral double ureter or of the contralateral ureter or bladder neck. Microscopic examination of the ureterocele reveals decreased numbers and abnormal orientation of muscle cells but a significant number of muscle cells are present.

REFERENCES

1. Ericsson, N.O.: Ectopic ureterocele in infants and children. Acta Chir. Scand., Suppl. *197*:8, 1954.
2. Stephens, F.D.: Congenital Malformations of the Rectum Anus, and Genitourinary Tracts. London, E & E Livingston Ltd., 1963.
3. Tanagho, E.A.: Embryologic basis for lower ureteral anomolies: A hypothesis, Urology, *7*:451, 1976.

637-A *(Campbell's, pp. 1424–1426; Fig. 34–70)*

The term preureteral vena cava is felt to be more anatomically correct than circumcaval ureter or retrocaval ureter because it more accurately implies that this anomaly develops from abnormal vascular, rather than ureteral, development. In this condition, the right ureter deviates medially and dorsal to the inferior vena cava, before coursing in front of the cava medial to lateral to resume a normal course distally. On excretory urogram, hydronephrosis and ureteral dilatation are noted up to the level of obstruction where a J or fish hook deformity is noted. This is the point where the ureter passes behind the cava. As stated, this anomaly develops from abnormal vascular development. Normally, the vena cava develops from the right side of a plexus of fetal veins. The right supracardinal and the lumbar portion of the right posterior cardinal veins atrophy. If, however, the lumbar portion of the right posterior cardinal vein persists and becomes dominant and the supercardinal vein atrophies, the ureter is trapped dorsally and becomes "circumcaval." Persistence of the ventral and dorsal right subcardinal veins with the right supracardinal vein results in a double vena cava. This can also trap and obstruct the right ureter but does not produce preureteral vena cava.

REFERENCES

1. Peisojovich, M.R., and Lutz, S.J.: Retrocaval ureter: A case report and successful repair with a new surgical technique. Mich. Med., *68*:1137, 1969.
2. Sasai, K., Sano, A., Imanaka, K., Nishizawa, S., Nagae, T., et al.: Right periureteric venous ring detected by computed tomography. J. Comput. Assist. Tomogr., *10*(2):349–351, 1986.

638-C *(Campbell's, pp. 1443–1444)*

A dysplastic kidney is a maldeveloped kidney which contains primitive structures. Dysplasia is a histologic diagnosis based on the finding of focal, diffuse, or segmentally arranged primitive ducts. The effected kidney may be of normal size and shape or may be small, malformed or cystic. All or only a portion of the kidney may be affected. The etiology of renal dysplasia is not known but is due to abnormal metanephric differentiation and evidence supports the theory that congenital obstruction plays a significant role. It is not clear, however, if obstruction must be present or if obstruction facilitates the dysplastic development of a metanephric blastema already deficient in mesenchyme. Finally, renal dysplasia may be suggested radiographically, but the diagnosis is confirmed on histologic examination only.

REFERENCES

1. Bernstein, J.: The morphogenesis of renal parenchymal maldevelopment (renal dysplasia). Pediatr. Clin. North Am., *18*:395, 1971.
2. Maizel, M., and Simpson, S.B., Jr.: Ligating the embryonic ureter facilitates the induction of renal dysplasia. Dev. Biol., Part B: 445, 1986.

639-E *(Campbell's, pp. 1443–1444; Fig. 35–1)*

As stated above, the diagnosis of renal dysplasia is based on histology only. Many features may be seen in a dysplastic kidney, but only the finding of primitive ducts lined by cuboidal or tall (often ciliated) columnar epithelium, surrounded by rings of connective tissue containing collagen but devoid of elastin confirms the diagnosis. All of the other features listed may be found, but they are not diagnostic.

REFERENCE

1. Ericsson, N.O., and Ivemark, B.I.: Renal dysplasia and pyelonephritis in infants and children I and II. Arch. Pathol., *66*:255 and *66*:264, 1958.

640-B *(Campbell's, pp. 1445–1448)*

Renal hypoplasia is a nonspecific condition consisting of a group of conditions sharing a common feature—an abnormally small kidney. Affected kidneys are not dysplastic but have a decreased number of calyces and nephrons. Three main types of renal hypoplasia are described—true hypoplasia, oligomeganephronia and segmental hypoplasia (also known as Ask-Upmark kidney).

True hypoplasia is a congenital condition in which the kidneys are histologically normal but of smaller size than normal. Clinically, these patients have no abnormalities or present with sequelae of renal insufficiency. Oligomeganephronia is a combination of a decreased number of nephrons and hypertrophy of each nephron. It is congenital but not familial and is generally bilateral. There may be multiple associated anomalies present and renal insufficiency is usually present at birth. Renal function may be stable for years but as the patient approaches adolescence creatinine clearance drops rapidly and proteinuria develops. Hemodialysis or transplantation is often required. Ask-Upmark kidney is segmental hypoplasia felt to result from reflux and ascending pyelonephritis. Like the other forms of hypoplasia it may present with proteinuria, renal insufficiency and small renal size on imaging studies, but unlike the other forms, severe hypertension is commonly present. None of the forms of renal hypoplasia are genetically inherited.

REFERENCES

1. Bernstein, J., Robbins, T.O., and Kissane, J.M.: The renal lesion of tuberous sclerosis. Semin. Diagn. Pathol., *3*:97, 1986.
2. Royer, P., Habib, R., Mathieu, H., et al.: L'hypoplasia renale bilaterale congenitale avec reduction due nombre et hypertrophie des nephrons chez l'enfant. Ann. Pediatr. (Paris), *38*:133, 1962.
3. Arant, B.S., Sotelo-Auila, C., and Bernstein, J.: Segmental "hypoplasia" of the kidney (Ask-Upmark). J. Pediatr., *95*:931, 1979.

641-C *(Campbell's, pp. 1448–1449)*

Renal hypodysplasia describes an abnormal kidney, which is smaller than normal and which contains primitive structures resulting from abnormal metanephric differentiation. This condition may be associated with a normal or abnormal ureteral orifice, urethral obstruction, ureterocele, or prune-belly syndrome. In a patient with posterior urethral valves two types of hypodysplasia develop. A less severe form with small subcapsular cysts and nearly normal renal function and a more severe form with larger, more widely distributed cysts and numerous islands of cartilage. The more severe form is associated with earlier onset and more severe reflux and obstruction. In these patients, the position of the ureteral orifice correlates well with the degree of hypodysplasia. A normally positioned orifice produces a hydronephrotic but histologically normal kidney. Slight lateral displacement results in hypoplasia and more pronounced lateral displacement produces hypodysplasia. This correlation appears to be independent of the presence or absence of reflux or the degree of urethral obstruction.

REFERENCES

1. Osathanondh, V., and Potter, E.L.: Pathogenesis of polycystic kidneys: Historical survey. Arch Pathol., *77*: 459, 1964.
2. Henneberry, M.O., and Stephens, F.D.: Renal hypoplasia and dysplasia in infants with posterior urethral valves. J. Urol., *123*:912, 1980.

642-A *(Campbell's, pp. 1450–1451)*

A number of classification systems of cystic diseases of the kidney exist. One of the more recent systems was created in 1987 by the Committee on Classification, Nomenclature and Terminology of the American Academy of Pediatrics Section on Urology. In this system, the various cystic disorders are primarily divided between genetic and nongenetic disease and then further classified according to clinical, radiologic, and pathologic features. This system recognizes seven genetically determined forms of renal cystic diseases: two types of polycystic kidney—autosomal recessive, or infantile, and autosomal dominant, or adult; two types of medullary cystic disease—juvenile nephronophthisis, which is autosomal recessive, and classic medullary cystic disease, which is autosomal dominant. The fifth type is congenital nephrosis which is autosomal recessive. Familial hypoplastic glomerulocystic disease is autosomal dominant. The final type is cystic disease accompanying multiple malformation syndromes. Medullary sponge kidney, on the other hand, is classified among the nongenetic diseases.

REFERENCE

1. Glassberg, K.I., and Filmer, R.B.: Renal dysplasia, renal hypoplasia and cystic disease of the kidney. *In* Kelalis, P.P., King, L.R., and Belman, A.B. (Eds.): Clinical Pediatric Urology. Philadelphia, W.B. Saunders Co., 1985, p. 922.

643-D *(Campbell's, pp. 1451–1453)*

Autosomal recessive polycystic kidney disease (RPK) or infantile polycystic kidney disease is a rare condition which affects about 1 in 40,000 newborns. This condition produces kidneys which retain their fetal lobulation and have a normal renal pelvis and ureter but have small subcapsular cysts visible when the capsule is removed. On histologic examination, dilated tubules can be seen radially arranged from the calyces to the capsule.

Clinically, the disease may be present at birth or slowly develop to present between ages 5 and 20. The usual course is progression to renal and hepatic failure with a slower rate of progression in patients who present later in life. All children with RPK have lesions in the periportal areas of the liver. Gross cysts are not found, but periportal fibrosis accompanied by proliferation, dilatation and branching of well differentiated bile ducts is seen. The other lesions listed are not seen more frequently in patients with RPK.

REFERENCES

1. Zerres, K., Hansmann, M., Mallman, R., et al.: Autosomal recessive polycystic kidney disease: Problems of prenatal diagnosis. Prenat. Diagn., *8*:215, 1988.
2. McGonigle, R.J.S., Mowat, A.P., Benwick, M., et al.: Congenital hepatic fibrosis and polycystic kidney disease: Role of portocaval shunting and transplantation in three patients. Q.J. Med., *50*:269, 1981.
3. Habib, R: Renal dysplasia, hypoplasia, and cysts. *In* Strauss, J. (Ed.): Pediatric Nephrology: Current Concepts in Diagnosis and Management. New York, Intercontinental Medical Book Corp., 1974, p. 209.

644-D *(Campbell's, p. 1453)*

Autosomal dominant (or adult) polycystic kidney disease is an important cause of renal failure. It accounts for over 9 per cent of the patients in the United States and Europe now on chronic hemodialysis. The trait has 100 per cent penetrance, so as an autosomal dominant trait, 50 per cent of an affected individual's offspring will be affected. The gene has been localized to the short arm of chromosome 16 and is known not to be the gene responsible for autosomal recessive polycystic kidney disease.

REFERENCES

1. Reeders, S.T., Breuning, M.H., Comey, G., et al.: Two genetic markers closely linked to adult polycystic kidney disease on chromosome 16. Br. Med. J., *292*:851, 1986.
2. Ramsey, M., Reeders, S.T., Thomason, P.D., et al.: Mutations for the autosomal recessive and autosomal dominant forms of polycystic kidney disease are not allelic. Hum. Genet., *79*:73, 1988.

645-A *(Campbell's, p. 1453)*

Autosomal dominant polycystic kidney (DPK) disease has been noted to have a number of associated anomalies. Cysts of liver, pancreas, spleen, and liver may be seen. Cardiovascular anomalies such as aneurysms of the circle of Willis and mitral valve prolapse have also been noted. Finally, colonic diverticula have been seen in association with DPK. Retinal angiomas, an anomaly associated with Von Hippel-Lindau disease, is not commonly seen with DPK.

646-E *(Campbell's, pp. 1459–1460)*

Juvenile nephronophthisis and medullary cystic disease are anatomically similar conditions producing progressive renal failure. In both conditions, it is believed that a defect in the tubular basement membrane is present and interstitial damage occurs secondary to leakage of Tamm-Horsfall protein. Interstitial nephritis, with round-cell infiltrates and tubular dilatation with atrophy, is almost always seen. Corticomedullary junction cysts are seen in most patients, particularly in those with medullary cystic disease.

Clinically, the diseases are similar in that both conditions cause polydipsia and polyuria. The polyuria is felt to be due to a severe renal tubular defect associated with an inability to conserve sodium. The polyuria is resistant to vasopressin and a large dietary sodium intake is often necessary. Hematuria and proteinuria are usually absent, but anemia, felt to be due to decreased production of erythropoietin, is seen. Renal failure is generally seen 5 to 10 years after initial presentation.

The two conditions differ in their pattern of inheritance and age of onset. Juvenile nephronophthisis is inherited as an autosomal recessive trait becoming manifest between ages 5 and 20. Medullary cystic disease is inherited in an autosomal dominant manner and presents in the third decade.

REFERENCES

1. Cohen, A.H., and Hoyer, J.R.: Nephronophthisis: A primary tubular basement membrane defect. Lab. Invest., *55*:584, 1986.
2. Mongeau, J.G., and Worthen, H.G.: Nephronophthisis and medullary cystic disease. Am. J. Med., *43*:345, 1987.
3. Contoni, A., Bomente, G., Coccoli, D., et al.: Familial nephronophthisis: A review and differential diagnosis. Clin. Pediatr., *25*:90, 1986.

647-B *(Campbell's, pp. 1461–1462)*

Tuberous sclerosis is a rare condition characterized by multiple malformations including renal cysts. It is inherited as an autosomal dominant trait in 15 to 20 per cent of cases. Clinically, it is described as part of a triad of epilepsy, mental retardation, and adenoma sebaceum (flesh-colored papules of angiofibroma) prevalent in the malar area. The hallmark central nervous system lesion is a superficial cortical hamartoma of the cerebrum with the appearance of a tuber or root.

Cerebellar hemangioblastomas are not associated with tuberous sclerosis. They are, however, associated with Von Hippel-Lindau diseases.

REFERENCE

1. Pampigliana, G., and Moynahan, E.J.: The tuberous sclerosis syndrome: Clinical and EEG studies in 100 children. J. Neurol. Neurosurg. Psychiatry., *39*:666, 1976.

648-D *(Campbell's, p. 1462)*

The kidneys of patients with tuberous sclerosis will display cysts, angiomyolipomas, or both. The cysts are difficult to detect clinically because they rarely exceed 3 cm in diameter. These cysts are of unique histologic type in that they have a lining of hypertrophic hyperplastic eosinophilic cells, with large, hyperchromatic nuclei and occasional mitoses. The cells will often aggregate into masses or tumorlets, and it is suspected that the lining of these cysts may evolve into renal cell carcinoma.

Renal failure is associated with tuberous sclerosis and may occur due to compression of the parenchyma by expanding cysts.

REFERENCES

1. Stillwell, T.J., Gomez, M.R., and Kelalis, P.P.: Renal lesions in tuberous sclerosis. J. Urol., *138*:477, 1987.
2. Stapleton, F.B., Johnson, D., Kaplan, G.W., et al.: The cystic renal lesion in tuberous sclerosis. J. Pediatr., *97*: 574, 1980.
3. Bernstein, J., and Landing, B.H.: Glomerulocystic kidney disease. Prog. Clin. Biol. Res., *305*:27, 1989.
4. Ibrahim, R.E., Weinberg, D.S., and Weidner, N.: Atypical cysts and carcinomas of the kidneys in the phacomatosis: A quantitative DNA study using static and flow cytometry. Cancer, *63*:148, 1989.

649-C *(Campbell's, pp. 1462–1464)*

Von Hippel-Lindau disease is a condition inherited as an autosomal dominant trait with 100 per cent penetrance. It is manifested by cerebellar hemangioblastomas; retinal angiomas; cysts of the pancreas, kidney and epididymis; pheochromocytoma; and renal cell carcinoma. Hepatic cysts are not associated.

Renal cysts are the most common associated malformations, and as in tuberous sclerosis, it appears that renal cell carcinoma develops from the cells lining these cysts. Renal ultrasound or CT is recommended as the study of choice to screen and follow patients with von Hippel-Lindau disease and to try to distinguish benign cysts from cancerous lesions. Annual or semiannual CT examinations are often advised. When cancer is identified, surgery should be as conservative as possible with local resection or partial nephrectomy being preferable, thereby sparing as much functional renal tissue as possible.

REFERENCES

1. Levine, E., Collins, D.L., Horton, W.A., et al.: CT screening of the abdomen in von Hippel-Lindau disease. AJR, *139*:505, 1982.
2. Ibrahim, R.E., Weingerg, D.S., and Weidner, N.: Atypical cysts and carcinomas of the kidneys in the phacomatosis: A quantitative DNA study using static and flow cytometry. Cancer, *63*:148, 1989.

650-E *(Campbell's, pp. 1465–1466)*

The multicystic kidney represents a severe form of dysplasia. The renal size is highly variable and often the normal reniform shape is lost. The etiology of this condition is not clear but it is felt by some to be an extreme form of hydronephrosis secondary to atresia of the ureter or renal pelvis. Other theories hold that failure of the union between the ureteric bud and metanephric blastoma leads to cystic dilatation of the latter; or that an ampullary abnormality in which the ampullae stop dividing early produces fewer generations of tubules which later become cystic.

Clinically, multicystic dysplasia is one of the most common causes of an abdominal mass in infants. The affected kidney is more commonly found on the left and slightly more often in males. In many cases, the contralateral upper tract is also abnormal and may be affected by ureteropelvic junction obstruction, obstructive megaureter, vesicoureteral reflux, and persistence of fetal folds within the ureter. The condition may be bilateral which is incompatible with survival. Complete ureteral duplication of the contralateral kidney is not commonly associated with multicystic dysplastic kidney.

REFERENCES

1. Felson, B., and Cussen, L.J.: The hydronephrotic type of congenital multicystic disease of the kidney. Semin. Roentgenol., *10*:113, 1975.
2. Osathanondh, V., and Potter, E.L.: Pathogenosis of polycystic kidney: Historical survey. Arch. Pathol., *77*: 459, 1964.

3. Green, L.F., Feinzaig, W., and Dahlin, D.C.: Multicystic dysplasia of the kidney: With special reference to the contralateral kidney. J. Urol., *105*:482, 1971.

651-B *(Campbell's, p. 1467)*

As stated previously, renal masses in infants most often represent either multicystic kidney disease or hydronephrosis. Distinguishing between the two is important because surgical intervention may be desirable to remove a nonfunctioning hydronephrotic kidney or to repair a ureteropelvic junction (UPJ) obstruction while a multicystic dysplastic kidney will generally be left in place. In most newborns, ultrasonography will be the first study performed. Three ultrasound features are diagnostic of multicystic kidney: (1) visible interfaces between cysts, (2) nonmedial location of larger cysts, and (3) absence of an identifiable renal sinus. Also, the cysts of a multicystic kidney will have haphazard distribution while those associated with UPJ obstruction will be organized around the periphery of the kidney with a large medial cyst or identifiable renal sinus. In more difficult cases, a dimercaptosuccinic acid (DMSA) renal scan may be useful due to the fact that hydronephrotic kidneys will generally have some evidence of function and multicystic dysplastic kidneys will not. Cortical thickening is not associated with multicystic dysplastic or hydronephrotic kidneys.

REFERENCE

1. Stuck, K.J., Koff, S.A., and Silver, T.M.: Ultrasonic features of multicystic dysplastic kidney: Expanded diagnostic criteria. Radiology, *143*:217, 1982.

652-A *(Campbell's, pp. 1467–1469)*

In the past, some multicystic kidneys were explored to rule out malignancy, and concern about the potential for malignant degeneration of a dysplastic kidney persists today. Reports of development of Wilms' tumor, renal cell carcinoma and embryonal tumor have been noted. Studies to define the risk of malignancy are currently in progress. Previous studies, however, have not supported a relationship between multicystic kidney and malignancy. One study estimated that one would have to remove 2000 multicystic kidneys to prevent one Wilms' tumor, while another study using flow cytometry on resected multicystic kidneys revealed no evidence of tetraploidy or aneuploidy as would be expected in a preneoplastic condition.

Hypertension has also been associated with multicystic kidney, but of nine cases reported since 1966, in only three did hypertension resolve after nephrectomy. The only clear risk factor associated with leaving a multicystic dysplastic kidney in place is the development of flank pain. When it occurs, this pain can be relieved by nephrectomy.

REFERENCES

1. Noe, H.N., Marshall, J.H., and Edwards, O.P.: Nodular renal blastema in the multicystic kidney. J. Urol., *127*:486, 1989.
2. Chen, Y.H., Stapleton, F.B., Roy, S., et al.: Neonatal hypertension from a unilateral multicystic dysplastic kidney. J. Urol., *133*:664, 1985.
3. Ambros, S.S.: Unilateral multicystic renal disease in adults. Birth Defects, *13*:349, 1976.

653-A *(Campbell's, pp. 1469–1472; Table 35–7)*

Multilocular cysts are not renal segments affected by multicystic kidney disease. They differ clinically, histologically and radiographically. Their association with malignancy is also quite different. While multicystic kidneys are rarely associated with malignancy, multilocular cysts are believed to be part of a spectrum of neoplasm with the benign multilocular cyst at one end and cystic Wilms' tumor at the other. Clinically, these lesions most likely present in males younger than 4 but in females older than 4 years. They generally present as asymptomatic masses in children but they often present with hematuria and abdominal pain in adults. Pyelonephritis is not part of the pathogenesis of this condition. Hypertension relieved after removal of a multilocular cyst has been reported but is not common. Due to its association with Wilms' tumor, the treatment for a multilocular cyst is nephrectomy.

REFERENCES

1. Wood, B.P., Muurahainen, N., Anderson, V.M., et al.: Multicystic nephroblastoma: Ultrasound diagnosis (with a pathologic-anatomic commentary). Pediatr. Radiol., *12*:43, 1982.
2. Madewell, J.E., Goldman, S.M., and Davis, C.J., Jr.: Multilocular cystic nephroma: A radiographic pathologic correlation of 58 patients. Radiology, *146*:309, 1983.

654-D *(Campbell's, pp. 1472–1474)*

Renal cysts are a common finding in both children and adults. They may present anytime from soon after birth to old age. The mean age of presentation in children is 4 years. Cysts rarely call attention to themselves and are usually discovered incidentally on sonography, CT, or urography being performed for another problem. They can, however, produce abdominal mass or pain and hematuria secondary to rupture into the pyelocalyceal system, hypertension due to segmental renal ischemia, or obstruction of calyces or the renal pelvis. Evidence of invasion or destruction of adjacent structures is indicative of an invasive or malignant process and is not consistent with the presence of a simple renal cyst.

REFERENCES

1. Lüscher, T.F., Wanner, C., Siegenthaler, W., et al.: Simple renal cyst and hypertension: Cause or coincidence? Clin. Nephrol., *26*:91, 1986.
2. Barloon, J.T., and Vince, S.W.: Caliceal obstruction owing to a large parapelvic cyst: Excretory urography, ultrasound and computerized tomography findings. J. Urol., *137*:270, 1987.

655-B *(Campbell's, p. 1473; Fig. 35–17)*

Ultrasonography is an excellent tool for the evaluation of renal cysts. The diagnosis of a benign simple cyst may be safely made when the following criteria are met: (1) sharply-defined, thin, distinct walls with smooth and distinct margins; (2) good transmission of sound waves through the cyst with consequent acoustic enhancement behind the cyst; (3) absence of internal echoes; and (4) spherical or slightly ovoid shape. When all of these criteria are met, the chances of malignancy being present are negligible. The presence of internal echoes or septa exclude the diagnosis of a simple cyst and may require further investigation to rule out an infectious or neoplastic etiology.

REFERENCES

1. Goldman, S.M., and Hartman, D.S.: The simple renal cysts. *In* Pollack, H.M. (Ed.): Clinical Urography. Philadelphia, W.B. Saunders Co., 1990, p. 1603.
2. Livingston, W.D., Collins, T.L., and Novick, D.E.: Incidental renal masses. Urology, *17*:257, 1981.

656-C *(Campbell's, pp. 1473–1474; Fig. 35–20)*

When the sonographic or CT criteria of a simple cyst are not met, conditions other than a simple cyst must be considered. In this setting, a complicated cyst (containing blood, pus, or calcifications) or cystic neoplasm must be ruled out and further studies may be needed. Cyst puncture for cytologic and chemical analysis of cyst fluid, with or without contrast injection, was popular in the past. This is required less often today due to improvements in sonography and CT. It is still indicated in cases of suspected infection, in the presence of low-level echoes on sonography but a classic cyst on CT, and with an equivocal lesion in a poor surgical candidate. MRI offers little information beyond that available from sonography or CT, but it is more specific in identifying the nature of the cyst fluid. A hemorrhagic cyst is identified by an extremely bright image on T2-weighted images due to the presence of methemoglobin. Also, Marotti and colleagues have shown that if the fluid has low signal intensity on T1-weighted images, the cyst is benign even if the wall is thick or septa are present.

REFERENCE

1. Marotti, M. Hricak, H., Fritzche, P., et al.: Complex and simple cysts: Comparative evaluation with MR imaging. Radiology, *162*:671, 1987.

657-E *(Campbell's, p. 1476)*

In 1986, Bosniak divided cysts and cystic lesions into four categories that have management implications. Type I cysts meet the CT and sonographic criteria of a single simple cyst and require no surgical treatment. Type II cysts are benign cystic lesions that are minimally complicated. They may contain five septations, small calcification, infection, or high density fluid and do not require surgery. Type III cysts are more complicated lesions with radiographic features also seen in malignancy. They will require surgical exploration or removal. Finally, Type IV cysts are cystic malignant tumors and are treated by radical nephrectomy.

REFERENCE

1. Bosniak, M.A.: The current radiological approach to renal cysts. Radiology, *158*:1, 1986.

658-A *(Campbell's, pp. 1476–1477)*

Medullary sponge kidney is a condition which, like the medullary cystic disease, juvenile nephronophthisis complex results in multiple medullary cysts. Unlike medullary cystic disease, medullary sponge kidney is not an inherited condition. The true incidence of this condition is not known due to the fact that a significant number of affected patients are asymptomatic and thus never identified. It has been estimated, however, to have an incidence of between 1 in 5000 and 1 in 20,000. The principal histologic finding is dilated intrapapillary collecting ducts and small medullary cysts. The cysts are lined by collecting duct epithelium and usually communicate with the collecting tubules.

REFERENCES

1. Bernstein, J., and Gardner, K.D., Jr.: Cystic disease of the kidney and renal dysplasia. *In* Walsh, P.C., Cittis, R.F., Perlmatter, A.D., et al. (Eds): Campbell's Urology, Ed. 5. Philadelphia, W.B. Saunders Co., 1986, p. 1760.
2. Bernstein, J.: A classification of renal cysts. *In* Gardner, K.D. Jr., and Bernstein, J. (Eds.): The Cystic Kidney. The Netherlands, Kluwer Academic Publishers, 1990, p. 147.

659-B *(Campbell's, pp. 1477–1478)*

The most common presentation of medullary sponge kidney is renal colic, followed by urinary tract infection, and gross hematuria. Any clinical presentation is generally not seen until after age 20. In many cases, the diagnosis is made when the patient undergoes intravenous pyelography for some unrelated problem. The urographic features consist of: (1) enlarged kidneys, possibly with calcification in the papillae; (2) elongated papillary tubules or cavities that fill with contrast; and (3) papillary contrast blush and persistent medullary opacification. In the absence of infection, the calculi found in these patients are generally composed of calcium oxalate either alone or in combination with calcium phosphate. The formation of these stones appears to be related to the fact that one third to one half of these patients have hypercalcuria due to a renal calcium leak, increased calcium absorption, and/or elevated parathyroid hormone levels.

REFERENCES

1. Kuiper, J.J.: Medullary sponge kidney. *In* Gardner, K.D. (Ed.): Cystic Disease of the Kidney. New York, John Wiley and Sons, 1976, p. 151.
2. Gedroyc, W.M.W., and Saxton, H.M.: More medullary sponge variants. Clin. Radiol., *39*:423, 1988.
3. Yendt, E.R.: Medullary sponge kidney, *In* Gardner, K.D., Jr., and Bernstein, J. (Eds.): The Cystic Kidney. The Netherlands, Kluwer Academic Publishers, 1990, p. 379.
4. Maschio, G., Tessitore, N., and D'Angelo, A.: Medullary sponge kidney and hyperparathyroidism: A puzzling association. Am. J. Nephrol., *2*:77, 1982.

660-D *(Campbell's, pp. 1479–1482)*

Acquired renal cystic disease (ARCD) is commonly seen in patients with end stage renal failure. The incidence of this condition overall appears to be about 34 per cent, but it varies from center to center and increases with the duration of chronic renal failure and time on dialysis. Initially ARCD was felt to be confined to patients receiving hemodialysis but it was later found to occur in patients receiving peritoneal dialysis and in patients with chronic renal failure who are being managed medically without any type of dialysis. In patients who successfully undergo renal transplantation, there is a regression of cysts. If the graft fails and the patient returns to dialysis, the cysts return. This finding of cyst regression and recurrence noted in the transplant patients suggests that there is some cystogenic or carcinogenic toxin of uremia, not removed by dialysis, which is responsible for the development of ARCD.

The importance of ARCD is twofold. First, these cysts may produce flank pain and/or hematuria from rupture of unsupported sclerotic vessels and bleeding into the retroperitoneum or collecting system. Second, there is a high incidence of benign and malignant renal tumors in patients with ARCD. Benign adenomas may occur in 20 to 25 per cent of patients while the incidence of renal cell carcinoma is estimated to be between 4 to 5.8 per cent.

REFERENCES

1. Thompson, B.J., Jenkins, D.A.S., Allan, P.L., et al.: Acquired cystic disease of the kidney: An indication for transplantation? Br. Med. J., *293*:209, 1988.
2. Miller, L.R., Soffer, O., Nasser, V.H., et al.: Acquired renal cystic disease in end stage renal disease: An autopsy study of 155 cases. Am. J. Nephrol., *9*:322, 1989.
3. Ishikowa, I., Yuri, T., Kitada, H., et al.: Regression of acquired cystic disease of the kidney after successful renal transplantation. Am. J. Nephol., *3*:310, 1983.
4. Gardner, K.D., and Evans, A.P.: Cystic kidneys: An enigma evolves. Am. J. Kidney Dis., *3*:403, 1984.

661-C *(Campbell's, pp. 1482–1485; Fig. 32–25)*

A calyceal diverticulum is a smoothly outlined intrarenal sac that communicates with the pelvicalyceal system by means of a narrow neck. They usually arise from the fornix of a calyx, most commonly an upper pole calyx. They are lined by a smooth layer of transitional epithelium and covered by renal cortex. Calyceal diverticula are generally asymptomatic and are discovered incidentally on intravenous urogram. They may produce symptoms due to infection or stone formation but seldom require surgical intervention. When indicated, percutaneous aspiration or stone retrieval are preferred over open surgery.

REFERENCES

1. Eshghi, M., Tuong, W., Fernandez, R., et al.: Percutaneous (endo) infundibulotomy. J. Endourol., *1*:107, 1987.
2. Hulbert, J.C., et al.: Percutaneous techniques for the management of caliceal diverticuli containing calculi. J. Urol., *135*:225, 1986.

662-B *(Campbell's, p. 1496)*

Sexual differentiation is a sequential process beginning with the establishment of chromosomal sex at fertilization, followed by development of gonadal sex, and culminating with the appearance of anatomic characteristics or phenotypic sex. The process of sexual differentiation does not begin immediately following fertilization. Phenotypic development of the human male and female urogenital tract is identical prior to the sixth to eighth week of development. After the eighth week, anatomic and physiologic development diverge to result in the formation of the male and female anatomy and hence, the development of phenotypic sex.

663-A *(Campbell's, pp. 1496–1497)*

As stated earlier, chromosomal sex is determined at the time of fertilization and the presence of a Y chromosome makes the fetus chromosomally male. The Y chromosome is the third smallest human chromosome and is felt to carry only a few functional genes. The undisputed function of the mammalian Y chromosome is to carry the genes that control testicular differentiation. The region of the Y chromosome thought to encode the human testis-determining factor (TDF) has been localized to the short arm of the Y chromosome between the centromere and the pseudoautosomal region. The presence of the TDF gene alone does not dictate that male development will occur. Other genes essential to normal male development are also located on the X chromosome, and autosomal genes are also essential for the development of both male and female phenotypes.

REFERENCES

1. Goodfellow, P.N., Ropers, H.H., and Davis, K.: Report of the X and Y committee, human gene mapping 8. Cytogenet. Cell Genet., *40*:296–352, 1985.
2. Page, D.C., Mosher, R., Simpson, E.M., et al.: The sex-determining region of the human Y chromosome encodes a finger protein. Cell, *51*:1091, 1987.
3. Wilson, J.D., and Goldstein, J.L.: Classification of hereditary disorders of sexual development. *In* Bergsma, D. (Ed.): Genetic Forms of Hypogonadism. Birth Defects Original Article Series, Vol. XI, 1975, pp. 1–16.

664-D *(Campbell's, p. 1497)*

The early stages of gonadal development are the same regardless of chromosomal sex. The gonadal ridges are formed during the fourth week of development by proliferation of the coelomic epithelium and condensation of the underlying mesenchyme. These primitive gonadal ridges are initially devoid of germ cells which prior to the second month of gestation are located in the endoderm of the yolk sac. During the second month, these cells migrate through the gut mesentery to the gonadal ridges. During migration, the germ cells undergo many mitotic divisions, expanding their numbers severalfold. By late in the fifth week of development, germ cell migration is complete but the male and female gonad remain indistinguishable. At this stage, the gonads are composed of three principal cell types: (1) germ cells, (2) supporting cells derived from the coelomic epithelium of the genital ridge, and (3) stromal (interstitial) cells derived from the mesenchyme of the gonadal ridge.

REFERENCES

1. Peters, H.: Migration of gonocytes into the mammalian gonad and their differentiation. Phil. Trans. R. Soc. Lond. (Biol.), *259*:91, 1970.

2. Witschi, E.: Migration of the germ cell of human embryos from the yolk sac to the primitive gonadal folds. Carnegie Contributions to Embryology, No. 209, *32*: 69, 1948.

665-C *(Campbell's, pp. 1497–1498; Fig. 36–4)*

Sexual differentiation of the gonads occurs after the gonadal ridges have formed and germ cell migration is complete. The first morphologic sign of sexual dimorphism in the gonads is the development of the primordial Sertoli cells and their aggregation into primitive spermatogenic cords in the fetal testis. Ovarian epithelial components, however, remain in irregular clusters around the primordial germ cells until the fourth month of gestation when the primitive granulosa cells organize around the dividing oocyte to establish the primordial follicle. Also around the seventh week, both testicular and ovarian endocrine differentiation begin to occur. The formation of müllerian-inhibiting substance is associated with the development of spermatogenic tubules and is the primordial hormone of the fetal testis. Shortly thereafter, Leydig's cells develop and begin to synthesize testosterone. Despite the lag in ovarian organization, ovarian estrogen synthesis occurs at approximately the same time as the onset of testosterone synthesis by the testis. The synthesis of testosterone and estrogen appears to involve the differential expression of relatively few of the many enzymes required, and primarily involves the expression of the rate limiting enzymes of the two synthesic pathways.

REFERENCES

1. Jost, A., and Magre, S.: Testicular developmental phases and dual hormonal control of organogenesis. *In* Serio, M., et al. (Eds.): Sexual Differentiation: Basic and Clinical Aspects. New York, Raven Press, 1984, pp. 1–15.
2. Gillman, J.: The development of the gonads in man, with a consideration of the role of fetal endocrines and the histogenesis of ovarian tumors. Carnegie Contributions to Embryology, No. 210, *32*:83, 1948.
3. Siiteri, P.K., and Wilson, J.D.: Testosterone formation and metabolism during male sexual differentiation in the human embryo. J. Clin. Endocrinol. Metab., *38*: 113, 1974.
4. George, F.W., and Wilson, J.D.: Conversion of androgen to estrogen by the human fetal ovary. J. Clin. Endocrinol. Metab., *47*:550, 1978.

666-E *(Campbell's, p. 1499; Fig. 36–5)*

The internal accessory organs of both sexes, as well as the renal collecting ducts, are derived from cells of the mesonephric kidney. The mesonephros develops during the fourth week of gestation from intermediate mesoderm. Tubules form within the substance of the mesonephros and later connect with a longitudinal mesonephric (wolffian) duct. At 6 weeks of development, the paramesonephric (müllerian) duct develops just lateral to the mesonephric duct. The caudal end of the paramesonephric duct becomes intimately associated with the developing mesonephric duct so that no basement membrane separates their epithelia. Paramesonephric duct development cannot occur in the absence of the mesonephric duct. By the seventh week of gestation, this duct system, mesonephric and paramesonephric, constitutes the phenotypically indifferent framework of the internal accessory organs of reproduction. As phenotypic differentiation occurs, the mesonephros proper gives rise to the epididymis. The mesonephric duct gives rise to the vas deferens and seminal vesicles. In the female, the mesonephric duct, after fusing with the caudal end of the paramesonephric duct, gives rise to the uterus and upper vagina. The fallopian tubes, however, arise from the cephalic end of the paramesonephric duct. This is not associated with the mesonephric duct and therefore not derived from cells of the mesonephric kidney.

REFERENCE

1. Gruenwald, P.: The relation of the growing müllerian duct to the wolffian duct and its importance for genesis of malformation. Anat. Rec., *81*:1, 1941.

667-C *(Campbell's, pp. 1498–1500)*

The initial event in the virilization of the male urogenital tract is the onset of paramesonephric duct regression. This coincides with the development of the spermatogenic cords in the fetal testis between 7 and 8 weeks of gestation and the production of müllerian-inhibiting substance. It is shortly after this time that Leydig's cells are noted, and production of testosterone begins by 9 weeks of gestation. Luteinizing hormone receptors have not been detected before 12 weeks of gestation. Around the time that testosterone production is noted, posterior migration of the genital swellings and fusion of the genital folds begin to ultimately form the scrotum and penile urethra, respectively.

668-B *(Campbell's, pp. 1500–1501; Figs. 36–7, 36–8)*

The transformation of the mesonephric or wolffian ducts into the male genital tract begins after müllerian duct regression has begun. The majority of the mesonephric tubules regress but those adjacent to the testis (epigenital tubules) lose their primitive glomeruli and establish contact with the developing rete and spermatogenic tubules to form the efferent ductules. The cranial segment of the wolffian duct atrophies and becomes the vestigial appendix epididymis. The portion of the duct immediately distal to the efferent ducts becomes elongated and convoluted to form the epididymis while the central portion forms thick muscular walls and becomes the vas deferens. The seminal vesicles develop as buds from the lower wolffian ducts at about 13 weeks of gestation. The terminal portions of the ducts between the developing seminal vesicles and the urethra become the ejaculatory ducts and the ampullae of the vas deferens. Despite undergoing almost complete regression, the cranial portion of the müllerian duct persists as the nonfunctional appendix testis and the extreme lower end persists as the prostatic utricle.

REFERENCES

1. Watson, E.M.: The development of the seminal vesicles in man. Am. J. Anat., *24*:395, 1918.
2. Glenister, T.W.: The development of the utricle and of the so-called "middle" or "median" lobe of the human prostate. J. Anat., *96*:443, 1962.

669-C *(Campbell's, p. 1501; Fig. 36–9)*

Testicular descent is a complex process. At 8 weeks of gestation, the testis and mesonephros are attached to the posterior abdominal wall by a broad peritoneal fold. As the mesonephros degenerates, the cranial portion of this fold also degenerates. The caudal end, however, persists as the caudal genital ligament and is continuous in the inguinal region with the gubernaculum, a band of mesenchyme extending into the genital swellings. The gubernaculum anchors the fetal testis to the inguinal region and probably serves to prevent upward movement of the testis during the rapid elongation of the trunk.

During the third month of gestation, a herniation of the coelomic cavity (processus vaginalis) forms on each side of the midline, through the ventral abdominal wall along the course of the gubernaculum. This herniation results from the development of pressure within the abdominal cavity. Enlargement of the processus vaginalis around the gubernaculum results in formation of an "inguinal canal." After the sixth month of gestation, the mesenchyme of the gubernaculum degenerates, and the testis slips through the inguinal canal assisted by abdominal pressure. The overall process is felt to be androgen-dependent. After the testes are within the scrotum, continued development of the abdominal musculature causes closure of the deep and superficial inguinal rings and obliteration of the processus vaginalis.

REFERENCES

1. Blackhouse, K.M.: Embryology of testicular descent and maldescent. Urol. Clin. North Am., 9:315, 1982.
2. Frey, H.L., Peng, S., and Rajfer, J.: Synergy of abdominal pressure and androgens in testicular descent. Biol. Reprod., *29*:1233, 1983.
3. George, F.W.: Development pattern of 5α-reductase activity in the rat gubernaculum. Endocrinology, *124*: 727, 1989.

670-A *(Campbell's, pp. 1501–1502; Figs. 26–8, 36–10)*

The female reproductive tract is formed from the müllerian ducts. The wolffian ducts persist only as the epoophoron in the mesovarium and occasionally as the Gartner ducts. The cephalic ends of the müllerian ducts form the fallopian tubes and the caudal portions fuse to form the body and cervix of the uterus. The uterus is initially divided by a septum but this subsequently degenerates and by 10 to 11 weeks of gestation, a single uterine cavity exists. Development of the vagina begins at around 9 weeks of gestation with the formation of a solid mass of cells (uterovaginal plate) between the caudal ends of the mullerian ducts and the dorsal wall of the urogenital sinus. The cells of the uterovaginal plate proliferate, increasing the distance between the developing uterus and urogenital sinus. Between 11 and 20 weeks of gestation, the caudal end of the vaginal plate forms a lumen and canalization occurs. The lumen of the vagina remains separated from the urogenital sinus by a thin membrane of mesoderm (hymen).

REFERENCES

1. O'Rahilly, R.: The development of the vagina in the human. *In* Blandau, R.J., and Bergsma, D. (Eds.): Morphogenesis and Malformation of the Genital System. Birth Defects Original Article Series. Vol. XIII, 1977, pp. 123–136.
2. Koff, A.K.: Development of the vagina in the human fetus. Carnegie Contributions to Embryology, No. 140, *24*:59, 1933.

671-E *(Campbell's, p. 1503)*

Regression of the müllerian ducts is the initial event in the virilization of the male urogenital tract. It begins at 8 to 9 weeks of gestation and is mediated by a large (>120 kD) dimeric glycoprotein that is secreted by fetal Sertoli cells. This protein has been purified, the complementary (c) DNA has been cloned, and the gene has been localized to the short arm of chromosome 19. This substance was initially thought to act locally to suppress müllerian duct development, but later studies have detected müllerian-inhibiting substance in young boys, but not girls, suggesting that it may act as a hormone.

REFERENCES

1. Josso, N.: Antimullerian hormone: New perspectives for a sexist molecule. Endocr. Rev., *7*:421, 1986.
2. Cate, R.L., Mattaliano, R.J., Mession, C., et al.: Isolation of the bovine and human genes for müllerian-inhibiting substance and expression of the human gene in animal cells. Cell, *45*:685, 1986.
3. Cohen-Haguenauer, O., Picard, J.Y., Mattéi, M.G., et al.: Mapping the gene for anti-müllerian hormone to the short arm of human chromosome 19. Cytogenet. Cell Genet., *44*:82, 1987.
4. Baker, M.L., Metcalfe, S.A., and Hutson, J.M.: Serum levels of müllerian-inhibiting substance in boys from birth to 18 years, as determined by enzyme immunoassay. J. Clin. Endocrinol. Metab., *70*:11, 1990.

672-D *(Campbell's, p. 1503)*

The precise mechanism of action of müllerian-inhibiting substance remains poorly understood. A few features of its action, however, are known. The two main features of müllerian duct regression are dissolution of the basement membrane and condensation of mesenchymal cells around the müllerian duct. One model proposes that müllerian-inhibiting substance acts by blocking phosphorylation of tyrosine residues on membrane proteins, possibly antagonizing the action of growth factors, such as epidermal growth factor.

REFERENCES

1. Trelstad, R.L., Hayashi, A., Hayashi, K., and Donahoe, P.K.: The epithelial-mesenchymal interface of the male rat müllerian duct: Loss of basement membrane integrity and ductal regression. Dev. Biol., *92*:27, 1982.
2. Ciagarroa, F.G., Coughlin, J.P., Donahoe, P.K., et al.: Recombinant human müllerian-inhibiting substance inhibited epidermal growth factor receptor tyrosine kinase. Growth Factors, *1*:179, 1989.

673-D *(Campbell's, pp. 1503–1504; Fig. 36–12)*

Virilization in the male fetus results from the action of androgen on specific target organs-the wolffian ducts, urogenital sinus, and external genitalia. Testosterone acts by entering target cells by passive diffusion down an activity gradient. Inside the cell, testosterone binds directly to specific high-affinity receptor proteins or undergoes 5α-reduction to dihydrotestosterone before binding to the androgen receptor. The hormone-receptor complex is then somehow transformed and acquires the capacity to bind with high affinity to specific receptor sites on the chromatin. As a consequence of binding to the target chromosome, an increase in transcription of specific messenger RNAs occurs, and new proteins are synthesized, giving rise to the phenotypic differentiation of the cell. No second messenger system appears to be involved.

REFERENCE

1. Evans, R.M.: The steroid and thyroid hormone receptor superfamily. Science, *240*:889, 1988.

674-B *(Campbell's, pp. 1504–1505)*

Virilization of the male genitalia requires the action of both testosterone and dihydrotestosterone. The enzyme 5α + reductase converts testosterone to dihydrotestosterone and is present in anlagen of the external genitalia (genital tubercle and swellings and urogenital sinus) prior to the onset of phenotypic differentiation. The wolffian duct, however, is incapable of converting testosterone to dihydrotestosterone until after male phenotypic differentiation is advanced and after the epididymis and seminal vesicle are formed. In humans with a hereditary deficiency of 5α-reductase, the external genitalia fail to virilize due to the inability to produce dihydrotestosterone. As a result, the penis and scrotum are incompletely or poorly developed. The wolffian derived structures–epididymis, vas deferens, and seminal vesicles–virilize normally. The testes are also structurally normal, but they may be undescended due to poor formation of the scrotum.

REFERENCES

1. Siiteri, P.K., and Wilson, J.D.: Testosterone formation and metabolism during male sexual differentiation in the human embryo. J. Clin. Endocrinol. Metab., *38*: 113, 1974.
2. Walsh, P.C., Madden, J.D., Harrod, M.J., et al.: Familial incomplete male pseudohermaphroditism, type 2: Decreased dihydrotestosterone formation in pseudovaginal perineoscrotal hypospadias. N. Engl. J. Med., *291*:944, 1974.

675-E *(Campbell's, pp. 1509–1518; Table 37–2)*

As outlined in Chapter 36, normal sexual differentiation is a sequential and orderly process; chromosomal sex determines gonadal sex, and gonadal sex, in turn, determines phenotypic sex. Disturbances of any step of this process may cause disorders of sexual differentiation. Disorders of chromosomal sex occur when the number or structure of the X or Y chromosomes is abnormal. In Klinefelter's syndrome, an extra X chromosome is present in the male. The common karyotype is either 47,XXY or 46,XY/47,XXY. In Turner's syndrome, a phenotypic female has any of several defects of the X chromosome and generally has a 45,XO karyotype. Mixed gonadal dysgenesis is a disorder in which phenotypically indeterminate infants have a testis on one side and a streak gonad on the other. Most patients have 45,X/46XY mosaicism. True hermaphroditism is a condition in which both an ovary and a testis or an ovotestis is present. Seventy percent of patients will have a 46,XX or 46,XY karyotype. The mechanism responsible for the gonadal asymmetry is unknown but is felt to be due to a genetic abnormality involving the X and Y chromosomes. Gonadal agenesis, on the other hand, is an abnormality of gonadal sex. The karyotype is always 46,XY and evidence of testicular function is evident but the testes fail or disappear before birth resulting in incomplete virilization.

REFERENCES

1. Jacobs, P.A., and Strong, J.A.: A case of human intersexuality having a possible XXY sex-determining mechanism. Nature, *183*:302, 1959.
2. Turner, H.H.: A syndrome of infantilism, congenital webbed neck, and cubitus valgus. Endocrinology, *23*: 566, 1938.
3. Sohval, A.R.: "Mixed" gonadal dysgenesis: A variety of hermaphroditism. Am. J. Hum. Genet., *15*:155, 1963.
4. van Niekerk, W.A., and Retief, A.E.: The gonads of human true hermaphrodites. Human Genet., *58*:117, 1981.

676-A *(Campbell's, pp. 1509–1512; Table 37–3)*

Klinefelter's syndrome is a disorder of men characterized by small, firm testes, varying degrees of impaired sexual maturation, azoospermia, gynecomastia, and elevated levels of urinary and plasma gonadotropins. The fundamental defect is the presence of an extra X chromosome in a male. The classic form has a karyotype of 47,XXY while the mosaic form commonly has a karyotype of 46,XY/47,XXY. This syndrome is the most common, major abnormality of sexual differentiation with an incidence of 1 in 500 males. The classic form of Klinefelter's syndrome is caused by meiotic nondisjunction of the chromosomes during gametogenesis. This mosaic form results from chromosomal mitotic nondisjunction after fertilization.

Clinically, these patients usually present after the time of expected puberty with infertility, gynecomastia or, occasionally, underandrogenization. In the classic form, damage to the seminiferous tubules and azoospermia are often found. The testes are small (less than 3.5 cm in length) and firm. Histologically, hyalinization of the tubules, absence of spermatogenesis, and increase in Leydig cells are often found. These patients also generally have an increased average body height as a result of an increased lower body segment. Gynecomastia ordinarily develops during adolescence and is generally bilateral and painless. Plasma testosterone levels average half that of normal and plasma and urinary levels of follicle-stimulating hormone (FSH) and luteinizing hormone (LH) are usually high. The incidence of hypospadias is not increased in these patients. It is increased, however, in patients with XX male syndrome, a syndrome with similar clinical features but different pathophysiology.

REFERENCES

1. Klinefelter, H.F. Jr., Reifenstein, E.C. Jr., and Albright, F.: Syndrome characterized by gynecomastia, aspermatogenesis without A-leydigism, and increased excretion of follicle-stimulating hormone. J. Clin. Endocrinol., *2*:615, 1942.
2. Jacobs, P.A., and Strong, J.A.: A case of human intersexuality having a possible XXY sex-determining mechanism. Nature, *183*:302, 1959.
3. Roe, T.F., and Alfi, O.S.: Ambiguous genitalia in XX male children. Report on two infants. Pediatrics, *50*: 55, 1977.

677-C *(Campbell's, pp. 1512–1515; Fig. 37–3)*

Gonadal dysgenesis is characterized by primary amenorrhea, sexual infantilism, short stature, multiple congenital anomalies, and bilateral streak gonads in a phenotypic female. The 45,X karyotype is most common but mosaic forms or 46,XX karyotype with structural abnormalities of the X chromosome may occur. This condition is also referred to as Turner's syndrome from the description of seven patients with sexual infantilism, short stature, congenital webbed neck, and cubitus valgus. The external genitalia are unambiguously female but immature, and no breast development occurs unless the patient receives exogenous estrogen. The internal urogenital tract consists of small but otherwise normal fallopian tubes and uterus and bilateral streak gonads located in the broad ligaments. Primordial germ cells are present transiently in the ovaries during embryogenesis but later disappear. At the age of expected puberty, the streaks contain only fibrous stroma with no identifiable follicles and ova. In response to the lack of functioning ovarian tissue, follicle-stimulating (FSH) and luteinizing hormone (LH) levels are markedly elevated after 10 years.

REFERENCES

1. Simpson, J.L.: Gonadal dysgenesis and sex chromosome abnormalities: Phenotypic-karyotypic correlations. *In* Vallet, H.L., and Porter, I.H. (Eds.): Genetic Mechanisms of Sexual Development. New York, Academic Press, 1979, p. 365.
2. Turner, H.H.: A syndrome of infantilism, congenital webbed neck, and cubitus valgus. Endocrinology, *23*: 566, 1938.
3. Singh, R.P., and Carr, D.H.: The anatomy and histology of XO human embryos and fetuses. Anat. Rec., *155*:369, 1966.

678-D *(Campbell's, pp. 1514–1515)*

Patients with Turner's syndrome characteristically are of short stature and the average adult height rarely exceeds 150 cm. The short stature is primarily due to a decrease in the lower segment height. Recombinant human growth hormone (hGH) has been given alone and with the anabolic steroid oxandrolone during childhood in an effort to increase the final adult height. A 3-year, randomized controlled study in 70 patients has shown that hGH by itself causes a significant but modest increase in height and that the addition of oxandrolone results in a more marked acceleration of growth over a 3-year period. Whether such therapy will permit a significant number of patients to achieve a "normal" adult height of greater than 150 cm is unclear.

REFERENCE

1. Rosenfeld, R.G., Hintz, R.L., Johnson, A.J., et al.: Three-year results of a randomized prospective trial of methionyl human growth hormone and oxandrolone in Turner syndrome. J. Pediatr., *113*:393, 1988.

679-B *(Campbell's, pp. 1515–1516)*

Mixed gonadal dysgenesis is a disorder in which phenotypic males or females have a testis on one side and a streak gonad on the other. Most have 45,X/46XY mosaicism, but many karyotypes have been noted. Two thirds of patients are reared as females, and most phenotypic males are incompletely virilized at birth. The majority exhibit some degree of ambiguous genitalia and, when present, the testis is usually located intra-abdominally. A uterus, vagina, and at least one fallopian tube are almost invariably present in both phenotypic males and females. In the older child or adult, the principal management consideration is the possibility of tumor development in the gonads. While the development of gonadoblastoma is most common in patients with mixed gonadal dysgenesis, the most common gonadal tumor in these patients is seminoma. The tumors may occur prior to puberty, develop most frequently in patients with a female phenotype who lack the somatic features typical of 45,X gonadal dysgenesis, and are more common in intra-abdominal testes than in streak gonads. As to which gonads will develop tumors, the following generalizations apply: (1) tumors develop in scrotal streak gonads but not in scrotal testes; (2) tumors developing in intra-abdominal testes are always associated with ipsilateral müllerian duct structures; and (3) tumors in streak gonads are always associated with tumor in the contralateral abdominal testis. It is therefore recommended that (1) all streak gonads be removed; (2) scrotal testes be preserved; and (3) intra-abdominal testes be excised unless they can be relocated in the scrotum and unless no ipsilateral mullerian duct structures are present.

REFERENCE

1. Sohval, A.R.: "Mixed" gonadal dysgenesis: A variety of hermaphroditism. Am. J. Hum. Genet., *15*:155, 1963.

680-A *(Campbell's, pp. 1516–1517)*

True hermaphroditism is a condition in which both an ovary and a testis or a gonad with histologic features of both (ovotestis) is present. To justify the diagnosis, there must be histologic documentation of both types of gonadal epithelium. The external genitalia display all gradations of the male to female spectrum and three fourths are sufficiently masculinized to be reared as males. Less than one tenth, however, will have normal male external genitalia. At puberty, signs of variable feminization and virilization develop–three fourths of patients develop significant breast enlargement, and about half menstruate. In phenotypic men, menstruation usually presents as cyclic hematuria. Ovulation occurs in approximately a fourth of patients. In phenotypic men, ovulation may occur as "testicular" or gonadal pain.

REFERENCE

1. Raspa, R.W., Subramaniam, A.P., and Romas, N.A.: True hermaphroditism presenting as intermittent hematuria and groin pain. Urology, *18*:133, 1986.

681-C *(Campbell's, p. 1518)*

The syndrome of pure gonadal dysgenesis is restricted to phenotypic females with gonads and genitalia identical to those with gonadal dysgenesis but who have normal height, few if any somatic anomalies, and either a uniform 46,XX or 46,XY karyotype. In these patients, a mutation prevents differentiation of the ovary or testis by an uncertain mechanism. As a result, bilateral streak gonads develop and female external genitalia are found but due to the lack of estrogen production sexual infantilism, primary amenorrhea, and failure of breast development are noted. These patients differ from those with Turner's syndrome, however, in that they achieve normal or greater than normal height.

682-E *(Campbell's, pp. 1519–1520; Fig. 37–6)*

A variety of syndromes result from hereditary defects in the enzymes of steroid hormone synthesis. Three enzymes are essential to the formation of glucocorticoids and androgens (20,22-desmolase, 3β-hydroxysteroid dehydrogenase, and 17α-hydroxylase). Two reactions are involved exclusively in androgen formation (17,20-desmolase and 17β-hydroxysteroid dehydrogenase). A defect in any of these enzymes leads to a deficiency of androgen synthesis and varying degrees of male pseudohermaphroditism. 11β-hydroxylase is the final enzyme used in synthesis of hydrocortisone. A defect in this enzyme leads to adrenal hyperplasia and either virilization in the female embryo or precocious masculinization in the male. This occurs due to compensatory increase in ACTH secretion, enhanced formation of adrenal steroids proximal to the enzymatic defect, and a secondary increase in androgen formation.

683-B *(Campbell's, pp. 1519–1521; Fig. 37–7)*

Congenital adrenal hyperplasia caused by 21-hydroxylase deficiency is the most common form of ambiguous genitalia in the newborn. Virilization is usually apparent at birth in the female. Severe deficiency of the enzyme is associated with salt loss due to inadequate production of cortisol and aldosterone, leading to severe salt wastage with anorexia, vomiting, volume depletion, and collapse, within the first few weeks of life. The genitalia may show hypertrophy and chordee of the clitoris, variable degrees of fusion of the labioscrotal folds, and virilization of the urethra. Rarely, the virilization is severe enough to cause development of a complete male penile urethra and prostate. The internal female structures and ovaries are unaltered so the vagina, uterus, and fallopian tubes will be present.

684-D *(Campbell's, pp. 1520–1521)*

A rare form of congenital adrenal hyperplasia associated with virilization of the external genitalia is 11β-hydroxylase deficiency. In this disorder, a block in hydroxylation at the 11-carbon results in cortisol deficiency, increased plasma ACTH levels with secondary increase in androstenedione and testosterone production, and accumulation of 11-deoxycortisol and deoxycorticosterone (DOC). Elevation of androgen levels, as in 21 hydroxylase deficiency, results in virilization of the external genitalia but has no effect on the internal genitalia. DOC is a potent mineralocorticoid. As a result of the accumulation of DOC, 11β-hydroxylase deficiency causes salt retention and hypertension rather than salt loss seen with 21-hydroxylase deficiency. Both 21-hydroxylase and 11β-hydroxylase deficiencies are inherited as autosomal recessive disorders.

685-E *(Campbell's, p. 1522; Fig. 37–8)*

Congenital absence of the vagina (müllerian agenesis) in combination with some form of abnormal or absent uterus (the Mayer-Rokitansky-Küster-Hauser syndrome) is second only to gonadal dysgenesis as a cause of primary amenorrhea. In most patients, this condition is found after the time of expected puberty because of failure to menstruate. Absence or hypoplasia of the vagina is found. The uterus may vary from almost normal, lacking only a conduit to the introitus, to the more characteristic rudimentary bicornuate cords with or without a lumen.

Renal, skeletal, or other congenital anomalies are common. About one third of patients have abnormal kidneys, most commonly agenesis or ectopy. Most cases are believed to be sporadic, but of the familial occurrences which have been reported, an autosomal dominant sex-limited mutation was felt to be present.

Vaginal agenesis can be treated by surgical and nonsurgical means, and successful pregnancies have been reported following corrective vaginal surgery in patients with normal uteri.

REFERENCES

1. Griffin, J.E., Edwards, C., Madden, J.D., et al.: Congenital absence of the vagina. The Mayer-Rokitansky-Küster-Hauser syndrome. Ann. Intern, Med., *85*:224, 1976.
2. Shokeir, M.H.K.: Aplasia of the müllerian system: Evidence for probable sex-limited autosomal dominant inheritance. *In* Summit, R.L., and Bergsma, D. (Eds.): *Differentiation and Chromosomal Abnormalities.* Birth Defects: Original Article Series, Vol. XIV, No. 6C. New York, Alan R. Liss, Inc., 1978, pp. 147–165.

686-A *(Campbell's, pp. 1522–1523; Fig. 37–6)*

Defective virilization of the male embryo (male pseudohermaphroditism) can result from defects in androgen synthesis, androgen action, and müllerian duct regression. Testosterone synthesis is abnormal in only 20 per cent of patients with male pseudohermaphroditism. Five defects in testosterone synthesis are known to cause incomplete virilization of the male embryo during embryogenesis. Three steps (20,22-desmolase, 3β-hydroxysteroid dehydrogenase, and 17α-hydroxylase) are common to the synthesis of other adrenal hormones as well. Consequently, their deficiency results in congenital adrenal hyperplasia as well as male pseudohermaphroditism. 17,20-desmolase and 17β-hydroxysteroid dehydrogenase are unique to the pathway of androgen synthesis, and their deficiency results in male pseudohermaphroditism only. 11-Hydroxylase is the final enzyme required for the production of hydrocortisone. Its deficiency results in congenital adrenal hyperplasia and female pseudohermaphroditism or precocious masculinization in the male.

REFERENCES

1. Campo, S., Monteagudo, C., Nicolau, G., et al.: Testicular function in prepubertal male pseudohermaphroditism. Clin. Endocrinol, *14*:11, 1981.
2. Campo, S., Stivel, M., Nicolau, G., et al.: Testicular function in postpubertal male pseudohermaphroditism. Clin. Endocrinol., *11*:481, 1979.
3. Savage, M.O., Chaussain, J.L., Evain, D., et al.: Endocrine studies in male pseudohermaphroditism in childhood and adolescence. Clin. Endocrinol., *8*:219, 1978.

687-B *(Campbell's, pp. 1523–1525; Fig. 37–6)*

In this patient, a male pseudohermaphrodite, a defect in androgen synthesis is evident due to the elevated level of the testosterone precursor androstenedione and the lack of virilization of the external genitalia. The blind ending vagina is suggestive of failure of development of müllerian structures indicating that müllerian inhibiting substance was present and active during sexual differentiation. This patient suffers from 17β-hydroxysteroid dehydrogenase deficiency. Inguinal or abdominal testes and virilized wolffian duct structures are present. The pubertal response to elevated gonadotropins results in elevated levels of androstenedione (the substrate of 17β-hydrosteroid dehydrogenase and a weak androgen), and the development of male secondary sex characteristics.

REFERENCE

1. Imperato-McGinley, J., Peterson, R.E., Stoller, R., and Goodwin, W.E.: Male pseudohermaphroditism secondary to 17β-hydroxysteroid dehydrogenase deficiency. Gender role change with puberty. J. Clin. Endocrinol. Metab. *43*:391, 1979.

688-C *(Campbell's, pp. 1525–1526; Table 37–5)*

5α-Reductase deficiency is a form of male pseudohermaphroditism. It is inherited in an autosomal recessive fashion and is characterized by (1) severe perineoscrotal hypospadias with a hooded prepuce, a ventral urethral groove, and opening of the urethra at the base of the phallus; (2) a blind vaginal pouch of variable size; (3) well-developed and histologically differentiated testes with normal epididymes, vasa deferentia, and seminal vesicles, and termination of the ejaculatory ducts into the blind ending vagina; (4) a female body habitus without female breast development but normal axillary and pubic hair; (5) an absence of female internal genitalia; and (6) a normal male plasma testosterone level and masculinization to a variable level at the time of puberty.

These findings are explained by the fact that various segments of the male genital tract differentiate under the influence of different hormones. Wolffian duct structures virilize under the influence of testosterone while derivatives of the urogenital sinus and anlage of the external genitalia virilize under the influence of dihydrotestosterone. In the presence of 5α-reductase deficiency, dihydrotestosterone is either not produced or is produced in abnormally low quantities. The external genitalia take on a more female appearance resulting in the findings described above. The müllerian duct derivatives regress normally because müllerian inhibiting substance is produced in normal amounts. Because testosterone itself is the hormone that regulates LH secretion, plasma LH level is minimally if at all elevated. As a result, testosterone and estrogen production rates are those of normal men, and gynecomastia does not develop.

REFERENCES

1. Imperato-McGinley, J., Peterson, R.E., Gautier, T., Sturla, E.: Androgens and the evolution of male-gender identify among male pseudohermaphrodites with 5-α-reductase deficiency. N. Engl. J. Med., *300*:1233, 1979.
2. Walsh, P.C., Madden, J.D., Harrod, M.J., et al.: Familial incomplete male pseudohermaphroditism, type 2. Decreased dihydrotestosterone formation in pseudovaginal perineoscrotal hypospadias. N. Engl. J. Med., *291*:944, 1974.

689-D *(Campbell's, pp. 1527–1530; Figs. 37–11, 37–12)*

Androgen receptor disorders may result in several distinct phenotypes but have similar endocrinology and pathophysiology. In all of these disorders, a decreased amount of apparently normal androgen receptor or a qualitatively abnormal androgen receptor is found. Plasma testosterone levels and rates of testosterone production by the testes are normal or higher than normal. The elevated rate of testosterone production is caused by the high mean plasma LH level, which, in turn, is due to defective feedback regulation caused by resistance to the action of androgen at the hypothalamic-pituitary level. Elevated LH concentration is probably also responsible for the increased estrogen production by the testes. Feminization occurs due to the lack of androgen action and elevated estrogen levels.

The different degrees of androgen resistance, coupled with variably enhanced estradiol production, results in different degrees of defective virilization and enhanced feminization. In complete testicular feminization, incomplete testicular feminization, Reifenstein syndrome, infertile male syndrome, and under virilized fertile male syndrome, a 46,XY Karyotype and some degree of androgen receptor abnormality are seen. Pure gonadal dysgenesis, as discussed earlier, has a 46,XX or 46,XY karyotype, bilateral streak gonads, and is restricted to female phenotypes. In both the 46,XX and 46,XY forms, the mutation prevents differentiation of the ovary and the testis, respectively, by an uncertain mechanism. The androgen receptors in the 46 XY patients are normal.

REFERENCES

1. Amrhein, J.A., Meyer, W.J., III, Jones, H.W., Jr., and Migeon, C.J.: Androgen insensitivity in man: Evidence

for genetic heterogeneity. Proc. Natl. Acad. Sci. USA, *73*:891, 1976.
2. Boyar, R.M., Moore, R.J., Rosener, W., et al.: Studies of gonadotropin-gonadal dynamics in patients with androgen insensitivity. J. Clin. Endocrinol. Metab., *47*: 1116, 1978.
3. MacDonald, P.C., Madden, J.D., Brenner, P.F., et al.: Origin of estrogen in normal men and women with testicular feminization. J. Clin. Endorinol. Metab., *49*: 905, 1979.

690-E *(Campbell's, p. 1527)*

Complete testicular feminization is the most common form of male pseudohermaphroditism and is the third most common cause of primary amenorrhea in phenotypic women. A phenotypic female is usually seen by a clinician because of either inguinal hernia (prepubertal cases) or primary amenorrhea (postpubertal cases). The development of the breasts after puberty, the general habitus, and the distribution of body fat are female in character. Axillary and pubic hair is normal, and facial hair is absent. The external genitalia are unambiguously female. The clitoris is normal or small. The vagina is short and blind-ending and may be absent or rudimentary. All internal genitalia are absent except for the gonads, which have histologic features of undescended testes. The testes may be located in the abdomen, along the course of the inguinal canal, or in the labia majora.

The major complication of undescended testes in this disorder, as in other forms of cryptorchidism, is the development of tumors. Testicular tumors rarely develop until after puberty. In these patients, the testes will respond to elevated LH levels and produce estradiol to stimulate normal pubertal growth spurts and successful feminization. As a result, castration is usually delayed until after puberty. Prepubertal castration is indicated if the testes are present in the inguinal region or in the labia majora and result in discomfort or hernia formation. After castration, suitable estrogen replacement is indicated.

REFERENCE

1. Hauser, G.A.: Testicular feminization. *In* Overzier, C. (Ed.): Intersexuality London, Academic Press, 1963, pp. 225–276.

691-D *(Campbell's, pp. 1530–1531)*

Persistent müllerian duct syndrome results in normal penile development and variable development of the vas deferens but, in addition, bilateral fallopian tubes, uterus, and upper vagina. These patients commonly present with inguinal hernias that contain the uterus. Cryptorchidism is common. Because the external genitalia are well developed and the patients masculinize normally at puberty, it is assumed that during the critical stage of embryonic sexual differentiation the fetal testes produced a normal amount of androgen. However, müllerian regression does not occur, possibly because of failure of the fetal testes to produce müllerian-inhibiting substance or possibly because of failure of the tissues to respond to this hormone.

The preservation of external male appearance and the maintenance of virilization are essential. A primary or staged orchiopexy should be performed. None of the reported patients has developed a malignancy in the uterus or vagina, and because the vas deferens is closely associated with the broad ligaments, the uterus and vagina should be left in place to avoid disruption of the vas deferens and consequently to preserve possible fertility.

REFERENCES

1. Guerrier, D., Tran, D., Vanderwinden, J.M., et al.: The persistent müllerian duct syndrome: a molecular approach. J. Clin. Endocrinal. Metab., *58*:46, 1989.
2. Sloan, W.R., and Walsh, P.C.: Familial persistent müllerian duct syndrome. J. Urol., *115*:459, 1976.

692-C *(Campbell's, pp. 1531–1532; Figs. 37–16, 37–17)*

Microphallus is a congenital disorder in which the penis is small but otherwise anatomically normal and, specifically, in which the urethra is that of a normal male. By most criteria it is defined as a penis that is below the 95 per cent confidence limits of penile size for age. In the newborn, stretched penile length less than 1.9 cm is usually considered microphallus. The condition is frequently associated with testicular maldescent.

Both the formation of the penile urethra and the phallic growth during embryogenesis are under the control of androgens. Formation of the urethra is complete by the end of the first trimester and differential growth of the phallus takes place during the second and third trimester. Microphallus is felt to be the consequence of defective androgen secretion during the second and third trimesters.

Evidence suggests that pituitary gonadotropins regulate testicuar androgen production during the last two trimesters but not between weeks 8 and 12, when the male urethra is formed. In keeping with this, some instances of microphallus are associated with hypogonadotropic hypogonadism. Others are associated with primary hypogonadism. Boys with hypogonadotropic hypogonadism will have low plasma gonadotropin levels and respond normally to standard challenge with human chorionic gonadotropin (hCG) by increasing plasma testosterone levels.

The initial management of microphallus is straightforward, namely, in patients younger that age 3 years, low-dosage, short-term systemic testosterone therapy causes penile growth so that most eventually reach the normal range. Sometimes, late treatment of previously unrecognized hypogonadotropic hypogonadism with systemic testosterone esters can have profound effects on penile size.

REFERENCES

1. Schonfeld, W.A., and Beebe, G.W.: Normal growth and variation in the male genitalia form birth to maturity. J. Urol., *48*:759, 1942.
2. Lee, P.A., Mazur, T., Danish, R., et al.: Micropenis. I. Criteria, etiologies, and classification. Johns Hopkins Med. J., *146*:156, 1980.
3. Guthrie, R.D., Smith, P.W., and Graham, C.B.: Testosterone treatment for micropenis during early childhood. J. Pediatr., *83*:247, 1973.

693-B *(Campbell's, p. 1533)*

Sexual ambiguity in the newborn constitutes a true medical emergency and assignment of the sex of rearing should be made as early as possible, preferably in the newborn nursery, but not before all necessary diagnostic procedures have been performed. While the infant is being evaluated, the family should be informed that the development of the external genitalia is incomplete and that additional studies are necessary before the correct gender assignment can be made. The procedures employed in the work-up include (1) a detailed history and physical examination; (2) an evaluation of chromosomal sex; (3) a biochemical evaluation of the urinary and plasma steroids before and after stimulation with hCG; (4) an evaluation of the urogenital sinus and internal duct structures utilizing endoscopy and radiography; (5) an exploratory laparotomy and gonadal biopsy; and (6) when available, an assessment of androgen action utilizing cultured skin fibroblasts.

The history taken should include a detailed family history and the mother should be questioned about virilizing signs and about ingestion of androgens, progestogens, or other drugs during pregnancy. The most important finding on physical examination is the presence of a gonad in the labioscrotal fold or scrotum. Because ovaries rarely descend, the presence of a palpable gonad excludes the diagnosis of female pseudohermaphroditism and limits the presumptive diagnosis to male pseudohermaphroditism, true hermaphroditism, or mixed gonadal dysgenesis.

694-A *(Campbell's, pp. 1534–1536; Fig. 37–19)*

The assignment of the sex of rearing of a child with ambiguous genitalia will have a great social impact on the future of the patient. Assignment of gender should be made as early as possible but not before all necessary diagnostic procedures and evaluation of the genital reconstruction potential have been completed. The major consideration in establishing the sex of rearing should be the achievement of functional genitalia. If the patient has an inadequate phallus, the individual should be reared as a female, regardless of the result of diagnostic tests. In the patient with an adequate phallus, however, as much information as possible should be obtained before a decision is made. It is in these patients that chromosomal sex, presence of gonads, histology of the gonads, biochemical evaluation, and potential for fertility become more important. If a functional phallus cannot be created and later virilized, the patient should be reared as a female, and therefore, should undergo any appropriate genital reconstruction, gonadectomy, and hormonal therapy.

REFERENCES

1. Donahoe, P.K.: The diagnosis and treatment of infants with intersex abnormalities. Pediatr. Clin. North Am., *34*:1333, 1987.
2. Osterling, J.E., Gearheart, J.P., and Jeffs, R.D.: A unified approach to early reconstructive surgery of the child with ambiguous genitalia. J. Urol., *138*:1079, 1987.
3. Pagon, R.A.: Diagnostic approach to the newborn with ambiguous genitalia. Pediatr. Clin. North Am., *34*:1019, 1987.

695-C *(Campbell's, p. 1537)*

As stated previously, gender assignment should be made as early as possible, preferably before the patient leaves the newborn nursery. Performing gender assignment early will minimize confusion about gender identity, role, or both for the parents and the affected individual. After a child has reached the period normally associated with well-differentiated psychosexual identity (1 1/2 to 2 years), reassignment of gender is unwise and should be undertaken only after careful psychiatric, social, and endocrinologic evaluations.

696-C *(Campbell's, pp. 1543–1544)*

Primordial germ cells migrate from the wall of the embryonic yolk sac along the dorsal mesentery of the hindgut and invade the genital ridges. These primordial germ cells secrete a protein under the regulation of a gene located on the short arm of the Y chromosome and cause the indifferent gonad to differentiate into the fetal testis by the seventh week of gestation. During the eighth week of gestation, the fetal testis secretes testosterone and müllerian inhibiting factor. The testosterone in turn causes the wolffian duct to differentiate into the male ductal system which forms the epididymis and vas deferens. Fetal Sertoli cells secrete müllerian inhibiting factor which causes regression of the müllerian ducts, leaving only the appendix testis as a remnant of the müllerian ductal system. The external genitalia develop between the 8th and 16th week of gestation under the influence of dihydrotestosterone which is converted from testosterone by the enzyme 5α-reductase. Between the 12th week and 7th month gestation, the process of testicular descent remains relatively dormant. Around the seventh month of gestation, the process rapidly resumes, and by the end of the eighth month of gestation, the testis has descended in the majority of cases.

697-D *(Campbell's, p. 1544)*

Cryptorchidism is relatively common in humans. Approximately 3.4 per cent of full-term infants are born with this condition and approximately 30.3 per cent of premature infants are born with an undescended testes. In the premature infant, birth may occur prior to normal testicular descent during the last trimester of gestation. Birth weight of the infant also influences the incidence of cryptorchidism, with smaller birth weights having a greater incidence.

698-C *(Campbell's, p. 1545)*

The incidence of cryptorchidism is approximately 0.8 per cent in the male adult population, as demonstrated in Baumrucker's study involving 10,000 U.S. army inductees. Other studies have noted similar incidences ranging anywhere from 0.7 per cent to slightly less than 1 per cent of the male adult population.

699-E *(Campbell's, pp. 1544–1545)*

Approximately 75 per cent of full-term cryptorchid testis and up to 95 per cent of premature cryptorchid testis spontaneously descend by 1 year of age. Furthermore, the majority of the testes that descend usually will do so in the first 3 months after birth. This is probably secondary to the elevated levels of androgen in the plasma during these first 3 months of life.

700-B *(Campbell's, p. 1545)*

At the time of inguinal exploration for cryptorchidism, approximately 3 to 5 per cent of the patients will have unilateral or bilateral anorchia. Around 10 per cent of patients with cryptorchidism have bilateral undescended testes.

701-A *(Campbell's, pp. 1545–1546)*

Although many theories have been developed concerning testicular descent, it is generally accepted that endocrine factors play the major role in promoting the descent of testis into the scrotum. The process of testicular descent is androgen mediated and regulated by pituitary gonadotropin. Mechanical forces may also contribute to the descent of the testis. The traction theory is based on the concept that the gubernaculum and/or the cremaster muscle pull the testis into the scrotum. The differential growth theory adheres to the concept that as the body wall grows, the testis is kept in proximity to the internal ring. The testis is then pulled into the scrotum by the relatively immobile gubernaculum as a result of rapid growth of the body wall during the last trimester of pregnancy. The intrabdominal pressure theory is based on the belief that the primary force causing the descent of testes from its intrabdominal location is caused by an increase in the intrabdominal pressure. The epididymal theory of testicular descent is based on the assumption that the differentiation and maturation of the epididymis induces testicular descent.

702-E *(Campbell's, pp. 1546, 1555)*

Cryptorchidism is associated with a wide variety of clinical syndromes and entities. Kallmann's syndrome results from deficient gonadotropin releasing hormone secretion from the hypothalamus. Cryptorchidism may be a presenting feature with this syndrome. Chromosomal abnormalities are also associated with the undescended testis. Klinefelter's syndrome, which is due to the presence of an extra X chromosome in the male, usually results in a sterile patient. Noonan's syndrome is the male counterpart of Turner's syndrome and results in a karyotype of XO. The majority of males with Noonan's syndrome have cryptorchidism and are usually infertile. Cystic fibrosis has been associated with a high incidence of congenital absence of the vas deferens and cryptorchidism. Von Hippel-Lindau disease is an autosomal dominant process manifested by retinal and cerebellar angioblastomas, cysts of the kidney, pancreas and epididymis, pheochromocytoma, and renal cell carcinoma.

703-A *(Campbell's, pp. 1546–1548)*

The cryptorchid testes can be classified as intrabdominal, canalicular, and ectopic. When the testis migrates away from its normal pathway of movement between the abdominal cavity and scrotum, it is then noted to be in an ectopic position. The most common ectopic location is the superficial inguinal pouch. Other major sites of ectopic testes are the perineum, femoral canal, suprapubic area, and contralateral scrotal compartment. The testicular ectopia is believed to be directly related to the development of the gubernaculum.

704-B *(Campbell's, p. 1549)*

Blind ending testicular vessels signify the absence of the testis on that side, and thus no further surgical exploration is necessary.

705-B *(Campbell's, pp. 1549–1550)*

The histologic alterations in the cryptorchid testis appear by 1 1/2 years of age and include smaller seminiferous tubules, fewer spermatogonia, and more peritubular tissue. These histologic abnormalities are more pronounced the further the testis resides from the bottom of scrotum and the longer the testis remains cryptorchid. Histologic changes have also been noted in the contralateral testis of a unilateral cryptorchid male. Electron microscopy has demonstrated ultrastructural changes in the seminiferous tubule which can occur as early as a second year of life and include degeneration of mitochondria, loss of ribosomes in the cytoplasm and smooth endoplasmic reticulum of the seminiferous tubule, and increase in collagen fibers in the spermatogonia and Sertoli cells.

706-C *(Campbell's, pp. 1550–1551)*

A strong association exists between neoplasia and cryptorchidism. The undescended testis is 35 to 48 times more likely to undergo malignant degeneration than the normal testis. Approximately 10 per cent of all testicular tumors arise from an undescended testis. An orchiopexy is recommended between the ages of 1 and 1 1/2 years since histologic and ultrastructural changes begin to occur at this early age. The location of the undescended testis also effects its malignant degeneration potential since an abdominal testis is four times more likely to undergo malignant degeneration than an inguinal testis. Seminoma followed by embryonal cell carcinoma are the two most frequent neoplasms encountered with cryptorchid testes.

707-A *(Campbell's, pp. 1551–1552)*

The undescended testes have an increased susceptibility to undergo torsion secondary to developmental anatomic abnormality between the testis and its mesentery. The incidence of torsion is greatest in the postpubertal period when the testis usually increases in size and thus is broader than its mesentery and more likely to twist on its stalk. Hernia sacs are found in greater than 90 per cent of patients with cryptorchidism. The processus vaginalis remains patent when the testis fail to descend and thus allows intraabdominal contents to enter the tunica vaginalis through the processus vaginalis and appear clinically as a hernia or hydrocele. Infertility is commonly associated with testicular maldescent. Generally the higher and longer the testis resides away from the bottom of the scrotum, the greater the likelihood of damage to the seminiferous tubules. The earlier the testis is brought down into the scrotum, the greater the potential for recovering spermatogenic activity. Spermatogenic activity may also be affected in the contralateral scrotal testis in the patient with unilateral cryptorchidism. Sperm counts are much lower than expected in men who have had successful unilateral orchiopexy and thus supports the hypothesis that there may be an inherent defect in both testes. In addition to the spermatogenic defect, the cryptorchid state may also affect the interstitial compartment of the testis, as demonstrated by inhibited testosterone synthesis. The cryptorchid state has also been associated with vasal and epididymal abnormalities. The epididymis may be extended in length, may undergo partial or total atresia, or may be totally disassociated from the testis. Similar abnormalities may be seen with the vas deferens.

708-B *(Campbell's, pp. 1553–1554)*

Medical therapy for undescended testis involves hormonal manipulation. Currently hCG and Gn-RH are two hormones utilized in hormonal therapy for undescended testis. hCG presumably via stimulation of Leydig's cells, results in increased plasma testosterone levels and thus promotes testicular descent. Gn-RH works under the premise that males with cryptorchidism have an abnormal hypothalamic–pituitary axis and thus increases LH levels to stimulate testicular descent. hCG is administered parenterally only and is given in doses varying from 3,000 I.U. to more than 40,000 I.U. Success rates with hCG vary between 14 and 50 per cent. Doses above 15,000 I.U. of hCG are associated with significant side effects including changes in testicular histology, alternations in bone age, and a transient increase in penile size. Gn-RH therapy is administered intranasally at a dose of 1.2 mg per day for 4 weeks. Success rates with Gn-RH therapy vary widely from 6 to 70 per cent. Although no side effects have been noted with intranasal Gn-RH therapy, approximately 10 per cent of patients relapse after 6 months of therapy.

709-C *(Campbell's, pp. 1555–1556)*

A hydrocele occurs in 6 per cent of full-term males. The hydrocele is a collection of fluid between the parietal and visceral layers of the tunica vaginalis and is usually secondary to a patent processus vaginalis. Most hydroceles resolve spontaneously within the first year of life secondary to the closure of the processus vaginalis. Testicular torsion or inguinal hernia must also be ruled out in the differential diagnosis of a scrotal mass. Surgical intervention is usually necessary after the first year of life if the hydrocele does not resolve.

710-D *(Campbell's, p. 1557)*

Extravaginal testicular torsion is most common during the newborn period, since this is the time in which the testis has just descended into the scrotum and the gubernaculum has not completely attached to the scrotal wall. This situation allows the testis and gubernaculum to freely rotate within the neonatal scrotum and thus the entire testis, epididymis, and tunica vaginalis may twist together in a vertical axis on the spermatic cord.

711-D *(Campbell's, pp. 1556–1558)*

Testicular torsion is possible at any age, however, it is most common during adolescence. The incidence is approximately 1 in 4,000 males less than the age of 25. Neonatal cases are rare. Testicular torsion can be either intravaginal or extravaginal. Intravaginal torsion, the more common form, occurs after puberty whereas extravaginal torsion occurs primarily in the neonate. The prognosis for torsion is good if the patient is operated on within 4 to 6 hours and contralateral orchidopexy is performed. The contralateral testis is pexed because of the possibility of delayed torsion. The differential diagnosis for testicular torsion includes acute epididymitis, strangulated hernia, hydrocele, testicular tumor, and torsion of testicular appendages. The appendix testis, a remnant of the müllerian duct, is the most common testicular appendage susceptible to torsion and can mimic true testicular torsion. The blue dot sign is characteristic of this entity. Doppler study and nuclear perfusion scan can aid in the diagnosis of testicular torsion; however, the history and physical examination will usually allow determination of the correct diagnosis.

712-E *(Campbell's, p. 1563)*

Maternal fetal sonography is performed in certain areas as a routine examination during pregnancy. In some countries, it is incorporated into the standard health care practice system as a mandatory procedure. In this country, there is no consensus about the need or cost-effectiveness of routine screening, but specific indications do exist for genitourinary evaluation in utero. Divergence from the expected fundal height for age is one indication. A reduction in the normal amount of amniotic fluid may be due to renal agenesis, dysgenesis, or severe obstructive uropathy. The finding of persistent breech presentation may also be associated with oligohydramnios and warrants further examination. Conversely, the presence of an increased amount of amniotic fluid (polyhydramnios) has also been reported to be associated with unilateral hydronephrosis and is reflected as an elevated height of the fundus compared with the height of the fundus for known gestational age. Maternal serum alpha-fetoprotein (AFP) has become a common screening test during pregnancy. Abnormally elevated AFP levels in mid-trimester are most commonly associated with neural tube defects, fetal deaths, or multiple fetuses. Elevated levels of AFP have also been reported with genitourinary anomalies and are, therefore, another indication for ultrasonography.

REFERENCES

1. Neal, R., and Andrassy, R.: Fetal surgery in utero. Tex. Med., *80*:40, 1984.
2. Broecker, B.H., Redwine, F.O., and Peters, R.E.: Reversal of acute polyhydramnios after fetal decompression. Urology, *31*:60, 1988.
3. Knootz, W.L., Seeds, J.W., Adams, N.J., et al.: Elevated maternal serum alpha-fetoprotein, second trimester oligohydramnios and pregnancy outcome. Obstet. Gynecol., *62*:301, 1983.

713-C *(Campbell's, p. 1564)*

The fetal genitourinary system can be observed at several different stages of development with reasonable clarity. The fetal kidney itself can be reliably detected after about 15 weeks of gestation. The images are not very clear, however, until about 20 weeks, at which time the internal renal architecture appears distinct. This change is presumably due to the deposition of fat in the perirenal space. Renal growth can be measured from that time on, and standards have been published for normal values according to gestational age.

REFERENCES

1. Lawson, T.L., Foley, W.D., Berland, L.I., and Clark, K.E.: Ultrasonic evaluation of fetal kidneys: Analysis of normal size and frequency of visualization as related to stage of pregnancy. Radiology, *138*:153, 1981.
2. Bowie, J.D., Rosenberg, E.R., Andreotti, R.F., et al.: The changing appearance of fetal kidneys during pregnancy. J. Ultrasound Med., *2*:505, 1983.

3. Jeanty, P., Dramaix-Wilmet, M., Elkhazen, N., et al.: Measurement of the fetal kidney growth on ultrasound. Radiology, *144*:159, 1982.

714-A *(Campbell's, pp. 1564–1565; Table 39–1)*

In a large series of patients with genitourinary defects detected in utero, the majority (87 per cent) had hydronephrosis. The remainder of the anomalies included multicystic dysplastic kidney, autosomal recessive polycystic kidney disease, renal agenesis, and hypodysplasia. Other abnormalities that have been described include bladder extrophy, adrenal hyperplasia, imperforate anus, cloacal abnormalities, neuroblastoma, mesoblastic nephroma, and genital abnormalities.

REFERENCE

1. Mandell, J., Blyth, B., Peters, C.A., et al.: The natural history of structural genitourinary defects detected in utero. Radiology, *178*:193, 1991.

715-B *(Campbell's, pp. 1565–1567; Fig. 39–3)*

When hydronephrosis is found on prenatal ultrasonography, a number of factors must be assessed. One must determine if the hydronephrosis is unilateral or bilateral, and, if bilateral, whether it is symmetric. The absence or presence of ureteral dilatation must be noted. The size of the fetal bladder, its emptying, and the presence or absence of posterior urethral dilatation should be noted. Determination of the presence or absence as well as relative volume of amniotic fluid should be noted as should the presence or absence of other anatomic abnormalities, the overall growth and development of the fetus, and its gender.

The diagnosis of posterior urethral valves can be made with relative assurance with findings of early onset bilateral hydroureteronephrosis; a thick-walled, slightly dilated bladder; incomplete bladder emptying; the suggestion of a dilated posterior urethra; and a male sex identification. Varying degrees of oligohydramnios may be present depending on the severity of the obstructing lesions.

REFERENCE

1. Mandell, J., Blyth, B., Peters, C.A., et al.: The natural history of structural genitourinary defects detected in utero. Radiology, *178*:193, 1991.

716-A *(Campbell's, p. 1570; Fig. 39–9)*

Maternal fetal ultrasonography has been noted to detect many anomalies in organ systems other than the genitourinary system. Tumors such as neuroblastoma, teratoma, and mesoblastic nephroma have been diagnosed prenatally. Anomalies in the exstrophy/cloacal/imperforate anus complex have also been diagnosed prenatally. Intraluminal intestinal calcifications seen in utero should immediately suggest the presence of an anorectal malformation. Diagnosis of congenital adrenal hyperplasia is not readily made with ultrasound, but it has been diagnosed by HLA typing, allowing fetal endocrine manipulation or therapeutic termination as potential options.

REFERENCES

1. Harris, R.D., Nyberg, D.A., Mack, L.A., et al.: Anorectal atresia: Prenatal sonographic diagnosis. AJR, *149*:395, 1987.
2. Mundell, J., Lillehie, C.W., Greene, M., et al.: Prenatal diagnosis of imperforate anus with rectourinary fistula: Dilated fetal colon with enterolithiasis. J. Pediatr. Surg., 1991.
3. Shalev, E., Weiner, E., and Zuckerman, H.: Prenatal ultrasound diagnosis of intestinal calcifications with imperforate anus. Acta Ostet. Gynecol., *65*:95, 1983.

717-D *(Campbell's, pp. 1570–1571)*

Based on routine ultrasound screening programs, the overall incidence of genitourinary defects appears to be between 0.2 and 0.9 per cent. In general, genitourinary anomalies represent 50 per cent of all sonographically detectable lesions. The postnatal outcome for identified fetal genitourinary anomalies, however, is difficult to assess. In several surveys, survival rate and postnatal treatment frequently are variable. The pre- and postnatal bias of the physicians and centers involved plays an important role in the variation seen in survival and surgical rates. Despite these variations, the outcome of these patients with genitourinary lesions is related to the occurence of nonrenal and renal anomalies. The strongest negative indicators of overall prognosis include early onset of severe renal parenchymal changes, oligohydramnios, severe nonrenal congenital anomalies, and bladder outlet obstruction. The majority of cases of hydronephrosis, even with bilateral involvement, fall within a moderate degree of obstruction and are not associated with these severe parameters. The overall prognosis for patients with other types of bilateral renal disease, whether it be hypoplasia, dysplasia, or cystic disease, is similarly linked to the presence of oligohydramnios.

REFERENCES

1. Scott, J.E.S., and Renwick, M.: Antenatal diagnosis of congenital abnormalities in the urinary tract. Br. J. Urol., *62*:295, 1987.
2. Avni, E.F., Rodesch, F., and Schulman, C.C.: Fetal uropathies: Diagnostic pitfalls and management. J. Urol., *134*:921, 1985.
3. Sholder, A.J., Maizels, M., Depp. R., et al.: Caution in antenatal intervention. J. Urol., *139*:1026, 1988.

718-B *(Campbell's, pp. 1571–1573)*

The natural consequence of the evolution of prenatal diagnosis in terms of sophistication and usage has been the issue of intervention before birth to reverse potentially life-threatening processes. The interest in intervention for congenital hydronephrosis began in the early 1980s. Percutaneous and open urinary diversion were reported as treatments for apparent bladder outlet obstruction with and without oligohydramnios. Despite early enthusiasm, the number of interventions reported has dramatically dropped over the past few years because the overall benefit of prenatal intervention for bladder outlet obstruction has been questioned. One of the major issues relates to the ability to prognosticate which fetuses might benefit from intervention. Some reports have indicated that aspirated fetal urinary electrolytes correlate well with ultimate outcome. Other indications for potential fetal renal function include sonographic findings related to the degree of echogenicity of the renal parenchyma and bladder refilling and emptying as a corollary to overall urine flow rate. The presence of oligohydramnios is the end stage of bladder outlet obstruction and implies a fairly far advanced degree of renal shutdown.

REFERENCES

1. Golbus, M.S., Harrison, M.R., Filly, R.A., et al.: In utero treatment of urinary tract obstruction. Am. J. Obstet. Gynecol., *142*:383, 1982.
2. Manning, F.A., Hill, L.M., and Platt, L.D.: Qualitative amniotic fluid volume determination by ultrasound: Antepartum detection of intrauterine growth retardation. Am. J. Obstet. Gynecol., *139*:254, 1981.
3. Crombleholme, T.M., Harrison, M.R., Golbus, M.S., et al.: Fetal intervention in obstructive uropathy: Prognostic indicators and efficacy of intervention. Am. J. Obstet. Gynecol., *162*:1239, 1990.
4. Mahoney, B.S., Filly, R.A., Callen, P.W., et al.: Fetal renal dysplasia: Sonographic evaluation. Radiology, *152*:143, 1984.

719-E *(Campbell's, pp. 1573–1575)*

Many of the issues of prenatal diagnosis are related to the fact that the parents and the physicians involved need to be informed of the congenital anomalies so that postnatal evaluation and treatment can commence. The issue as to which studies should be performed and when they should be performed remains open to debate. The authors do not feel that ultrasound examination needs to be performed immediately unless bladder outlet obstruction is suspected. For example, in the presence of marked bilateral hydronephrosis and a thick-walled bladder on prenatal ultrasound examination, postnatal evaluation, especially in the male infant, should be performed within the first 24 hours of life. Neonatal oliguria may mask a moderately obstructive lesion and is also an indication for early postnatal evaluation. If an abnormality other than bladder outlet obstruction is suspected, ultrasonography may be delayed. Also, preterm delivery, in and of itself, is not an indication for radiographic evaluation of the genitourinary system.

REFERENCES

1. Laing, F.C., Burke, V.D., Wing, V.W., et al.: Postpartum evaluation of fetal hydronephrosis: Optimal timing for follow-up sonography. Radiology, *152*:423, 1984.
2. Keating, M.A., and Retik, A.B.: Management of the dilated obstructed ureter. Urol. Clin. North Am., *17*: 291, 1990.

720-C *(Campbell's, pp. 1576–1577)*

Autosomal recessive polycystic kidney disease is being extensively investigated and a mouse model has been identified and described for 10 years. It has permitted detailed investigation of the pathogenesis of renal cysts in tissue culture. This work suggests that cystogenesis may be related to a sodium-potassium ion pump in the tubular cells. Others have described basement membrane changes, disordered regulation of epidermal growth factor gene expression, and induction of the c-*myc* proto-oncogene in polycystic mice. Other work has focused on gene mapping and has localized the gene to mouse chromosome 12.

REFERENCES

1. Preminger, G.M., Koch, W.E., Fried, F.A., et al.: Murine congenital polycystic kidney disease: A model for studying development of cystic disease. J. Urol., *127*: *556*, 1982.
2. Holthöfer, H., Kumpulainen, T., and Rapola, J.: Polycystic disease of the kidney: Evaluation and classification based on nephron segment and cell-type specific markers. Lab. Invest., *62*:363, 1990.
3. Davisson, M.T., Guay-Woodford, L.M., Harris, H.W., and D'Eustachio, P.: The mouse polycystic kidney disease mutation (cpk), is located on proximal chromosome 12. Genomics, *9*:778, 1991.

721-D *(Campbell's, p. 1578)*

The prenatal kidney is undergoing rapid growth and development with formation of new structures as well as significant structural and functional maturation of previously formed elements. The fetal kidney is in an environment where the placenta performs virtually all of the dialysis of the fetal circulation. The principal activity of the fetal kidney is growth and development rather than function. Renal blood flow is greatly reduced in the fetal kidney, being 3 per cent of cardiac output at 20 weeks of gestation versus 20 to 30 per cent postnatally. The oxygen tension is markedly reduced and the hormonal environment is different in the fetal kidney. While atrial natriuretic peptide levels are distinctly higher in the fetus, the sensitivity of the fetal kidney to its natriuretic effects is less.

REFERENCES

1. Rudolph, A.M., and Heyman, M.A.: Circulatory changes during growth in the fetal lamb. Circ. Res., *26*:289, 1970.
2. Robillard, JE., Nakamura, K.T., Varille, V.A., et al.: Ontogeny of the renal response to natriuretic peptide in sheep. Am. J. Physiol., *254*:F634, 1988.
3. Smith, F.G., and Robillard, J.E.: Pathophysiology of fetal renal disease. Semin. Perinatol., *13*:305, 1989.

722-D *(Campbell's, p. 1578)*

Multiple animal models have been created to study both the effects of prenatal renal obstruction and the effects of surgical and medical treatments to overcome this obstruction. Early obstructions have been induced in the chick embryo at the metanephric stage, which allows investigation of the production of renal dysplastic lesions. These models have the advantage of permitting manipulation very early in renal development. Congenital obstruction may be produced in the fetal rabbit kidney as early as 23 days out of 32 days in gestation. The rabbit kidney continues glomerulogenesis until age 2 weeks postnatally, which has made it attractive for consideration of the effects of obstruction on nephrogenesis. The opossum, a marsupial, has recently be used to study congenital obstruction. Opossum pups are "born" into the marsupium of the mother at a developmental stage approximately equivalent to 8 weeks of gestation in the human. At this point, metanephric development is just beginning. Obstructions induced several days later are comparable to those at the 12th to 14th week in the human. This system has the advantage of not requiring surgical violation of the uterus, which may precipitate preterm labor. Finally, the fetal sheep has been used for many years to investigate the fetal kidney. This animal offers the advantage of having a long gestation similar to that of the human, as well as being manipulable for experimental preparations without excessive fetal loss. Multiple procedures may be performed on a given fetal sheep to explore the dynamics of renal response to obstruction.

REFERENCES

1. Berman, D.J., and Maizels, M.: The role of urinary obstruction in the genesis of renal dysplasia: A model in the chick embryo. J. Urol., *128*:1091, 1982.
2. McVary, K., and Maizels, M.: Urinary obstruction reduces glomerulogenesis in the developing kidney: A model in the rabbit. J. Urol., *142* (Part 2):646, 1989.
3. Steinhardt, G.F., Vogler, G., Salinas-Madrigal, L., and LaRegina, M.: Induced renal dysplasia in the young pouch opossum. J. Pediatr. Surg., *23*:1127, 1988.
4. Peters, C.A., Whitcomb, W., Kozakewich, H., et al.: The fetal kidney: Morphologic responses to obstruction and decompression. J. Urol., *143*:253A, 1990.

723-E *(Campbell's, p. 1578)*

The response of the fetal kidney to obstruction can be completely distinct from that in the postnatal animal. This has been proven by clinical observation and in experimental animals. Postnatally induced obstruction has never been reported to produce changes consistent with renal dysplasia or to produce the growth effects seen with prenatally obstructed kidneys. The response of the fetal kidney to obstruction is determined to various degrees by (1) the time of onset of obstruction during gestation, (2) the duration of the obstruction, and (3) the severity of the obstruction. The status of the contralateral kidney has also been shown to have a significant role in the response of the affected kidney to obstruction.

REFERENCE

1. Beck, A.D.: The effect of intra-uterine urinary obstruction upon the development of the fetal kidney. J. Urol., *105*:784–789, 1971.

724-A *(Campbell's, pp. 1578–1580)*

Postnatal renal functional assessment following prenatal obstruction has been carried out in a number of models. The nature of the defects observed reflects those seen clinically in the postnatal period in the child with obstructive uropathy, including reduced glomerular filtration, impaired acid excretion, and reduced sodium and water reabsorption. Postnatal renal blood flow in congenital obstruction has not been evaluated extensively. In a model of spontaneous congenital obstruction in the rat, renal blood flow has been demonstrated to be an important factor in the renal response to obstruction. In prenatally induced partial ureteral obstruction, reductions in blood flow were demonstrated. It remains unclear whether these changes in blood flow are a secondary phenomenon or are directly related to the causes of the functional impairments.

REFERENCES

1. Hawtrey, C.E., VanVoohis, B., and Robillard, J.E.: Experimental congenital unilateral hydronephrosis in fetal lambs, an anatomic and physiologic assessment (Abstract 66). J. Urol., *133* (Part 2): 130A, 1985.
2. Hutcheon, R.A., Kaplan, B.S., and Drummond, K.N.: Distal renal tubular acidosis in children with chronic hydronephrosis. J. Pediatr., *89*:372, 1976.
3. Boineau, F.G., Vari, R.C., and Lewy, J.E.: Reversible vasoconstriction in rats with congenital unilateral hydronephrosis: Pediatr. Nephrol., *1*:498, 1987.

725-C *(Campbell's, pp. 1580–1581; Figs. 39–15, 39–16)*

Experimentally, renal structural abnormalities have been produced with prenatal obstruction in various animal models. Impaired nephrogenesis has been reported in the fetal rabbit and this effect was apparently reversed with early postnatal decompression. Renal obstruction in the opossum has produced histologic dysplasia but due to the fact that the opossum pup's kidneys are not on placental dialysis, it is not clear how this model correlates with other mammals. Dysplastic changes have been reported in fetal sheep kidneys with early gestational obstruction. This dysplasia is characterized by primitive ductal epithelium, peritubular mesenchymal collars, cystic changes, and disorganized architecture. In the avian kidney, similar results were only achieved with obstruction in combination with mesenchymal stripping. In utero compensatory hypertrophy has been induced and documented with prenatal nephrectomy and in the setting of unilateral prenatal obstructive uropathy. The actual mediators effecting the changes seen in prenatal obstructive uropathy remain unknown but hydrostatic pressure appears to be involved. Alterations in renal blood flow and inflammatory and immunologic responses are also felt to play a role.

REFERENCES

1. McVary, K., and Maizels. M.: Urinary obstruction reduces glomerulogenesis in the developing kidney: A model in the rabbit. J. Urol., *142* (Part 2):646, 1989.
2. Gonzalez, R., Reinberg, Y., Burke, B., Wells, T., and Vernier, R.L.: Early Bladder outlet obstruction in fetal lambs induces renal dysplasia and the prune-belly syndrome. J. Pediatr. Surg., *25*:342, 1990.
3. Moore, E.S., deLeon, L.B., Weiss, L.S., et al.: Compensatory renal hypertrophy in fetal lambs. Pediatr. Res., *13*:1125, 1979.
4. Peters, C.A., Whitcomb, W., Kozakewich, H., et al.: The fetal kidney: Morphologic responses to obstruction and decompression. J. Urol., *143*:253A, 1990.

726-A *(Campbell's, pp. 1581–1583; Figs. 39–17, 39–18)*

The effect of congenital bladder outlet obstruction may be seen perinatally in terms of the renal and pulmonary injury. This effect may continue long after the correction of the obstruction in the form of bladder dysfunction. A variety of patterns of bladder dysfunction are seen in the postobstructive bladder, yet it is unclear what differentiates these patterns in terms of etiology. In a model of complete early gestational bladder outlet obstruction, a marked increase in the mass of bladder smooth muscle is seen. Morphometric data suggest this is mostly muscle cell hypertrophy, but it is possible that some degree of hyperplasia is present. Connective tissue elements are increased to a lesser degree than the smooth muscle mass. Patterns of collagen subtypes within the bladder have also been shown to be altered in human cases of prenatal obstruction. The ratio of myosin heavy chain isoforms, which have been well described to progress in a predictable fashion during development, and which may have physiologic consequences, are affected by in utero obstruction. A prematurely accelerated pattern is seen. The levels of muscarinic cholinergic receptors are also affected by prenatal bladder outlet obstruction. No significant change in receptor density was seen with obstruction, however, despite a marked increase in the amount of smooth muscle mass. Ultrasonography of affected individuals reveals a bladder wall thicker than normal for age.

REFERENCES

1. Peters, C.A., Bolkier, M., Bauer, S.B., et al.: The urodynamic consequences of posterior urethral valves. J. Urol., *144*:122, 1990.
2. Dator, D.P., Peters, C.A., Retik, A.B., and Mandell, J.: The effect of congenital bladder obstruction on bladder smooth muscle nuclear number and size. J. Urol., *145*:218A, 1991.
3. Kim, K.M., Kogan, B.A., and Massas, C.A.: Collagen and elastin in the obstructed fetal bladder. J. Urol., *146*:528, 1991.
4. McConnell, J.D., Lin, V.K., and Cher, M.L.: Myosin heavy chain expression in bladder obstruction (Abstract 78): *In* Programs and Abstracts of Neurourology and Urodynamics, the 20th Meeting of the International Continence Society, 1990.

727-B *(Campbell's, pp. 1583–1585; Figs. 39–19, 39–20)*

The relationship of congenital uropathies to maldevelopment of the lungs has been recognized for nearly 40 years. The relationship of the kidney and amniotic fluid to pulmonary development has been investigated in several model systems. In the rabbit, oligohydramnios has been produced by bladder outlet obstruction as well as by amniotic shunting. In both situations, in the last third of gestation, lung size is decreased. Work with guinea pigs has shown that lung growth and development are modulated by lung fluid dynamics. Increased lung growth can be produced by retention of the lung fluid with tracheal ligation, providing support to the concept of a simple mechanical factor relating the kidneys and lungs through the amniotic fluid.

It remains to be explained why a significant impairment of lung growth in humans can be induced by kidney damage that occurs in the first trimester, before the absence of urine would produce oligohydramnios. In cases of renal agenesis or bilateral dysplasia, airway branching is diminished. Embryologically, branching is known to occur only up to 14 weeks of gestation, a time when the kidneys have not yet begun to contribute significantly to the amniotic fluid volume. This finding raises the strong possibility of a very specific kidney factor being necessary for normal lung airway branching.

The most detailed experimental models used to investigate the clinically relevant relationship of the kidney and lung have employed fetal sheep. Pulmonary hypoplasia has been produced by creation of a bladder outlet obstruction during the last one third of gestation. More significant impairment of pulmonary development is noted when obstruction is created earlier in gestation. It has also been shown that, with in utero decompression of these obstructive lesions, partial prevention of pulmonary hypoplasia and completion of structural maturity can be accomplished.

REFERENCES

1. Nakayama, D.K., Glick, P.L., Harrison, M.R., et al.: Experimental pulmonary hypoplasia due to oligohydramnios and its reversal by relieving thoracic compression. J. Pediatr. Surg., *18*:347, 1983.
2. Scurry, J.P., Adamson, T.M., and Cussen, L.J.: Fetal lung growth in laryngeal atresia and tracheal agenesis. Aust. Paediatr. J., *25*:47, 1989.
3. Clemmons, J.J.W.: Embryonic renal injury. A possible factor in fetal malnutrition. (Abstract), Pediatr. Res., *11*:404, 1977.
4. Harrison, M.R., Nakayama, D.K., Noall, R.A., and deLorimer, A.A.: Correction of congenital hydronephrosis in utero: II. Decompression reverses the effects of obstruction on the fetal lung and urinary tract. J. Pediatr. Surg., *17*:965, 1982.

728-B *(Campbell's, p. 1590)*

The neonate is generally considered a newborn within the first month life. About two thirds of all infant deaths occur during the first year. The neonatal period is the most critical time, and most deaths within the neonatal period occur on the first day. From 10 to 15 per cent of neonatal deaths are a result of gross genital malformations. Autopsies in stillborn infants and neonates show a 17 per cent incidence of one or more urologic abnormalities.

729-E *(Campbell's, pp. 1590–1591)*

A family history of fetal wastage or chromosomal abnormality such as translocation increases the likelihood of fetal malformation. Oligohydramnios is associated with obstructive uropathy, renal agenesis and purine belly syndrome and Polyhydramnios are associated with neonatal ovarian cyst. Bleeding, particularly in the first trimester, is associated with an increased risk of congenital malformation. Illnesses such as rubella on diabetes, drug administration during pregnancy, and intrauterine growth retardation are associated with abnormalities. The effect of age on increased risk of malformations is clear, but increased risk, including perinatal mortality, is identified beyond the age of 35.

730-A *(Campbell's, pp. 1591–1593)*

Approximately 0.9 per cent of all babies are born with a single umbilical artery. About 28 per cent of infants with a single umbilical artery who die have genitourinary malformations. Some have suggested that surviving infants with a single umbilical artery and should be evaluated for urologic malformation.

REFERENCE

1. Bryan, E.M., and Koler, H.G.: The missing umbilical artery: II. Pediatric follow-up. Arch. Dis. Child., *50*: 714, 1975.

731-D *(Campbell's, p. 1593)*

Examination of the newborn can give clues to the existence of urologic abnormalities. The classic Potter's facies is characterized by large, low-set flabby ears and widely spaced eyes and is seen in renal agenesis, prune belly syndrome, and bilateral multicystic kidneys. Abnormalities of the external ear may signal the presence of uropathy. Widely spaced nipples are associated with multiple urologic defects. Deficiency of abdominal musculature is a reliable indication of prune belly uropathy and cryptorchidism.

732-C *(Campbell's, pp. 1593–1595)*

Despite the theoretical advantages of fetal intervention, the efficacy of in utero decompression remains unproven and investigational. Early fetal obstructive uropathy appears to result in irreversible dysplasia, and in utero decompression at 20 weeks has failed to prevent renal dysplasia or pulmonary hypoplasia. The rate of diagnostic error is as high as 30 to 40 per cent, and early delivery should not be performed in the fetus with unilateral hydronephrosis. The most common obstructive lesion is ureteropelvic junction obstruction.

733-C, 734-D *(Campbell's, pp. 1595–1599)*

One half or more of neonatal abdominal masses arise from the kidney. Hydronephrosis, most frequently the result of uteropelvic junction obstruction, is the most common cause, followed by multicystic kidney. Work-up includes physical examination, excretory transillumination and abdominal ultrasonography. Excretory urography is often limited by poor contrast excretion in the neonate. While excretory urography had been considered the most important diagnostic tool, it is being subplanted by real time abdominal ultrasonography. Sonographic criteria for the diagnosis of multicystic dysplastic kidney include the presences of interfaces between cysts, nonmedical location of the largest cysts, absence of identifiable renal sinus, multiple noncommunicating cysts, and the absence of a parenchymal rim. When the differential diagnosis between multicystic kidney and hydronephrosis remains in doubt, radionuclide renal scan will generally make the diagnosis.

735-A *(Campbell's, pp. 1600–1601)*

The increased use of umbilical artery catheters in monitoring neonates has increased the incidence of renal artery thrombosis.

Hematuria is often the first sign of renal artery thrombosis. Other causes of hematuria include drugs such as indomethacin, quinone, and 8-quinolinol as well as renal calculi following furosemide administration. Additional findings in neonatal hematuria include renal vein thrombosis, obstructive uropathy, polycystic kidney disease, sponge kidney, and rarely, Wilms' tumor.

736-E *(Campbell's, p. 1601)*

Arterial hypertension is rare in neonates, and requires prompt evaluation to prevent complications such as congestive heart failure and cerebrovascular accidents. The most common cause of hypertension in the neonate is coarctation of the aorta. Renal artery thrombosis is a relatively common and urgent renal cause of neonatal hypertension. Adrenal hemorrhage, adrenogenital syndrome, and, rarely, pheochromocytoma, Cushing's disease, primary hyperaldosteronism, and neuroblastomas cause neonatal hypertension.

737-D *(Campbell's, pp. 1601–1602)*

More than 90 per cent of neonates will void within the first 24 hours. A weak urinary stream, especially with a palpable lower abdominal mass, may be caused by posterior urethral valves. A distended bladder may be the initial sign of neurologic deficit. Drugs administered to the mother may affect bladder function. Magnesium sulfate or ritodrine, for example, may result in transient bladder atony requiring catheterization.

738-B *(Campbell's, pp. 1602–1605)*

Obstructive uropathy is the usual cause of neonatal ascites, and urine is the most common fluid found. The most common cause of urinary ascites is the presence of posterior urethral valves, and therefore urinary ascites are seven times more common in boys. Ureteropelvic junction obstruction is second most common cause. Abdominal ultrasonography should confirm the presence of ascites and provide an initial evaluation of the urinary tract. In about 85 per cent of cases, the etiology can be determined.

739-B, 740-C *(Campbell's, pp. 1605–1607)*

Hydronephrosis is the most common cause of a neonatal abdominal mass and one of the most common abnormalities requiring surgical correction. The most common site of obstruction is the ureteropelvic junction. Ultrasonography and radionuclide studies are most important in diagnosis, but excretory urography and even retrograde pyelograms are still necessary in selected cases. Indications for surgical correction in the neonate include bilateral ureteropelvic junction obstruction and an obstructive kidney contributing less than 40 per cent of overall function by renal scan.

741-A *(Campbell's, pp. 1607–1608)*

Multicystic dysplastic kidney, classified as Potter type II, is associated with atresia of the ureter. It is the second most frequent cause of neonatal abdominal mass, and is now most commonly diagnosed in utero by prenatal ultrasonography. Although previously these kidneys were removed, many reports now advocate conservative management with long-term surveillance.

The multicystic kidney may undergo spontaneous involution, but infrequently pain, infection, hypertension, or neoplasia may develop. Up to 33 per cent of patients will have an associated urologic anomaly including contralateral renal agenesis, horseshoe kidney, contralateral ureteropelvic junction obstruction, megaureter, or reflux.

742-E, 743-E *(Campbell's, pp. 1608–1610)*

The clinical features of renal vein thrombosis include renal enlargement, hematuria, thrombocytopenia, anemia, acidemia, nonfunction on intravenous urography, proteinuria, and shock/sepsis. It occurs most frequently in the first 2 weeks of life. Sluggish renal perfusion due to low blood pressure associated with normal neonatal polycythemia predispose to renal vein thrombosis, especially if combined with trauma, dehydration or infection. Up to 20 per cent of cases are bilateral. Primary renal vein thrombosis, which occurs suddenly in a previously healthy neonate, has a better prognosis than secondary renal vein thrombosis which results from a known cause such as dehydration. Abdominal ultrasonography is most helpful in establishing the diagnosis. Treatment includes hydration, correction of electrolyte imbalance, and antibiotics. Heparinization and low dose streptokinase administration have been used successfully. Nephrectomy is rarely necessary and should be done only for difficult-to-control hemorrhage or infection. Caval thrombectomy may be required in bilateral renal venous thrombosis.

744-D, 745-D, 746-C *(Campbell's, pp. 1610–1613)*

Small hemorrhages in the adrenal glands are found in up to 2 per cent of infant autopsies, but massive adrenal hemorrhage is rare. Conservative management is appropriate for most neonates.

Predisposing features include prolonged labor, traumatic delivery and possible resuscitation efforts. Possible risk factors include large birth weight, perinatal anoxia, bradycardia, sepsis, and hypoprothrombinemia.

Clinical features include flank mass, signs of blood loss, jaundice and urinary infection or sepsis. Azotemia may be present. Microscopic hematuria is frequent. The most useful diagnostic test is abdominal ultrasound.

747-A *(Campbell's, p. 1613)*

Wilms' tumor is the most common renal tumor in childhood, but in the neonate, congenital mesoblastic nephroma is the predominant tumor. These tumors have a benign course and therefore the hazards of treatment for Wilms' tumor should be avoided. These tumors typically present as an incidental palpable mass and have ultrasonographic and pyelographic features of a solid renal mass. Although the tumor may recur locally, distant metastasis is exceedingly rare and radiation and chemotherapy are not indicated.

748-D *(Campbell's, pp. 1614–1616)*

Vaginal atresia, inherited as a autosomal recessive, is the most common cause of hydrometrocolpos, although imperforate hymen can produce vaginal obstruction. Fluid retention in the uterus and vagina, resulting from secretion of cervical glands, is a rare cause of abdominal mass in a neonate. Hydrometrocolpos typically produces a large firm mass arising from the pelvis. Ureteral obstruction with hydronephrosis commonly occurs. Examination of the introitus may reveal imperforate hymen, but more commonly vaginal atresia is present. Imperforate anus or cloacal anomalies as well as ambiguous genitalia may be associated features. Treatment is by simple incision for imperforate hymen. Vaginal pull through operation for vaginal atresia is generally required. Inadequate treatment can result in sepsis and death.

749-C *(Campbell's, p. 1621)*

Enuresis is defined as an involuntary discharge of urine. The term is often used alone, imprecisely, to describe wetting that occurs only at night during sleep. It is more accurate, however, to refer to nighttime wetting as nocturnal enuresis and to distinguish it from daytime wetting, or diurnal enuresis. The age at which enuresis becomes inappropriate depends on the statistics of developing urinary control, the pattern of wetting, and the sex of the child. Approximately 15 per cent of normal children still wet at night at age 5 years. Nocturnal enuresis occurring after the age of 5 or by the time the child enters grade school is generally considered a cause for concern. With a spontaneous resolution rate of about 15 per cent per year, 99 per cent of children are dry by the age of 15 years.

REFERENCE

1. Forsythe, W.I., and Redmond, A.: Enuresis and spontaneous cure rate: Study of 1129 enuretics. Arch. Dis. Child., *49*:259, 1974.

750-B *(Campbell's, pp. 1621–1622)*

The development of urinary control is a gradual process normally occuring over the first three to four years of life. In the infant, micturition occurs spontaneously as a spinal cord reflex. Even in the newborn, the periurethral striated muscles that compose the voluntary (external) urinary sphincter are fully integrated into the voiding reflex so that as the bladder fills, the urinary sphincter constricts progressively to prevent incontinence. During micturition, the striated muscle sphincter relaxes reflexly to allow low-pressure bladder emptying. During the first year of life, the number of voidings per day is fairly constant at about 20. Over the next 2 years, the frequency of urinations per day decreases to about 11, while the mean voided volume increases nearly fourfold. This reduction in voiding frequency is due to a growth-related increase in bladder capacity that is proportionately greater than is the increase in urine volume produced. In addition to an increase in bladder capacity, the child must develop voluntary control of both the periurethral striated sphincter and direct volitional control over the spinal micturition reflex to prevent involuntary detrusor contractions. Control of the external sphincter is usually accomplished by age 3 years, while control of the spinal micturition reflex occurs by age 4 years.

REFERENCES

1. Goellner, M.H., Ziegler, E.E., and Fomon, S.J.: Urination during the first three years of life. Nephron., *28*:174, 1981.

2. Nash, D.E.E.: The development of micturition control with special reference to enuresis. Ann. R. Coll. Surg. Engl., *5*:318, 1949.

751-A *(Campbell's, p. 1622)*

The development of urinary control fits into an orderly scheme of overall bowel and bladder control. This follows a typical sequence of development: (1) control of bowel function of night; (2) control of bowel function by day; (3) control of bladder function by day; and (4) finally, after a lag of several months or more, control of bladder function by night. This sequence of achieving urinary control is malleable and can be overridden by external forces. Consequently, there is a marked individual variability in the age of achieving nighttime urinary control.

REFERENCE

1. Stein, Z.M., and Susser, M.W.: Social factors in the development of sphincter control. Dev. Med. Child Neurol., *9*:692, 1967.

752-E *(Campbell's, pp. 1622–1623)*

A number of urodynamic factors have been studied in enuretic children. The single most important static urodynamic observation in these children is a reduced bladder capacity, often less than 50 per cent of the expected normal. The disturbance reducing bladder capacity is functional rather than anatomic. Under anesthesia, these patients have a normal bladder capacity. These children also appear to have uninhibited bladder contractions. Initial studies noted uninhibited contractions in more than 50 per cent of unselected patients, but current studies using provocative tests aimed at eliciting uninhibited contractions note a much higher incidence of 78 to 84 per cent. The finding of uninhibited bladder contractions is also seen during urodynamic studies performed during sleep. Sleep cystometrograms recorded from enuretics show spontaneous bladder contractions that are more frequent and of greater amplitude than those of controls. If concomitant electromyography is performed, it is found that during spontaneous bladder contractions, enuretics have a silent pelvic floor and associated sleep wetting. In nonenuretics, pelvic floor muscle activity signaled arousal; the patients awoke and voided voluntarily.

REFERENCES

1. Wu, H.H.H., Chen, M.-T., Lee, Y.-H.: Urodynamics studies and primary nocturnal enuresis. Chin. Med. J. (Taipei), *41*:227–232, 1988.
2. Troup, C.W., and Hodgson, N.B.: Nocturnal functional bladder capacity in enuretic children. J. Urol., *129*:132, 1971.
3. Mahoney, D.T., Laferte, R.O., and Blais, D.J.: Studies on enuresis: IX. Evidence of a mild form of compensated detrusor hyperreflexia in enuretic children. J. Urol., *126*:520, 1981.
4. Norgaard, J.P., Hansen, J.H., and Willdschiotz, G.: Cystometrics in children with nocturnal enuresis. J. Urol., *141*:1156, 1989.

753-D *(Campbell's, pp. 1623–1624)*

Nocturnal and diurnal enuresis represent an arrest in development because both occur normally in young children. A developmental cause for enuresis is supported by the observation that a number of nonorganic disturbances, such as social factors and stress, can modify the attainment of urinary control and influence the timing and duration of enuresis. Bed wetting is more common in lower socioeconomic groups. In families undergoing stress, the likelihood of enuresis occurring is increased threefold. An increased prevalence of enuresis has been found in children from deprived environments, from broken homes, and with a history of temporary institutional habitation. There has also been a significantly higher proportion of bed wetting observed in children who are delayed in walking and in talking, and a significant number of children with primary enuresis display retardation in skeletal maturation (bone age), which may reflect delayed maturation of regulatory central nervous system functions.

Abnormalities in sleep patterns, while not fully associated with delayed development, have been associated with enuresis. Historically, enuresis has been considered a disorder of sleep and more precisely a consequence of deep sleep. More recent controlled sleep research studies, however, indicate that children with enuresis sleep no more deeply than do normals and that a proportion of enuretics actually wet during very light sleep or while awake. Thus it appears that enuretic sleep patterns are not appreciably different from the sleep patterns of normal children, and that most enuretics do not wet as a consequence of sleeping too deeply.

REFERENCES

1. Essen, J., and Peckhan, C.: Nocturnal enuresis in childhood. Dev. Med. Child Neurol., *18*:577, 1976.
2. Miller, F.J.W., Court, S.D.M., Walton, N.G., and Knox, E.G.: Growing-up in Newcastle upon Tyne. London, Oxford University Press, 1960.
3. Mimouni, M., Schuper, A., Mimouni, F., et al.: Retarded skeletal maturation in children with primary enuresis. J. Pediatr., *144*:234–235, 1985.
4. Ritvo, E.R., Ornitz, E.M., Gottlieb, F., et al.: Arousal and non-arousal enuretic events. Am. J. Psychiatry, *126*:115, 1969.

754-A *(Campbell's, p. 1626)*

It is often difficult to pinpoint the etiologic factor of enuresis and to eliminate the symptoms. Most children with enuresis do not have an organic lesion and those who do are readily detected by routine evaluation. A careful history, physical examination, and urinalysis with culture are needed for all children with bed wetting and are all that is needed for the child with purely nocturnal enuresis. Routine radiographic studies such as intravenous pyelography or voiding cystourethrography, are not indicated for enuretics who have a normal physical examination, a negative urine, and no obvious neuropathy. In the vast majority of enuretics, the diagnostic yield from cystourethroscopy is nil, thus endoscopic evaluation is unwarranted. Retrograde urethrograpy, likewise, is not useful. In patients with diurnal enuresis, normal history and physical examination no evidence of neuropathy, and negative urine, urinary tract anatomy should be screened. This can be accomplished noninvasively and satisfactorily with an ultrasound examination of the kidneys, ureters, and bladder before and after voiding. Any positive findings can be pursued with conventional urologic studies.

REFERENCE

1. American Academy of Pediatrics, Committee on Radiology: Excretory urography for evaluation of enuresis. Pediatrics, *65*:644, 1980.

755-C *(Campbell's, p. 1627)*

Therapy for enuresis has evolved along two lines: pharmacologic therapy and modification of behavior. Overall, the effectiveness of anticholinergic drug therapy has been disappointing with an effectiveness in the range of 5 to 40 per cent. In some series, therapy was inappreciably different from placebo. These drugs have been shown to increase functional bladder capacity in patients with enuresis but in 59 per cent of patients, clinical improvement does not follow. Because these agents are very useful in eliminating uninhibited contractions, they may be effective for subgroups of enuretics with this urodynamic disturbance. Anticholinergics have been found to be very effective (87.5 per cent) in treating enuretic patients with symptoms of bladder hyperactivity, such as urgency, frequency, and day and night incontinence, and highly effective (90.6 per cent) in those with proven uninhibited bladder contractions. The success rate was much less (50 per cent) in patients with pure nocturnal enuresis and was only 11 per cent in those with normal cystometrograms.

REFERENCES

1. Lovering, J.S., Tallett, S.E., and McKendry, J.B.J.: Oxybutynin efficacy and the treatment of primary enuresis. Pediatrics, *82*:104–106, 1988.
2. Johnstone, J.M.S.: Cystometry and evaluation of anticholinergic drugs in enuretic children. J. Pediatr. Surg., *7*:18, 1972.
3. Kass, E.J., Piokno, A.C., and Montealegre, A.: Enuresis: Principles of management and result of treatment. J. Urol., *121*:794, 1979.

756-D *(Campbell's, p. 1627)*

Reduction of urine output at night is theoretically attractive for treating bed wetting but simply limiting fluids or using diuretics during the daytime to produce relative dehydration at night has not been effective. Manipulation of antidiuretic hormone (ADH) levels, however, has proven to be effective. Measurements of urinary and serum ADH demonstrate an absence or reversal of the normal circadian rhythm in enuretics who have lower than normal excretion levels of ADH during the night. With the development of desmopressin (DDAVP), an analog of vasopressin, wide potential application for treating enuresis became available. This drug can be given nasally, has no pressor or smooth muscle activity in the effective dose range, and has an effect lasting 7 to 10 hours. It may also be given in oral form.

In double-blind studies, DDAVP has been shown to be more effective than placebo in treating enuresis. It has been reported to achieve a 30 to 60 per cent reduction in wet nights and up to a 50 per cent cure rate. The usual clinical dose ranges between 20 and 40 μg and responses are dose dependent. Better results have occurred in older children. Unfortunately, this drug is relatively expensive and, upon discontinuation, less than one third of cured patients stay dry.

REFERENCES

1. Norgaard, J.P., Rittig, S., and Djurhuus, J.C.: Nocturnal enuresis: An approach to treatment based on pathogenesis. J. Pediatr., *114*:705–710, 1989.
2. Klauber, G.T.: Clinical efficacy and safety of desmopressin in the treatment of nocturnal enuresis. J. Pediatr., *114*:719–722, 1989.
3. Miller, K., Goldberg, S., and Atkin, B.: Nocturnal enuresis: Experience with long-term use of intranasally administered desmopressin. J. Pediatr., *114*:723–726, 1989.

757-B *(Campbell's, pp. 1627–1628)*

The tricyclic antidepressants, and specifically, imipramine, are probably the most effective and most widely studied of all antienuretic agents. Imipramine has proved to be significantly effective in large numbers of well-controlled clinical studies. Overall, enuresis can be cured in more than 50 per cent of children and will be improved in another 15 to 20 per cent. Discontinuation of medication, however, will cause up to 60 per cent of patients to relapse.

Imipramine possesses several pharmacologic actions on the central and peripheral nervous systems that could be responsible for its effect in enuresis. Its peripheral effects include (1) weak anticholinergic activity (which is ineffective in abolishing uninhibited detrusor contractions); (2) direct in vitro antispasmodic activity on bladder smooth muscle that is inapparent at clinically effective antienuretic doses; and (3) a complex effect on sympathetic input to the bladder, which prevents norepinephrine action on alpha receptors and enhances its effect on beta receptors by inhibiting norepinephrine reuptake. Combined, these peripheral actions of imipramine produce significant increases in bladder capacity. Imipramine effects on the central nervous system include its antidepressant activity and its action on sleep. It is unlikely that the antineuretic effect is related to antidepressant activity because the time course on enuresis is immediate, whereas the effect on depression requires higher dosage and is often develayed for a period of time. Imipramine significantly alters sleep patterns by decreasing the time spent in REM sleep and increasing the time spent in light NREM sleep. In sleep studies, imipramine can be shown to reduce the total number of wetting episodes, but it does not appreciably alter the time at which wetting occurs. Despite the lack of a clear explanation as to how the central and peripheral effects of imipramine promote antienuresis, it continues to be the mainstay of pharmacologic therapy.

REFERENCES

1. Blackwell, B., and Currah, J.: The psychopharmacology of nocturnal enuresis. *In* Kolvin, I., Mackeith, R.C., and Meadows, S.R. (Eds.): Bladder Control and Enuresis. London, W. Heinmann Medical Books Ltd., 1973, pp. 231–237.

2. Diokno, A.C., Hyndman, C.W., Hardy, D.A., and Lapides, J.: Comparison of actions of imipramine (Tofranil) and propantheline (Probanthine) on detrusor contractions. J. Urol., *107*:42, 1982.
3. Labay, P., and Boyarsky, S.: The action of imipramine on the bladder musculature. J. Urol., *109*:385, 1973.
4. Rapoport, J.L., Mikkelsen, E.J., Zavodil, A., et al.: Childhood enuresis. II, Arch. Gen. Psychiatry, *37*: 1146, 1980.

758-B *(Campbell's, pp. 1628–1629)*

As stated previously, treatment for enuresis has evolved along two main lines, pharmacologic therapy and modification of behavior. Modification of behavior has met with varying degrees of success but certain specific approaches, when determinedly applied to a motivated child, produce the most effective rate of sustained cure and should be considered a first-line approach to the management of enuresis. Bladder training, or so called retention control training, was developed as specific therapy for the reduced functional bladder capacity that characterizes most enuretics. As a cure for enuresis, however, this method has not met with great success and does not appear to significantly decrease bed wetting in many children. An alternative behavior modification technique is responsibility reinforcement. The components of a successful responsibility reinforcement program include motivation, reward, response shaping, and reinforcement. The program aims to motivate the child to assume both the responsibility for wetting and the credit for dryness. The results of these programs are difficult to evaluate on a controlled basis because better results are seen with all therapies when the child takes an active rather than a passive role. For selected children, improvement may be more rapid and the relapse rate lower with responsibility reinforcement than with other types of programs.

At least four randomized controlled trials have shown that conditioning therapy is the most effective means of eliminating bed wetting. In this method, a sensor detects when the child voids and an alarm sounds. The child is awakened, turns off the alarm, then gets up and completes voiding in the toilet. The success of this system has been explained by classical conditioning theory. Not only has this method been shown to be superior to other forms of behavior modification, in controlled studies, this system is superior to drug therapy with imipramine and DDAVP.

REFERENCES

1. Kimmel, H.D., and Kimmel, E.C.: An instrumental conditioning method for the treatment of enuresis. J. Behav. Ther. Exp. Psychiatry, *1*:121, 1970.
2. Marshall, S., Marshall, H.H., and Lyon, R.P.: Enuresis: An analysis of various therapeutic approaches. Pediatrics, *52*:813, 1973.
3. Moffatt, M.E.K,, Kato, C., and Pless, I.B.: Improvements in self-concept after treatment of nocturnal enuresis: Randomized controlled trial. J. Pediatr., *110*: 647–652, 1987.

759-A *(Campbell's, p. 1630)*

Enuresis occurring in adults is seen in two contexts: persistent, primary enuresis, which occurs in more than 1 per cent of the population; and adult onset enuresis. Unlike the situation in children, a high proportion (greater than 70 per cent) of adults with persistent primary enuresis will display overt urodynamic abnormalities, generally in the form of uninhibited bladder activity. It is a matter of clinical judgment in each case to determine the need for and the extent of investigation in excess of the evaluation used for childhood enuresis. Patients will usually require a thorough anatomic evaluation as well as a careful neurologic and urodynamic study. It is noteworthy, however, that caffeine withdrawal significantly reduces bed wetting in adult enuretics, suggesting that caffeine intake should first be reduced before other forms of treatment are initiated.

REFERENCES

1. Miller, F.J.W., Knox, E.G., and Brandon, S.: Children who wet the bed. *In* Kolvin, I., MacKeith, R.C., and Meadow, S.R. (Eds.): Bladder Control and Enuresis. London, W. Heinemann Medical Books. Ltd., 1973, pp. 47–52.
2. Torrens, M.J., and Collins, C.D.: The urodynamic assessment of adult enuresis. Br. J. Urol., *47*:433, 1975.
3. Edelstein, B.A., Keaton-Brasted, C., and Burd, M.M.: Effects of caffeine withdrawal on nocturnal enuresis, insomnia, and behavioral restraints. J. Consult. Clin. Psychol., *52*:857–862, 1984.

760-E *(Campbell's, pp. 1634–1636; Fig. 42–3)*

The functional assessment of the lower urinary tract is an essential element in the evaluation of a child with suspected neurogenic vesical dysfunction. A complete urodynamic evaluation includes uroflometry with measurement of the post-void residual. Urethral pressure profilometry is sometimes obtained. A careful cystometrogram using a rectal balloon catheter to measure intra-abdominal pressure is then performed followed by having the patient void to measure voiding pressure.

External urethral sphincter electromyography (EMG) may be recorded using a 24-gauge concentric needle electrode inserted perineally in males or paraurethrally in females. This needle is advanced into the skeletal muscle component of the sphincter and individual motor unit action potentials are recorded. Alternatively, perineal or abdominal patch electrodes, or anal plugs have been used to record the bioelectric activity in the sphincter muscle.

REFERENCES

1. McGuire, E.J., Woodside, J.R., Borden, T.A., and Weiss, R.M.: The prognostic value of urodynamic testing in myelodysplastic patients. J. Urol., *126*:205, 1981.
2. Blaivas, J.G., Labib, K.B., Bauer, S.B., and Retik, A.B.: A new approach to electromyography of the external urethral sphincter. J. Urol., *117*:773, 1977.
3. Blaivas, J.G., Labib, K.B., Bauer, S.B., and Retik, A.B.: Changing concepts in the urodynamic evaluation of children. J. Urol., *117*:777, 1977

761-E *(Campbell's, p. 1635)*

When performing a cystometrogram, it has been shown that rapid filling rates may yield falsely low levels of detrusor compliance and minimize uninhibited contractions. In an attempt to avoid this, the bladder may be filled

In an attempt to avoid this, the bladder may be filled slowly with saline solution warmed to 37°C. The rate of bladder filling is set by determining the child's predicted bladder capacity: average capacity (ml)=[age (years) + 2] × 30, and dividing by 10. Thus the average bladder capacity for an 8 year old is estimated to be (8+2) × 30 or 300 ml and the rate of filling would be 30 ml/min. When it is important to determine very mild degrees of hypertonicity, even slower rates of filling may be employed.

REFERENCES

1. Joseph, D.B., and Duggan, M.L.: The effects of fast and slow saline infusion on hypertonicity and peak/leak pressure during cystometrogram evaluation of infants and children with myelodysplasia. J. Urol., 1991.
2. Turner-Warwick, R.T.: Some clinical aspects of detrusor dysfunction. J. Urol., *113*:539, 1975.
3. Koff, S.A.: Estimating bladder capacity in children. Urology, *21*:248, 1983.

762-D *(Campbell's, p. 1637)*

The most common etiology of neurogenic bladder dysfunction in children is secondary to abnormal spinal column development. Myelodysplasia is an all-inclusive term used to describe the various abnormal conditions of the vertebral column that affect spinal cord function. More specific labels regarding each abnormality include the following. Spina bifida is a condition in which the vertebral neural arches fail to close, exposing the contents of the spinal canal posteriorly. The contents of the canal may or may not protrude through the opening. A meningocele occurs when just the meninges extend beyond the confines of the vertebral canal without any neural elements contained inside of it. A myelomeningocele implies that neural tissue, either nerve roots and/or portions of the spinal cord, have evaginated with the meningocele. A lipomyelomeningocele denotes that fatty tissue has developed with the cord structures and both are protruding into the sac.

763-B *(Campbell's, pp. 1637–1638)*

Myelomeningocele accounts for more than 90 per cent of all the open spinal dysraphic states. Most spinal defects occur at the level of the lumbar vertebrae, with the sacral thoracic and cervical areas affected in decreasing order of frequency. Usually, the meningocele is made up of a flimsy covering of transparent tissue, but it may be open and leaking cerebrospinal fluid. It is for this reason that urgent repair is necessary with sterile precautions being followed in the interval between birth and closure. In 85 per cent of affected children, there is an associated Arnold-Chiari malformation in which the cerebellar tonsils have herniated down through the foramen, obstructing the fourth ventricle and preventing the cerebrospinal fluid from entering the subarachnoid space surrounding the brain and spinal cord. This defect may have profound effects on the brain stem and pontine center, which are involved in control over lower urinary tract function.

REFERENCE

1. Bauer, S.B., Labib, K.B., Dieppa, R.A., et al.: Urodynamic evaluation in a boy with myelodysplasia and incontinence. Urology, *10*:354, 1977.

764-C *(Campbell's, p. 1638)*

In a newborn with a significant neurospinal dysraphism, it would be best to perform urodynamic testing immediately after the baby is born to determine the degree of voiding dysfunction and to determine the most appropriate method of management. The risk of spinal infection and the exigency for closure, however, have not made this a viable option. Renal ultrasonography and a measure of residual urine are performed as early as possible after birth, either before or immediately after the spinal defect is closed. Urodynamic studies are delayed until it is safe to transport the child to the urodynamic suite and place him on his back or side for the test. In the interim, bladder emptying may be accomplished by having the patient void spontaneously, use of the Credé maneuver, or using clean intermittent catheterization (CIC). If the patient cannot void spontaneously, the Credé maneuver is initially performed instead of CIC, but CIC must be used if the postvoid residual urine is elevated (generally greater than 5 ml in a newborn) after Credé voiding. Completion of the evaluation with excretory urogram or renal ultrasonography and renal scan to reassess the upper urinary tract and a voiding cystourethrogram and urodynamic study to evaluate the lower urinary tract are performed once the spinal closure has healed sufficiently. The results of these studies will dictate which method of bladder emptying is ultimately most appropriate.

765-A *(Campbell's, pp. 1639–1640; Figs. 42–5, 42–6)*

Urodynamic studies in the newborn period have shown that 57 per cent of myelodysplastic infants have bladder contractions. Approximately 43 per cent have an areflexic bladder; compliance during bladder filling is either good (25 per cent) or poor (18 per cent) in this subgroup. EMG assessment of the external urethral sphincter demonstrates an intact sacral reflex arc with no evidence of lower motor neuron denervation in 47 per cent of newborns, whereas partial denervation is seen in 24 per cent and complete loss of sacral cord function is noted in 29 per cent.

Combining bladder contractility and external sphincter activity results in three categories of lower urinary tract dynamics: synergic, dyssynergic with and without detrusor hypertonicity, and complete denervation. Categorizing lower urinary tract function in this way has been extremely useful because it has revealed which children are at risk for urinary tract changes, which should be treated prophylactically, which need close surveillance, and which can be followed at greater intervals. Of newborns with dyssynergy, 71 per cent had, on initial assessment or on subsequent studies, urinary tract deterioration within the first 3 years of life; whereas only 17 per cent of synergic children and 23 per cent of completely denervated individuals developed similar changes. The infants in the synergic group who deteriorated did so only after they converted to a dyssynergic pattern. The children with complete denervation deteriorated after developing outlet obstruction due to fibrosis of the skeletal muscle component of the external sphincter.

REFERENCES

1. Bauer, S.B., Hallet, M., Khoshbin, S., et al.: The predictive value of urodynamic evaluation in the newborn with myelodysplasia. JAMA, *152*:650, 1984.

2. Spindel, M.R., Bauer, S.B., Dyro, F.M., et al.: The changing neuro-urologic lesion in myelodysplasia. JAMA, *258*:1630, 1987.
3. Sidi, A.A., Dykstra, D.D., and Gonzalez, R.: The value of urodynamic testing in the management of neonates with myelodysplasia: A prospective study. J. Urol., *135*:90, 1986.
4. Bauer, S.B.: Early evaluation and management of children with spina bifida. *In* King., L.R. (Ed.): Urologic Surgery in Neonates and Young Infants. Philadelphia, W.B. Saunders Co., 1988, pp. 252–264.

766-A *(Campbell's, pp. 1641–1642)*

The neurologic lesion in myelodysplasia is a dynamic disease process with changes taking place throughout childhood especially in early infancy, and then at puberty, when the linear growth rate accelerates again. When a change is noted on neurologic, orthopedic, or urodynamic assessment, radiologic investigation of the central nervous system often reveals (1) tethering of the spinal cord, (2) a syrinx or hydromyelia of the cord, (3) increased intracranial pressure due to a shunt malfunction, or (4) partial herniation of the brain stem and cerebellum. Children with completely intact or partially denervated sacral cord function are particularly vulnerable to progressive changes. Today, magnetic resonance imaging (MRI) is the test of choice because it reveals excellent anatomic details of the spinal column and central nervous system. It is not, however, a functional study, and when used alone, it cannot provide exact information with regard to a changing neurologic lesion.

REFERENCES

1. Epstein, F.: Meningocele: Pitfalls in early and late management. Clin. Neurosurg., *30*:366, 1982.
2. Spindel, M.R., Bauer, S.B., Dyro, F.M., et al.: The changing neuro-urologic lesion in myelodysplasia. JAMA, *258*:1630, 1987.
3. Begger, J.H., Meihuizen de Regt, M.J., Hogen Esch, I., et al.: Progressive neurologic deficit in children with spina bifida aperta. Z. Kinderchir., *41*(Suppl. 1): 13, 1986.

767-D *(Campbell's, pp. 1643–1644)*

The indications for antireflux surgery in patients with myelodysplasia are not very different from those for children with normal bladder function. These indications include the following: (1) recurrent symptomatic urinary tract infection while on adequate antibiotic therapy and appropriate catheterization techniques, (2) persistent hydroureteronephrosis despite effective emptying of the bladder and lowering of intravesical pressure, (3) severe reflux with an anatomic abnormality at the ureterovesical junction, and (4) reflux persisting into puberty. In addition, children with any grade of reflux who are being considered for implantation of an artificial urinary sphincter or any other procedure designed to increase bladder outlet resistance should have the reflux corrected at the time or before the antiincontinence surgery.

768-C *(Campbell's, pp. 1644–1645)*

Urinary continence is becoming an increasingly important issue to deal with at an early age as parents try to mainstream their handicapped children. Initial attempts at achieving continence include CIC and drug therapy designed to maintain low intravesical pressure and a reasonable level of urethral resistance. If initial attempts with CIC and oxybutynin fail to achieve continence, urodynamic testing should be performed. If urodynamic testing reveals that urethral resistance is inadequate to maintain continence because there is either a failure of the sphincter to react to increases in abdominal pressure or a drop in resistance with bladder filling, then alpha-sympathomimetic agents are added to the regimen; phenylpropanolamine is the most effective drug in this regard. Surgery becomes a viable option when this program fails to achieve continence. In general, this alternative is not undertaken until the child is about 5 years of age and ready to start school. Urethral and bladder neck resistance can be improved by a number of techniques. These include bladder neck reconstruction using the Young-Dees and Leadbetter procedures, or the Kropp procedure. Other techniques include fascial sling operations to suspend the bladder neck or implantation of an artificial urinary sphincter. Generally, medical therapy should be allowed to fail prior to proceeding with one of the surgical alternatives. Finally, if detrusor hypertonicity or uninhibited contractions persist, they also should be treated with appropriate medical or surgical management.

REFERENCES

1. Dees, J.E.: Congenital epispadias with incontinence. J. Urol., *62*:513, 1949.
2. Kropp, K.A., and Angwafo, F.F.: Urethral lengthening and reimplantation for neurogenic incontinence in children. J. Urol., *135*:533, 1986.
3. McGuire, E.J., Wang, C.C., Usitalo, H., and Savastano, J.: Modified pubovaginal sling in girls with myelodysplasia. J. Urol., *135*:94, 1986.
4. Barrett, D.M., and Furlow, W.L.: The management of severe urinary incontinence in patients with myelodysplasia by implantation of the AS791/792 urinary sphincter devise. J. Urol., *128*:44, 1982.

769-B *(Campbell's, p. 1646)*

Sexuality in the myelodysplasia population is becoming an increasingly important issue to deal with as more and more individuals are reaching adulthood and wanting to either marry or have meaningful long-term relationships with the opposite sex. In one study, researchers interviewed a group of teenagers and reported that at least 28 per cent of them had one or more sexual encounters, whereas almost all had a desire to marry and ultimately bear children. Another study revealed that 70 per cent of myelodysplastic women were able to get pregnant and have an uneventful pregnancy and delivery, although urinary incontinence in the latter stages of gestation and cesarean section were common in many. In the same study, 17 per cent of males claimed they were able to father children but it is more likely for males to have problems with erectile and ejaculatory function because of the frequent neurologic involvement of the sacral spinal cord. Reproductive function in the female, which is under hormonal control, is not affected.

Sexual maturation of myelodysplastic boys and girls also differs somewhat. Boys reach puberty at an age similar to that for normal males. In the female, however, breast development and menarche start as much as 2 years earlier than usual. The etiology of this hormonal surge is uncertain, but it may be related to pituitary function changes in girls secondary to their hydrocephalus.

REFERENCES

1. Cromer, B.A., Enrile, B., McCoy, K., et al.: Knowledge, attitudes and behavior related to sexuality in adolescents with chronic disability. Dev. Med. Child Neurol., *32*:602, 1990.
2. Cass, A.S., Bloom, B.A., and Luxenberg, M.: Sexual function in adults with myelomeningocele. J. Urol., *136*:425, 1986.
3. Hayden, P.: Adolescents with meningomyelocele. Pediatr. Rev., *6*:245, 1985.

770-E *(Campbell's, pp. 1646–1648; Fig. 42–15)*

Certain congenital defects affect the formation of the spinal column but do not result in an open vertebral canal. These lesions may have no outward signs, but in more than 90 per cent of these children, a cutaneous abnormality overlying the lower spine is found. This abnormality may vary from a small dimple or skin tag to a tuft of hair, a dermal vascular malformation, or a very noticeable subcutaneous lipoma. When these children are evaluated in the newborn or early infancy period, the majority have a perfectly normal neurologic examination. Urodynamic testing is also generally normal but will reveal abnormal lower urinary tract function in about one third of the babies under the age of 1 1/2 years. In contrast, practically all individuals over 3 years of age who have not been operated on or who have been belatedly diagnosed as having occult dysraphism will have an upper motor neuron lesion or a lower motor neuron lesion on urodynamic testing (92 per cent), neurologic signs of lower extremity dysfunction, or absent perineal sensation and back pain.

REFERENCES

1. James, C.M., and Lassman, L.P.: Spinal dysraphism: Spinal bifida occulta. E. Norwalk, CT, Appleton-Lange, 1972.
2. Anderson, F.M.: Occult spinal dysraphism: A series of 73 cases. Pediatrics, *55*:826, 1975.
3. Keating, M.A., Rink, R.C., Bauer, S.B., et al.: Neurourologic implications of changing approach in management of occult spinal lesions. J. Urol., *140*:1299, 1988.
4. Yip, C.M., Leach, G.E., Rosenfeld, D.S., et al.: Delayed diagnosis of voiding dysfunction: Occult spinal dysraphism. J. Urol., *124*:694, 1985.

771-D *(Campbell's, pp. 1648–1649; Fig. 42–18)*

As stated earlier, newborns with occult spinal dysraphism generally have a normal neurologic examination, but one third will have abnormal lower urinary tract function on urodynamic testing. If affected children are identified and treated with laminectomy, removal of the intraspinal process, and release of any cord tether, stabilization and improvement of neurologic abnormalities may occur. In children without detectable abnormality, early intervention will give a degree of protection from subsequent cord tethering, which seems to be a frequent occurrence when the lesion is not treated expeditiously in infancy. Consequently, in addition to MRI, urodynamic testing should be conducted in everyone who has a questionable skin or bony abnormality of the lower spine. This combination provides an anatomic and functional evaluation of the lower cord, thereby maximizing the chance of detecting a significant cord lesion.

REFERENCES

1. Foster, L.S., Kogan, B.A., Cogan, P.H., and Edwards, M.S.B.: Bladder function in patients with lipomyelomeningocele. J. Urol., *143*:984, 1990.
2. Tami, S., Yamada, S., and Knighton, R.S.: Extensibility of the lumbar and sacral cord: Pathophysiology of the tethered cord in cats. J. Neurosurg., *66*:116, 1987.
3. Campobasso, P., Galiani, E., Verzerio, A., et al.: A rare cause of occult neuropathic bladder in children: The tethered cord syndrome. Pediatr. Med. Chir., *10*:641, 1988.
4. Hall, W.A., Albright, A.L., and Brunberg, J.A.: Diagnosis of tethered cord by magnetic resonance imaging. Surg. Neurol., *30*(Suppl. 1):60, 1988.

772-B *(Campbell's, pp. 1649–1651; Figs. 42–19, 42–20, 42–21)*

Sacral agenesis has been defined as absence of part or all of two or more lower vertebral bodies. The etiology of this condition is still uncertain, but teratogenic factors may play a role because insulin-dependent mothers have a 1 per cent chance of giving birth to a child with this disorder. Conversely, 16 per cent of children with sacral agenesis have an affected mother. Oftentimes, the mothers may only have gestational insulin-dependent diabetes. The disease was reproduced in chicks when their embryos were exposed to insulin. Maternal insulin-antibody complexes have been noted to cross the placenta, and their concentration in the fetal circulation is directly correlated with macrosomia. It is possible that a similar cause-and-effect phenomenon is occurring in sacral agenesis.

REFERENCES

1. Guzman, L., Bauer, S.B., Hallet, M., et al.: The evaluation and management of children with sacral agenesis. Urology, *23*:506, 1983.
2. Passarge, E., and Lenz, K.: Syndrome of caudal regression in infants of diabetic mothers: Observations of further cases. Pediatrics, *37*:672, 1966.
3. White, R.I., and Klauber, G.T.: Sacral agenesis: Analysis of twenty-two cases. Urology, *8*:521, 1976.
4. Menon, R.K., Cohen, R.M., Sperling, M.A., et al.: Transplacental passage of insulin in pregnant women with insulin-dependent diabetes mellitus. N. Engl. J. Med., *323*:309, 1990.

773-C *(Campbell's, pp. 1650–1653; Fig. 42–23)*

Imperforate anus is a condition that can occur alone or as part of a constellation of anomalies that has been called the VATER or VACTERL syndrome. This mnemonic stands for all the organs that can possibly be affected. V = vertebral, A = anal, C = cardiac, TE = tracheoesophageal fistula, R = renal, and L = limb. Urinary incontinence is not common unless the spinal cord is involved or the pelvic floor muscles and/or nerves are injured during the imperforate anus repair. A VCUG and an ultrasound of the spine and kidneys are obtained in the neonatal period in all children, regardless of the level of rectal atresia, once the child has either stabilized or had a colostomy performed. As with occult dysraphism, any hint of abnormality on these studies or the presence of a lower midline skin lesion overlying the spine warrants an MRI and, if the radiologic images demonstrate an abnormality, urodynamic studies. These studies serve two functions: (1) they provide a reason to explore and treat any intraspinal abnormality in order to improve the child's chances at becoming continent of both feces and urine, and (2) they provide a baseline for comparison if incontinence should become a problem in the future.

REFERENCES

1. Barry, J.E., and Auldist, A.W.P: The Vater syndrome. Am. J. Dis. Child., *128*:769, 1974.
2. Karrer, F.M., Flannerty, A.M., Nelson, M.D. Jr., et al.: Anal rectal malformations: Evaluation of associated spinal dysraphic syndromes. J. Pediatr. Surg., *23*:45, 1988.
3. Tunnel, W.P., Austin, J.C., Barnes, T.P., and Reynolds, A.: Neuroradiologic evaluation of sacral abnormalities in imperforate anus complex. J. Pediatr. Surg., *22*:58, 1987.
4. Barnes, P.D., Lester, P.D., Yamanashi, W.S., and Prince, J.R.: MRI in infants and children with spinal dysraphism. Am. J. Radiol., *147*:339, 1986.

774-C *(Campbell's, pp. 1652–1654; Tables 42–6, 42–7, and 42–8)*

Cerebral palsy is a nonprogressive injury to the brain in the perinatal period that produces a neuromuscular disability or a specific symptom complex of cerebral dysfunction. Its incidence is approximately 1.5 per 1000 births but may be increasing because many smaller and younger premature infants are surviving in intensive care units. It is usually due to a perinatal infection or a period of anoxia or hypoxia that affects the central nervous system. Despite having delayed gross motor development, abnormal fine motor performance, altered muscle tone, abnormal stress gait, and exaggerated deep tendon reflexes, most children with cerebral palsy develop total urinary control. Often times continence is achieved at a later than expected age. Urodynamic evaluation is reserved for children who appear trainable and do not seem to be hampered too much by their physical impairment, but who have not achieved continence by late childhood or early puberty. In a study of 57 patients with cerebral palsy undergoing urodynamic evaluation, 86 per cent had a picture of partial upper motor neuron type of dysfunction with exaggerated sacral reflexes, detrusor hyperreflexia, and/or detrusor-sphincter dyssynergia, even though they manifested voluntary control over voiding. Around 11 per cent, however, may show evidence of both upper and lower motor neuron denervation with detrusor areflexia or abnormal motor unit potentials on sphincter EMG.

REFERENCES

1. Naeye, R.I., Peters, E.C., Bartholomew, M., and Landis, R.: Origins of cerebral palsy. Am. J. Dis. Child., *143*:1154, 1989.
2. Nelson, K.B., and Ellenberg, J.H.: Antecedents of cerebral palsy. N. Engl. J. Med., *315*:81, 1986.
3. Decter, R.M., Bauer, S.B., Khoshbin, S., et al.: Urodynamic assessment of children with cerbral palsy. J. Urol., *138*:1110, 1987.

775-A *(Campbell's, pp. 1654–1655)*

Traumatic spinal injuries are rarely encountered in children. When an injury does occur, it is most likely to happen as a result of a motor vehicle accident, a gunshot wound, or a diving accident. It has also occurred iatrogenically following surgery to correct scoliosis, kyphosis, or other intraspinal processes as well as congenital aortic anomalies or patent ductus arteriosus. Newborns are particularly prone to hyperextension injuries during high forceps delivery. The lower urinary tract dysfunction that ensues is not likely to be an isolated event; rather, it is usually associated with loss of sensation and paralysis of the lower limbs. Radiologic investigation of the spine may not reveal any bony abnormality even though momentary subluxation of osseus structures due to elasticity of vertebral ligaments can result in neurologic injury. Myelography and computed tomography (CT) will show swelling of the cord below the level of the lesion. The lesions will often be transient and although sensation and motor function in the lower extremities may be restored relatively soon, the dysfunction involving the bladder and rectum may persist for a considerable period of time.

If urodynamic evaluation is performed in these patients, differing results will be found in the immediate postinjury period from those found in later evaluation. Immediately after the injury, a period of spinal shock ensues and results in a lower motor neuron type lesion with detrusor areflexia. Most cases resolve completely as edema of the cord in response to the injury subsides, leaving no permanent damage. Most permanent traumatic injuries, when they occur, will result in an upper motor neuron type lesion resulting in detrusor hyperreflexia and detrusor-sphincter dysergia.

REFERENCES

1. Adams, C., Babyn, P.S., and Logan, W.J.: Spinal cord birth injury: Value of computed tomographic nyelography. Pediatr. Neurol., *4*:109, 1988.
2. Pollack, J.F., Pang, D., and Sclabassi, R.: Recurrent spinal cord injury without radiographic abnormalities in children. J. Neurosurg., *69*:177, 1988.
3. Iwatsubo, E., Iwakawa, A., Koga, H., et al.: Functional recovery of the bladder in patients with spinal cord injury-prognosticating programs of an aseptic intermittent catheterization. Acta Urol., Japonica, *31*: 775, 1985.
4. Fanciullacci, F., Zanollo, A., Sandri, S., and Catanzaro, F.: The neuropathic bladder in children with spinal cord injury. Paraplegia, *26*:83, 1988.

776-A *(Campbell's, p. 1655)*

Enuresis is defined as inappropriate voiding at an age when urinary control is expected. The evaluation of the incontinent child is detailed in Chapter 41, but briefly it begins with a comprehensive history and physical examination, a detailed neurologic examination, and characterization of the wetting episodes. Further studies will be indicated based on the results of this initial evaluation. The indications for performing urodynamic studies are as follows: any suspicion of a neurologic condition, diurnal incontinence with no associated pathology, nocturnal enuresis in a pubertal child who is resistant to conventional therapy, fecal and urinary incontinence at any age, persistent voiding difficulties long after an infection has been treated, recurrent urinary tract infection despite continuous antibiotics, and bladder trabeculation or "sphincter spasm" on voiding cystography. A girl who voids normally but is constantly damp both day and night should be evaluated for an ectopic ureter. Thus an excretory urogram or renal ultrasound should be performed instead of urodynamics.

777-B *(Campbell's, pp. 1656–1657; Fig. 42–27)*

An inflammatory reaction in the bladder wall may produce irritability that affects the sensory threshold and increases the need to void sooner than anticipated. If the detrusor muscle is affected as well, the increased irritability may lead to instability of the muscle and eventually to poor compliance. When the child attempts to hold back urination because it is either painful or inappropriate to void, he or she may actually tighten, or partially or intermittently relax the external sphincter during voiding, producing a form of outflow obstruction and disrupting the laminar flow pattern that normally exists.

Start-and-stop voiding leads to recurrent infection because bacteria can be carried back up into the bladder from the meatus as a result of the "milk back" phenomenon occurring within the urethra when urination is interrupted in this manner. Theoretically, if unrecognized or left untreated in young girls, this condition may become the forerunner of interstitial cystitis seen in many adult females.

REFERENCES

1. Mayo, M.E., and Burns, M.W.: Urodynamic studies in children who wet. Br. J. Urol., *65*:641, 1990.
2. Hansson, S., Hjalmas, K., Jodal, U., and Sixt, R.: Lower urinary tract dysfunction in girls with untreated asymptomatic or covert bacteriuria. J. Urol., *143*:333, 1990.
3. VanGool, J.D., and Tanagho, E.A.: External sphincter activity and recurrent urinary tract infection in girls. Urology, *10*:348, 1977.
4. Webster, G.D., Koefoot, R.B., and Sihelnik, S.: Urodynamic abnormalities in neurologically normal children with micturition dysfunction. J. Urol., *132*:74, 1984.

778-D *(Campbell's, p. 1657)*

Detrusor hyperreflexia may be the cause of diurnal enuresis in some children. During bladder filling, capacity may be reached sooner than expected, at which time a normal detrusor contraction occurs with a sustained relaxation of the sphincter and complete emptying of the bladder. Some children will not be able to suppress this contraction even though the bladder has not been filled to capacity. These findings may be the result of a cerebral insult, however mild, in the neonatal period; but, more commonly, they are linked to delayed maturation of the reticulospinal pathways and the inhibitory centers in the mid-brain and cerebral cortex. On occasion, children with profound constipation develop uninhibited contractions of the bladder and urinary incontinence secondary to them. The etiology of this condition is unclear, but treatment of the bowel distention has resulted in a dramatic improvement in the bladder dysfunction.

REFERENCES

1. MacKeith, R.L., Meadow, S.R., and Turner, R.K.: How children become dry. *In* Kolvin, I., MacKeith, R.L., Meadow, S.R. (Eds.): Bladder Control and Enuresis. Philadelphia, J.B. Lippincott Co., 1973, pp. 3–15.
2. Yeats, W.K.: Bladder function is normal micturition. *In* Kolvin, I., MacKeith, R.C., and Meadow, S.R. (Eds.): Bladder Control and Enuresis. Philadelphia, J.B. Lippincott Co., 1973, pp. 28–41.
3. O'Regan, S., Yazbeck, S., and Schick, E.: Constipation, unstable bladder, urinary tract infection syndrome. Clin. Nephrol., *5*:154, 1985.
4. O'Regan, S., Yazbeck, S., Hamburger, B., and Schick, E.: Constipation: A commonly unrecognized cause of enuresis. Am. J. Dis. Child., *140*:260, 1986.

779-E *(Campbell's, p. 1657)*

Children with long-standing symptoms of daytime frequency, urgency, or sudden incontinence and squatting, in addition to nocturia and/or enuresis, may have detrusor hyperreflexia. Vincent's curtsy, characteristic posturing by these children in an attempt to prevent voiding, is a commonly described behavior pattern. Oftentimes, the child's parents or siblings relate a history of delayed control over micturition. The child's physical examination may be normal, but hyperactive deep tendon reflexes in the lower or upper extremities, ankle clonus, posturing with a stress gait, or difficulty with tandem walking or mirror movements (similar motion in the contralateral hand when the individual is asked to rapidly pronate and supinate one hand) may be evident. X-ray evaluation usually reveals no abnormality other than a mildly trabeculated or thick-walled bladder. Urodynamic studies demonstrate uninhibited contractions of the bladder during filling, which the child may or may not sense or abolish by increasing the activity of the external urethral sphincter.

REFERENCES

1. Kondo, A., Kobayashi, M., Otani, T., et al.: Children with unstable bladder: Clinical and urodynamic observation. J. Urol., *129*:88, 1983.
2. Vincent, S.A.: Postural control of urinary incontinence: The curtsy sign. Lancet., *2*:631, 1966.
3. Bauer, S.B., Retik, A.B., Colodny, A.H., et al.: The unstable bladder of childhood. Urol. Clin. North Am., *7*: 321, 1980.
4. Rudy, D.C., and Woodside, J.R.: Non-neurogenic bladder: The relationship between intravesical pressure and the external sphincter EMG: Neurourol. Urodynam., *10*:169–176, 1991.

780-C *(Campbell's, pp. 1659–1660; Figs. 42–30, 42–31)*

Most children void four to five times per day and defecate daily or at least every other day. Some children, primarily girls, may void only twice a day, once in the morning and again at night. These children have learned to withhold micturition for extended periods of time. Often they only void enough to relieve the pressure to urinate and do not empty their bladder completely. The infrequent voiding and incomplete emptying produce an ever-increasing bladder capacity and a diminished stimulus to urinate. Often the problem is diagnosed following a voiding cystourethrogram when a larger-than-normal capacity (for age) is noted and the residual urine volume on initial catheterization is measured. In addition, cystogram usually reveals a smooth-walled bladder without reflux.

Urodynamic studies demonstrate a very large capacity, highly compliant bladder. Sphincter EMG reveals normal motor unit potentials at rest and normal responses to various sacral reflexes, bladder filling, and attempts at emptying. The urinary flow rate may be intermittent with sudden peaks coinciding with straining, or it may be normal but short-lived secondary to an unsustained detrusor contraction. Unless strongly encouraged, the child will not completely empty his or her bladder during voiding.

REFERENCES

1. DeLuca, F.G., Swenson, O., Fisher, J.H., and Loutfi, A.H.: The dysfunctional "lazy" bladder syndrome in children. Arch. Dis. Child., *37*:117, 1962.
2. Webster, G.D., Koefoot, R.B., and Sihelnik, S.: Urodynamic abnormalities in neurologically normal children with micturition dysfunction. J. Urol., *132*:74, 1984.
3. Bauer, S.B., Retik, A.B., Colodny, A.H., et al.: The unstable bladder of childhood. Urol. Clin. North Am., *7*: 321, 1980.

781-A *(Campbell's, pp. 1661–1664; Fig. 42–32, 42–33)*

Some children have an apparent "syndrome" of voiding dysfunction that mimics neuropathic bladder disease, but which may be a learned disorder. It is produced by active contraction of the sphincter during voiding, which creates a degree of outflow obstruction. These children have urgency, urge and/or stress incontinence, infrequent voluntary voiding, intermittent urination associated with straining, recurrent urinary tract infection, and irregular bowel movements with fecal soilage in-between times. What is most striking is the similarity in the pattern of family dynamics. The parents, especially the father, tend to be domineering, exacting, unyielding, and intolerant of weakness or failure.

Radiologic evaluation reveals profound changes within the urinary tract. Hydroureteronephrosis with or without pyelonephritic scarring from recurrent infection occurs in two thirds of children. About 50 per cent have severe vesicoureteral reflux. Nearly every child has a grossly trabeculated, large-capacity bladder with a considerable post void residual urine volume. Spinal canal imaging with magnetic resonance has failed to reveal any intraspinal processes as a cause for the voiding dysfunction in these children.

REFERENCES

1. Bauer, S.B., Retik, A.B., Colodny, A.H., et al.: The unstable bladder of childhood. Urol. Clin. North Am., *7*: 321, 1980.
2. Allen, T.D., and Bright, T.C.: Urodynamic patterns in children with dysfunctional voiding problems. J. Urol., *119*:247, 1978.
3. Hinman, F.: Non-neurogenic bladder (the Hinman Syndrome) fifteen years later. J. Urol., *136*:769, 1986.

782-D *(Campbell's, pp. 1669–1670)*

The most reliable urine specimens are obtained in infants and small children by suprapubic aspiration. Bag specimens usually reflect perineal and rectal flora and usually are helpful only if the culture is negative. It is difficult to obtain a midstream specimen in this age group. Urethral catheterization is better than the bag specimen but may introduce some urethra flora into the bladder with this. The suprapubic aspiration is performed by introducing a 21-gauge needle 1 to 2 cm above the pubic symphysis until the bladder is entered.

783-B *(Campbell's, p. 1670)*

Urinary tract infections in children are all complicated by definition. They are categorized as either first infection, unresolved bacteriuria during therapy, bacterial persistence at an anatomic site, and reinfections. Periurethral colonization is not a reason for urinary tract infection to persist, although it does contribute to recurrent infections. Inadequate therapy and bacterial resistance will result in persistent infections. Inadequate urinary drug concentrations due to poor renal concentration or GI absorption also result in persistent infection. Multiple organisms are also difficult to eradicate. Usually, a persistent infection can be effectively treated by choosing the appropriate antibiotic after cultine and sensitivity studies.

784-A *(Campbell's, p. 1670)*

Urinary tract infections are more common in boys than girls during the first few months of life. Otherwise they are more common in girls of all age groups. Bacteriuria is present in about 2 per cent of boys in their first year of life and 0.7 per cent in girls. After that the ratio is reversed and it is more common in girls.

785-A *(Campbell's, pp. 1670–1672)*

Host factors contributing to bacteriuria include periurethral colonization, age, immune status, blood group antigen receptors, reflux, sex, and genitourinary anomalies. The P1 blood group antigen as well as ABO, Lewis, and secretor phenotypes all appear to increase the risk of urinary tract infection and bacteriuria. Reflux and any other anomalies also have a higher incidence of bacteriuria. Children with recurrent UTI and bacteriuria have lower urinary concentration in secretory IgA than others. P-fimbriae are markers of bacterial virulence and are related to the infecting organism rather than to the host.

786-C *(Campbell's, p. 1672)*

It is very difficult clinically to differentiate cystitis from pyelonephritis in children. Of patients presenting with flank pain and fever, only 46 per cent had upper tract infection. When patients had bladder symptoms, 15 per cent still had upper tract infections. Additionally, 17.5 per cent of asymptomatic bacteriuria was localized to the upper tracts. A fever greater than 38°C is the best correlated sign or symptom, although it does not correlate strongly either. Therefore, the entire clinical picture must be looked at and a judgment decision made in most cases.

787-E *(Campbell's, pp. 1672–1673)*

There are five grades of reflux according to the international reflux study classification: Grade I, reflux into the ureter only; Grade II, into ureter renal pelvis and calices; Grade III, dilatation of ureter and renal pelvis with no or minimal forniceal blunting; Grade IV, moderate dilatation of the ureter and pelvis with blunting of the formices; Grade V, gross dilation of the ureter and pelvis with absence of the papillary impression. Reflux probably occurs because of more lateral position of the orifice and a short submucosal tunnel. It may also be affected by immature bladder dynamics. The incidence is 0.4 to 1.8 per cent in asymptomatic patients and the incidence decreases with age.

788-D *(Campbell's, p. 1673)*

Twenty-one to fifty-seven per cent of children with bacteriuria subsequently are found to have reflux. This generally resolves with age and conservative therapy. When infections are prevented, 87 per cent of Grade I, 63 per cent at Grade II, 53 per cent of Grade III, and 33 per cent of Grade IV reflux will resolve over a 3-year time period.

789-C *(Campbell's, pp. 1674–1675)*

The combination of vesicourcteral reflux and bacteriuria can result in renal scarring. Seventeen per cent of children with bacteriuria on screening urine cultures have renal scarring. Scarring may occur with symptomatic or asymptomatic infections at the same rate. About 60 per cent of children with renal scarring will have vesicoureteral reflux. The higher the grade of reflux, the greater the risk of scarring. Children under 5 years are particularly vulnerable to scarring. After 10 years of age, infections are rarely associated with scarring. If early antibiotic therapy is initiated within the first few days, the acute suppurative response to bacteria is prevented and renal scarring occurs less often.

790-E *(Campbell's, p. 1675)*

When infection and reflux occur together, the four factors which influence development of renal scarring are: intrarenal reflux, the pressure or water-hammer effect of reflux, host immune response to infection and reflux, and the individual's age. Females are more likely to have infections and reflux, although once infection and reflux are present, there is no difference between the sexes as far as who develops scars.

791-C *(Campbell's, p. 1676)*

Hypertension develops in 10 to 20 per cent of children with reflux uropathy. This occurs regardless of the degree of scarring present. The etiology is not well understood and is felt to be most likely related to the renin-angiotensin system.

792-D *(Campbell's, pp. 1676–1677)*

If there is significant injury to the kidneys, then progressive renal deterioration may develop. This may occur despite the fact that there are no further urinary tract infections. Proteinuria greater than 1 g per day is strongly correlated with progressive deterioration in renal function. Theories implicate progressive renal damage from hyperfiltration by the remaining nephrons, or progressive immunologic damage to the kidney by an autoimmune mechanism involving Tamm-Horsfall protein. The progressive renal damage may occur long after reflux or infections have ceased.

793-D *(Campbell's, pp. 1677–1678)*

The prevalence of bacteriuria in pregnant women is the same as that in nonpregnant women. If bacteriuria is left untreated in pregnant women, the incidence of pyelonephritis developing is between 13 and 65 per cent. The incidence of pyelonephritis may be related to the development of hydronephrosis, which is secondary to mechanical obstruction and possibly to elevated progesterone levels causing smooth muscle atony of the urinary tract. Pregnant patients with reflux probably have similar incidences of pyelonephritis during pregnancy when compared to patients without reflux. There is no strong evidence that reflux prior to conception increases the incidence of pyelonephritis during pregnancy.

794-A *(Campbell's, p. 1679)*

Children may develop hemorrhagic cystitis with frequency, urgency, and dysuria. It is commonly associated adenovirus 11 and *E. coli*. Urine cultures show no growth in 60 per cent, adenovirus 11 in 14 per cent, adenovirus 21 in 3 per cent, and *E. coli* in 17 per cent. Radiographic work-up should still be done for hematuria to eliminate other causes in these cases.

795-E *(Campbell's, p. 1681)*

Prophylactic agents ideally should have low serum levels with high urinary levels and minimal effect on the fecal flora. They should cover the common organisms causing urinary tract infections and should be well tolerated and low in cost. Nitrofurantoin has been used for a long period of time in doses of 1 to 2 mg/kg once a day. Side effects include acute allergic pneumonitis, neuropathy, and liver damage. Long-term problems have been associated with pulmonary fibrosis. It should not be used in children with glucose-6-phosphate dehydrogenase deficiency as it can cause hemolysis. Cephalexin used in doses of 1/4 teaspoon/kg per day is very effective prophylaxis. Trimethoprim is unique in that it is secreted into the vaginal fluid and decreases vaginal colonization. It should not be given in the first few months of life as it can cause hyperbilirubinemia. Nalidixic acid or other quinolones are not recommended in children because of the potential interference with cartilage development.

796-B *(Campbell's, pp. 1681–1682)*

Renal scarring can take up to 2 years to evolve after an episode of pyelonephritis. Therefore, if the patient has remained infection free yet some scarring develops in this time period, it would still be reasonable to continue medical therapy. Multiple breakthrough infections while on prophylaxis, poor compliance with medical therapy, no resolution of reflux after many years on prophylaxis, necessary open bladder surgery for other reasons, or significant progression of renal scarring while on prophylaxis are all reasons to proceed with surgical therapy for reflux.

PART XI

PEDIATRIC UROLOGIC SURGERY

CHAPTERS 44 THROUGH 54

DIRECTIONS: Each question below contains suggested responses. Select the ONE BEST response to each question.

797. Which of the following statements concerning the ureterovesical junction is *false*?
   A. The ureter is composed of longitudinal and spiral muscle fibers; at the ureteral hiatus of the bladder only the spiral muscle fibers continue into the intravesical ureter.
   B. As the intravesical ureteral muscle fibers pass from the hiatus to its orifice, the fibers decussate, passing medially to form Mercier's bar and inferiorly to form Bell's muscle (the borders of the superficial trigone).
   C. The adventitia of juxtavesical ureter has a superficial and deep periureteral sheath, the superficial derived from the bladder and the deep derived from the ureter.
   D. A plane of cleavage called the space of Waldeyer separates the superficial and deep periureteral sheaths.

798. The most important mechanism preventing vesicoureteral reflux is:
   A. A peristaltic pressure of the extravesical ureter between 25 and 30 mm Hg
   B. A resting pressure in the bladder between 7 and 15 mm Hg is enough to compress the submucosal ureter
   C. The length of the intravesical ureter relative to its diameter
   D. The cystoscopic appearance of the ureteral orifice (cone, stadium, horseshoe, golf hole)

799. Which of the following statements is *false*?
   A. The incidence of reflux in healthy children is less than 1 per cent.
   B. Reflux is found in 30 per cent of siblings of children with known reflux.
   C. Reflux is 10 times more common in white female infants than black female infants.
   D. Reflux has an autosomal dominant mode of inheritance.

800. Match the following grades of reflux to the corresponding (International Grading System):
   A. Grade I
   B. Grade II
   C. Grade III
   D. Grade IV
   E. Grade V

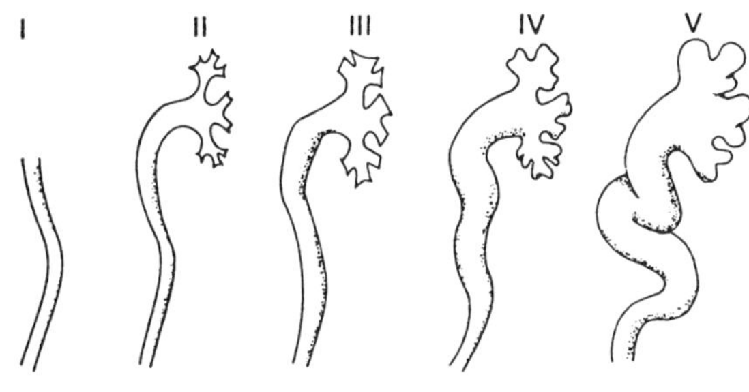

801. Relative indications for early surgery for reflux include all of the following EXCEPT:
   A. Grade IV–V reflux
   B. A lateral, golf hole, or horseshoe orifice with a short (2–5 mm) or absent intravesical ureter
   C. Noncompliance with long-term prophylactic antibiotics
   D. Recurrent infection or progressive renal scarring
   E. Clinical presentation of reflux after reaching the teen years

802. Which one of the following statements is *false*?
   A. An abnormal ureteral bud site on the wolffian duct may result in obstruction and abnormal development or dysgenesis.
   B. The position at which the ureteral bud contacts the metanephric blastema determines the quality of the kidney that results (normal vs. dysplastic).
   C. Only refluxing units with abnormal orifice sites contain dysplastic elements.
   D. Sterile reflux is the primary cause of renal scarring.
   E. Primary reflux is determined by the site of the ureteral bud formed at 4 weeks gestation.

803. All the following are associated with, cause, or serve as a marker for reflux nephropathy EXCEPT:
   A. Intrarenal reflux
   B. Phagocytosis of bacteria by neutrophils with liberation of toxic superoxide
   C. Tamm-Horsfall protein
   D. Sterile vesicoureteral reflux
   E. Infected urine with vesicouretheral reflux

804. Which of the following is not associated with secondary reflux or a known predisposition for reflux?
   A. Urethral valve

B. Neurogenic bladder
C. Ureteral duplication
D. Bladder infection (cystitis)

805. Which statement concerning the resolution/persistence of reflux is *false*?

A. The rate of resolution of reflux is about 20 per cent in each 2-year period throughout childhood.
B. Reflux is more likely to resolve in those without recurrent infections.
C. If the submucosal tunnel (intravesical ureter) is 5 mm or greater, there is a 55 to 60 per cent chance that reflux will resolve spontaneously.
D. About 15 per cent of cases with refluxing submucosal tunnel <2 mm will resolve spontaneously.

806. Which of the following statements is *false*?

A. Chronic glomerulonephritis is the most common finding in hypertensive children followed in frequency by pyelonephritic scarring.
B. Hypertension is not necessarily related to renal failure but is probably associated with vascular lesions within the kidney.
C. Elimination of reflux prior to development of focal scars protects against the possible future development of hypertension.
D. Hypertension is not caused by nor associated with pyelonephritic scarring if the peripheral renin activity is low.
E. Removal of a scarred renal segment cures hypertension in many cases.

807. In the female with an ectopic ureter, all of the following statements are true EXCEPT:

A. Incontinence may be seen.
B. Ectopic ureters are more commonly seen with a single renal unit (i.e., no ureteral duplication).
C. Ectopic ureters may empty into the bladder neck, proximal urethra, distal urethra, or vestibule.
D. Ectopic ureter may insert into müllerian structures, such as the cervix or uterus.

808. All of the following statements are true concerning the presentation and evaluation of ectopic ureters EXCEPT:

A. The most common presentation is urinary tract infection.
B. Ectopic ureters can present with abdominal mass or hydronephrosis on antenatal ultrasound.
C. Reflux may be demonstrated into an ipsilateral lower pole ureter, and the ectopic ureter may reflux during active voiding occasionally.
D. IVP may show the "classic" drooping lilly lower pole renal unit with 10 to 12 calyces.
E. IVP will usually show a functioning but dilated upper pole segment and identify the site of ureteral opening/insertion.

809. The most appropriate treatment for ectopic ureter with very poorly functioning upper pole segment and grade II lower pole ureteral reflux is:

A. Upper pole nephrectomy and partial ureterectomy leaving the ureteral stump open after it is decompressed.
B. Same as A, but with lower pole ureteral reimplantation.
C. Observation with suppressive antibiotics.
D. Upper pole nephrectomy and complete excision of upper pole ureter.
E. Reimplantation of upper and lower pole ureters together with a common sheath reimplantation.

810. Which of the following statements concerning ectopic ureters in boys is *false*?

A. The most common presentation is with urinary tract infection.
B. Ectopic ureter commonly presents with continuous incontinence without sphincter abnormality.
C. The ectopic ureter will open into the proximal urethra (not distal to the veramontanum), bladder neck, seminal vesicle, vas deferens, or, rarely, the rectum.
D. Ectopic ureter is more common in girls than boys, but is more often associated with a single renal unit/ureter in boys.
E. Boys with ectopic ureters may present with epididymoorchitis.

811. The rare finding of bilateral single system ectopic ureters can be associated with all of the following EXCEPT:

A. Agenesis of the bladder and urethra
B. Bilateral dysplastic kidneys
C. Dilated, refluxing ureters
D. A wide, poorly defined, incompetent bladder neck and sphincter
E. A large volume, poorly contractile bladder that often empties poorly

812. All of the following statements concerning ureteroceles are true EXCEPT:

A. Ureteroceles may be orthotopic or ectopic.
B. Ectopic ureteroceles are more common in females than males.
C. Ureteroceles may prolapse into the urethra and cause bladder outlet obstruction.
D. Ureteroceles are always obstructing.
E. A ureterocele is a cystic dilatation of the terminal ureter within the bladder, urethra, or both.

813. A cecoureterocele is a:

A. Wide-mouthed ureterocele
B. Ureterocele that empties into the cecum or colon
C. Ureterocele where the ureteral lumen extends distal to the ureteral orifice beneath the submucosa
D. Blind-ending ureterocele without a demonstrable ureteral orifice

814. The radiographic evaluation of ureteroceles should always include which TWO of the following studies?

A. MRI
B. IVP
C. Ultrasound
D. VCUG
E. CT scan

815. The initial treatment in most children with small ectopic ureteroceles associated with a nonfunctioning or poorly visualized upper renal segment should include which one of the following?

A. Upper pole nephrectomy and complete ureterectomy
B. Upper pole nephrectomy and complete ureterectomy if there is low-grade reflux into the ipsilateral lower pole ureter
C. Observation on prophylactic antibiotics
D. Upper pole nephrectomy and partial ureterectomy decompressing the ureterocele and leaving the distal ureter open
E. Upper pole nephrectomy and total ureterectomy with lower pole ureteral reimplantation

816. In rare cases of ureterocele where upper pole function appears good, consideration should be given to all of the following procedures EXCEPT:

A. Ureteroureterostomy with partial ureterectomy
B. Pyeloureterostomy with partial ureterectomy
C. Excision of ureterocele and common sheath reimplantation, especially if significant (high-grade) lower pole ipsilateral reflux is present
D. Total nephroureterectomy

817. All of the following statements are true about the exstrophy–epispadias complex EXCEPT:

A. Prenatal ultrasound findings of an empty bladder, low-set umbilicus, and a mass of echogenic tissue overlying the lower abdominal wall are suggestive of classic bladder exstrophy.
B. Infants born with bladder exstrophy and epispadias are generally sickly, premature babies with numerous coexisting anomalies.
C. Bladder exstrophy and epispadias affect more males than females.
D. Infants of younger mothers tend to develop bladder exstrophy more often.
E. Offsprings of individuals with bladder exstrophy have a 500-fold greater risk of inheriting the trait than the general population.

818. Which statement concerning the embryology of bladder development is *false*?

A. In the exstrophy–epispadias complex, abnormal overdevelopment of the cloacal membrane prevents medial mesodermal ingrowth and results in impaired abdominal wall development, pubic diastasis, and failed medial fusion of the genital tubercles.
B. Downgrowth of the urorectal septum divides the cloaca into a urogenital sinus anteriorly and anorectal canal posteriorly.
C. The cloacal membrane is a bilaminar layer composed of endoderm and mesoderm.
D. At 5 weeks of gestation, the cloacal membrane reaches its greatest dimension, then regresses in size thereafter.
E. Mesenchymal ingrowth between the layers of the cloacal membrane results in the formation of the lower abdominal muscles and the pelvic bones.

819. The incidence of bladder exstrophy is between ____ and ____ live births:

A. 1 in 1,000 and 1 in 5,000
B. 1 in 5,000 and 1 in 10,000
C. 1 in 10,000 and 1 in 50,000
D. 1 in 50,000 and 1 in 75,000
E. 1 in 100,000 and 1 in 200,000

820. Variants of the exstrophy–epispadias complex include all the following EXCEPT:

A. Prune-belly syndrome
B. Pseudoexstrophy
C. Superior vesical fissure
D. Cloacal exstrophy
E. Duplicate exstrophy

821. Significant urinary tract abnormalities occur in all of the following EXCEPT:

A. Superior vesical fissure
B. Epispadias
C. Classical bladder exstrophy
D. Cloacal exstrophy
E. Pseudoexstrophy

822. Which statement about the skeletal defects characteristic of the exstrophy–epispadias complex is *false*?

A. Pubic diastasis is present in all cases of exstrophy.
B. Lateral, inferior separation of the innominate bones occurs in severe cases of cloacal exstrophy.
C. Outward rotation of the innominate bones is usually the only skeletal abnormality associated with epispadias.
D. The waddling gait develops secondary to internal rotation of the lower extremities and requires orthopedic intervention for correction.
E. Outward rotation of the innominate and pubic bones occurs in cases of classic bladder exstrophy.

823. Which statement regarding male genital defects associated with exstrophy is *true*?

A. The penis is shortened secondary to abnormally short corpora cavernosa.
B. Gender reassignment is necessary in the majority of cases.
C. The cavernous nerves are displaced medially.
D. Fertility is impaired secondary to testicular dysfunction, impotence, and undescended testes.
E. The vas deferens and ejaculatory ducts are normal.

824. Vesicoureteral reflux occurs in nearly ____ of cases after closure of the exstrophied bladder:

A. 10 per cent
B. 25 per cent
C. 50 per cent
D. 75 per cent
E. 100 per cent

825. Primary functional bladder closure is contraindicated in all of the following conditions EXCEPT:

A. Exstrophy with ectopic bowel
B. Exstrophied bladder with 3 ml capacity at birth
C. Small bladder patch with poor elasticity contractility
D. High grade hydronephrosis
E. Penile-scrotal duplication

826. Which statement concerning the use of osteotomies in exstrophy patients is *false*?
   A. The majority of infants undergoing primary bladder closure within 72 hours of birth require an osteotomy.
   B. Disadvantages of the bilateral posterior iliac osteotomy include the need to turn the patient from prone to supine positions intraoperatively and poor mobility of the pubis.
   C. Improved symphyseal approximation reduces midline abdominal closure tension, thus lowering dehiscence rates.
   D. Continence rates are improved when osteotomies are performed at the time of bladder closure.
   E. An osteotomy allows for penile lengthening by bringing the corpora cavernosa closer together.

827. Which statement about primary bladder closure for bladder exstrophy is *false*?
   A. Rotational paraexstrophy skin flaps are used to reconstitute the urethral groove.
   B. Urethral catheterization for 2 weeks postoperatively is mandatory to maintain patency of the neourethra.
   C. The primary goal is to convert exstrophy into complete epispadias with incontinence.
   D. Partial detachment of the corpora cavernosa from the inferior pubic rami facilitates penile lengthening.
   E. A transverse incision of the urethral plate is made when the male urethral groove is of inadequate length.

828. Complications associated with ureterosigmoidostomy include all the following EXCEPT:
   A. Pyelonephritis
   B. Hypochloremic acidosis
   C. Rectal incontinence
   D. Increased malignancy potential
   E. Ureteral obstruction

829. Which statement regarding the association of exstrophy and malignant processes is *false*?
   A. The majority of carcinomas identified in patients with bladder exstrophy is adenocarcinoma.
   B. The exstrophied bladder has a 10× greater potential to undergo malignant degeneration.
   C. The mean latency period for the development of intestinal adenocarcinoma following ureterointestinal anastomosis is 10 years.
   D. Squamous cell carcinoma and rhabdomyosarcoma occur in exstrophied bladders.
   E. Chronic irritation and infection induce metaplastic transformation, including cystitis granularis, a premalignant lesion.

830. Which statement concerning sexual function and fertility in exstrophy patients is *true*?
   A. Cervical and uterine prolapse occur commonly following pregnancy in women with bladder exstrophy.
   B. Libido in the male exstrophy patient is low.
   C. The majority of the exstrophy patients are impotent due to damaged neurovascular bundles.
   D. Following functional bladder closure, the majority of male exstrophy patients demonstrate normal sperm counts.
   E. Spontaneous vaginal delivery is contraindicated in female exstrophy patients.

831. The incidence of cloacal exstrophy ranges between ____ and ____ live births:
   A. 1/10,000, 1/50,000
   B. 1/100,000, 1/200,000
   C. 1/200,000, 1/400,000
   D. 1/500,000, 1/750,000
   E. 1/1,000,000, 1/2,000,000

832. Of the following statements concerning epispadias, which one is *false*?
   A. The incidence in males is 1/117,000 and in females is 1/484,000.
   B. A dorsal chordee is almost always associated with epispadias.
   C. Penile epispadias is the most common form.
   D. Ureterovesical reflux occurs in 30–40 per cent of cases.
   E. Urinary incontinence is greater in penopubic than either glandular or penile epispadias.

833. Which of the following statements concerning congenital bladder diverticula is *false*?
   A. This entity almost always occurs in males.
   B. Ehlers-Danlos syndrome has been associated with it.
   C. Congenital diverticula are usually multiple in nature.
   D. Intravenous urography is not the diagnostic study of choice.
   E. Congenital diverticula are usually larger than those associated with neurogenic bladders or lower tract obstruction.

834. All of the following are true concerning urachal abnormalities EXCEPT:
   A. A large urachal diverticulum is frequently seen in patients with prune-belly syndrome.
   B. Bladder outflow obstruction is usually the cause for an acquired patent urachus.
   C. The malignancy most commonly associated with urachal cyst is adenocarcinoma.
   D. Peritonitis is a potentially serious complication associated with infected urachal cysts.
   E. Adequate therapy for a patent urachus is simple incision and drainage.

835. The organism most commonly cultured from an in fected urachal cyst is:
   A. *Escherichia coli*
   B. *Staphylococcus epidermis*
   C. *Candida albicans*
   D. *Staphylococcus aureus*
   E. *Pseudomonas aeruginosa*

836. All of the following statements are true concerning the embryologic development of the GU tract EXCEPT:
   A. At 5 weeks gestation, the genital, urinary, and gastrointestinal tracts all empty into a common chamber known as the cloaca.
   B. "Cloaca" is the Latin word for sewer.
   C. At the sixth week of gestation, the urorectal septum divides the cloaca into a posterior gastrointestinal canal and an anterior urogenital sinus.

D. The paired paramesonephric ducts give use to the ureteral buds and in males give rise to the epididymis, seminal vesicles, and vas deferens.

837. In females with cloacal abnormalities, the anatomic variations are more complex because:

A. Females tend to present later and develop more early complications.
B. In males, the urorectal convergence tends to be lower or more distal and therefore more easily repaired.
C. Men just don't understand women.
D. In females, the genital tract (uterus, vagina) is interposed between the bladder and rectum and makes for a greater variety and complexity of possible malformations.

838. In females, all of the following locations for entry of the rectum into the cloaca are seen EXCEPT:

A. The posterior margin of the vaginal introitus
B. Anterior to the urogenital sinus on the perineum
C. At the base of the vaginal septum (where one exists)
D. Into the vagina or bladder
E. On the perineum, but anteriorly displaced and separated from the vagina/urogenital sinus by only a thin membrane instead of the normal perineal body

839. Common presentation and findings in a female with severe cloacal deformity usually include all of the following EXCEPT:

A. Abdominal distention
B. Abnormal perineal anatomy
C. Plain film radiographs demonstrating a large fluid filled structure
D. Hydronephrosis on ultrasound
E. Sepsis

840. Components of the initial therapy and subsequent repair of cloacal malformations include all of the following EXCEPT:

A. Early diverting colostomy
B. Urogenital sinus x-rays to evaluate the anatomy of the malformation
C. A thorough endoscopic evaluation under anesthesia
D. Repair of all rectal, vaginal, and urologic abnormalities by 3–6 months of age
E. Intermittent catheterization of the sinus in an attempt to decompress the lower urinary tract

841. Principles of correction for cloacal abnormalities include all of the following EXCEPT:

A. Cloacal preoperative evaluation, including x-ray and endoscopic studies to identify the anatomy
B. Thorough cleansing of the distal limb of the colostomy to prevent gross soilage during reconstruction
C. Waiting until puberty to attempt functional vaginal reconstruction
D. Separation of the urinary, genital, and rectal systems followed by reconstruction to create a separate bladder/urethra, functional vagina (possibly using bowel to bring the vagina to the perineum), and construction of a perineal body with pull through of rectum through perineum and closure of levator ani muscles appropriately around the rectal pull through
E. Complete sterile prep of abdomen/back and lower extremities so that repositioning from prone, lithotomy, supine, and jackknife positions may be used as needed

842. All of the following are part of the "classic" prune-belly syndrome EXCEPT:

A. Congenital absence, deficiency, or hypoplasia of the abdominal musculature
B. Bilateral cryptorchidism
C. Hypospadias
D. Large hypotonic bladder
E. Dilated and tortuous ureters

843. All of the following statements concerning the abdominal wall defect in prune-belly syndrome are true EXCEPT:

A. In older children, the abdominal wall has a characteristic pot belly appearance instead of the classic wrinkled appearance.
B. Surgical repair of the abdominal wall defect is an important component to help with improved drainage of the kidneys and efficient bladder emptying.
C. The abdominal muscle is often patchy and asymmetric, being characteristically absent in the lower and medial abdomen with the upper rectus and lateral portion of the obliques developed.
D. Wound healing generally proceeds normally despite poor muscle and fascia, with dehiscence being rare.
E. The flanks often bulge with the thorax showing costal flaring. Poor abdominal and thoracic muscle support leads to an ineffective cough and predisposes to respiratory infections.

844. All of the following are true statements concerning the kidneys in prune-belly syndrome EXCEPT:

A. Hydronephrosis is the general rule, but may be less than anticipated by the degree of ureteral dilatation.
B. Renal dysplasia is common and often asymmetric, but can vary from normal function to bilateral severely dysplastic kidneys and renal failure.
C. The degree of renal dysplasia is often more severe in patients with associated urethral stenosis, megaurethra, or imperforate anus.
D. Severely dysplastic kidneys should be surgically removed due to a high association with renal cell carcinoma.

845. All of the following statements are true concerning the ureters in prune-belly syndrome EXCEPT:

A. Ureteral orifices are characteristically ectopic, most commonly being located in the posterior urethra or sphincteric region.
B. Histologically, the ureters may display fibrosis and a scarcity of muscle.
C. Ureters are tortuous and dilated, with the lower ureter usually most severely affected.
D. Ureterovesical junction is markedly abnormal, with reflux being present in most cases.
E. Ureteral peristalsis is often poor.

846. Which of the following statements concerning the bladder with prune belly syndrome is *true*?

A. The bladder is typically hypertrophied and of small volume.
B. Urodynamic studies invariably show abnormal pressure flow profiles.
C. The dome of the bladder is tethered to the abdominal wall at the umbilicus and often bulges to give the appearance of a pseudodiverticulum.
D. The urachus is almost always patent.
E. The trigone and bladder neck are usually normal.

847. All of the following statements concerning prune-belly complex are true EXCEPT:

A. Congenital megaurethra (scaphoid) may be seen.
B. Bilateral cryptorchid testes demonstrate normal histology for age.
C. Most with this syndrome have intestinal malrotation and infrequently imperforate anus (usually associated with urethral atresia).
D. Erection and orgasm are normal and most patients with prune-belly syndrome are fertile.
E. The prostatic urethra is usually dilated and tapers to a relatively or functionally narrow point in the membranous urethra.

848. Prune-belly syndrome is associated with all of the following EXCEPT:

A. Cardiac abnormalities in 10 per cent of cases, including ventricular septal defects, atrial septal defects and tetralogy of Fallot.
B. Orthopedic deformities ranging from club foot and congenital hip dislocation to severe lower extremity defects.
C. CNS lesions in 50 per cent of cases, including seizures and mental retardation.
D. Pulmonary hypoplasia (secondary to oligohydramnios), which may be complicated by pneumothorax, pneumomediastinum, and even death by respiratory failure.
E. Renal agenesis, rarely.

849. All of the following are true concerning the initial presentation, evaluation and treatment of prune-belly syndrome EXCEPT:

A. The initial clinical diagnosis is usually easily made due to the classic abdominal wall appearance.
B. Ultrasound evaluation of the kidneys, ureters, and bladder during the first few days of life should be done.
C. Cardiac and pulmonary evaluation are the most immediate concerns after birth.
D. An IVP and VCUG should be done in all neonates within the first week to ten days of life to evaluate function, drainage, and reflux.
E. The creatinine will be normal at birth but should be checked regularly over the first week to ten days of life.

850. All of the following are appropriate treatment recommendations in prune-belly syndrome EXCEPT:

A. Patients in category III with stable renal function may be placed on observation and prophylactic antibiotics, monitoring renal function and urine cultures.
B. Aggressive surgical reconstruction in category II patients to allow better upper tract drainage, prevent reflux, and aid in bladder emptying has produced increased long-term survival.
C. Recurrent infection or deteriorating renal function may require urinary diversion, preferably vesicostomy, but loop ureterostomies are occasionally necessary.
D. Stasis due to dilatation and poor peristalsis of the ureters may require ureteral tapering and reimplantation of the proximal ureter (the only frequently normal appearing ureteral segment) if there is renal deterioration (progressive hydronephrosis or increasing creatinine).

851. All of the following statements are true concerning development of the urethra EXCEPT:

A. Bulbous and penile urethral development are uniquely male and entirely dependent on androgen action for differentiation.
B. The urorectal septum at 6 weeks gestation divides the cloaca into rectal and urogenital sinus portion (the posterior urethra).
C. There is no androgen effect on the posterior urethra since it is present in both males and females.
D. The urethral plate tubularizes to form the anterior urethra.
E. Abnormally low androgen production or end organ insensitivity due to insufficient receptor number or function will result in incomplete tubularization of the anterior urethra.

852. Which of the following types of posterior urethral valves is felt not to exist as a clinical entity?

A. Type I urethral valves (described as an obstructing membrane radiating distally from the verumontanum anteriorly to the membranous urethra where it is fused in the midline).
B. Type II posterior urethral valves (described as folds radiating in a cranial direction from the verumontanum to the posterolateral aspect of the bladder neck).
C. Type III posterior urethral valves (represent incomplete dissolution of the urogenital membrane and are described as a ringlike membrane with a central pinpoint opening distal to the verumontanum).

853. All of the following are classic presentations of posterior urethral valves EXCEPT:

A. A newborn with palpable abdominal and flank masses (bladder and hydronephrotic kidneys).
B. A newborn with respiratory distress requiring positive pressure ventilation, possibly complicated by pneumomediastinum or pneumothorax (pulmonary hypoplasia).
C. Acute abdomen from bowel obstruction secondary to mass effect of distended bladder.
D. A prenatal ultrasound showing bilateral hydronephrosis and bladder distention.
E. Classic features of Potter's syndrome including dysmorphic facial features, fetal growth retardation, positional limb deformities and pulmonary hypoplasia.
F. A 3-week-old infant with urosepsis, dehydration, failure to thrive, severe electrolyte abnormalities, and a dribbling urinary stream.

854. Which of the following statements concerning renal function in patients with posterior urethral valves is *false*?

A. Renal parenchymal dysplasia is common, tends to be microcystic in nature in the peripheral cortical zone, and its degree is the single most important predictor of ultimate renal function.
B. The ultimate goal is to maximize and preserve glomerular filtration by relief of high intravesical and intraureteral pressures, prevention of infection and perhaps glomerulosclerosis associated with hyperfiltration and hypertension.
C. A nadir creatinine of <2.0 reliably predicts long-term stable renal function without surgical intervention.
D. Anatomic conditions that appear to be associated with generally better renal function during fetal development are massive unilateral VUR, large bladder diverticula, and urinary ascites, each serving as a "pop off" valve for high intraluminal pressures.
E. High ureteral pressures effect the distal nephron first, causing a concentrating defect (acquired nephrogenic diabetes insipidus) and resulting in a fixed high output of dilute urine regardless of hydration status, making dehydration and electrolyte disturbances common.

855. All of the following are true statements concerning posterior urethral valves (PUV) EXCEPT:

A. Hydronephrosis and massive ureteral dilatation and tortuousity are common.
B. Vesicoureteral reflux is found in >95 per cent and is thought to be secondary reflux due to high intravesical pressures, development of paraureteral diverticula and loss of ureterovesical valvular competence.
C. Lasix renogram or Whitaker test (pressure perfusion test) may be necessary to evaluate persistent/progressive hydroureteronephrosis with deteriorating renal function (to determine whether it is due to true vesicoureteral dysfunction [rare], ineffective ureteral peristalsis, or elevated intravesical pressures from a fixed high urinary flow rate).
D. 25 per cent of patients with PUVs will have abnormal bladder function typically manifested by incontinence and thought to be secondary to an unstable noncompliant bladder.
E. After relief of obstruction, gradual but significant decrease in hydronephrosis generally occurs and vesicourethral reflux will resolve in approximately one third of patients.

856. Initial management of patients with posterior urethral valves suspected after prenatal ultrasound include all of the following EXCEPT:

A. Ultrasound to confirm hydronephrosis, bladder thickening/distention, and posterior urethral dilitation
B. Urethral catheter or suprapubic drainage of the bladder as an initial method to decompress the urinary tract
C. Monitoring for and treating electrolyte and acid-base abnormalities and observing the serum creatinine trend for the first week after birth
D. A VCUG to evaluate for vesicoureteral reflux in the first few days of life and early ureteral reimplantation for severe reflux
E. Primary endoscopic valve ablation/incision in the first 1–2 weeks in an otherwise healthy (non-septic/acidotic) newborn

857. All of the following statements are true concerning surgical management of posterior urethral valves EXCEPT:

A. If simple valve ablation/incision results in stable renal function and a creatinine of 1.0 mg/dl or less, an indefinite period of observation (with or without antibiotic prophylaxis) is indicated.
B. In children with nadir creatinines of 1.8 mg/dl or higher, a temporizing urinary diversion with bilateral cutaneous ureterostomies or elective vesicostomy is indicated to decompress the upper tracts during the first few months of life while the kidney is still growing new nephrons.
C. Prenatal intervention with placement of vesicoamniotic shunts has been proven to improve ultimate renal function and effectively prevent the potentially fatal hypoplastic lung syndrome.
D. Prenatal variables that predict poor postnatal renal function are moderate to severe oligohydramnios, increased echogenicity (suggesting dysplasia) or a frankly cystic kidney, and abnormal fetal urinary chemistries, including sodium > 100 mEq/L, chloride > 90 mEq/L, osmolarity > 210 mOsm, and urinary output < 2 ml/hr.

858. All of the following statements are true regarding anterior urethral obstruction EXCEPT:

A. It is more common than posterior urethral valves.
B. Lesions can include congenital diverticulum of the urethra anterior urethral valves, valvular obstruction of the fossa novicularis and, rarely, cystic dilatations of Cowper's glands (syringoceles).
C. The most common variety—anterior urethral valves—is actually a ventral diverticulum that may fill with voiding and occlude urinary flow.
D. Syringoceles (cystic dilatation of Cowper's glands) are usually inconsequential findings, but if large can rarely cause obstruction and should be treated with endoscopic unroofing.
E. Obstructing anterior urethral diverticula are best demonstrated on voiding cystourethrogram and, when they present with urosepsis or severe renal insufficiency, should be managed initially in the same manner as posterior urethral valves with transurethral or percutaneous suprapubic tube drainage for stabilization.

859. All of the following statements are true concerning megalourethra EXCEPT:

A. While megalourethra may be an isolated finding, it is often associated with upper tract abnormalities and therefore upper tract imaging is indicated in all cases.
B. Isolated megalourethra is not an obstructing lesion but cosmetic repair by trimming the excess urethra and creating a normal caliber urethra is indicated.
C. In scaphoid megalourethra, the anatomic abnormality is isolated to the corpus cavernosum.

D. In the fusiform megalourethra variety, there is a variable defect in the corpus cavernosum along with the corpus spongiosum and urethral defects.
E. If the corpora cavernosa are severely deficient, it may be appropriate to consider change of sex of rearing in the newborn period.

860. All of the following statements are true concerning urethral duplication EXCEPT:

A. Most urethral duplications occur in the same sagittal plane (one on top of the other) with the rarer side-by-side duplex urethra being associated with bladder duplication and complete penile duplication.
B. In the dorsal variety, the normal urethra is ventral and ends on the glans with a normal meatus while the duplication opens in an epispadiac position with or without dorsal chordee.
C. In the dorsal variety of duplication, the dorsal abnormal segment of urethra extends proximally beneath the pubic symphysis before reaching the bladder, but may rarely join the urachus.
D. In dorsal duplications, bladder neck and sphincter are malformed and excision of the epispadiac urethra alone will rarely cure the incontinence.
E. Ventral duplications may be complete with both originating at the level of the bladder, but more commonly they bifurcate at the level of the prostatic urethra with a hypospadiac accessory meatus.

861. All of the following statements regarding hypospadias and penile anatomy are true EXCEPT:

A. The more distal the meatus, the more likely will the ventral penile surface be shortened and curved by chordee.
B. The dorsal neurovascular bundle lies deep to Buck's fascia in the groove between the corpora cavernosa.
C. The prepuce is deficient ventrally and forms a dorsal hood.
D. The fibrous tissue found with chordee replaces Buck's fascia and the dartos fascia.
E. The dartos fascia is superficial to Buck's fascia.

862. The most common anomaly (ies) associated with hypospadias is (are):

A. Myelomeningocele
B. Imperforate anus
C. Undescended testes and inguinal hernia
D. Anomalies of the upper urinary tract
E. Cardiac anomalies

863. The intersex states that must be ruled out in a child with severe hypospadias include all the following EXCEPT:

A. Adrenogenital syndrome
B. Klinefelter's syndrome
C. Mixed gonadal dysgenesis
D. Incomplete male pseudohermaphroditism, type I
E. True hermaphroditism

864. The most common type of hypospadias is:

A. Chordee without hypospadias
B. Perineal
C. Midshaft
D. Penoscrotal
E. Glanular and subcoronal

865. All of the following statements are true regarding urethroplasty and skin coverage during surgical treatment of hypospadias EXCEPT:

A. Vascularized flaps of preputial or penile skin may be mobilized for the urethroplasty.
B. The key to success with a free graft is coverage of the graft with well-vascularized skin.
C. Skin adjacent to the meatus may be tubularized for the neourethra.
D. Free skin grafts for urethroplasty should be split-thickness rather than full-thickness.
E. Scrotal flaps may be used when there are deficiencies of the penile skin.

866. The most important factor when considering use of the standard meatal advancement and glanuloplasty (MAGPI) is:

A. Mobility of the dorsal prepuce
B. Skin thickness over the dorsal urethra
C. Mobility of the distal urethra
D. Mobility of the glans
E. Mobility of the ventral penile skin

867. Most surgeons feel that the ideal age for hypospadias repair is:

A. Less then 3 months
B. 6 to 18 months
C. 2 to 5 years
D. 5 to 8 years
E. 10 to 13 years

868. All of the following statements regarding postoperative care after hypospadias repair are true EXCEPT:

A. Prophylactic antibiotics are essential in avoiding wound infection.
B. Poor wound healing is primarily due to ischemic flaps.
C. A compression dressing left for 2 to 3 days is the best method for controlling edema and hematoma formation.
D. Postoperative erections in postpubertal patients can be catastrophic and may be managed with amyl nitrite.
E. A urethral stent allows sealing of the suture lines without leakage of urine outside the neourethra.

869. All of the following are true regarding management of late complications after hypospadias repair EXCEPT:

A. The most common error in urethrocutaneous fistula closure is failure to recognize a concomitant diverticulum or distal stricture.
B. The use of scrotal tissue for urethroplasty may lead to postpubertal stone formation and encrustation.
C. Ventral tunical deficiency may be replaced with strips of paratesticular tunica vaginalis.
D. Strictures after urethroplasty are effectively managed with cold-knife urethrotomy.
E. Balanitis xerotica obliterans is a devastating complication after hypospadias repair.

870. Complex redo hypospadias is the most difficult hypospadias surgery. Which one of the following statements is *false*?

A. These patients usually present with a combination of problems, including curvature, fistula, and stricture.

B. Genital skin flaps are preferred when available.
C. When penile skin is not available, extragenital (inner arm, inguinal skin, or postauricular) flaps are the optimal urethral replacement.
D. The main complication with bladder mucosa grafts is meatal eversion and irritation.
E. If the urethral gap is less than 5 cm, buccal mucosa is the preferred graft material.

871. The procedure best suited for a hypospadias patient in which the ventral skin is very thin or who has a mid or distal shaft hypospadias without chordee is the:

A. Mathieu procedure
B. Devine-Horton flip-flap procedure
C. Mustarde procedure
D. Onlay island flap
E. Glans approximation procedure

872. All of the following statements about normal development of the male genitalia are true EXCEPT:

A. The genital tubercle differentiates into the glans penis, the genital swellings become the scrotum, and the genital folds became the shaft of the penis.
B. Differentiation of the external genitalia occurs between 9 and 13 weeks gestation.
C. After birth, gonadotropin levels are low and stay at their low baseline until puberty.
D. If there is an abnormality in testosterone production, a 5α-reductase enzyme defect, or an androgen receptor defect, the genital tubercle becomes the clitoris, the genital folds become labia minora and the genital swellings become the labia majora.

873. External genital anomalies are associated with all of the following EXCEPT:

A. Anorectal malformations (cloacal) in up to one half
B. Boys with tracheoesophageal fistula or atresia
C. Robinow syndrome
D. Prune-belly syndrome
E. Prader-Willi syndrome

874. All of the following are true statements concerning penile torsion or lateral curvature of the penis EXCEPT:

A. Penile torsion is almost always rotation counterclockwise (to the left) with the penis generally normal otherwise, although there is occasionally an associated hooded prepuce or mild hypospadias.
B. Lateral curvature of the penis is due to overgrowth or hypoplasia of one corporal body.
C. Penile torsion is primarily of cosmetic concern and correction is generally unnecessary if rotation is less than 60 to 90 degrees from midline.
D. Both penile torsion and lateral curvature of the penis may be corrected with a modified Nesbit type procedure.
E. Even with severe lateral curvature the penis may appear normal when flaccid.

875. Which of the following statements concerning micropenis is *true*?

A. Micropenis in a term newborn infant is defined as being less than 4.0 cm in length.
B. As a rule, the corporal bodies are severely hypoplastic, the scrotum is normal, and the testes are descended.
C. Differentiation of male external genitalia is complete by the 12th week of gestation and requires normal testosterone production controlled by fetal luteinizing hormone.
D. The most common etiologies of micropenis are hypogonadotrophic hypogonadism, hypergonadotrophic hypogonadism (primary testicular failure), and idiopathic micropenis.
E. During the second and third trimester, growth of the penis is stimulated by fetal testicular testosterone which is stimulated by maternal chorionic gonadotropin.

876. All of the following are true of aphallia EXCEPT:

A. The usual appearance is that of a well-developed scrotum with descended testes and the anus is generally anteriorly displaced.
B. There is no identifiable penile shaft.
C. The urethra generally opens cephalad to the scrotum.
D. Associated malformations include occasional cryptorchidism, vesicoureteral reflux, horseshoe kidney, renal agenesis, imperforate anus, musculoskeletal and cardiopulmonary abnormalities.
E. Gender reassignment is recommended in the newborn with bilateral orchiectomy and feminizing genitoplasty and later/staged construction of a neovagina.

877. Which one of the following statements concerning diphallia is *false*?

A. Diphallia is a very rare anomaly that exhibits a spectrum from a small accessory penis to complete duplication.
B. Each phallus has only one corporal body.
C. The phalli are generally of unequal size.
D. Associated anomalies are common and include hypospadias, bifid scrotum, bladder duplication, and anal and cardiac abnormalities.
E. All patients should be evaluated for upper tract abnormalities, such as renal agenesis or ectopia.

878. The following are true statements concerning penoscrotal transposition (scrotal engulfment) EXCEPT:

A. It is frequently associated with penoscrotal, scrotal, or perineal hypospadias with chordee.
B. The penoscrotal transposition may be partial or complete.
C. It is felt to be due to improper migration of the genital tubercle.
D. When associated with severe hypospadias, a transverse preputial island flap hypospadias repair is usually done in a staged fashion with later scrotoplasty to avoid devascularization of the island flap.

879. All of the following are common etiologies of interlabial masses in children EXCEPT:

A. Paraurethral cyst
B. Imperforate hymen
C. Prolapsed ureterocele
D. Urethral inflammatory polyp
E. Labial adhesions

880. The following are true concerning vaginal anomalies of vertical fusion EXCEPT:

A. They result from either an abnormality in caudal development of the müllerian duct and/or canalization of the vaginal plate with typically normal fallopian tubes and ovaries.
B. An abnormality in the wolffian duct system can lead to abnormal differentiation of the müllerian ductal system (female genital system).
C. Clinically, vertical fusion abnormalities result in a rudimentary uterus without a lumen and/or vaginal agenesis.
D. Diagnosis is most common within the first year of life.
E. Vaginal agenesis is the second most common cause of primary infertility in women after gonadal dysgenesis.

881. All of the following are true concerning müllerian disorders of medial fusion EXCEPT:

A. Medial fusion defects can result in partial or complete uterovaginal duplication ranging from a bicornuate uterus to uterus didelphys (complete uterine and vaginal duplication).
B. Associated renal anomalies are rare with complete uterovaginal duplication.
C. Often one side of a duplex system is obstructed, which may present at puberty with cyclic abdominal pain and apparently normal menses.
D. A vaginal septum may be treated with transvaginal incision.

882. Indications for orchiopexy include all of the following EXCEPT:

A. Retractile testis despite treatment with gonadotropin-releasing hormone analogs
B. Possible preservation of fertility
C. Simpler diagnosis of testicular malignancy in the future
D. Cosmetic benefits
E. Psychologic benefits

883. Which of the following statements concerning orchiopexy is *false*?

A. The incision should be made in a skin crease just lateral to the pubic tubercle over the inguinal canal.
B. The external oblique fascia is incised in the direction of its fibers with care not to injure the ilioinguinal nerve.
C. If the testis is identified in the canal, the gubernaculum testis is divided and the spermatic cord is mobilized to the level of the internal ring, which usually will allow adequate length for the testis to be placed into the scrotum.
D. If a blind-ending vas deferens is found, there will be no testes and the case can be terminated.
E. After adequate length has been obtained, the testis is pexed with nonabsorbable suture or placed into a dartos pouch to prevent it from retracting back into the inguinal canal.

884. Bilateral nonpalpable testes may be appropriately managed in all of the following ways EXCEPT:

A. Laparoscopy to determine if the testicles are present or not
B. Observation for 2 to 3 years with repeat examination every 6 months
C. Bilateral inguinal and abdominal exploration with orchiopexy if the testes are identified
D. hCG stimulation test

885. All of the following are true statements concerning the exploration and treatment in a child presenting with unilateral torsion of the testis EXCEPT:

A. Emergent exploration via a scrotal incision, detorsion, and examination of the testis are indicated.
B. Testes that are obviously necrotic should be removed.
C. If good color does not return to the testis (persistent ischemia), the testis should be removed.
D. If good color returns to the testis, it should be secured to the scrotum with nonabsorbable suture at 3 points on the medial aspect of the upper pole (least vascular area).
E. The contralateral hemiscrotum is entered and the contralateral testis fixed in a similar fashion.

886. All of the following statements concerning varicocele repair are true EXCEPT:

A. Massive size, pain, or ipsilateral testicular growth retardation are indications for surgical repair.
B. High ligation via small transverse incision medial to the anterior superior iliac crest and incision of the external oblique (with retraction of internal iliac muscle) allows direct visualization of the gonadal vessels.
C. Low ligation has a lower recurrence rate than high ligation.
D. Low ligation via hernia type incision with opening of the external oblique fascia and isolation of the spermatic cord allows identification and ligation of the spermatic veins.
E. Optical magnification, Doppler probe identification of the spermatic artery to aid in its preservation, and venograms are recommended by some to help identify all the veins and help preserve the artery.

887. Inguinal orchiectomy/exploration is indicated in which of the following cases?

A. Older child with loculated hydrocele
B. Classic unilateral torsion in a newborn
C. Scrotal pain when physical exam cannot exclude a testis tumor
D. An antenatal infarcted testis which is atrophic
E. Definite testicular appendix torsion

888. All of the following statements concerning exploration for possible testis tumor are true EXCEPT:

A. A testis tumor should always be approached inguinally.
B. The external oblique fascia is opened over the inguinal canal and the spermatic cord isolated with care taken not to injure the ilioinguinal nerve.
C. After the testis is delivered into the wound, a rubber shod or vascular clamp should be placed across the vascular pedicle.
D. If a testicular mass is present, a high ligation of the vas deferens and vascular pedicle is indicated (radical orchiectomy).

889. Which of the following statements concerning hydrocele/hernia repair in infants is *false*?

A. A simple hydrocele may be observed for 9–12 months and may resolve spontaneously.
B. Nonincarcerated infant hernias may be observed for up to 1 year of age and may resolve spontaneously.
C. The hernia sac may usually be isolated and divided without opening the external oblique fascia.
D. The tunica vaginalis over the testis should be incised with or without excision of excess tunica or bottle-neck procedures before being replaced in the scrotum.

890. The options for treatment of undescended testis (if adequate length cannot be obtained without excessive tension to place the testis into the scrotum) include all of the following EXCEPT:

A. Autotransplantation
B. Staged orchiopexy
C. Placement of a testicular prosthesis, leaving the testis secured as distal in the inguinal canal as possible
D. Gonadal vessel transection and Fowler-Stephens orchiopexy
E. Orchiectomy for a small dysgenetic or atrophic testis

891. Elements of the Fowler-Stephens orchiopexy include all of the following EXCEPT:

A. An extended inguinal incision to allow proper exposure for mobilization
B. Ligation of the spermatic vessels at the level of the internal ring
C. Avoiding excessive dissection of the vas and distal spermatic artery
D. Preservation of the peritoneum medial to the distal spermatic vessels and vas deferens
E. Clamping the spermatic artery and demonstrating preserved blood flow to the testis with either intravenous fluorescein dye or demonstrating arterial bleeding from a small testicular biopsy site

892. The most important factor in appropriate management of infants with ambiguous genitalia is:

A. Correct identification of chromosomal sex
B. Appropriate assignment of gender
C. Rapid assessment of hormonal abnormalities
D. Reassurance of parents
E. Accurate identification of male or female gonads

893. The most important factor in determining embryologic development of the testis is:

A. The maternal hormonal environment
B. The X chromosome
C. The Y chromosome
D. Testis determining factor
E. Testosterone

894. During normal development of the male internal reproductive ductal system, the fate of the paramesonephric ducts is determined by:

A. Müllerian inhibitory substance
B. Testosterone
C. Testis determining factor
D. The X chromosome
E. The Y chromosome

895. Normal development of the mesonephric ductal system in the male is determined by:

A. Müllerian inhibitory substanace
B. Testosterone
C. Testis determining factor
D. The X chromosome
E. The Y chromosome

896. In the absence of any gonadal influence, ongoing development of the internal reproductive ductal system will result in:

A. Regression of both the mesonephric and paramesonephric ducts
B. Normal development of both the mesonephric and paramesonephric ducts
C. Normal development of the mesonephric duct and regression of the paramesonephric duct
D. Regression of the mesonephric duct and normal development of the paramesonephric duct
E. A phenotypically normal male

897. During male embryologic development, normal formation of the external genitalia is dependent on all of the following EXCEPT:

A. Secretory products of Sertoli cell
B. Testosterone
C. 5α-Reductase
D. Dihydrotestosterone
E. Androgen receptors

898. The most common category of intersex is:

A. Microphallus
B. True hermaphroditism
C. Mixed gonadal dysgenesis
D. Male pseudohermaphroditism
E. Female pseudohermaphroditism

899. The most common etiology of female pseudohermaphroditism is:

A. Progesterone administered during pregnancy
B. Virilizing ovarian tumors
C. Idiopathic
D. Congenital adrenal hyperplasia
E. Virilizing adrenal tumors

900. The most common form of congenital adrenal hyperplasia is:

A. 21-Hydroxylase deficiency
B. 17-Hydroxylase defiency
C. 11β-Hydroxylase deficiency
D. 3β-Hydroxysteroid dehydrogenase defiency
E. 5α-Reductase defiency

901. A major distinguishing feature of the 11β-hydroxylase defiency form of congenital adrenal hyperplasia is:

A. More severe virilization
B. Less severe virilization
C. Adrenal insufficiency
D. Salt and water retention leading to hypertension
E. Feminization in males

902. The genetic pattern found in most patients with mixed gonadal dysgenesis is:

A. 46XX
B. 46XY
C. 45XO

D. 47XYY
E. 45XO/46XY

903. Patients with mixed gonadal dysgenesis and intraabdominal gonads should undergo early gonadectomy because:

A. Gonadal identification is important for sex assignment.
B. Hormones from intraabdominal gonads may complicate development in the assigned sex.
C. Malignant degeneration is common.
D. Intrabdominal torsion may cause surgical emergency.
E. The development of autoimmunity may result in impaired infertility.

904. Testicular feminization syndrome is caused by:

A. A form of congenital adrenal hyperplasia
B. Chromosomal mosaicism
C. Absent testis determining factor
D. Deficient androgen receptor binding
E. 5α-Reductase deficiency

905. Pseudovaginal perineoscrotal hypospadias is caused by:

A. A form of congenital adrenal hyperplasia
B. Chromosomal mosaicism
C. Absence of testis determining factor
D. An androgen receptor deficiency
E. 5α-Reductase deficiency

906. Hernia uteri inguinalis is caused by:

A. 5α-Reductase deficiency
B. Defective androgen receptor binding
C. Chromosomal mosaicism
D. Defective paramesonephric duct regression
E. A form of congenital adrenal hyperplasia

907. True hermaphroditism is defined as:

A. XX/XY chromosomal mosaicism
B. Genital ambiguity with gonadal tissue of both sexes present
C. Genital ambiguity alone
D. The presence of internal reproductive ducts of both sexes
E. The ability to function in both sexual roles

908. Assignment of sex in an infant with intersex should be based on:

A. Chromosomal sex
B. Gonadal sex
C. Functional anatomic potential
D. The parents' desire
E. Prospects for fertility

909. The optimal time for genital reconstruction for patients with intersex is:

A. Neonatal period
B. Age 18 months to 3 years
C. Age 6
D. Pubertal period
E. Adulthood

910. Of the following, the most correct description of appropriate management of the enlarged clitoris in patients with female pseudohermaphroditism is:

A. Clitorectomy should be performed in the neonatal period.
B. Clitorectomy should be performed at age 18 months to 3 years.
C. The enlarged clitoris will regress to a normal size with steroid replacement.
D. The enlarged clitoris causes no functional disability and requires no therapy.
E. Clitoral recession and reduction should be performed after maximum spontaneous regression due to steroid replacement.

911. The minimal phallic length in the male newborn regarded as adequate to allow male sex assignment is:

A. 0.5 cm
B. 1 cm
C. 1.5 cm
D. 2.5 cm
E. 5 cm

912. All of the following statements regarding long-term results of intersex management are true EXCEPT:

A. Revisional vaginoplasty may be necessary.
B. Fertility is possible in some patients with congenital adrenal hyperplasia.
C. Noncompliance with steroid replacement is a common problem.
D. Caesarean sections are common in females with congenital adrenal hyperplasia.
E. Psychosexual problems are often severe.

913. All of the following are true statements concerning malignancies in children EXCEPT:

A. Neuroblastoma is the second most common malignant tumor of infancy and after brain tumors (the most common malignant solid tumor of childhood); >50 per cent present at less than 2 years of age.
B. Wilms' tumor is the most common malignant neoplasm of the urinary tract in children (80 per cent of solid GU tumors in children under age 15) with peak presentation between ages 3 and 4 years.
C. The most common prepubertal testis tumor is choriocarcinoma.
D. Surgical cure can be expected for the vast majority of stages I and II neuroblastomas, whereas stages III and IV (excluding IV-S) have a dismal prognosis despite aggressive combination therapy.
E. Sarcomas are the fifth most common solid tumor of childhood after CNS tumors, lymphomas, neuroblastomas, and Wilms' tumor.

914. All of the following are true concerning Wilms' tumor EXCEPT:

A. An abnormality in the 11p gene may be important in the pathogenesis of Wilms' tumor.
B. Wilms' tumor results from abnormal differentiation of the metanephric blastema without normal differentiation into tubules and nephrons.
C. The majority of patients with Wilms' tumor have one or more other congenitalanomalies.
D. Up to 15 per cent of long-term survivors of Wilms' tumor have a second malignancy and include sarcomas, adenocarcinomas and leukemias.

915. All of the following statements regarding Wilms' tumor presentation are true EXCEPT:

A. Three quarters of cases present with an abdominal mass and increasing abdominal girth.

B. The peak age of presentation is between 3 and 4 years, with 75 per cent being diagnosed between one and five years of age.
C. Most children with Wilms' tumor appear sick or toxic on presentation.
D. Physical examination usually reveals a firm smooth, nontender unilateral abdominal mass.
E. Acute onset of pain with fever, abdominal mass, anemia, and hypertension suggest Wilms' tumor with subcapsular hemorrhage.

916. Which one of the following statements concerning Wilms' tumor types and histology is *true*?

A. Anaplasia, clear cell, and rhabdomyosarcoma are unfavorable histologic types.
B. Multilocular cyst, congenital mesoblastic nephroma, and rhabdoid tumor are the favorable histologic types.
C. Rhabdoid tumor has the worst prognosis of all cell types (80 per cent die from tumor).
D. Multilocular cyst is treated by excision (nephrectomy) and chemotherapy.

917. The principles of treatment for Wilms' tumor include all of the following EXCEPT:

A. A generous incision, with careful evaluation of the contralateral kidney and biopsy of suspicious lesions
B. Ligation of the renal artery and vein prior to mobilization of the tumor
C. Primary resection of tumor en bloc, including portions of the colon, duodenum, liver, pancreas, stomach, and/or vena cava to obtain tumor-free margins
D. Evaluation of the liver, periaortic, and hilar lymph nodes with biopsy of suspicious lesions and only then evaluation of the mass for resectability

918. Important prognostic indicators in Wilms' tumor include all of the following EXCEPT:

A. Histology
B. The presence of hematogenous metastasis
C. The age of the patient
D. Lymph node involvement
E. Local tumor extension

919. Which of the following statements concerning neuroblastoma is *false*?

A. It originates from the cells of the neural crest in the adrenal cortex.
B. Ganglioneuroma is the benign counterpart to neuroblastoma.
C. Neuroblastoma histologically is one of the small round cell tumors of childhood.
D. Ganglioneuroblastoma is intermediate between the benign ganglioneuroma and the malignant neuroblastoma.
E. Neuroblastoma may excrete catecholamines and may be identified on bone marrow aspirates.

920. Presentation of neuroblastoma may commonly include all of the following EXCEPT:

A. A firm, irregular, nontender abdominal mass that often extends across the midline
B. Unexplained fever, general malaise, anorexia, weight loss, irritability, bone pain, and pallor secondary to anemia in those with widespread metastatic disease
C. The incidental finding of a mass/renal obstruction in the evaluation for childhood UTI
D. Paravertebral tumors originating from the sympathetic chain may grow through the intervertebral foreman causing neurologic symptoms of cord compression
E. Presacral tumors arising from the organ of Zuckerkandl may present with urinary frequency, urgency, or urinary retention secondary to extrinsic bladder compression

921. All of the following are part of the routine evaluation of a child with abdominal mass suspected of having neuroblastoma EXCEPT:

A. Laboratory evaluation including urinalysis, CBC, coagulation profile, LFTs and urinary vanillylmandelic acid, and homovanillic acid (catecholamine metabolites)
B. Bone marrow aspiration
C. Imaging with intravenous pyelogram and ultrasound or CT scan to assess the kidney and for tumor extension/metastasis
D. MRI to evaluate for renal vein/vena caval involvement
E. Chest x-ray and skeletal survey

922. All of the following are poor prognostic indicators of survival with neuroblastoma EXCEPT:

A. Elevated serum ferritin levels
B. Older age at presentation
C. Stage IV-S disease
D. Adrenal site of origin versus cervical, mediastinal, pelvic, or nonadrenal abdominal tumors
E. DNA index of one by flow cytometry

PART XI

PEDIATRIC UROLOGIC SURGERY

CHAPTERS 44 THROUGH 54

ANSWERS

797-A *(Campbell's, pp. 1689–1690)*

Answers B, C, D, and E are correct statements concerning the ureter and ureterovesical junction. A is incorrect in that only the longitudinal muscle fibers of the distal ureter continue into the intravesical ureter and on to the trigone.

798-C *(Campbell's, p. 1690)*

The length of the intravesical ureter relative to its diameter is the single most critical factor in preventing reflux. All the other factors mentioned are of only secondary importance.

799-D *(Campbell's, pp. 1690–1691)*

Reflux is not inherited in an autosomal dominant fashion. Most investigators believe there is a polygenic or multifactorial mode of inheritance.

800-E *(Campbell's, pp. 1694–1695)*

International 5 grade staging of reflux.

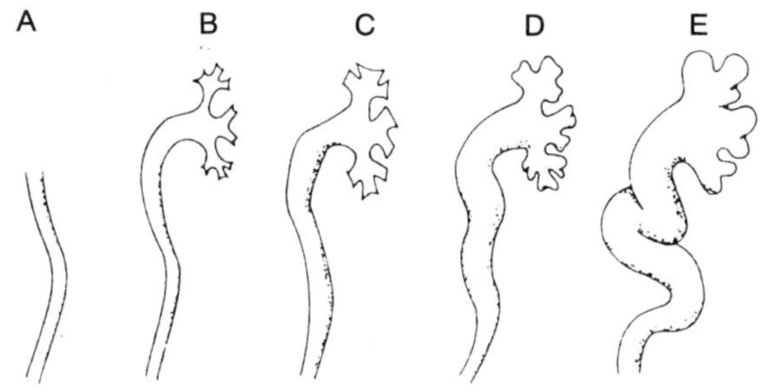

801-E *(Campbell's, p. 1696)*

A to D are all relative indications for surgical therapy early after diagnosis. E is false; presentation in the teen years is not in itself an indication for surgery.

802-D *(Campbell's, pp. 1697–1698)*

All statements are true except D. Sterile reflux is not responsible for renal scarring. A renal scar is secondary to focal tissue loss and requires infection to induce the cascade of events leading to tissue destruction. Sterile reflux has been shown to cause scars in the pig model when intravesical pressures are very high, analogous to the situation of some neurogenic bladders and valve bladders (Ransley and Risdon).

803-C *(Campbell's, pp. 1701–1702)*

Intrarenal reflux is the means by which bacteria reach the interstitium—it occurs primarily in the upper and lower poles subtended by compound papillae. Superoxide is lethal to tubular epithelial cells; enzymatic blockage of its formation prevents renal scarring in dogs and monkeys. Sterile reflux is a marker for a patient at risk for scarring if infection occurs. Reflux of infected urine delivers bacteria to the compound papillae where intrarenal reflux occurs.

804-C *(Campbell's, pp. 1698–1699)*

Ureteral duplication in and of itself may or may not be associated with reflux. Complete ureteral duplication is common but most do not reflux. If reflux is present with a duplicated system, it is generally the lower pole ureter (which inserts more posteriorly and laterally into the bladder) that refluxes (Meyer-Weggart law). Partial ureteral duplication is rarely associated with reflux. Infection in children appears to be a marker for reflux since the incidence in infected children is 30 to 60 per cent, while it is only 0.4 per cent in the screening population. Patients with bladder outlet obstruction (urethral valves) or elevated intravesical pressure secondary to neurogenic bladder are predisposed to secondary vesicoureteral reflux.

805-B *(Campbell's, p. 1705)*

Reflux is as likely to resolve in those with recurrent infections as in those without infections.

806-D *(Campbell's, p. 1706)*

Glomerulonephritis is the most common cause of hypertension in children, followed by pyelonephritic scarring. Elimination of reflux prior to the development of renal scarring (or an infection that will later give rise to renal scarring) should protect against infection, subsequent renal scarring, and hypertension. Scarring is probably related to hypertension due to vascular lesions and subsequent production of renin. Low peripheral renin does not eliminate focal renin hypersecretion. When segmental vein renins are elevated, removal of scarred upper poles may alleviate hypertension.

807-B *(Campbell's, pp. 1743–1744)*

An ectopic ureter opens anywhere except on the trigone. In females with ectopic ureters, the sites of ureteral opening/insertion can include bladder neck, proximal or distal urethra, vestibule, vagina, uterus, cervix, or rarely the rectum. The müllerian sites of openings are the vagina (including müllerian duct cysts), uterus, and cervix. Since ureteral openings in females can be distal to the urethral sphincter, continuous or intermittent incontinence or persistent vaginal discharge may be seen. Ectopic ureters are more commonly seen with ureteral/renal duplication in females than with single ureters.

REFERENCE

1. Tanagho, E.A.: Embryologic basis for lower ureteral anomalies: A hypothesis. Urology, 7:451–464, 1976.

808-D *(Campbell's, pp. 1744–1746)*

The most common presentation for ectopic ureters is urinary tract infection in young children, although they occasionally are diagnosed by prenatal ultrasound or as a palpable mass from large upper pole hydronephrosis. Reflux is common in the lower pole ureter, with over one half refluxing. X-ray findings on IVP can include lateral displacement of the lower pole segment by the upper pole hydronephrosis, fewer calyces than expected (<8) on the side with ureteral duplication, non- or poorly visualized upper pole segment, and the lower pole ureter may be scalloped and tortuous secondary to a markedly dilated upper pole pelvis and collecting system and ureter. The dilated ureter is clearly extravesical with a thick septum of bladder muscle between the bladder lumen and ureteral lumen, which contrasts with a ureterocele where the septum is very thin.

809-A *(Campbell's, pp. 1746–1751)*

The most common clinical scenario is infection, a poorly functioning upper pole segment with distal upper pole ureteral obstruction, with or without lower pole reflux. If the lower pole reflux is low grade (not grade IV or V), upper pole nephrectomy and partial ureterectomy (leaving the ureteral stump open) is the preferred treatment. (Only one third of patients will require a second surgery for reflux or to deal with distal stump complications.) With upper pole reflux, the entire upper pole ureter must be excised. Antibiotic prophylaxis is not indicated and reimplantation of both ureters is inappropriate since one is not likely to regain significant upper pole function, and reimplantation of the lower pole ureter risks reflux or obstruction in a previously normal system.

810-B *(Campbell's, pp. 1751–1754)*

Ectopic ureter is not as common in boys as it is in girls, but boys more commonly have a nonduplicated system (ureter). Because all the sites of the ureteral opening are proximal to the external sphincter (in contrast to females), continuous incontinence is not seen in the absence of sphincteric dysfunction. The common sites of ectopic ureteral openings in boys are the bladder neck and proximal urethra. Less commonly the ureter may open into the seminal vesical or vas deferens (higher ureteral bud formation) or, very rarely, the rectum.

811-E *(Campbell's, pp. 1752–1754)*

Bilateral single system (single ureter) ectopia is very rare. Embryologically, the portion of the urogenital sinus between the orifices of the wolffian duct and the ureter develops into the bladder neck musculature. This development does not take place if both ureters remain in the position of the wolffian duct orifice (high ureteral bud). There is therefore no development of the trigone and the base of the bladder and a wide, poorly defined incompetent bladder neck results. Rarely, there can be associated agenesis of the bladder and urethra which may not be compatible with life. The kidneys are commonly dysplastic with dilated refluxing ureters. The bladder is commonly of small capacity. After ureteral reimplantation and bladder neck reconstruction, the bladder volume will often increase, but augmentation cystoplasty may ultimately be indicated.

812-D *(Campbell's, p. 1754)*

A ureterocele is defined as a cystic dilatation of the distal ureter within the bladder, urethra, or both, and can be orthotopic or ectopic. Ectopic ureteroceles are more common in females by a 2:1 ratio than in boys and can occasionally prolapse into the urethra causing bladder outlet obstruction. They may prolapse all the way out the urethral meatus in females. Ureteroceles are not always obstructing and can represent an incidental/insignificant finding if asymptomatic and without hydronephrosis.

813-C *(Campbell's, p. 1757)*

Classification of ectopic ureteroceles includes: (1) stenotic ectopic ureteroceles (40 per cent), characterized by a small orifice located on the superior or inferior surface of the distal end of the ureterocele; (2) sphincteric ectopic ureteroceles (40 per cent), which terminate within the internal sphincter, and those orifices may be normal or large and may open in the posterior urethra in males or even distal to the sphincter in females; (3) cecoureterocele (rare, <5 per cent), where the ureteral lumen extends distal to the ureteral orifice in the urethral submucosa, and where the orifice communicates with the bladder lumen, is large and as a rule incompetent; (4) blind ectopic ureteroceles (rare, <5 per cent) with atrophy of the portion of the ureter distal to the ureterocele and with no orifice; and (5) nonobstructive ectopic ureterocele (rare, <5 per cent) with terminal expansion of the ureter and a large ureteral orifice in the bladder.

814-B,D *(Campbell's, pp. 1759–1762)*

A CT scan or MRI should not be routinely used to evaluate ureteroceles, hydronephrosis, or obviously cystic renal structures. The ultrasound may be used as the initial screening modality or may on prenatal ultrasound start the evaluation for hydronephrosis and suggest ureterocele by the thin-lined dilatation at the bladder bed. The required studies are the IVP to assess the contralateral renal unit, to evaluate for single versus duplicate ureters on the side of the ureterocele, and to demonstrate the presence of the distal ureteral dilatation (cobrahead). At times, the obstructed upper pole system will be non-visualized but may displace the upper pole laterally or be associated with the drooping lilly lower pole system. A VCUG should be obtained with dilute contrast and may demonstrate reflux into an ipsilateral lower pole ureter (or rarely into the ureterocele ureter), show the ureterocele as a bladder filling defect, or demonstrate contralateral reflux.

815-D *(Campbell's, p. 1763)*

In most cases where an ectopic ureterocele is associated with a poor or nonfunctioning upper pole segment and low grade or no lower pole segment reflux (and a normal contralateral kidney), an upper pole nephrectomy with partial ureterectomy should be the treatment of choice. The distal ureteral stump should be decompressed and left open. In two thirds of cases, no further surgery on the distal ureter/bladder neck will be required. Lower pole reflux may resolve on its own, but it is also possible that reflux can start in a previously non-refluxing system. If high-grade lower pole reflux exists, it is less likely to resolve, and distal ureterectomy should be undertaken with lower pole ureteral reimplantation, either initially or as a staged procedure.

816-D *(Campbell's, pp. 1768–1769)*

All of the answers are possible options except D. Preservation of functioning renal tissue is a primary goal in reconstructive genitourinary surgery.

817-B *(Campbell's, pp. 1773–1775, 1777–1778, 1812)*

The exstrophy-epispadias complex includes bladder exstrophy, cloacal exstrophy, and epispadias. In both bladder exstrophy and epispadias, males are more commonly affected than females. The male:female ratio of bladder exstrophy ranges from 2:1 to 6:1. The male:female ratio of epispadias varies between 3:1 and 5:1. The risk of recurrence of bladder exstrophy in a given family is approximately one in one hundred. The risk of bladder exstrophy in the offspring of individuals with bladder exstrophy and epispadias is one in 70 live births, a 500-fold greater incidence than in the general population. Fetal ultrasound allows for the prenatal diagnosis of exstrophy. Findings consistent with exstrophy include an empty bladder, low set umbilicus, and a mass of echogenic tissue overlying the lower abdominal wall. Bladder exstrophy also tends to occur more often in infants of younger mothers. In general, infants born with bladder exstrophy and epispadias are robust, full-term babies with the anomalous development confined to structures adjacent to the cloacal membrane.

818-C *(Campbell's, pp. 1772–1773)*

The common embryological defect in the exstrophy-epispadias complex is failure of the cloacal membrane to be reinforced by ingrowth of mesoderm. The cloaca is that portion of the gut caudal to the opening of the allantoenteric diverticulum. The cloaca itself is separated from the outside by a thin plate of tissue called the cloacal membrane which is bilaminar in nature consisting of ectodermal and endodermal layer. The cloacal membrane reaches its greatest dimension at five weeks of gestation and then regresses in size. Mesenchymal ingrowth between the ectodermal and endodermal layers of the cloacal membrane results in formation of the lower abdominal muscles and the pelvic bones. After mesenchymal ingrowth occurs, downgrowth of the urorectal septum divides the bladder into a urogenital sinus anteriorly and anorectal canal posteriorly. Marshall and Muecke's theory for the embryology of the exstrophy-epispadias complex is that the basic defect is an abnormal overdevelopment of the cloacal membrane, thus blocking the ingrowth of mesenchymal tissues. The persistent cloacal membrane in turn inhibits medial fusion of the genital tubercles and thus leaves the urethra and bladder open to the ventral abdominal walls. The variant of the exstrophy-epispadias complex that results is determined by the timing of the rupture of the cloacal defect. Other theories concerning the embryology of the exstrophy-epispadias complex postulate an abnormal medial fusion of the genital tubercles caudally below the cloacal membrane, or abnormal caudal insertion of the body stalk resulting in failure of intraposition of mesenchymal tissue in the midline.

REFERENCE

1. Hinman, F. Jr.: Atlas of Urological Anatomy. Philadelphia, WB Saunders Co., 1993, pp. 310–328, 1993.

819-C *(Campbell's, p. 1773)*

Classic bladder exstrophy is a rather rare event with an estimated incidence between 1 in 10,000 and 1 in 50,000 live births.

820-A *(Campbell's, pp. 1776–1777)*

The exstrophy-epispadias complex involves a spectrum of anomalies related by a common fault in their embryogenesis. Pseudoexstrophy is characterized by the classical musculoskeletal defects of exstrophy. However, no major defect in the urinary system has been noted. Superior vesical fissures have the same musculoskeletal defects as those in the classic bladder exstrophy. However, the persistent cloacal membrane opens only at the uppermost portion. Duplicate exstrophy occurs when a superior vesicle fissure opens but there is later fusion to the abdominal wall and a portion of the bladder elements remains outside. Prune-belly syndrome is characterized by the absence or hypoplasia of the abdominal muscles, distension of the bladder, ureters, renal pelvis, and cryptorchidism and does not share the same defect in embryogenesis as the others in the exstrophy-epispadias complex.

REFERENCE

1. Hinman, F. Jr.: Atlas of Urological Anatomy. Philadelphia, WB Saunders Co., 1993, p. 100.

821-E *(Campbell's, p. 1775)*

Pseudoexstrophy, a variant of the exstrophy-epispadias complex, shares the characteristic musculoskeletal defects of the exstrophy anomaly. However, no major defect in the urinary tract is noted. It is theorized that in pseudoexstrophy the mesodermal migration is interrupted only in the superior aspect and thus allows formation of the genital tubercle.

822-D *(Campbell's, pp. 1778–1781)*

Pubic diastasis is characteristic of all cases of the exstrophy-epispadias complex. This is due to the outward rotation of the innominate bone along both sacroiliac joints. Usually the only skeletal abnormalities present in epispadias is this outward rotation of the innominate bones. On the other hand, classic bladder exstrophy is associated with outward rotation of the pubic rami at their junction with the ischial and iliac bones in addition to the outward rotation of the innominate bones. In severe cases of cloacal exstrophy, a lateral separation of the innominate bones inferiorly is present in addition to the other skeletal defects. The waddling gait develops secondary to the external rotation of the lower extremities resulting from the posterolateral position of the acetabula. Although noted when ambulating, the waddling gait corrects itself and leaves no orthopedic problems thereafter.

823-E *(Campbell's, pp. 1782–1783)*

The male genital defects associated with exstrophy are quite severe. Although the individual corpus cavernosum is of normal caliber, the penis appears foreshortened because of the wide separation of the crural attachments, prominent dorsal chordee, and shortened urethral groove. An acceptable penile length can be achieved surgically with relief of the dorsal chordee, lengthening of the urethral groove, and mobilization of the crurae in the midline. Rarely, the patient will have a very small or dystrophic penis and thus should be considered for gender reassignment. Since there is lateral displacement of the cavernous nerves which supply autonomic innervation for the corpus cavernosum, potency is preserved in the majority of male exstrophy patients. Although testicular function has not been comprehensively studied, fertility is usually not impaired. Furthermore, testes frequently appear undescended; however, they are usually retractile in nature and thus do not require orchiopexy. The vas deferens and ejaculatory ducts are normal provided that they are not injured iatrogenically during surgical reconstructive procedures. Female congenital defects include shortened urethra and vagina, bifid clitoris, divergent labia and mons pubis, and stenotic vaginal orifice. The uterus, fallopian tubes, and ovaries are normal.

824-E *(Campbell's, pp. 1783–1784)*

Nearly 100 per cent of patients have vesicoureteral reflux after closure of an exstrophied bladder. The ureters have abnormal course terminations secondary to downward and lateral displacement of the ureters by the enlarged and unusually deep peritoneal pouch of Douglas between the bladder and rectum. The distal segment of the ureter approaches the bladder from a point inferior and lateral to the orifice and thus enters the bladder with little or no obliquity. Reimplantation of the ureter is necessary subsequently.

825-B *(Campbell's, pp. 1785–1786)*

Conditions that preclude primary closure of the bladder in an exstrophy infant include penile-scrotal duplication, ectopic bowel within the exstrophied bladder, small bladder patch, and significant hydronephrosis. Size and functional capacity of the detrusor muscle are important considerations in the eventual success of functional closure. The exstrophied bladder that is estimated at birth to have a capacity of 3 ml or more and demonstrates elasticity and contractility may be expected to develop a useful size capacity following successful closure.

826-A *(Campbell's, pp. 1787–1790)*

The benefits of performing an osteotomy in conjunction with the functional closure of an exstrophy bladder include: facilitation of abdominal wall closure; penile lengthening; and improved continence. Symphyseal approximation reduces midline abdominal closure tension and thus reduces the dehiscence rate, too. The posterior bilateral iliac osteotomy and the anterior bilateral transverse innominate osteotomy are currently being used for the exstrophy patient. Poor mobility of the pubis, the occasional delayed union or malunion of the ilium, and the need to turn the patient from the prone to supine position intraoperatively are some of the drawbacks to the posterior approach. The anterior transverse osteotomy, similar to the Salter osteotomy used for congenital hip dislocation, necessitates the use of external fixation with Buck's traction. Modified Bryant's traction can also be used postoperatively to immobilize patients after osteotomy and functional bladder closure. Usually within the first 72 hours of birth, functional bladder closure can be accomplished without an osteotomy because of the malleability of the pelvic ring. Occasionally osteotomies are necessary in the first 72 hours of life if the pubic diastasis is unduly wide or if the pelvis is not malleable.

827-B *(Campbell's, pp. 1789–1795)*

During primary bladder closure for the exstrophied bladder, a transverse incision of the urethral plate may be necessary when the male urethral groove is of inadequate length. Lateral skin incisions allow rotation of paraexstrophy skin flaps to cover the elongated penis if the urethral groove has been transected. Further penile lengthening is achieved by exposing the corpora cavernosa bilaterally and freeing the corpora from their attachments to the suspensory ligaments and the anterior part of the inferior pubic rami. Following closure of the exstrophied bladder, drainage is maintained by suprapubic catheterization. The urethra, however, is not stented in order to avoid pressure necrosis or the accumulation of infected secretions in the neourethra. Ureteral stents provide drainage during the first two weeks after the closure of the bladder. Thus the primary goal of bladder closure is to convert exstrophy into complete epispadias and incontinence.

828-B *(Campbell's, p. 1806)*

Not all children born with bladder exstrophy are candidates for staged functional bladder closure. Historically, ureterosigmoidostomy was the first urinary diversion to be utilized in this patient group. Ureterosigmoidostomy has the advantage of lacking an abdominal stoma; however, there are serious potential complications including pyelonephritis, hyperchloremic acidosis, rectal incontinence, ureteral obstruction, and late development of malignancy.

829-B *(Campbell's, pp. 1807–1808)*

The extended survival of patients with bladder exstrophy has uncovered the association of malignant processes with bladder exstrophy. About 80 per cent of carcinomas identified in exstrophied bladders are adenocarcinomas. Squamous cell carcinoma, rhabdomyosarcoma, and undifferentiated carcinoma account for the remainder. The prevalence of adenocarcinoma in exstrophied bladders is approximately 400-fold greater than that of normal bladders. Metaplastic transformation secondary to chronic irritation, infection and obstruction can give rise to premalignant lesions such as cystitis granularis. Adenocarcinoma of the colon adjacent to ureterointestinal anastomosis in exstrophy patients has also been reported. The risk of adenocarcinoma of the colon in exstrophy patients following ureterosigmoidostomy is 7,000 times that of the general population in patients 25 years of age or under. The mean latency interval from the time of ureterointestinal anastomosis to the diagnosis of intestinal tumor is 10 years.

830-A *(Campbell's, p. 1808)*

Male exstrophy patients are usually infertile. Sperm counts are usually low in men who have had primary bladder closure. This is probably attributable to iatrogenic injury of the verumontanum during functional closure and to retrograde ejaculation. Libido in exstrophy patients is normal and the erectile mechanism is usually intact. Female exstrophy patients have successfully delivered via vaginal or cesarean section. The main complication following pregnancy in the female exstrophy patient is cervical and uterine prolapse.

831-C *(Campbell's, p. 1808)*

Cloacal exstrophy represents one of the most severe congenital anomalies compatible with intrauterine viability. This is exceedingly rare and occurs in approximately 1 in 200,000 to 400,000 live births.

832-C *(Campbell's, pp. 1812–1813)*

Epispadias in males is classified according to the position of the dorsally displaced urethral meatus. It occurs in 1 out of 117,000 males and in one out of 484,000 females. Penopubic epispadias is the most common form, followed by penile and glandular epispadias in that order. Urinary incontinence is observed in the majority of penopubic epispadias and less in penile and glandular epispadias. A dorsal chordee is nearly always associated with epispadias. Epispadias in females is characterized by bifid clitoris, flattening of the mons, and separation of the labia. Anomalies associated with epispadias include vesicoureteral reflux which has been reported to be around 30 to 40 per cent.

833-C *(Campbell's, pp. 1814–1815)*

Congenital bladder diverticula unassociated with posterior urethral valves or neurogenic bladder are rare. This entity is almost exclusively seen in male patients. Characteristically these congenital diverticula are solitary and round and found in smooth walled bladders. They are generally larger than those associated with neurogenic bladders or lower tract obstructive anomalies. Upper tract imaging using intravenous pyelography is not the diagnostic study of choice and they are rarely detected on these studies. An association with Ehlers-Danlos syndrome has been noted in patients with congenital bladder diverticulum. All reported cases of congenital bladder diverticula associated with Ehlers-Danlos syndrome have been in males.

834-E *(Campbell's, pp. 1815–1818)*

Urachal abnormalities include patent urachus, urachal cyst, external urachal sinus, and urachal diverticulum. Patent urachus may be either congenital or acquired. The congenital form is a rare anomaly and can be either a vesicoumbilical fistula or persistence of the patent urachus with a partially distended bladder. On the other hand, an acquired patent urachus in the adult is usually a urinary umbilical fistula that results from bladder outflow obstruction. A urachal cyst may form within the isolated urachal canal if the lumen is enlarged from epithelial desquamation and degeneration. A urachal cyst may permit bacterial infection, and peritonitis may occur if there is rupture into the peritoneal cavity. Usually a urachal diverticulum is small and minimally contractile and thus does not require treatment. However, large urachal diverticula are frequently seen in patients with prune-belly syndrome and thus require resection. Adequate therapy for a patent urachus requires excision of all anomalous tissue with a cuff of bladder. Simple drainage of a urachal cyst is associated with recurrent infection in 30 per cent of the cases and late occurrence of adenocarcinoma, too.

835-D *(Campbell's, p. 1817)*

Staphylococcus aureus is the most common organism cultured from infected urachal cyst. Usually the signs and symptoms of a loculated infected urachal cyst include lower abdominal pain, fever, disturbed micturition, and midline hypogastric tenderness.

836-D *(Campbell's, p. 1822)*

Answers A, B, and C are all true statements concerning embryologic development of the genitourinary tract and the Latin derivation of cloaca. It is the mesonephric or wolffian duct which gives rise to the ureteral bud and develops into the vas deferens, seminal vesical and epididymis. The paramesonephric ducts in females give rise to the fallopian tubes, uterus, and upper vagina.

837-D *(Campbell's, pp. 1922–1825)*

Males and females both tend to present early with abdominal distention, and the distribution between high and low convergence of the urorectal tracts is equal between the sexes.

Females are somewhat more complex due to the presence of the vagina and uterus between the bladder and the rectum. The rectum may enter anterior or posterior to the vagina, into the vagina, or the vagina and rectum can enter the bladder. The vagina can vary from having a septum to complete duplication of the vagina with two cervices and uteri. In short, in females there are three sets of structures that intercommunicate, while in males there are only two sets of structures (the rectum and urethra) in need of surgical repair.

838-B *(Campbell's, p. 1825)*

The most common site for the rectovaginal fistula is the posterior margin of the vaginal orifice or at the base of a vaginal septum. It may also be confluent with the vagina, bladder, or have a fistulous tract from dilated colon high in the pelvis just behind the uterus, with the fistulous tract running the full length of the vagina to meet the urogenital sinus. The rectal opening can rarely be anterior to two separate or a single vagina (transposed) but the rectum is not seen anterior to the urethra or urogenital sinus.

839-E *(Campbell's, pp. 1826–1827)*

Most female infants with severe cloacal anomalies present at birth or soon after with abdominal distention and are discovered to have an abnormal perineum suggestive of imperforate anus/cloacal abnormality. There is routinely hydronephrosis, with or without vesicoureteral reflux and commonly there is a large fluid-filled structure in the pelvis. While this structure could possibly be the bladder, it is much more likely to be a large vagina filled with urine. Catheterization of the urogenital sinus will usually result in catheterization of the vagina and decompression. It is often difficult or impossible to catheterize the urethra without cystoscopy as it frequently enters the urogenital sinus at a very anterior sharp angle. While infection or sepsis are possible with cloacal abnormalities, they are not common presentations.

840-D *(Campbell's, pp. 1826–1828)*

A diverting colostomy is the initial step in treatment once a severe cloacal abnormality is diagnosed. A thorough radiographic and endoscopic evaluation are mandatory before any attempt at reconstruction or repair is considered. Sinograms, IVP, and ultrasound may all be useful x-rays. MRI of the LS spine should be done if there is a neurologic deficit due to the high association of tethered cord in these patients. During the endoscopic examination, the use of a feeding tube to inject contrast into the different tracts may be helpful. Intermittent catheterization of the UGS may allow the lower urinary tract to empty better even though one frequently only enters a large fluid filled vagina. Most nonemergent reconstruction should be delayed to age 1 year or more, when the infant is better able to stand a long major reconstructive procedure.

841-C *(Campbell's, pp. 1828–1830)*

Selection C is incorrect. A, B, D, and E are true principles regarding correction of cloacal abnormalities.

842-C *(Campbell's, p. 1851)*

Prune-belly syndrome, also known as triad syndrome, is a complex of abnormalities including an abdominal wall muscular deficit, large hypoplastic bladder with or without patent urachus, dilated tortuous ureters, and bilateral cryptorchidism. While hypospadias has been described, and megalourethra is common, neither constitutes part of the "classic" syndrome.

843-B *(Campbell's, p. 1869)*

Abdominal wall reconstruction is predominantly a cosmetic procedure with no functional effect on renal or bladder function.

844-D *(Campbell's, pp. 1852–1853)*

Hydronephrosis and renal dysplasia are the two renal abnormalities typically associated with the syndrome. With severe renal dysplasia, if oligohydramnios and pulmonary hypoplasia are not lethal, the degree renal function/failure may determine the prognosis. The renal dysplasia may be unilateral, bilateral or the kidneys may be histologically normal. In patients with associated lower urinary tract anomalies such as megaurethra, urethral stenosis, and imperforate anus, the degree of renal dysplasia has a tendency to be more severe. There is no evidence to suggest that a higher rate of renal malignancy is associated with the renal dysplasia in the prune-belly syndrome.

845-A *(Campbell's, p. 1853)*

All of the statements are true except A concerning the location of the ureteral orifices. The usual location of the ureteral orifices is very lateral and posterior in association with a large and at times enormous trigone. Reflux is common and fluoroscopic studies often show poor peristalsis.

846-C *(Campbell's, p. 1853)*

The bladder in prune-belly syndrome is typically very large with a thick wall and is attached to the anterior abdominal wall at the umbilicus. There is often a pseudodiverticulum at the dome and the urachus may be patent, especially if bladder outflow obstruction exists. The trigone is large and on occasions enormous with the bladder neck being wide, relaxed, and ill defined. Urodynamic studies in many are normal, while some have reported finding elevated detrusor pressures relative to the flow rate.

847-D *(Campbell's, pp. 1854–1855)*

All of the statements are true except D. Erection and orgasm are normal in prune-belly syndrome, but due to the abnormal bladder neck and dilated prostatic urethra retrograde ejaculation is common and no cases of fertility have been documented.

848-C *(Campbell's, p. 1855)*

All are true statements associated with prune-belly syndrome except C. Neurologic lesions are not common with prune-belly syndrome.

849-D *(Campbell's, p. 1858)*

Statement D is false. If the ultrasound shows significant hydronephrosis and ureteral dilatation, an IVP may be considered, but if the infant voids well, and has a stable normal creatinine, prophylactic antibiotics and avoidance of instrumentation of the urinary tract (VCUG) is recommended. Also, intravenous contrast is poorly concentrated in the kidneys in the first 2 to 3 weeks of life. A combination of ultrasound, nuclear renal scans, and intravenous pyelograms can usually give adequate evaluation. If surgery is indicated due to urinary tract infections or deteriorating renal function, a VCUG may be indicated before planning an operative course. Often cardiac and pulmonary complications require immediate evaluation and treatment after birth and must delay initial urologic evaluation. Creatinine is normal at birth (mothers renal function), but the creatinine should be monitored over the first week when creatinine will reflect the neonates renal function.

850-B *(Campbell's, pp. 1861–1856)*

The patients in category II (see below) may do well with no or minimal intervention. Urinary diversion may be required in selected patients with renal deterioration and recurrent infections. There is no proof that aggressive surgical intervention (without the indications of renal deterioration or recurrent infection) improves long-term survival.

Categories of Prune-Belly Syndrome

- I Oligohydramnios, pulmonary hypoplasia or pneumothorax. May have urethral obstruction, club foot, or patent urachus.
- II Typical external features and uropathy of the full-blown syndrome but no immediate risk to survival.

May have mild or unilateral renal dysplasia. May or may not develop urosepsis or gradual azotemia.

III External features may be mild or incomplete. Uropathy is less severe and renal function is stable.

851-C *(Campbell's, p. 1872)*

A, B, D, and E are true statements about urethral developments. Statement C is false. Although the posterior urethra develops in the male and female, androgen does affect the posterior urethra in the male. It is involved in development of the prostate and genital ducts (seminal vesical and vas deferens), which are intimately involved with posterior urethral anatomy.

852-B *(Campbell's, pp. 1872–1874)*

While type II posterior urethral valves were described by Hugh Hampton Young in the initial classification of posterior urethral valves, they are now accepted as a nonobstructing anatomical variant, and it is agreed that type II posterior urethral valves do not exist as a clinical entity.

853-C *(Campbell's, pp. 1876–1877)*

All are true statements except C. Acute abdomen due to bowel obstruction is not generally found with posterior urethral valves and no gastrointestinal malformations are associated with the defect. Ascites may be seen and infected ascites associated with renal fornix extravasation and transudation of retroperitoneal urine across the thin permeable peritoneum. Even when empty, the thick walled bladder may be palpable in the lower abdomen. Toddlers may present with UTIs or voiding dysfunction and school aged boys (the least common age of presentation) will have voiding dysfunction, most commonly incontinence, as their presenting symptoms.

854-C *(Campbell's, pp. 1878–1879)*

A nadir creatinine of <1.0 is associated with good long-term prognosis *after* ablation of posterior urethral valves. A, B, D, and E are true statements.

855-B *(Campbell's, pp. 1879–1882)*

All statements are true except B. VUR is present in only 30 to 50 per cent at presentation with PUVs.

856-D *(Campbell's, pp. 1882–1883)*

With reflux being found in one third to one half of infants with posterior urethral valves, it is recommended that antibiotic prophylaxis be started empirically. Monitoring electrolytes, acid-base, and creatinine with appropriate fluid and antibiotic therapy, if indicated for infection, should be routine. If the infant is ill or septic, valve ablation should be delayed. While initial upper tract studies such as ultrasound or IVP are useful as a baseline, the authors recommend *not* repeating the voiding cystourethrogram until a couple of months after valve ablation since reflux is common and any surgical repair should not be considered unless there is progressive upper tract dilatation with deterioration of renal function or recurrent infections.

857-C *(Campbell's, pp. 1883–1884)*

Prenatal intervention has not been shown to affect outcome, and risks early labor, amniotic infection, and hemorrhage. There is no way to reliably differentiate severe bilateral VUR or prune-belly syndrome from posterior urethral valves. Statements A and D are true, and the consideration of decompressive diversion for patients with nadir creatinines >1.8 is complicated. The goal of long-term, gradual improvement in renal function by maximizing renal growth and drainage has been suggested to be superior with cutaneous ureterostomies over cutaneous vesicostomies. The downside is that the child is still committed to reconstructive surgery following cutaneous ureterostomies.

858-A *(Campbell's, p. 1886)*

All are true statements concerning urethral obstruction except A. Posterior urethral valves are much more common than anterior urethral obstruction.

859-C *(Campbell's, p. 1888)*

Megalourethra is a nonobstructing urethral dilatation of the penile urethra, which may be isolated or associated with upper tract abnormalities. In the scaphoid variety, the corpus spongiosum/urethra is the only abnormality, whereas the fusiform variety is associated with the typical corpus spongiosum defect and a variable defect in the corpus cavernosum. With the fusiform variety, rarely the cavernosal defect may be so severe that a functional phallus is not possible and gender reassignment may be appropriate. Usually a circumcision incision with degloving of the penis will allow resection of the excess urethra and reconstruction of a normal-caliber urethra.

860-D *(Campbell's, pp. 1888–1889)*

A, B, C, and E are all true statements concerning urethral duplication. Statement D is false. With dorsal urethral duplication the ventral "normal" urethra is associated with a normal bladder neck and sphincter mechanism, and therefore simple excision of the urethral duplication will provide most with continence.

861-A *(Campbell's, p. 1893)*

Hypospadias is a congenital defect of the penis, resulting in incomplete development of the anterior urethra. The abnormal urethral opening may be found anywhere along the shaft of of the penis or on the perineum. The more *proximal* the meatus, the more likely will the ventral surface appear shortened and curved by chordee. Hypospadias results in various degrees of urethral and corpus spongiosum deficiency. The fibrous tissue found with chordee replaces Buck's fascia and the more superficial dartos fascia. The skin over the ventral surface is thin. The prepuce is deficient ventrally and forms a dorsal hood over the glans.

862-C *(Campbell's, p. 1895)*

The most common anomalies associated with hypospadias are undescended testes and inguinal hernia. This is probably a reflection of a common endocrinologic etiology. Although one would not expect an increase in other urinary abnormalities due to different fetal developmental timing and stimuli for formation, some authors report more urinary abnormalities than normal in boys with hypospadias. Nevertheless, most feel that routine excretory urography is not justified due to the low incidence of other urinary abnormalities.

863-B *(Campbell's, pp. 1895–1896)*

In severe forms of hypospadias, especially with cryptorchism, the diagnosis of intersex must be ruled out. The intersex states that must be ruled out in a child with hypospadias include the following: (1) adrenogenital syndrome; (2) mixed gonadal dysgenesis; (3) incomplete male pseudohermaphroditism, type I (Reifenstein syndrome); (4) incomplete male pseudohermaphrodism, type II; (5) true hermaphroditism; and (6) micropenis. Buccal smears and karyotype are not routinely necessary, but in the newborn with hypospadias and nonpalpable testes, they become essential. In general, the presence of palpable scrotal testes can be taken as evidence of the patient being a genetic male. Klinefelter's syndrome is one of the most common forms of hypogonadism and infertility. The invariable clinical features of Klinefelter's syndrome in adults are a male phenotype, small firm testes, and azoospermia.

REFERENCE

1. Kelais, P.P., King L.R., and Belman, A.B.: Clinical Pediatric Urology, 3rd ed. Philadelphia, WB Saunders Co., 1992, p. 623.

864-E *(Campbell's, p. 1894)*

Anterior hypospadias comprises approximately 50 per cent of the cases. The most common lesion presents with a proximal glanular or subcoronal meatus, a glanular distal groove, and a transverse web resulting in deflection of the urinary stream. Middle and posterior hypospadias represent 30 and 20 per cent of cases, respectively.

REFERENCE

1. Duckett: AUA Update Series, Vol. XII, Lesson 17.

865-D *(Campbell's, pp. 1900–1901)*

Once the urethroplasty has been accomplished, coverage of the ventral surface can usually be achieved by mobilization of penile and preputial skin. Free skin grafts should be full-thickness rather than split-thickness because of the tendency of split-thickness grafts to contract. Because the free graft must be revascularized, the key to success is perfect skin cover of the graft with well-vascularized dorsal preputial and penile skin. Scrotal skin may be transposed to the penis when penile skin is deficient, but this is used mainly in adults and for secondary procedures.

866-C *(Campbell's, p. 1902)*

The decision to use the standard MAGPI procedure depends on the mobility of the urethra. This is tested with fine forceps and distal traction on the lateral lips of the meatus. If immobile, a proper advancement cannot be achieved because the distal glans must then be brought proximally to meet the meatus, giving the glans a depressed or flattened appearance.

867-B *(Campbell's, p. 1912)*

Most surgeons feel that age 6 to 18 months is the ideal time for repair in order to minimize the emotional effect of this surgery. This time frame is chosen to reduce the effects of separation anxiety and genital awareness. Generally, the penis with hypospadias is of sufficient size at 3 months to accomplish this surgery and anesthesia risks are reduced after 3 months of age.

868-A *(Campbell's, p. 1913)*

Attention to details that will avoid complications during and after surgery is paramount. To avoid wound infection, well-prepared skin should be ensured; however, prophylactic antibiotics have little value in avoiding wound infection. Diversion of urine (e.g., urethral stent) is intended to allow sealing of the suture lines and sufficient healing to avoid leakage of urine into the tissues outside the neourethra. Edema occurs to some degree in most hypospadias repairs. A compression dressing left for 2 to 3 days is effective in controlling edema and hematoma formation. Poor wound healing after hypospadias is primarily due to ischemic flaps. Postoperative erections in the postpubertal patient may disrupt suture lines and are best controlled with amylnitrate pulvules.

869-D *(Campbell's, p. 1914)*

Common complications after hypospadias repair include residual chordee, meatal stenosis, urethral diverticula, urethrocutaneous fistula, and urethral stricture. Urethral stenosis and stricture are most likely the results of poor vascularity of a flap or graft or contraction at a suture line. A thin stricture occurring within 3 months of surgery may respond to dilatation or incision by urethrotomy, but only a small percentage of late strictures respond to such manipulation. Generally, strictures require excision and reanastomosis. Symptoms of a stricture in the very young child include a dribbling stream and straining to void. Often UTI is the first sign of a problem. Evaluation includes observation of stream, urethrography, and endoscopy.

870-C *(Campbell's, p. 1914)*

Redo hypospadias patients usually present with a combination of problems, including curvature, fistulas, and stricture. Using available genital skin as flaps is preferred when possible, however, when there is no penile skin available, bladder mucosa grafts are the optimal urethral replacement. However, if the urethral gap is less than 5 cm, then buccal mucosa is the preferred graft material. The main complication of bladder mucosa grafts is that the mucosa does not withstand the irritation at the skin surface and eversion occurs. Meatal dilatation on a daily basis may help avoid this complication.

REFERENCE

1. Duckett, J.: AUA Update Series, Vol. XII, Lesson 17.

871-D *(Campbell's, p. 1905)*

An onlay island flap is the procedure of choice if there is no chordee, but the meatus is too proximal for a Mathieu procedure or the ventral skin is too thin for a flap. These conditions require a procedure to replace the ventral urethra. The onlay island flap is an extremely versatile procedure which is useful for both mid or distal shaft hypospadias.

872-C *(Campbell's, p. 1920)*

All are true statements concerning development of the male genitalia except C. At birth the inhibitory effect of maternal estrogens on the pituitary is released. This results in a surge in gonadotropins and subsequent surge in testosterone resulting in penile growth during the first six months of life. The penis grows much more slowly during the rest of childhood until puberty and gonadotropins are low until then.

873-D *(Campbell's, p. 1921)*

Anorectal or cloacal malformations in boys may be associated with hypospadias, penile duplication, micropenis, and scrotal deformity. In females with imperforate anus, anomalies include bicornuate uterus, uterus didelphys, hypoplastic uterus, vaginal septum, vaginal agenesis, imperforate hymen, and absence of the lower third of the vagina.

Boys with tracheoesophageal fistula or esophageal atresia may have hypospadias (6 per cent), penile agenesis, penoscrotal transposition, and scrotal agenesis or malformation.

Robinow's syndrome consists of hemihypertropy and small genitalia.

Prader Willi's syndrome is believed to be secondary to a hypothalamic defect. These patients are usually obese, retarded, hypotonic, short in stature, and have microphallus or ambiguous genitalia. Prune-belly syndrome is not usually associated with abnormal external genitalia.

874-D *(Campbell's, pp. 1923–1924)*

Lateral curvature may often only be demonstrable with the penis in the erect state. Significant lateral curvature may be corrected with a modified Nesbit procedure (in which ellipses of tunica albuginea are excised from the site of maximal curvature to straighten the penis. Care to avoid injury to the neurovascular bundles and artificial erection to assure adequate correction are critical).

Mild penile torsion is corrected by degloving the penile skin and simply rearranging the skin on the shaft of the penis. Severe torsion may also require lysis of fibrous bands at the base of the penis. If still rotated, a nonabsorbable suture may be placed through the lateral aspect of the base of the corpora cavernosum on the side opposite the direction of rotation (generally the right side) and fixing it to the pubic symphysis dorsal to the penile shaft.

875-D *(Campbell's, pp. 1924–1925)*

Micropenis is defined as a penis less than 2.5 cm in length with the ratio of length to circumference usually normal. The corporal bodies are only occasionally found to be severely hypoplastic with the scrotum typically fused but hypoplastic and the testes frequently undescended. Differentiation and growth of the penis requires testicular testosterone, which is driven by *maternal* chorionic gonadotropin during the first trimester and *fetal* luteinizing hormone during the second and third trimester.

876-C *(Campbell's, pp. 1925–1926)*

All statements are true except C. The urethra generally is found on the anal verge adjacent to a small skin tag and in others opens onto the scrotum.

877-B *(Campbell's, p. 1926)*

All statements are true except B. The two phalluses may either have a single or two corporal bodies.

878-C *(Campbell's, pp. 1927–1928)*

All statements are true except C. The genital tubercle is the precursor of the glans penis. The defect in scrotal engulfment is felt to be due to incomplete, or failure of, the normal inferomedial migration of the genital swellings which become the scrotum.

879-E *(Campbell's, pp. 1930–1931)*

Urethral prolapse represents eversion of the urethral mucosa and may respond to local application of estrogen cream and sitz baths but may occasionally require excision of the prolapsed mucosa and closure of the urethral mucosa to the introital mucosa. Paraurethral cysts usually regress spontaneously over 1 to 2 months but occasionally may need to be incised.

Imperforate hymen with hydrocolpos presents as a white/gray bulging interlabial mass with the retained vaginal secretions (up to a liter) trapped behind the intact hymen. Simple incision of the hymen allows normal drainage of secretions.

Uterovaginal prolapse is rare and associated with meningomyelocele. The anomaly results from denervation of the levator ani with subsequently poor pelvic support. It may resolve spontaneously or mechanical support may be needed.

Labial adhesions do not present as a mass.

880-D *(Campbell's, pp. 1934–1929)*

All statements concerning vertical fusion defects of the müllerian duct are true except D. The diagnosis is generally made at puberty in the evaluation of girls with amenorrhea. The external genitalia are normal, and either the vagina is absent or there is a shallow pouch 2 to 3 cm in depth.

881-B *(Campbell's, p. 1936)*

All the statements are true except B. In complete duplication, it is common to have one hemivagina obstructed resulting in unilateral hydrometrocolpos. The obstructed hemivagina and bicornate uterus are almost always associated with ipsilateral renal agenesis.

882-A *(Campbell's, p. 1939)*

All are true indications for orchiopexy with undescended testicle except A. There is rarely an indication to perform an orchiopexy for a retractile testis. The exceptions are intermittent pain or significantly reduced size of the retractile testis.

883-D *(Campbell's, p. 1939)*

All are true statements except D. A blind ending vas is often associated with an absent testis on that side, but the blind-ending gonadal vessels must be identified in the inguinal canal or retroperitoneum to ensure the absence of the testes.

884-B *(Campbell's, p. 1944)*

All answers are true except B. While 6 months to a year of observation is appropriate, definitive treatment should be undertaken before the patient is 2 years old in the hope of possible preservation of fertility. Either laparoscopy or bilateral inguinal exploration are appropriate depending on the surgeon's preference or experience. With persistent bilateral nonpalpable testis and otherwise normal male external genitalia, a baseline testosterone followed by administration of chorionic gonadotropin stimulating hormone is recommended. If the baseline gonadotropin levels are elevated and there is no testosterone increase in response to the hCG, there is no testis present and exploration is not warranted.

885-C *(Campbell's, p. 1946)*

All are true statements except C. If not obviously necrotic (dead) but with persistent ischemia, the testis should be pexed in the scrotum and preserved. While spermatogenesis may very well never return, the testis may retain normal hormonal function.

886-C *(Campbell's, pp. 1947–1948)*

All are true statements except C. There is no adequate proof to support the idea that there is a significant difference in long-term recurrence rate between high and low ligation.

887-C *(Campbell's, p. 1949)*

An older child with loculated hydrocele may be approached via a scrotal incision. A classic torsion also is generally approached via a scrotal incision. An atrophic testis and a definite torsion of the appendix testis may not require exploration but should be approached via a scrotal incision if surgery is necessary.

888-C *(Campbell's, pp. 1949–1950)*

All statements are true except C. After the external oblique fascia is opened, the vascular pedicle is atraumatically clamped before the testis is mobilized.

889-B *(Campbell's, p. 1946)*

All are true except B. While a hydrocele should be observed up to one year for spontaneous resolution, a true hernia should be treated on an urgent (not necessarily emergent) basis with contralateral exploration being debated by many if no clinical hernia/hydrocele is present.

890-C *(Campbell's, pp. 1939–1944)*

Option C is false. All of the other options are valid, but the testis may be at some increased risk for carcinoma and needs ultimately to be removed or brought down into the scrotum where it can at least be intermittently examined.

891-B *(Campbell's, pp. 1941–1942)*

All features of the classic Fowler-Stephens orchiopexy are true except B. The spermatic vessels should be divided as high in the retroperitoneum as possible to preserve as many of the communications with the vasal and cremasteric vessels as possible.

892-B *(Campbell's, p. 1951)*

Appropriate assignment of gender as soon as possible after birth is the most important factor in management of neonates with the intersex state. Procrastination and temporary or inappropriate gender assignment at birth may lead to psychosexual developmental abnormalities with permanent consequences. Electrolyte abnormalities should be closely monitored as well.

893-D *(Campbell's, p. 1951)*

The testis-determining factor located on the Y chromosome is the most important factor determining testicular development. In the absence of this factor, testicular differentiation does not occur, and an ovary is formed at the end of the first trimester.

894-A *(Campbell's, p. 1951)*

Müllerian inhibitory substance, a glycoprotein produced by Sertoli cells in the fetal testis, acts locally to cause regression of the paramesonephric ductal system, which in the female becomes the fallopian tubes, uterus, and upper vagina.

895-B *(Campbell's, p. 1951)*

Testosterone, secreted by the Leydig cells of the fetal testis, acts locally on the mesonephric duct to induce formation of the epididymis, vas deferens, and seminal vesicle.

896-D *(Campbell's, pp. 1951–1952)*

In the absence of müllerian inhibitory substance and testosterone secreted by the fetal testis, the mesonephric ducts regress and the paramesonephric ducts develop into fallopian tubes, uterus, and upper vagina.

897-A *(Campbell's, p. 1952)*

Development of the male external genitalia and urogenital sinus is dependent on 5-alpha reductase, an enzyme that converts testosterone to dihydrotestosterone, which in turn binds with androgen receptor to effect molecular changes that result in virilization.

898-E *(Campbell's, p. 1953)*

Female pseudohermaphroditism occurs when a genetic female (XX chromosomal pattern) is exposed to excessive androgens in utero, and is the most common category of intersex.

899-D *(Campbell's, p. 1953)*

Congenital adrenal hyperplasia accounts for 60 per cent of children with ambiguous genitalia. This condition is caused by an hereditary deficiency of one of several enzymes necessary for normal adrenal steroidogenesis, which results in increased ACTH secretion and abnormally high levels of adrenal steroid precursors that have androgenic effects.

900-A *(Campbell's, pp. 1953–1954)*

Around 95 per cent of patients with congenital adrenal hyperplasia have 21-hydroxylase deficiency. This occurs in two forms, mild and severe. The severe form can cause adrenal insufficiency in the first weeks after birth.

901-D *(Campbell's, p. 1954)*

11-Beta-hydroxylase deficiency results in increased formation of desoxycorticosterone, a steroid that promotes sodium retention and leads to hypertension.

902-E *(Campbell's, p. 1954)*

Normal karyotypes are usual in true hermaphroditism, testicular feminization, and 5-α reductase deficiency; 45XO is typical for Turner's syndrome. The most common genetic pattern in patients with mixed gonadal dysgenesis is the mosaic 45XO/46XY. This is the second most common cause of ambiguous genitalia after congenital adrenal hyperplasia.

903-C *(Campbell's, p. 1955)*

Intra-abdominal gonads in patients with mixed gonadal dysgenesis have a high rate of malignant degeneration with formation of seminoma or gonadoblastoma. Because tumors may occur in early childhood, early gonadectomy is recommended. Malignant degeneration is common whenever a dysgenetic testis and a Y chromosome coexist.

904-D *(Campbell's, p. 1955)*

Testicular feminization syndrome is caused by deficient androgen receptor binding. This form of intersex is usually diagnosed at puberty during investigation of amenorrhea, and occurs in phenotypically normal females.

905-E *(Campbell's, p. 1955)*

Pseudovaginal perineoscrotal hypospadias is caused by deficiency of 5-alpha reductase, which is necessary for normal development of male external genitalia.

906-D *(Campbell's, p. 1955)*

Defective paramesonephric duct regression, perhaps caused by inadequate müllerian inhibitory substance function, leads to hernia uteri inguinalis. In this condition, phenotypic males are found to have a rudimentary uterus and fallopian tubes, usually during inguinal exploration for cryptorchidism or hernia.

907-B *(Campbell's, p. 1955)*

True hermaphroditism is defined as genital ambiguity with gonadal tissue of both sexes. It is rare compared to other causes of genital ambiguity. In the lateral type of hermaphroditism, there is a testis on one side and an ovary on the other; unilateral hermaphroditism has an ovotestis on one side and a normal contralateral gonad; the bilateral type has an ovotestis on both sides. Most true hermaphrodites have a large phallus and are assigned a male sex.

908-C *(Campbell's, p. 1955)*

Assignment of sex should be based on functional anatomic potential. Because construction of a functional phallus is more difficult than that of an adequate vagina, female sex assignment is appropriate for the majority of patients with intersex.

909-B *(Campbell's, p. 1956)*

Genital reconstruction should be accomplished before the age of sexual awareness (age 3–3½). Surgery during the neonatal period sacrifices the spontaneous phallic regression that occurs in female pseudohermaphrodite patients with steroid replacement. Surgery at about 18 months of age is optimal for many patients, although in situations where there is significant parental anxiety regarding ambiguous genitalia, earlier surgery can be considered.

910-E *(Campbell's, p. 1957)*

Clitorectomy should never be performed during genital reconstruction because of the resultant cosmetic deficits and sexual dysfunction. Although steroid replacement does result in clitoral regression, this is usually not complete enough to avoid the need for surgical revision. The best strategy is to allow for maximal spontaneous diminution in clitoral size and then perform surgical revision.

911-D *(Campbell's, p. 1961)*

A phallus of less than 2.5 cm stretched length in the neonate is likely to be inadequate for satisfactory function in the male sex assignment. Systemic testosterone administration can be used to assess growth response. If an inadequate phallus is present, female sex assignment should be strongly considered.

912-E *(Campbell's, p. 1965)*

Intersex patients have typically achieved satisfactory psychosexual development and have experienced erotic attraction that is concordant with sex assignment in the neonatal period.

913-C *(Campbell's, pp. 1967, 1988, 1997, 2003)*

All statements are true except C. The most common ALL type in testis tumors of prepubertal boys is yolk sac carcinoma (also known as endodermal sinus tumor, orchidoblastoma, embryonal adenocarcinoma, infantile adenocarcinoma, and testicular adenocarcinoma with clear cells).

914-C *(Campbell's, p. 1968)*

Only a small minority of patients with Wilms' tumor, approximately 15 per cent, have another congenital defect. Aniridia is found in 1.1 per cent with Wilms' tumor (U.S. 0.000027 in the general population) and is part of the WAGR syndrome: *W*ilms' tumor, *A*niridia, *G*enitourinary anomalies, and *R*etardation. Parahemihypertrophy is seen in 2.9 per cent of those with Wilms' tumor and is associated with an increased incidence of other cancers including embryonal carcinomas and especially adrenocortical carcinomas and hepatoblastomas. The Beckwith-Wiedemann syndrome consists of visceromegaly involving the adrenal cortex, kidneys, liver, pancreas, and gonads. Omphalocele, hemihypertrophy, microcephaly, mental retardation, and macroglossia may also be present. Musculoskeletal anomalies are seen in 3 per cent of Wilms' tumor patients and there is a 30-fold increase in the incidence of neurofibromatosis. Genitourinary anomalies are seen in 4.4 per cent, most commonly including renal hypoplasia, ectopia, fusions, duplications, cystic disease, hypospadias, cryptorchidism, and pseudohermaphroditism.

915-C *(Campbell's, pp. 1976–1977)*

Most children with Wilms' tumor appear well in contrast to neuroblastoma where the child usually *looks* sick. Other occasional findings include hypertension in 25 to 63 per cent secondary to renal compression and subsequent production of renin or direct production of renin from the tumor itself. Rare cases of Wilms' tumor are associated with polycythemia secondary to erythropoietin production by the tumor. Even more rare presentations include varicocele, hernia, enlarged testis, congestive heart failure secondary to arteriovenous shunting within the tumor or caval or atrial tumor thrombus, Cushing's syndrome, and hydrocephalus secondary to brain metastasis.

916-C *(Campbell's, pp. 1971–1975)*

Anaplasia, clear cell, and rhabdoid tumor are the unfavorable histologic tumor types. Multilocular cyst, congenital mesoblastic nephroma, and rhabdomyosarcoma tumor are the favorable histologic cell types. Multilocular cysts are treated adequately with simple excision alone and are considered benign tumors. Congenital mesoblastic nephroma tends to have local infiltration rather than the classic pseudocapsule and has a uniformly benign course. Rhabdomyomatous nephroblastoma is characterized by the presence of fetal striated muscle and is a rare but favorable histologic type. Only 10 per cent of Wilms' tumor are of unfavorable histology but account for 60 per cent of deaths. Anaplastic is more common in older children. It is defined as having a three-fold variation in nuclear size with hyperchromatism and abnormal mitotic figures. Rhabdoid tumor makes up only 2 per cent of Wilms' tumors but is the most lethal type with an 82 per cent death rate. The cells are large and uniform with large nuclei and prominent nucleoli. Cytoplasmic eosinophilic inclusions appear to be fibrils under microscopy but are not actually muscle and the demonstration of striated muscle actually excludes the diagnosis of rhabdoid tumor.

917-C *(Campbell's, pp. 1978–1980)*

All treatments are true except C. A limited resection of bowel or liver may be indicated, but heroic efforts to resect all tumor is not justified. In a right-sided mass with vena-caval invasion from thrombus, the cava may be resected to the level of the hepatic veins because the left kidney has adequate collaterals via the gonadal and adrenal veins. No improvement in survival has been demonstrated by radical node dissection if nodes are positive.

918-C *(Campbell's, p. 1981)*

Although younger patients are more likely to have favorable histology, in any given patient, age is not a good prognosticator of outcome. Histology is the most important single variable. Unfavorable histology is associated with higher recurrence and death rates. Beckwith, on the other hand, believes age is prognostically important and that even rhabdomyomatous Wilms' in older patients do poorly.

Hematogenous metastasis (with lung being the most common, followed by liver, bone, and brain) is important to detect. Aggressive chemotherapy dramatically improves survival for these patients. In NWTS-II, negative nodes were associated with 82 per cent survival versus 54 per cent in those with positive nodes.

Local tumor extension with invasion into or through the pseudocapsule, or with vascular or renal sinus invasion is associated with a higher local recurrence rate, which can be reduced by radiation of the tumor bed.

A subgroup of patients with postrelapse survival at three years of 40 per cent was identified with five favorable characteristics: (1) favorable histology tumors that recurred only in the lung; (2) local recurrence in the abdomen when no postoperative radiation was given; (3) originally stage I tumors; (4) tumors originally treated with only two drugs; and (5) recurrence 12 months or more after diagnosis.

919-A *(Campbell's, pp. 1987–1988)*

All statements are true but A. While neuroblastoma does arise from cells of neural crest origin, it is from the adrenal medulla—it also may arise from anywhere along the sympathetic chain including head and neck (7 per cent), chest (13 per cent), pelvis (4 per cent), and abdominal nonadrenal (18 per cent). The adrenal is the single most common primary site with 37 per cent of neuroblastomas originating in the adrenal gland.

920-C *(Campbell's, pp. 1988–1989)*

All statements are true except C. Neuroblastoma is rarely an incidental finding. In contrast to Wilms' tumor, which usually presents with a unilateral, smooth mass in an otherwise healthy appearing child, the child with neuroblastoma frequently looks sick, with one or more of the features listed in answer B.

921-D *(Campbell's, pp. 1991–1993)*

Renal vein and/or vena caval tumor is not seen with neuroblastoma, although external compression with anterior caval displacement may be seen. MRI is rarely preferable to ultrasound and/or CT scan. Anemia and occasionally thrombocytopenia and coagulopathy are seen. Neuroblastoma is an APUD tumor (*a*mine *p*recursor *u*ptake and *d*ecarboxylation) and may secrete catecholamines which may produce paroxysmal attacks of sweating, pallor, headaches, hypertension, palpitations, and flushing. Vasoactive intestinal peptide (VIP) has also been reported as a product of these APUD tumors and may cause intractable watery diarrhea and hypokalemia. Bone marrow aspiration should be done in all patients with suspected neuroblastoma. About 70 per cent have metastasis at presentation and 50 per cent have positive bone marrow aspirates. Chest x-ray is routinely done in search of a thoracic mass, as is a skeletal survey in search of bone metastases.

922-C *(Campbell's, pp. 1994–1995)*

Stage IV-S is a favorable prognostic sign. It is a unique form of disseminated disease of infancy with metastatic disease limited to the skin (bluish subcutaneous nodules), liver, or bone marrow. The tumor in this group usually regresses spontaneously with long-term survival of approximately 80 per cent.

Serum ferritin is elevated in 40 to 50 per cent with stage III or IV disease. Survival in stage III disease is 76 per cent with normal serum ferritin versus 23 per cent if it is elevated. For stage IV disease, survival is 27 per cent versus 3 per cent. Age is inversely proportional to survival. In the Breslow and McCann study, survival is 74 per cent in infants under one year of age and 26 per cent and 12 per cent for those 12 to 23 months and those over the age of 2 years, respectively.

The DNA index by flow cytometry is of prognostic significance. An index of one rarely occurs in low stage disease. In disseminated disease an index of one is associated with a poorer response to cyclophosphamide and doxorubicin.

Stage is an important prognostic indicator and is independent of age at diagnosis and site of tumor.

Stage and prognosis charts are shown below. Two-year survival without evidence of relapse is usually equivalent to cure.

Stage		Survival
Stage 0	Neuroblastoma in situ	80% 2-year survival
Stage I	Tumor confined to the organ or structure of origin	80% 2-year survival
Stage II	Tumors extending in continuity beyond organ or structure of origin but not crossing midline; ipsilateral regional nodes may be involved	80% 2-year survival
Stage III	Tumors extending in continuity beyond midline; regional lymph nodes may be involved bilaterally	37% 2-year survival ↑ Ferritin 23% NL ferritin 27%
Stage IV	Distant mets involving bones, bone marrow, brain, skin, liver, lung soft tissues, or distant lymph nodes	5–7% 2-year survival ↑ Ferritin 3% NL Ferritin 27%
Stage IV-S	Patients who would be classified as stage I or II but have remote spread of tumor to one or more of the following sites: liver, skin, or bone marrow (without radiographic evidence of bone mets on skeletal survey); usually do not have elevated serum ferritin or E-rosette inhibitory factor	80%

Treatment	Surgery	Adjunctive Treatment
Stage I	Simple surgical removal en bloc.	Neither chemotherapy nor radiation have been shown to enhance survival.
Stage II	Removal of adjacent organs is not justifiable with the exception of adjacent kidney with adrenal neuroblastoma.	Same as for Stage I.
Stage III/IV	Radical surgery appears to offer no benefit for long-term survival.	XRT-for large or painful nets 1000–2000 cGy. Chemo- 4-6 drug combination chemo (cyclophosphamide, doxorubicin, cisplatin are the most effective single agents). No one combination has improved survival greatly or been shown to be superior.

PART XII

RENAL DISEASES OF UROLOGIC SIGNIFICANCE

CHAPTERS 55 THROUGH 57

DIRECTIONS: Each question below contains suggested responses. Select the ONE BEST response to each question.

923. Atherosclerotic renal artery disease:

A. Accounts for one third of all renovascular hypertension
B. Begins as a proliferation of myointimal cells in the intima and rarely involves the ostium of the renal artery
C. Is associated with reversal of hypertension after surgical correction less often than in patients with fibromuscular disease
D. Usually involves only the renal arteries
E. Is rarely progressive and may be controlled medically without threat of renal deterioration

924. The most common of the fibromuscular diseases is:

A. Intimal fibroplasia
B. Fibromuscular hyperplasia
C. Perimedial fibroplasia
D. Medial fibroplasia
E. Takayasu's aortitis

925. Renin is released from the juxtaglomerular apparatus in response to all the following stimuli EXCEPT:

A. Low renal perfusion pressure
B. A high chloride or sodium concentration in the distal convoluted tubule
C. Adrenergic stimulation of beta-1 receptors in the JG cells
D. Increase in cylic adenosine monophosphate (cAMP)
E. Decreased cellular calcium

926. Activation of the angiotensin II receptor results in all of the following EXCEPT:

A. Vasoconstriction
B. Sodium retention
C. Release of aldosterone
D. Release of catecholamines
E. Increased production of renin

927. The diagnosis of renovascular hypertension is predicated on all the following EXCEPT:

A. The demonstration of a physiologically significant decrease in renal blood flow to one or both kidneys
B. Hypersecretion of renin from the more ischemic kidney
C. Agiographic demonstration of renal arterial disease
D. The absence of renin secretion from the contralateral kidney
E. Lowering of blood pressure on removal of the source of hyperreninemia or on blockage of the renin-angiotensin system

928. All of the following are clinical features suggesting that renovascular hypertension may be present EXCEPT:

A. Hyperkalemia
B. Abrupt onset of severe or malignant hypertension
C. Poor response of hypertension to standard diuretic therapy or antiadrenergic agents.
D. Cigarette smoking
E. Age of onset of hypertension: less than 25 years or greater than 45 years

929. Advantages of the single-dose captopril test over peripheral plasma renin activity include all the following EXCEPT:

A. Patients may remain on beta-blockers.
B. It has a specificity of 95 per cent and sensitivity of 100 per cent.
C. Patients may remain on diuretics.
D. There is no need for a 24-hour urine sodium collection if patients have been on a normal or high salt diet.
E. The exclusion value is 100 per cent.

930. The gold standard in identifying which kidney is the cause of abnormal renin secretion is:

A. Single-dose captopril test
B. Differential renal vein renin determination
C. Intravenous urogram
D. Captopril renogram
E. Angiography

931. In which of the following renal vein renin patterns would surgical correction most likely be curative?

A. Left renal vein-12; right renal vein-9; IVC-6
B. Left renal vein-12; right renal vein-6; IVC-6
C. Left renal vein-15; right renal vein-15; IVC-12
D. Left renal vein-5; right renal vein-5; IVC-4

932. All of the following are true regarding medical management of renovascular hypertension EXCEPT:

A. Blood pressure is more effectively controlled with a converting enzyme inhibitor than with

standard triple therapy (a diuretic, beta-blocker, and vasodilator).
B. Effective control of blood pressure does not protect against deterioration of renal function.
C. Patients with bilateral renal artery stenosis or renal artery stenosis in a solitary kidney are best managed by converting enzyme inhibitors.
D. All patients with renovascular hypertension treated pharmacologically must have routine evaluations of renal function and size.
E. Angiotensin converting enzyme inhibitors are 90 per cent effective in controlling blood pressure in patients with renovascular hypertension.

933. The ideal patient for percutaneous transluminal renal artery angioplasty has:

A. Diffuse atherosclerosis primarily involving the aorta
B. Total occlusion of the renal artery
C. Multiple branch lesions, particularly at vessel bifurcations
D. Ostial stenosis
E. Fibromuscular dysplasia

934. The patient with atherosclerotic vascular disease best suited for angioplasty has:

A. Bilateral renal artery stenoses
B. Total renal artery occlusion
C. Unilateral, nonosteal, nonoccluded lesion
D. Diffuse involvement of the aorta with a unilateral osteal lesion
E. Stenosis at the bifurcation of branch vessels

935. For a renal arterial lesion to be functionally significant and lead to renovascular hypertension, the arterial lumen must be reduced by approximately:

A. 10 per cent
B. 30 per cent
C. 50 per cent
D. 70 per cent
E. 90 per cent

936. A 42-year-old hypertensive woman undergoing evaluation for possible renovascular hypertension has a "string of beads" appearance at renal arteriography. The most likely arterial pathology is:

A. Atherosclerosis
B. Intimal fibroplasia
C. Fibromuscular hyperplasia
D. Medial fibroplasia
E. Perimedial fibroplasia

937. The most characteristic abnormality during excretory urography in patients with renovascular hypertension is:

A. Poor visualization of collecting system
B. Extrinsic vascular impression
C. Enlarged kidney
D. Delayed excretion of contrast
E. Early excretion of contrast

938. The recommended screening test for renovascular hypertension in a 35-year-old woman with moderate hypertension and a normal physical examination is:

A. Plasma renin activity
B. Single-dose captopril test
C. Differential renal vein renin
D. Hypertensive excretory urogram
E. Captopril renogram

939. The glomerular filtration rate (GFR) may be measured by determining renal clearance of a substance that is filtered but not absorbed or secreted. Based on the following data, what is the GFR using inulin?

Plasma inulin conc: 0.5 mg/dl	Urine volume: 135 ml
Urine inulin conc: 80 mg/dl	Time: 270 min
Plasma creatinine: 0.8 mg/dl	Urine rate: 30 ml/hr

A. 100 ml/min
B. 120 ml/min
C. 80 ml/min
D. 115 ml/min
E. 64 ml/min

940. Which of the following statements concerning creatinine is *false*?

A. Creatinine is freely filtered at the glomerulus and is not reabsorbed throughout the tubules or collecting duct.
B. Creatinine secretion accounts for 10 per cent of total creatinine excretion.
C. Creatinine is produced at a fairly constant rate and provides an index of total body muscle mass.
D. Cimetidine enhances tubular creatinine secretion.
E. Trimethoprim inhibits tubular creatinine secretion.

941. What is the maximal urine osmolality (mOsmol/kg) and obligate solute excretion (mOsmol/day) for a 70-kg man?

A. 600 mOsmol/kg and 300 mOsmol/day
B. 800 mOsmol/kg and 500 mOsmol/day
C. 1000 mOsmol/kg and 500 mOsmol/day
D. 1000 mOsmol/kg and 800 mOsmol/day
E. 600 mOsmol/kg and 1000 mOsmol/day

942. The most common cause of acute renal failure (ARF) is:

A. Acute tubular necrosis
B. Urinary obstruction
C. Myocardial infarction
D. Acute glomerulonephritis
E. Prerenal azotemia

943. All of the following statements concerning acute tubular necrosis (ATN) are true, EXCEPT:

A. ATN induced by radiocontrast is typically oliguric in nature.
B. Oliguric ATN has an associated mortality of 40–50%.
C. Aminoglycoside induced ATN is usually nonoliguric and develops 5–7 days after initiating therapy.
D. Renal ischemia is the most common predisposing cause of ATN.
E. Nonoliguric ATN has an associated mortality of 20%.

944. All of the following substances may cause ATN EXCEPT:

A. Cisplatin
B. Amphotericin
C. Acyclovir

D. Chloroquine
E. Ethylene glycol

945. All of the following statements concerning the pathogenesis of ATN are true EXCEPT:

A. Maintenance factors in ischemic ATN are primarily tubular.
B. Tubular obstruction from sloughed brush border membranes, cellular debis, and Tamm-Horsfall protein, appears to be the most important maintenance factor in ATN.
C. Experimental models indicate injury occurs primarily in the proximal tubules and possibly in the ascending limb of Henle.
D. On the cellular level, ischemic events lead to lipid peroxidation and membrane injury which is followed by an influx of calcium into the tubular cell and eventually cell necrosis.
E. Backleak of glomerular filtrate during ATN improves perfusion and recovery.

946. Efforts to ameliorate ischemic ATN might reasonably include all of the following EXCEPT:

A. Administration of loop diuretics prior to the ischemic event, if it is anticipated
B. Administration of calcium channel blockers after the ischemic insult
C. Administration of atrial natriuretic factor
D. Papaverine administration after the ischemic event
E. Avoidance of even mild hypotensive episodes following the development of ATN

947. Acute interstitial nephritis may be caused by all of the following medications EXCEPT:

A. Methicillin
B. Isoniazid
C. Phenytoin
D. Fenoprofen
E. Captopril

948. With prerenal azotemia urinanalysis shows the following EXCEPT:

A. High specific gravity
B. Few red blood cells
C. Few hyaline casts
D. Many cellular components
E. Hypertonic urine

949. With acute tubular necrosis, urinalysis may show each of the following EXCEPT:

A. White blood cell casts
B. Isotonic urine
C. Coarse granular casts
D. Tubular-epithelial cells
E. Tubular epithelial cell casts

950. In the differential diagnosis of acute renal failure, each of the following statements is true EXCEPT:

A. Heavy proteinuria with hematuria and red blood cell casts suggests acute glomerulonephritis.
B. Eosinophilia suggests acute interstitial nephritis.
C. A renal failure index, RFI=(Urine Na)×(Plasma Cr/Urine Cr), greater than 2 indicates prerenal azotemia.
D. White blood cell casts suggest pyelonephritis, acute glomerulonephritis, or acute interstitial nephritis.
E. A BUN creatinine ratio (BUN/serum Cr) greater than 20 indicates prerenal azotemia, increased catabolism, or possibly urinary obstruction.

951. Which of the following statements concerning imaging modalities in the evaluation of acute renal failure (ARF) is *false*?

A. Gallium scans definitively make the diagnosis of interstitial nephritis as a cause of ARF.
B. Magnetic resonance spectroscopy of the ^{31}P isotope shows promise for the differential diagnosis of ARF.
C. A 20 per cent false positive rate is found when ultrasonography is used to diagnose urinary obstruction.
D. Radiocontrast studies other than retrograde or antegrade pyelography have little place in the evaluation of ARF.
E. Nuclear studies enable the measurement of glomerular filtration rate and the evaluation of tubular secretion.

952. In experimental models, each of the following treatments may improve the course of ARF EXCEPT:

A. Mannitol infusion
B. ATP-$MgCl_2$ infusion
C. Verapamil
D. Nifedipine
E. Aldosterone

953. In the management of acute renal failure, which of the following statements is *false*?

A. High doses of loop diuretics may be used to convert oliguric to nonoliguric ATN.
B. When conversion of the patient with ATN from an oliguric to a nonoliguric state occurs, mortality is diminished and renal recovery hastened.
C. Low-dose dopamine (2.5 μg/kg/min) may increase the number of patients who respond to high dose loop diuretics.
D. Nonconservative management (dialysis) is the standard of care when BUN levels are above 100 mg/dl.
E. Indications for dialysis or hemofiltration include fluid and electrolyte imbalances that are refractory to conservative measures and the development of uremic signs and symptoms.

954. Regarding the diagnosis, prevention, and treatment of electrolyte abnormalities secondary to ARF, which of the following statements is *false*?

A. The administration of intravenous glucose and insulin rapidly causes a shift of potassium from the extracellular compartment to the intracellular compartment; however, this effect is short-lived.
B. When severe ECG alterations due to hyperkalemia are noted, intravenous calcium chloride or calcium gluconate (9.6 mEq of calcium) should be administered immediately.
C. When severe hyperkalemia is present, the ECG tracing may appear as a sine wave.
D. Sodium polystyrene sulfonate is useful to bind phosphate orally and may prevent hyperphosphatemia.

E. Magnesium-containing antacids or cathartics must be avoided.

955. All of the following statements are true concerning focal and segmental glomerulosclerosis (FSGS) EXCEPT:

A. FSGS typically presents with nephrotic syndrome and hypertension, and usually progresses to chronic renal insufficiency.
B. IgM, IgG, complement, and fibrin may be found in scars of the focal and segmentally scarred glomeruli, although immune complexes are not thought to be a factor in the pathogenesis of FSGS.
C. The histologic entity of FSGS has been associated with intravenous drug abusers and with patients with acquired immunodeficiency syndrome.
D. FSGS usually afflicts older children or young adults.
E. Corticosteroids are useful in delaying the development of end-stage renal disease from FSGS.

956. Which of the following statements concerning focal proliferative glomerulonephritis (FPGN) is *false*?

A. Microscopic hematuria and recurrent episodes of gross hematuria are noted with FPGN.
B. FPGN is characterized by mesangial proliferation.
C. IgG, IgM, and/or IgA deposits are seen within the mesangium.
D. If deposits are primarily composed of IgA, this form of FPGN is known as Berger's disease.
E. FPGN affects adults in their third and fourth decades.

957. Which of the following statements concerning diffuse proliferative glomerulonephritis (DPGN) is *false*?

A. Poststreptococcal glomerulonephritis due to group A streptococci is a form of DPGN, and develops 2 to 4 weeks following skin infection.
B. Light microscopy of renal tissue with DPGN shows swollen congested glomeruli with proliferation and exudation.
C. Gamma interferon has been shown to decrease the duration and improve the prognosis of DPGN.
D. On electron microscopy, massive subepithelial deposits known as "humps" are seen which consist of electron-dense substances.
E. DPGN due to streptocooci has a good prognosis, but remains an important cause of ESRD because of the high frequency of poststreptococcal DPGN.

958. Which of the following statements concerning rapidly progressive glomerulonephritis (RPGN) is *false*?

A. Epithelial crescents are not seen on light microscopy.
B. RPGN is characterized by a presentation similar to acute glomerulonephritis but proceeds to chronic renal failure within weeks to months.
C. Antiglomerular basement membrane antibody (anti-GBM) formation may be seen with RPGN.
D. When RPGN with anti-GBM antibodies is associated with pulmonary hemorrhage, the disease is referred to as Goodpasture's syndrome.
E. When anti-GBM antibodies occur with RPGN, plasma exchange, cytotoxic agents, and corticosteroids are thought to be helpful.

959. Conditions or diseases that may cause the development of chronic renal failure include all of the following EXCEPT:

A. Autosomal dominant polycystic kidney disease
B. Medullary sponge kidney
C. Systemic lupus erythematosus
D. Polyarteritis nodosa
E. *Schistosoma haematobium* infection

960. Each of the following statements concerning uremia and uremic syndrome is true EXCEPT:

A. Some of the manifestations of uremic syndrome are autonomic neuropathy, pericardial effusion, seizures, and cardiomyopathy.
B. Uremic bleeding has been associated with a deficiency of von Willebrand factor multimers.
C. The middle molecule theory of uremia suggests that molecules with molecular weights in the 1,000 to 10,000 dalton range are responsible for uremia.
D. Desmopressin acetate (DDAVP) may reverse uremic coagulopathy.
E. The small solute theory of uremia best accounts for most uremic manifestations.

961. Which of the following statements concerning the use of a dipstick for hematuria screening is *false*?

A. Dipsticks are very sensitive and miss only 1 per cent of patients with microscopic hematuria.
B. Vitamin C can cause false-negative results.
C. Hypochlorite can cause false-positive results.
D. Hemoglobin from red blood cells catalyzes the conversion of the dipstick indicator by hydrogen peroxide and changes the color of the dipstick.
E. The test detects intact red blood cells, free hemoglobin, and myoglobin.

962. Glomerular hematuria is caused by all of the following disorders EXCEPT:

A. Alport syndrome
B. Systemic lupus erythematosus
C. Hemolytic uremic syndrome
D. Schönlein-Henoch purpura
E. Thrombotic thrombocytopenic purpura

963. Which statement concerning IgA nephropathy (Berger's disease) is *false*?

A. 25 per cent of patients develop renal insufficiency.
B. The typical clinical presentation is recurrent episodes of gross hematuria following an upper respiratory tract infection.
C. The presence of IgA deposits is pathognomonic for the disease.
D. Old age at onset, consistent proteinuria, and hypertension are poor prognostic indicators.
E. A viral etiology has been implicated in some cases.

964. Which is the best urine specimen for detecting and quantitating red blood cells in the urine?

A. 24-hour collection
B. First-voided overnight specimen
C. Second-voided overnight specimen

D. Midday voided specimen
E. Postprandial specimen

965. All of the following statements are true about sickle-cell nephropathy EXCEPT:

A. Papillary necrosis is a common complication and can result in serious renal dysfunction.
B. Hematuria is usually from the left kidney.
C. Sickle-cell disease occurs in approximately 8 per cent of blacks.
D. Intravenous distilled water, sodium bicarbonate, mannitol, loop diuretics, and ϵ-aminocaproic acid are used in the treatment of hematuria associated with the disease.
E. Lasix prophylaxis can prevent recurrent episodes of hematuria.

966. A 65-year-old male in the intensive care unit with a diagnosis of a transmural myocardial infarction suddenly complains of severe right flank pain and gross hematuria. An intravenous urogram reveals nonvisualization of the right kidney. What is the most likely cause?

A. Renal cell carcinoma
B. Renal vein thrombosis
C. Acute pyelonephritis
D. Renal artery thrombosis
E. Renal arteriovenous fistula

967. Renal infarction is characterized by all of the following EXCEPT:

A. Leukocytosis
B. Elevated serum glutamic-oxaloacetic transaminase
C. Elevated serum glutamic-pyruvic transaminase
D. Elevated lactate dehydrogenase
E. Elevated alkaline phosphatase

968. Which statement concerning the management of renal artery thrombosis is true?

A. Unilateral thrombosis is best managed by conservative, nonoperative anticoagulation therapy.
B. Bilateral thrombosis is best managed by emergent surgical thrombectomy or embolectomy performed within a few hours after occlusion, or else significant renal function is lost in the majority of patients.
C. Intra-arterial fibrinolytic therapy is ineffective in the majority of patients.
D. Transluminal recanalization does not result in significant recovery of renal function.
E. High-dose corticosteroids should be started promptly.

969. Renal arteriovenous fistulas are characterized by all of the following EXCEPT:

A. Approximately 75 per cent of patients have a continuous abdominal or flank bruit.
B. Congenital fistulas account for the vast majority of renal arteriovenous fistulas.
C. Percutaneous needle biopsies account for over 40 per cent of acquired fistulas.
D. Acquired fistulas usually appear as solitary communications between artery and vein.
E. The majority of postbiopsy fistulas require no intervention.

970. A neonate, severely dehydrated from prolonged diarrhea, has bilateral flank masses and gross hematuria. Ultrasonography reveals an enlarged, hypoechoic kidney. The most likely etiology is:

A. Bilateral ureteropelvic junction obstruction
B. Infantile polycystic disease
C. Bilateral renal artery thrombosis
D. Bilateral renal vein thrombosis
E. Bilateral Wilms' tumor

971. Which of the following statements concerning renal vein thrombosis in the adult is *false*?

A. Surgical thrombectomy is the most effective therapy.
B. It is usually unilateral.
C. Renal venography is the definitive diagnostic study.
D. Anticoagulation therapy should be initiated as soon as the diagnosis is made.
E. There is a higher incidence in patients with nephrotic syndrome due to membranous glomerulonephritis.

972. Which statement regarding proteinuria is *false*?

A. In healthy adults, the normal daily protein excretion is 200 mg.
B. For any given rate of protein excretion, the concentration of protein in a single voided sample of urine varies inversely with urine flow.
C. The maximum level of protein excretion in children is 140 mg/m^2 of body surface area per day.
D. Gross hematuria can cause false-positive dipstick results.
E. Highly alkaline urine (pH > 8) can cause false-negative dipstick results.

973. The colorimetric dipsticks used for screening proteinuria react preferentially with:

A. Tamm-Horsfall protein
B. Serum globulins
C. Bence Jones protein
D. Immunoglobulin
E. Serum albumin

974. Normal composition of urine protein is ____ serum albumin, ____ serum globulins, and ____ tissue proteins:

A. 0%, 50%, 50%
B. 10%, 50%, 40%
C. 20%, 40%, 40%
D. 30%, 20%, 50%
E. 30%, 30%, 40%

975. Tubular proteinuria is associated with all of the following conditions EXCEPT:

A. Fanconi's syndrome
B. Cadmium poisoning
C. Lead poisoning
D. Diabetes mellitus
E. Mercury poisoning

976. The normal protein/creatinine (in mg/mg) ratio in a single urine sample is:

A. <0.2
B. 0.5
C. 1.0
D. 2.0
E. >2.0

977. Acute renal failure occurs in ____ per cent of multiple myeloma patients:
A. 0–5
B. 5–10
C. 10–15
D. 15–20
E. 20–25

978. Creatinine is produced by muscle cells at a constant rate of:
A. 1 mg/kg/day
B. 10 mg/kg/day
C. 20 mg/kg/day
D. 30 mg/kg/day
E. 40 mg/kg/day

979. Which statement concerning analgesic nephropathy is *false*?
A. Phenacetin and aspirin can cause renal papillary necrosis and chronic interstitial nephritis.
B. There is an increased incidence of transitional cell carcinoma associated with analgesic nephropathy.
C. The total amount of analgesic consumed is unrelated to the degree of renal function impairment.
D. Women between the ages of 30 and 50 are predominantly affected.
E. More than 80 per cent of patients who stop abusing analgesics will frequently show an improvement or at least a slowing of renal function deterioration.

980. Nonsteroidal anti-inflammatory drugs have the potential for significant nephrotoxicity by all of the following mechanisms EXCEPT:
A. Decreased synthesis of renal prostaglandin E_2
B. Impaired renin secretion
C. Allergic interstitial nephritis
D. Enhanced tubular water reabsorption
E. Impaired tubular sodium reabsorption

981. In patients with normal renal function, the incidence of nephrotoxicity from intravenous pyelography is:
A. 0.2 per cent
B. 0.6 per cent
C. 1.2 per cent
D. 2 per cent
E. 5 per cent

982. A 40-year-old man, taking lithium carbonate for his bipolar disorder, has polydipsia and polyuria (10 liters/day). His serum osmolality is 315 mOsm/kg and urine osmolality is 200 mOsm/kg. Following the administration of exogenous ADH, there is no appreciable increase in the urine osmolality. What is the most likely etiology?
A. Neurogenic diabetes insipidus
B. Psychogenic polydipsia
C. Diabetes mellitus
D. Nephrogenic diabetes insipidus
E. Mannitol ingestion

983. Papillary necrosis is associated with all of the following conditions EXCEPT:
A. Type 2 renal tubular acidosis
B. Diabetes mellitus
C. Sickle-cell disease
D. Phenacetin abuse
E. Pyelonephritis

PART XII

RENAL DISEASES OF UROLOGIC SIGNIFICANCE

CHAPTERS 55 THROUGH 57

ANSWERS

923-C *(Campbell's, pp. 2019–2020, 2038)*

Atherosclerosis of the renal arteries is common and accounts for 60 to 70 per cent of lesions that cause renovascular hypertension. These lesions usually occur in the proximal 2 cm of the renal artery including the aorta (ostial lesions) and begin as a proliferation of myointimal cells in the intima. Total reversal of hypertension following correction is less common than in patients with fibromuscular disease, as these patients often have diffuse atherosclerotic disease and essential hypertension. Hypertension of renal origin is frequently difficult to manage medically, and most lesions are progressive making careful follow-up of renal function and size of utmost importance.

924-D *(Campbell's, pp. 2021–2022)*

Fibromuscular diseases of the renal artery are responsible for one third of cases of renovascular hypertension. Medial fibroplasia is the most common fibrous lesion, constituting 75 to 80 per cent of the total and characteristically occurring in women between the ages of 20 to 50 years. Takayasu's aortitis is a rare chronic sclerosing aortitis that may involve the renal arteries.

925-B *(Campbell's, pp. 2025–2026)*

Renin is primarily released in response to (1) a low renal perfusion pressure in the afferent arteriole (baroreceptor mechanism); (2) *a low* chloride (or sodium) concentration in the filtrate reaching the distal convoluted tubule (macula densa mechanism); and (3) adrenergic stimulation of beta–1 receptors in the juxtaglomerular cells. Changes in renin secretion induced by all these stimuli are mediated by changes in intracellular calcium or cAMP. Thus, an increase in cytosolic calcium suppresses renin release, and an increase in cAMP increases renin release. Converse relationships also pertain.

926-E *(Campbell's, pp. 2024–2025)*

Most of the actions of angiotensin II are directed toward maintenance or increase of blood pressure. This control is accomplished through both its direct effect as a vasoconstrictor and its effect on sodium and volume. It activates the zone glomerulosa of the adrenal gland to increase the production of aldosterone and increases sodium reabsorption. Angiotensin II also has a direct sodium retaining effect, acting at the ascending limb of the loop of Henle. Mechanisms that serve to dampen the system are feedback-inhibiting loops which *inhibit* renin release. These are mediated by aldosterone-induced sodium retention, volume expansion, increased blood pressure, and angiotensin II's direct inhibition of renin release.

927-C *(Campbell's, pp. 2027–2036)*

The angiographic finding of a stenosed renal artery is insufficient evidence on which to diagnose renovascular hypertension. This only detects anatomic vascular disease and the functional significance of the lesion must still be demonstrated. Rather, the diagnosis of renovascular hypertension is predicated on (1) the demonstration of a physiologically significant decrease in renal blood flow to one or both kidneys, (2) hypersecretion of renin from the more ischemic kidney, (3) the absence of renin secretion from the contralateral kidney, and (4) lowering of the blood pressure on removal of the source of hyperreninemia, or on blockage of the renin-angiotensin system.

REFERENCE

1. Sosa, R.E., and Vaughan, E.D.: AUA Update, Vol. VIII, Lesson 18, p. 140.

928-A *(Campbell's, pp. 2027–2028)*

There are no pathognomonic clinical characteristics that lead to a reliable diagnosis; however, a number of clinical features should arouse suspicion that renovascular hypertension may be present. The only laboratory finding of importance is *hypokalemia.* The low potassium level is due to secondary hyperaldosteronism; however, this is present in less than 20 per cent of patients with renovascular hypertension. The average age of essential hypertension is 31 ± 10 years. Children and young adults usually will have fibromuscular disease, whereas adults over 45 years are more likely to have atherosclerosis. While essential hypertension usually presents with a "labile" phase before mild hypertension becomes established, renovascular hypertension often first appears as moderate to severe hypertension. Seventy-four per cent of patients with fibromuscular renal artery stenosis and 88 per cent of those with atherosclerotic disease smoke. Probably the most typical feature is that it responds poorly to diuretics and often only transiently to antiadrenergic drugs.

929-C *(Campbell's, pp. 2029–2032)*

The single-dose captopril test appears to accurately separate patients with renovascular hypertension from those with essential hypertension. It has a specificity of 95 per cent and sensitivity of 100 per cent as well as the highest predictive and exclusion values of the screening tests. Patients can remain on beta-blockade if the PRA >1 ng/ml/hr and a 24 hour urine collection is not necessary.

930-B *(Campbell's, pp. 2028–2036)*

Differential renal vein renin determinations remain the gold standard in identifying which kidney is the cause of abnormal renin secretion. Hypersecretion of renin serves as the primary criterion for the diagnosis of renovascular hypertension and the second criterion is the absence of renin secretion from the contralateral or noninvolved kidney. The single-dose captopril test is an excellent screening test but does not identify the involved kidney. The intravenous urogram has a false-positive rate of 13 per cent and a false-negative rate of 22 per cent, making it an unreliable test. The captopril renogram, in theory, not only screens for renovascular hypertension, but also identifies the involved kidney, however, the predictive value of this test does not yet approach that of renal vein renin determinations. Angiography is only capable of providing anatomic information and not the functional significance of a lesion.

931-B *(Campbell's, p. 2035)*

In essential hypertension at all levels of renin secretion, the renin level in each renal vein is about 25 per cent greater than either the peripheral arterial or the venous level (C & D). In curable renovascular hypertension, the active kidney is solely responsible for maintaining the peripheral renin levels. Hence the increment is 50 per cent (0.5) and becomes progressively greater as renal blood flow is reduced (B). Unequal bilateral renin secretion indicates bilateral disease and decreases the chance of cure following corrective unilateral surgery (A). The inferior vena caval (IVC) renin and plasma renin activity are the same (V-IVC/IVC).

932-C *(Campbell's, p. 2038)*

Angiotensin converting enzyme inhibitors are the most potent antihypertensive drugs in the treatment of patients with renovascular hypertension and are nearly 90 per cent effective in controlling blood pressure in these patients. The major concern with medical management is not blood pressure control, but maintenance of renal function, and all patients should have serial tests of renal function and size. In patients with bilateral renal artery stenosis or renal artery stenosis in a solitary kidney, treatment with ACE inhibitors may allow dramatic decreases in renal function to occur.

REFERENCE

1. Vaughan, E.D., and Sosa, R.E.: AUA Update, Vol. VIII, Lesson 36.

933-E *(Campbell's, p. 2038)*

The ideal patient for percutaneous transluminal angioplasty (PTA) is one with unilateral disease, positive renin indices and fibromuscular dysplasia or nonosteal nonoccluded atherosclerotic renal artery stenosis. Patients with diffuse atherosclerosis, total occlusion, multiple branch lesions and ostial lesions are less likely to respond to angioplasty.

934-C *(Campbell's, p. 2038)*

Unilateral, nonosteal, nonoccluded atherosclerotic renal artery stenoses are the most suitable lesions for treatment with PTA. The other lesions are all associated with a lower success rate, although an occasional patient will have long-term success.

935-D *(Campbell's, p. 2019)*

The identification of an anatomic renal arterial lesion in a hypertensive patient is not proof of functional significance. Arterial narrowing of 70 per cent may be necessary to reduce renal blood flow sufficiently to initiate the pathophysiologic events of renovascular hypertension.

936-D *(Campbell's, p. 2021)*

Medial fibroplasia produces a "string of beads" appearance at renal arteriography. This is the most common of the fibrous arterial lesions, constituting 75 to 80 per cent of the total.

937-D *(Campbell's, pp. 2028–2029)*

The "hypertensive" excretory urogram, with a rapid sequence of films taken during the first four minutes after contrast injection, has been used as a screening test for renovascular hypertension. Positive findings include decreased renal size, delayed excretion of contrast and hyperconcentration of contrast on delayed films because of increased absorption of water. A high false-negative rate has reduced use of this test.

938-A *(Campbell's, p. 2037)*

The initial screening test for renovascular hypertension should be measurement of peripheral plasma renin activity, indexed for urinary sodium excretion. If this demonstrates high renin, differential renal vein renins can be determined for confirmation of renovascular hypertension and identification of the affected side. The single-dose captopril test can be performed in patients with normal plasma renin in whom renovascular hypertension is still suspected. See Fig. 55–23.

939-C *(Campbell's, p. 2045)*

The glomerular filtration rate may be measured by determining renal clearance of a substance that is filtered but not absorbed or secreted. In the calculation of renal clearance, a steady-state plasma concentration of the substance is needed as well as a steady-state urine concentration of the substance. Additionally, the urine flow rate is needed. The renal clearance of such a substance is then calculated by multiplying the urine concentration of the substance times the flow rate and dividing by the plasma concentration of the substance. Inulin is a polysaccharide substance neither reabsorbed nor secreted within the tubules or collecting ducts and is thus an ideal substance for measuring glomerular filtration rate. When one calculates the renal clearance of inulin according to the data given, the correct answer is 80 cc per minute. This is obtained by dividing the urine inulin concentration of 80 mg/dl by the plasma inulin concentration of 0.5 mg/dl and multiplying by the urine rate which is 30 ml/hr which must be divided by 60 to obtain a rate based on minutes.

940-D *(Campbell's, p. 2046)*

Creatinine is a nitrogenous compound that is a breakdown product of creatine. Creatinine is generated at a constant rate and is dependent on the amount of total creatine in the body, which is an index of total body muscle mass. Daily creatinine production is nearly constant. Creatinine is freely filtered at the level of the glomerulus and is not reabsorbed; however, it is secreted slightly. Creatinine secretion accounts for 10 per cent of the total creatinine excretion. Both cimetidine and trimethoprim inhibit tubular creatinine secretion. When these medications are on board the renal clearance of creatinine correlates closely with glomerular filtration rate as measured by other compounds such as inulin.

941-C *(Campbell's, p. 2046)*

Normal kidneys can concentrate urine to produce a maximal urine osmolality of approximately 1,000 mOsm/kg. In a 70 kg man, the approximate obligate solute excretion is 500 mOsm/day. Therefore, a urine flow rate of approximately 500 ml/day is required for maintainance of solute balance and reductions in urine output below this are referred to as oliguria.

942-E *(Campbell's, p. 2046)*

The most common cause of acute renal failure is prerenal azotemia.

943-B *(Campbell's, pp. 2047–2048)*

Acute tubular necrosis (ATN) may develop from several etiologies; however, the most common predisposing cause is renal ischemia. ATN is classified as oliguric or nonoliguric and oliguric ATN has an associated mortality of 60 to 80 per cent while nonoliguric ATN has an associated mortality of 20 per cent. Aminoglycoside-associated ATN is usually nonoliguric and develops 5 to 7 days after initiation of therapy. Usually patients who develop ATN secondary to aminoglycosides have underlying chronic renal insufficiency. Radiocontrast-induced ATN is also more likely in patients who have chronic renal insufficiency, such as those with long-standing diabetes. Radiocontrast-induced ATN is usually oliguric in nature.

REFERENCES

1. Anderson, R.J., Linas, S.L., Berns, A.S., et al.: Nonoliguric acute renal failure. N. Engl. J. Med., *296*:1134, 1977.
2. Stott, R.B., Cameron, J.S., Ogg, C.S., and Bewick, M.: Why the persistently high mortality in acute renal failure. Lancet, *2*:75, 1972.
3. Appel, B.B.: Aminoglycoside nephrotoxicity. Am. J. Med., *159*:427, 1990.
4. Schrier, R.W., and Shapiro, J.I.: Drug-induced acute renal failure. *In* Serono Symposium on Acute Renal Failure. New York, Raven Press, 1985, p. 242.

944-D *(Campbell's, p. 2048)*

ATN may be caused by amphotericin, acyclovir and cisplatinum. These drugs typically result in renal potassium and magnesium wasting that can persist for long periods. Ingestion of ethylene glycol or anti-freeze is also known to cause ATN. Chloroquine has not been reported to be a significant cause of ATN.

945-E *(Campbell's, pp. 2048–2049)*

Ischemia is the most common insult giving rise to ATN; however, once ATN has developed, maintenance factors are primarily tubular. Tubular obstruction appears to be the most important maintenance mechanism and this develops when sloughed brush border membranes, cellular debris, and Tamm-Horsfall protein build up in the tubules causing obstruction. Glomerular filtrate backleak is also felt to be a maintenance factor in some experimental models. In experimental models of ischemic ATN, the major site of injury is the proximal tubule. It has been theorized, however, that the ascending limb of Henle survives on the edge of anoxia because of its blood supply and is at greatest risk for ischemia. In experimental models, this segment clearly can show transport related injury and may be a factor in the development of ATN. The development of cellular debris in the tubules is no doubt a result of cell necrosis from ischemia. Important events which lead to cellular destruction include lipid peroxidation and membrane injury which allows an influx of calcium into the tubular cell leading to cell necrosis.

REFERENCES

1. Levinsky, N.G.: Pathophysiology of acute renal failure. N. Engl. J. Med., *296*:1453, 1977.
2. Burke, T.J., Cronin, R.E., Duchin, K.L., et al.: Ischemia and tubule obstruction during acute renal failure in dogs: Mannitol in protection. Am. J. Physiol., *238*: F305, 1980.
3. Schrier, R.W., and Conger, J.D.: Acute renal failure: Pathogenesis, diagnosis and management. *In* Schrier, R.W. (Ed.): Renal and Electrolyte Disorders. Boston, Little, Brown & Co., 1986, p. 423.
4. Venkatachalam, M.A., Bernard, D.B., Donohoe, J.F., and Levinsky, N.G.: Ischemic damage and repair in the rat proximal tubule: Differences among the S1, S2 and S3 segments. Kidney Int., *14*:31, 1978.
5. Brezis, M., Rosen, S., Silva, P., and Epstein, F.H.: Transport activity modifies thick ascending limb damage in the isolated perfused kidney. Kidney Int., *25*:65, 1984.

946-D *(Campbell's, p. 2049)*

Osmotic or loop diuretics, when given before ischemic insults, appear to reduce the severity of ischemic ATN in experimental models. This effect may be due to increased tubular pressures and flows which decrease tubular obstruction. Calcium channel blockers may have a protective effect on cells in the area of ischemia by reducing cytosolic calcium overload which as previously discussed may lead to cell necrosis. Atrial natriuretic factor may also have some calcium-channel blocking cellular effect and does give protection in experimental models of acute renal failure. Once acute tubular necrosis has developed, mild hypotensive episodes may lead to increasing insult to the ischemic area and prolong the course of ATN or cause progression. Papaverine administration is not reported as a therapy in the treatment of ATN.

REFERENCES

1. Burke, T.J., Cronin, R.E., Duchin, K.L., et al.: Ischemia and tubule obstruction during acute renal failure in dogs: Mannitol in protection. Am. J. Physiol., *238*: F305, 1980.
2. Burke, T.J., Arnold, P.E., Gordon, J.A., et al.: Protective effect of intrarenal calcium membrane blockers before or after ischemia. J. Clin. Invest., *74*:1830, 1984.
3. Shapiro, J.I., Cheung, C., Itabashi, A., et al.: The protective effect of verapamil on renal function after warm and cold ischemia in the isolated perfused rat kidney. Transplantation, *40*:596, 1985.
4. Nakamoto, M., Shapiro, J.I., Chan, L., and Schrier, R.W.: The in vitro and in vivo protective effect of atriopeptin III in ischemic acute renal failure in the rat. J. Clin. Invest., *80*:698, 1987.

947-B *(Campbell's, p. 2048)*

Medications which may induce acute interstitial nephritis are listed in Table 56–3. Common groups in this table include penicillins and cephalosporins as well as rifampicin, trimethoprim and sulfa derivatives. Seizure medications including phenytoin, carbamazepine and phenobarbital are also listed, as are the antihypertensives captopril and alpha methyldopa. Isoniazid is metabolized in the liver and is not reported to give rise to acute interstitial nephritis.

948-D *(Campbell's, p. 2050)*

Urinalysis may be very useful in the differential diagnosis of acute renal failure. With prerenal azotemia urine is concentrated; therefore, it is hypertonic and has a high specific gravity. Red blood cells are not necessarily seen on urinalysis unless there is another disease process giving rise to them. Few hyaline casts may be noted; however, there should not be a significant number of such casts and minimal cellular components should be noted in the urine. Therefore, answer D is incorrect.

949-A *(Campbell's, p. 2050)*

Again, the urinalysis is useful in the differential diagnosis of acute renal failure. With acute tubular necrosis, tubules are not able to concentrate urine and urine is isotonic. Both tubular-epithelial cells and casts of tubular-epithelial cells may be observed in the urine. Additionally, coarse granular casts and other cellular debris may be seen in the urine. White blood cell casts are not associated with ATN.

950-C *(Campbell's, pp. 2050–2051)*

In the differential diagnosis of acute renal failure, white blood cell casts indicate acute pyelonephritis, acute interstitial nephritis or acute glomerular nephritis. Acute glomerular nephritis is usually associated with high urine protein concentrations as well as hematuria and red blood cell casts. The presence of eosinophilia on differential blood count suggest acute interstitial nephritis. An elevation in BUN/serum creatinine ratio greater than 20 indicates prerenal azotemia as well as increased catabolism. This may also indicate early urinary obstruction. The renal failure index is calculated by multiplying the urine sodium and the plasma creatinine and dividing by the urine creatinine. When this quantity is less than 1, it indicates prerenal azotemia.

REFERENCE

1. Shapiro, J.I., and Anderson, R.J.: Urinary diagnositic indices in acute renal failure. Am. Kidney Found. Nephrol. Lett., *1*:13, 1984.

951-A *(Campbell's, p. 2050)*

Renal ultrasound has become an important initial screening study in the evaluation of acute renal failure. Dilation of the collecting system seen on ultrasound is a sensitive test for obstruction; however, it has a 20 per cent false-positive incidence for diagnosing obstruction. Additionally, with the ultrasound unit, Doppler studies can be performed to verify renal blood flow. Nuclear renal scans allow the measurement of renal perfusion as well as glomerular filtration rate and the evaluation of tubular secretion and are very useful in the evaluation of acute renal failure. Due to radiocontrast nephro-toxicity, studies which use intravenous radiocontrast have little place in the evaluation of acute renal failure. When the collecting system does need to be evaluated, retrograde or antegrade studies can be performed. Gallium scans will detect the presence of inflammation within the kidney but are relatively non-specific and answer A is, therefore, incorrect. Magnetic resonance spectroscopy using the phosphorous isotope shows promise for differential diagnosis of acute renal failure; however, this remains experimental.

REFERENCE

1. Chan, L., and Shapiro, J.I.: NMR in the investigation and differential diagnosis of acute renal failure. Ann. NY Acad. Sci., *508*:420, 1987.

952-E *(Campbell's, p. 2051)*

Osmotic diuretics as well as loop diuretics may improve the course of acute renal failure. Again, this is felt to be due to increasing flow through the tubules and relieving tubular obstruction. When ATP-magnesium chloride is given to supplement the adenine nucleotide pool, the course of ATN may be improved. Calcium channel blockers including verapamil, diltiazem and nifedipine may have a protective effect on the ischemic cells in preventing the buildup of intracellular calcium. Aldosterone is not reported to improve the course of acute renal failure.

REFERENCES

1. Siegel, N.J., Avison, M.J., Reilly, H.F., et al.: Enhanced recovery of renal ATP with post ischemic infusion of ATP-$MgCl_2$ determined by P-31 NMR. Am. J. Physiol., *245*:F530, 1983.
2. See references listed for answer to question 946.

953-B *(Campbell's, pp. 2052–2053)*

Presently, data support the use of high-dose loop diuretics in ATN to convert from an oliguric state to a nonoliguric state, making fluid management easier. However, when this conversion is achieved, mortality is not diminished and renal recovery is not hastened. Uncontrolled studies indicate that renal dose dopamine may indeed increase the number of patients who respond to loop diuretics. Nonconservative management, dialysis, is indicated when fluid and electrolyte balances occur that are refractory to conservative measures or when uremic signs and symptoms develop. The present standard of care indicates that when the BUN reaches a level of 100, dialysis should be employed.

REFERENCES

1. Bailey, R.R., Natale, R., Turnbull, I., and Linton, A.L.: Protective effect of furosemide in acute tubular necrosis and acute renal failure. Clin. Sci. Mol. Med., *45*:1, 1973.
2. Graziani, G., Cantaluppi, A., Casati, S., et al.: Dopamine and furosemide in oliguric acute renal failure. Nephron, *37*:39, 1984.

954-D *(Campbell's, pp. 2052–2053)*

Patients with acute renal failure develop electrolyte abnormalities including acidosis, hyperkalemia, hypermagnesemia, hyperphosphatemia, and hypercalcemia. Hyperkalemia is the most common, most dangerous electrolyte abnormality seen with acute renal failure. When the serum potassium value has reached a level of 6.0 mEq/L or greater, an electrocardiogram should be performed. Early changes on the electrocardiogram consist of peaking or cannonball T waves. Following this, the amplitude of the P wave decreases and then widening of the QRS complex is seen. The EKG may resemble a sinusoidal wave when severe hyperkalemia develops. Alterations on the electrocardiogram due to hyperkalemia warrant intravenous therapy. In severe cases, intravenous calcium chloride or calcium gluconate should immediately be administered in the quantity of 9.6 mEq of calcium. Calcium opposes the electrophysiologic effects of potassium and the effect seen after administration of calcium lasts approximately 20 to 30 minutes. Other therapies which may cause a rapid drop in serum potassium levels include the administration of intravenous glucose and insulin which leads to a shift of potassium from the extracellular compartment to the intracellular compartment, and the administration of bicarbonate which leads to a shift of hydrogen ion into the extracellular compartment while potassium is exchanged and driven into the intracellular compartment. This therapy, again, only temporizes and buys time during hyperkalemia until a more definitive treatment such as dialysis or the administration of potassium-binding resins is implemented. Sodium polystyrene sulfonate is used to bind potassium and may lower serum potassium levels several hours after administered orally or per rectum. Answer D is, therefore, incorrect. Finally, antacids or cathartics which contain magnesium may lead to dangerous hypermagnesemia and their administration should be avoided during renal failure.

955-E *(Campbell's, pp. 2055–2056)*

Focal and segmental glomerulosclerosis (FSGS) is a primary renal disease that causes chronic renal insufficiency and chronic renal failure. It typically afflicts older children and young adults but may occur at any age. Patients usually develop nephrotic syndrome and become hypertensive. Focal and segmental scarring of the glomeruli are seen on light microscopy and electron scanning microscopy. When the glomerular scars are analyzed, IgM, IgG, complement, and fibrin may be found in them. However, the pathogenesis of this disease is not felt to be caused by immune complexes. Presently, there is no effective therapy for FSGS although hypertension is aggressively treated.

956-E *(Campbell's, p. 2056)*

Focal proliferative glomerulonephritis (FPGN) affects older children and adolescents. Microscopic hematuria and recurrent episodes of gross hematuria are seen with FPGN. The development of marked proteinuria or renal insufficiency is a poor prognostic sign. However, in the absence of these features, progression to chronic renal failure is uncommon. FPGN is characterized by mesangial proliferation and expansion and depositis of IgG, IgM and/or IgA are noted within the mesangium. When these deposits primarily consist of IgA, the disease is referred to as Berger's disease or IgA nephropathy. There is no therapy that definitely affects the natural history of Berger's disease.

957-C *(Campbell's, p. 2056)*

Diffuse proliferative glomerulonephritis (DPGN) is a histologically defined renal disease that manifests with acute nephritic syndrome. Light microscopy shows swollen, congested glomeruli with proliferation and exudation. Cellular crescents may be seen and if they are extensive the prognosis is worse. Immunoflouresence shows a "lumpy, bumpy" distribution of IgM, IgG, and C3. Electron microscopy shows massive subepithelial deposits called "humps" which consists of electron dense substances. The most well-known form of DPGN is that caused by group A streptococci which is known as poststreptococcal glomerulonephritis. This usually develops 2 to 4 weeks following infection and generally has a benign course with good prognosis. There is no known therapy for poststreptococcal DPGN. Because of the high frequency of DPGN due to streptococci, this remains an important cause of end-stage renal disease. Interferon is not reported to affect the course of DPGN.

958-A *(Campbell's, p. 2057)*

Rapidly progressive glomerulonephritis (RPGN) is a clinical syndrome with a presentation similar to acute glomerulonephritis but with progressive development of chronic renal failure. Chronic renal failure usually occurs within weeks to months of development of RPGN. Pathophysiology of RPGN may be due to vasculitis and also to the development of antiglomerular basement membrane antibody formation. When RPGN is seen with antiglomerular basement membrane antibodies and is associated with pulmonary hemorrhage, the disease is referred to as Goodpasture's syndrome. When antiglomerular basement membrane antibodies are present, plasma exchange as well as cytotoxic agents and corticosteroids are thought to be helpful in the arrest of progression of RPGN. On light microscopy, numerous epithelial crescents are seen.

REFERENCES

1. Kincaid-Smith, P.: Plasmapheresis in rapidly progressive glomerulonephritis. Am. J. Med., *65*:564, 1978.

959-B *(Campbell's, pp. 2057–2059)*

Schistosoma haematobium infection may be the leading cause of chronic renal failure worldwide and is related to strictures of the collecting system and obstructive uropathy. Polyarteritis nodosa is a vasculitis which affects predominantly middle-sized muscular arteries. Renal involvement occurs in 80 to 90 per cent of afflicted patients and may lead to chronic renal insufficiency and renal failure. In patients with systemic lupus erythematosus, symptomatic renal disease develops in 50 per cent. Finally, autosomal dominant polycystic kidney disease, also known as adult polycystic disease, is noted to cause chronic renal failure; however, it has considerable variability in its manifestation. Other systemic diseases that cause chronic renal failure are listed in Table 56–7 of *Campbell's Urology* on p. 2058.

960-E *(Campbell's, pp. 2051, 2054, 2060–2061)*

Manifestations of uremia are listed in Table 56–4 on p. 2051 of *Campbell's Urology* and include autonomic neuropathy, pericardial effusion, cardiomyopathy, seizures, pleuritis, uremic pneumonitis, as well as bleeding disorders and gastrointestinal complaints. Uremic bleeding has been associated with the deficiency of von Willebrand factor multimers. When desmopressin acetate (DDAVP) is administered, it causes the release of von Willebrand factor multimers from endothelial cells and this may reverse uremic coagulopathy. Three theories exist concerning the pathogenesis of uremic symptoms which are the small solute theory, the middle molecule theory and the trade off hypothesis. In the small solute theory, it is proposed that small molecules such as urea and creatinine produce uremic symptoms; however, no well-characterized small solute accounts for the majority of uremic signs and symptoms. In the middle molecule theory of uremia, molecules with molecular weights in the range of 1,000 to 10,000 daltons are supposed to be responsible for uremia; however, no such middle molecules responsible have been identified. In the trade-off hypothesis, hormones are supposed to accumulate in above-normal plasma concentrations and, although homeostasis is maintained, these high concentrations are toxic to cellular and organ functions and give rise to uremia.

961-A *(Campbell's, p. 2065)*

Hematuria is defined as the excretion of abnormal quantities of erythrocytes in the urine. For routine urinalysis, a dipstick is often used to screen for hematuria. The test is based on the principle that hemoglobin from red blood cells will catalyze the conversion of the indicator on the dipstick by hydrogen peroxide and change the color of the dipstick. Besides detecting intact red blood cells, free hemoglobin and myoglobin are also detected. False-positive results may occur if oxidizing agents such as hypochlorite are present. False-negative results may also occur if large amounts of reducing agents such as vitamin C are present. Although dipsticks are widely used for screening purposes, they are not sufficiently sensitive because approximately ten per cent of patients with microscopic hematuria are missed.

962-E *(Campbell's, pp. 2066–2068)*

Hematuria can be of glomerular or nonglomerular origin. Erythrocytes originating from glomerular diseases are commonly dysmorphic. On the other hand, erythrocytes originating from a nonglomerular lesion are commonly isomorphic in nature. Alport syndrome, systemic lupus erythematosus, hemolytic uremic syndrome, and Henoch-Schönlein purpura are disorders manifested by glomerular hematuria. Thrombotic thrombocytopenic purpura, on the other hand, is a disorder associated with nonglomerular hematuria. Nonglomerular hematuria, furthermore, is associated with tubulointerstitial, renovascular, and systemic disorders. Other disorders associated with glomerular hematuria include IgA nephropathy, focal segmental proliferative glomerulonephritis, Goodpasture's syndrome, and poststreptococcal glomerulonephritis. Hypercalciuria, hyperuricosuria, and other bleeding disorders may cause nonglomerular hematuria.

963-C *(Campbell's, pp. 2066–2068)*

IgA nephropathy (Berger's disease) accounts for approximately 30 per cent of patients with glomerular hematuria. Recurrent episodes of gross hematuria after an upper respiratory tract infection or exercise is the typical presentation of the disease. The condition is most common in children and young adults. The prognosis is generally good, with renal insufficiency developing in only approximately 25 per cent of patients. However, old age at onset, heavy consistent proteinuria, and hypertension are indicators of a poor prognosis. Pathologically, deposits of IgA, IgG, and β_1 c-globulin are found on mesangial cells. However, IgA and IgG mesangial deposits are found in other forms of glomerulonephritis as well; hence, the presence of IgA deposits is not truly pathognomonic of the disease. Because gross hematuria frequently follows an upper respiratory tract infection, viral antigens have been implicated in some cases. Although no evidence of any beneficial effects of therapy has been shown, clinical and laboratory evaluation are essential because of similarities to other systemic diseases such as systemic lupus erythematosus, Goodpasture's syndrome, and Wegener's granulomatosis.

964-B *(Campbell's, p. 2065)*

A first-voided overnight urine specimen is ideal for detecting and quantitating red blood cells. On the other hand, urine specimens that are obtained after a patient has eaten may become alkaline and thus contain lysed red blood cells. Timed urine collections may be required for definitive assessment of renal functions, proteinuria, and electrolyte abnormalities.

965-C *(Campbell's, pp. 2068–2069)*

Sickle-cell nephropathy occurs in patients with both sickle-cell traits and sickle-cell disease. Sickle-cell trait occurs in approximately 8 per cent of blacks whereas sickle-cell disease affects approximately 1 in 600. The major renal disturbances associated with sickle-cell nephropathy are hematuria, polyuria, renal failure, and thrombotic complications that may lead to the nephrotic syndrome. Although the mechanism of hematuria is not clear, it presumably results from increased sickling and sludging of blood in the medulla and papillae, leading to extravasation of red blood cells, ischemia, and papillary necrosis. Cystoscopy and intravenous urography can be used to localize the site of bleeding, which is usually from the left kidney. Initial treatment for the hematuria include rest and IV hydration. In addition, other techniques including intravenous distilled water, sodium bicarbonate, mannitol, loop diuretics, and ε-aminocaproic acid have also been used to treat hematuria. If hematuria persists despite conservative treatment, arterial embolization, or segmental or total nephrectomy may be required. Recurrent episodes of hematuria may be diminished by regular administration of oral furosemide. A common complication of sickle-cell nephropathy is papillary necrosis. This can rarely result in serious deterioration of renal function.

966-D *(Campbell's, p. 2069)*

Occlusion of the main renal arteries most commonly results from emboli associated with mitral stenosis and atrial fibrillation, artificial heart valves, subacute bacterial endocarditis, or mural thrombi associated with myocardial infarction. Other sources of thrombus include aortic plaque, inflammatory vascular disorders, and also following blunt abdominal trauma or manipulation of the aorta during angiography or surgery. Clinically, the patients may present with sudden, sharp, persistent pain in the flank or upper abdomen, nausea, vomiting, and fever. However, most patients will be symptom free. Radiographically, an intravenous urogram will show absence of visualization of all or part of the kidney. Radionuclide imaging demonstrates nonperfusion of the kidney. Renal arteriography can be used to confirm the diagnosis.

967-C *(Campbell's, p. 2069)*

Renal infarction characteristically causes a rapid rise in the serum glutamic-oxaloacetic transaminase levels, which returns to normal within 3 to 4 days followed by a striking elevation of lactate dehydrogenase which remains elevated for as long as two weeks. Serum alkaline phosphatase levels may be slightly increased. Leukocytosis may be present. Elevated serum glutamic-pyruvic transaminase levels are not a characteristic laboratory finding associated with renal infarction.

968-A *(Campbell's, pp. 2069–2070)*

Early management of renal artery thromboembolism is determined by degree of renal involvement, duration of involvement, and cause of the occlusion. In cases with bilateral renal artery thrombi, surgical thrombectomy or embolectomy performed within a few hours after the occlusion has shown good results; however, significant return of renal function has been documented in patients operated on as long as 15 to 43 days following occlusion. Reports indicate that transluminal recanalization or dissolution by intra-arterial fibrinolytic agents can result in significant recovery of renal function. Unilateral thrombosis, on the other hand, warrants a conservative approach because the contralateral kidney will continue to function, and recovery of function on the ischemic side has been reported. Anticoagulation therapy should be instituted promptly to prevent further propagation of clot into the renal artery or embolization of other organs. High dose corticosteroid therapy has no place in the management of renal artery thrombosis.

969-B *(Campbell's, p. 2070)*

Renal arteriovenous fistulas can be either congenital or acquired. Congenital fistulas account for only one fourth of all arteriovenous fistulas and present as distinct, tortuous, coiled vascular channels grouped in clusters, with multiple communications between arteries and veins on angiography. Acquired arteriovenous fistulas usually appear as solitary communications between artery and veins, account for almost 75 per cent of all fistulas, and are posttraumatic in origin. Over 40 per cent of acquired fistulas occur after a percutaneous needle biopsy. Other causes for acquired fistula include penetrating or blunt abdominal trauma, partial nephrectomies, and tumor invasion into adjacent veins. Approximately 75 per cent of affected patients have a continuous abdominal or flank bruit. Management of arteriovenous fistulas is based upon the cause and associated symptoms. Most congenital fistulas are small, asymptomatic, and of little clinical importance. Similarly, approximately 95 per cent of postbiopsy fistulas heal spontaneously in 1 to 18 months. Surgical intervention includes embolization techniques, partial nephrectomy, or total nephrectomy.

970-D *(Campbell's, pp. 2070–2071)*

Renal vein thrombosis in infants may arise bilaterally in association with severe dehydration due to diarrhea or vomiting or with severe plasma hyperosmolarity related to angiography. The intralobular, or arcuate veins, are usually affected. Clinically, acute thrombosis is associated with severe flank pain, hypertension, shock, and gross or microscopic hematuria. Intravenous urography may show an enlarged kidney, which usually, though not always, excretes contrast material. Ultrasonography during the acute phase shows an enlarged, hypoechoic kidney and thrombus in the renal vein. The best management for renal vein thrombosis in infancy is rehydration. Results with emergent thrombectomy and fibrinolytic agents have also been favorable.

971-A *(Campbell's, pp. 2070–2072)*

In adults, renal vein thrombosis is frequently unilateral and it is usually associated with the nephrotic syndrome due to membranous glomerulonephritis. Another cause includes invasion of renal veins by tumor or retroperitoneal disease. Whether renal vein thrombosis is the cause or consequence of the nephrotic syndrome is questionable. Increased renal venous pressure secondary to congestive heart failure or after surgical ligation of the renal vein can produce proteinuria. However, the nephrotic syndrome is a hypercoagulable state and thrombotic events are common. Although intravenous urography and ultrasonography are helpful in the diagnosis of renal vein thrombosis, the definitive diagnostic study is renal venography. Initial management of renal vein thrombosis includes anticoagulation therapy as soon as the diagnosis is made. On the other hand, surgical removal of the clot from the renal vein is neither possible nor helpful because thrombosis of intrarenal channels is most likely present.

972-A *(Campbell's, pp. 2072–2073)*

The detection of proteinuria raises the question of renal disease and may indicate an underlying renal glomerular, vascular, or tubulointerstitial disease. In healthy adults approximately 80 to 150 mg of protein are excreted daily. The maximum level in small children is 140 mg/m per meter squared of body surface area per day. For any given rate of protein excretion, the concentration of protein in a single voided sample of urine will vary inversely with urine flow. The concentration of protein in normal urine usually does not exceed 10 to 20 mg/dl; thus, higher concentrations imply the existence of proteinuria. On the other hand, in patients with dilute urine, significant proteinuria may be present with concentrations well below 20 mg/dl. Proteinuria can be detected by either turbidimetric (protein precipitations) or colorimetric (dipstick) methods. False-positive or false-negative test results can occur with either method. False negative colorimetric dipstick test can occur when urine is highly alkalinized (pH >8) or following contamination with antiseptics such as chlorhexidine or benzalkonium chloride. Highly concentrated urine in a dehydrated patient or gross hematuria can result in false-positive results.

973-E *(Campbell's, p. 2073)*

A colorimetric dipstick is impregnated with tetrabromphenol blue which reacts preferentially with serum albumin and changes color in its presence. It is relatively insensitive to serum globulin, Bence Jones protein, and other tissue protein such as Tamm-Horsfall protein. The intensity of the shade of green is proportional to the concentration of protein in the urine. The reagent strips are generally sensitive to total protein concentrations as low as 20 mg/dl.

974-E *(Campbell's, p. 2073)*

Normal composition of urine protein is about 30 to 40 per cent serum albumin, 30 per cent serum globulin, and 40 per cent tissue proteins. This profile can be altered by both physiologic and pathologic conditions that affect filtration, reabsorption, or excretion of urine protein.

975-D *(Campbell's, pp. 2073–2074)*

Tubular proteinuria is defined as the appearance in the urine of normally filtered protein as a result of impaired tubular reabsorption. Examples of tubular proteinuria include Fanconi's syndrome and cadmium, lead, or mercury poisoning. On the other hand, diabetes mellitus can give rise to glomerular proteinuria which is the most common type of proteinuria. This is caused by increased glomerular capillary permeability to protein. Other examples of glomerular proteinuria include systemic lupus erythematosus, lipoid nephrosis, or any other glomerulopathy associated with a systemic illness.

976-A *(Campbell's, p. 2073)*

The determination of a protein/creatinine ratio in a single urine sample obtained during normal daytime activity can support the 24-hour urine collections in a clinical quantitation of proteinuria. In the presence of stable renal function, a ratio of less than 0.2 is within normal limits. However, a ratio of more than 3.5 suggests nephrotic range proteinuria.

977-B *(Campbell's, pp. 2074–2075)*

Multiple myeloma is a neoplastic transformation of plasma cells leading to the production and secretion of abnormal and unique immunoglobulin protein. Renal dysfunction may take a variety of forms, including acute renal failure, chronic failure, and tubular disorders, related to the type of myeloma. IgG, IgA, and light chain disease myeloma exist. Acute renal failure occurs in approximately 5 to 10 per cent of myeloma patients and is precipitated by intravenous or retrograde urography, dehydration, hypercalcemia, hyperuricemia, or pyelonephritis. Regardless of the cause, the prognosis is poor in those patients that develop acute renal failure, with a 60 to 75 per cent mortality.

978-C *(Campbell's, p. 2076)*

The creatinine clearance provides a simple and reliable means for estimating GFR and thus the status of renal function. Creatinine is produced at a constant rate by muscle cells. The breakdown of creatinine occurs at a rate of approximately 20 mg/kg/day. The plasma concentration and daily urine creatinine excretion remains relatively constant if lean body mass is not changed appreciably.

979-C *(Campbell's, p. 2077)*

Correlation between chronic analgesic abuse, interstitial nephritis, papillary necrosis, and chronic renal failure is now widely recognized. Large doses of phenacetin and aspirin, especially in combination, may cause renal papillary necrosis and chronic interstitial nephritis. The degree of renal function impairment is dose dependent, and a total of 2 kg of phenacetin alone is considered the minimal amount that will cause nephropathy. Analgesic nephropathy is predominantly seen in women between the ages of 30 and 50. Intravenous urography or retrograde pyelography will demonstrate bilateral renal papillary necrosis that involves all the calyceal groups. Although no effective treatment is available, more than 80 per cent of patients who stop abusing analgesics will frequently show an improvement or at least a slowing of deterioration in renal function. The presence of hematuria should be carefully investigated and cytologic studies performed regularly because of an increased incidence of transitional cell carcinoma.

980-E *(Campbell's, pp. 2077–2078)*

Nonsteroidal anti-inflammatory drugs have the potential for significant nephrotoxicity and can produce a wide spectrum of nephrotoxic syndromes. The mechanisms by which nonsteroidals can affect renal function include decreased synthesis of renal prostaglandin E_2, allergic interstitial nephritis, impaired renin secretion, and enhanced tubular water and sodium reabsorption. Patients usually recover baseline renal function within several days of discontinuing therapy with nonsteroidals.

981-B *(Campbell's, p. 2078)*

Radiographic contrast media nephropathy is defined as an acute deterioration in renal function associated with intravascular exposure to these agents. Among hospitalized patients with normal renal function, the incidence of nephrotoxicity from intravenous pyelography is 0.6 per cent and 2 per cent following major angiography. Predisposing factors include preexisting renal insufficiency, diabetes mellitus, age older than 55 years, dehydration, hypertension, peripheral vascular disease, proteinuria, hyperuricemia, and recent nephrotoxic drug exposure. Renal failure is usually abrupt, with oliguria beginning shortly after the injection of contrast material and persisting for 2 to 4 days. The renal failure is reversible in most patients; however, dialysis may be required, and permanent renal failure may occur in some patients with severe pre-existing renal insufficiency. The use of new nonionic, less hyperosmolar contrast agents may also reduce the risk of nephropathy in high-risk patients.

982-D *(Campbell's, pp. 2078–2079)*

Polyuria is generally defined as a urine volume of 2500 ml or more per day. Polyuria can be caused by various etiologies including compulsive water drinking due to psychogenic factors, inadequate vasopressin secretion (neurogenic diabetes insipidus), diminished response of the renal tubule to vasopressin (nephrogenic diabetes insipidus), or osmotic diuresis owing to excessive endogenous or exogenous solutes. The patient in this case demonstrates nephrogenic diabetes insipidus which can be idiopathic or acquired. The acquired type may be caused by obstructive uropathy, sickle-cell disease, potassium depletion, hypercalcemia, chronic pyelonephritis, and drugs such as lithium or amphotericin B. The urine is usually hypotonic and the plasma osmolality is usually high normal. The diagnosis is established by demonstrating inability to concentrate urine despite an appropriate osmotic stimulus, followed by the administration of exogenous ADH. Treatment consists of correcting the underlying cause if possible and the administration of chlorothiazide coupled with a low sodium diet. In patients with psychogenic polydypsia, who are usually female, urine osmolality is generally hypotonic to the plasma osmolality, which is usually normal. In patients with neurogenic diabetes insipidus (which is sometimes seen as a consequence of brain tumor, after head trauma, or following pituitary ablation for acromegaly), the plasma osmolality is in the high normal range, urine osmolality is hypotonic, and plasma levels of ADH are undetectable. Polyuria due to osmotic diuresis is seen in association with diabetes mellitus, after relief of obstructive uropathy, and transiently with mannitol or radiographic contrast media infusion. These patients will usually show isotonic or slightly hypertonic urine osmolality.

983-A *(Campbell's, pp. 2079–2080)*

Papillary necrosis is the consequence of toxic or ischemic injury to the renal papillae with resultant ischemic necrosis. Common conditions associated with it are diabetes mellitus, urinary obstruction, pyelonephritis, sickle-cell disease, and analgesic abuse. Papillary necrosis is the pathologic description of a lesion most frequently diagnosed by radiologic criteria and is not a clinical entity. The most common presentation of papillary necrosis is the insidious onset of renal failure; however, some patients will present with renal colic and hematuria secondary to ureteral obstruction from sloughed papilla. The calyceal deformities of renal papillary necrosis may be divided into two forms, medullary and papillary. In the medullary form, there is central necrosis of the tip of the pyramid and a round or oval cavity occurs. In the papillary form, there is necrosis of the larger portions of the entire papilla and the resulting defect is triangular in shape. Management includes relief of ureteral obstruction, treatment of infection, rehydration, and removal of any causative agents.

PART XIII

URINARY LITHIASIS

CHAPTERS 58 THROUGH 62

DIRECTIONS: Each question below contains suggested responses. Select the ONE BEST response to each question.

984. The predominant site of urinary calculi in developing, preindustrialized countries is the:
   A. Renal calyx
   B. Renal pelvis
   C. Ureter
   D. Bladder
   E. Urethra

985. With regard to the epidemiology of stone disease, all of the following statements are true EXCEPT:
   A. The incidence of stone disease in men is 3 times that of women.
   B. Stone disease occurs primarily in the third, fourth, and fifth decades of life.
   C. Stone disease is more prevalent in blacks than other races.
   D. In children, male and female incidence of stone disease is equal.
   E. Stone disease is common in individuals of Northern European ancestry.

986. The highest incidence of stone disease in the United States is in:
   A. New England
   B. Midwest
   C. Southwest
   D. Southeast
   E. West

987. In the physical chemistry of stone formation, spontaneous nucleation of crystals occurs:
   A. At concentrations less than solubility product
   B. At concentrations between the solubility product and formation product
   C. In the metastable zone
   D. At concentrations above the formation product
   E. At all concentrations of crystallizable substances

988. The deposition of one type of crystal upon the surface of another crystal of different chemical composition but similar lattice structure is called:
   A. Crystal growth
   B. Aggregation
   C. Nucleation
   D. Matrix formation
   E. Epitaxy

989. The smallest stone that can obstruct the lumen of the ureter has a diameter of:
   A. 1 mm
   B. 2 mm
   C. 3 mm
   D. 4 mm
   E. 5 mm

990. All of the following have been suggested as possible inhibitors of stone formation EXCEPT:
   A. Substance A
   B. Citrate
   C. Magnesium
   D. Pyrophosphate
   E. Zinc

991. All of the following symptoms/signs are typical of renal colic EXCEPT:
   A. Costovertebral angle pain that radiates anteriorly
   B. Pain in the testicle
   C. Nausea and vomiting
   D. Pain relief obtained in supine position with knees flexed
   E. Urinary frequency and urgency

992. In the patient with stone disease, all of the following statements are true EXCEPT:
   A. Gross or microscopic hematuria is always present.
   B. Pyuria may occur in the absence of infection.
   C. The presence of cystine, uric acid or calcium oxalate crystals may indicate the type of calculus ultimately found.
   D. Urinary pH may provide a clue to the type of stone found.

993. Approximately what percentage of stones are sufficiently radiodense to be visualized on a KUB film?
   A. 10 per cent
   B. 40 per cent
   C. 50 per cent
   D. 90 per cent
   E. 100 per cent

994. All of the following types of urinary calculi are radiolucent EXCEPT:
   A. Uric acid
   B. Matrix
   C. 2,8-Hydroxyadenine
   D. Cystine
   E. Xanthine

995. Complete ureteral obstruction by a stone will cause at least some irreversible renal damage by:
   A. 24 hours
   B. 2 weeks

C. 4 weeks
D. 6 weeks
E. 8 weeks

996. Of the 5 major types of renal calculi, the most common is:

A. Calcium oxalate
B. Calcium phosphate
C. Triple phosphate
D. Uric acid
E. Cystine

997. The type of calculus seen most often in hyperparathyroidism is:

A. Calcium magnesium ammonium phosphate
B. Calcium oxalate
C. Calcium phosphate
D. Cystine
E. Uric acid

998. Xanthogranulomatous pyelonephritis (replacement lipomatosis) can occur in kidneys damaged by calculi and is most often associated with infection caused by:

A. *E. coli*
B. *Staphylococcus epidermidis*
C. *Proteus mirabilis*
D. *Klebsiella*
E. *Enterobacter*

999. The most important factor in the formation of uric acid calculi is:

A. Concentration of uric acid in urine
B. Volume of urine
C. Limited solubility of uric acid in acidic solutions
D. Excessive dietary intake of purines
E. Presence of gout

1000. Patients with ileostomies are at increased risk for urinary calculi composed of:

A. Uric acid
B. Calcium oxalate
C. Cystine
D. Calcium phosphate
E. 2,8-Hydroxyadenine

1001. The most common complication associated with D-penicillamine therapy, limiting its use for cystine stone disease, is:

A. Leukopenia
B. Gastrointestinal distress
C. Lowering of the seizure threshold
D. Sexual dysfunction
E. Allergic reaction with arthralgia, rash and nephrotic syndrome

1002. All of the following bacteria are capable of producing urease and potentially causing infection stones EXCEPT:

A. *E. coli*
B. *Staphylococcus epidermidis*
C. *Proteus mirabilis*
D. *Pseudomonas*
E. *Klebsiella*

1003. The actions of parathormone on the kidney are to:

A. Increase calcium and phosphorous absorption
B. Decrease calcium and phosphorus absorption
C. Increase calcium and decrease phosphorus absorption
D. Increase phosphorus and decrease calcium absorption
E. Increase calcium and decrease phosphorus absorption, promote production of active vitamin D

1004. Patients with normal urinary tract anatomy and no past history of calculus disease who then develop regional ileitis are at risk for urinary calculi of the following composition:

A. Calcium phosphate
B. Struvite
C. Calcium oxalate
D. Uric acid
E. Cystine

1005. Indicated medical therapy for renal leak hypercalciuria is:

A. Oral citrates
B. Magnesium oxide or gluconate
C. Cellulose phosphates or neutral phosphates
D. Allopurinol
E. Thiazide diuretics

1006. Stones may rarely form from which anti-hypertensive medication?

A. Hydrochlorothiazide
B. Propranolol
C. Captopril
D. Triamterene
E. Procardia

1007. The most important etiologic factor for bladder calculi in the developed world is:

A. Hypercalciuria
B. Urinary tract infection
C. A foreign object in urine
D. Urine pH
E. Bladder outlet obstruction

1008. The most common type of bladder calculus found in the United States is:

A. Calcium oxalate
B. Calcium phosphate
C. Ammonium acid urate
D. Struvite
E. Cystine

1009. Prostatic calculi are usually formed of:

A. Calcium oxalate
B. Calcium phosphate
C. Struvite
D. Uric acid
E. Cystine

1010. Which of the following concerning the mechanism of stone fracture by shock waves is *true*?

A. When the shock (pressure) wave strikes the stone, it is split into compressive and tensile components, of which the compressive component is reflected toward the source.
B. Disintegration begins at the center of the stone due to cavitation.
C. Shear forces from reflected pressure wave components give rise to stone disintegration at the surface nearest the source.
D. A high-pressure gradient due to a reflected ten-

sile wave and continuing compressive wave leads to disintegration at both proximal and distal stone surfaces.
E. When the stress tensor is greater than unity at the stone surface, disintegration occurs.

1011. Which one of the following statements concerning shock wave generators and their application to lithotripsy is *false*?

A. The electromagnetic generator produces a shock wave by rapid magnetic repulsion of a metal plate within a tube.
B. In the piezoelectric lithotriptors, the shock wave is generated by ceramic elements excited by a high frequency high voltage pulse.
C. Cardiac arrhythmias are not induced by piezoelectric shock generators.
D. With spark gap generators, discharge must coincide with the refractory period of the heart to avoid dysrhythmias.
E. Shock waves generated by explosion of lead azide pellets are focused with an acoustic lens in the microexplosive lithotripter (Yachiyoda Company).

1012. Studies of tissue subjected to lithotripter shock waves show all of the following EXCEPT:

A. Free plasma hemoglobin increases linearly with the number of shocks when whole blood is subjected to lithotripsy.
B. Cavitation effects from shock waves appear to be responsible for tissue injury, and these effects may increase with increasing frequency of shock wave exposure.
C. In tissue culture, viability of both proximal and distal tubular cells subjected to shock waves appears to be related to the number of shock waves and not the energy of the wave (kV).
D. Bacterial viability is decreased when bacterial cultures are subjected to 2,000 shocks at 22 kV.
E. When in vitro models of renal cell carcinoma are subjected to shock waves, a significant decrease in cell viability is seen.

1013. All of the following effects on animal organs have been observed after lithotriptor shock wave treatment focused directly on the organ specified EXCEPT:

A. Massive hemoptysis in rats after a single shock wave to the thorax
B. Epiphyseal growth plate abnormalities in immature rats, with 17 per cent of treated rats exhibiting shortened extremities
C. Complete devastation of chick embryos
D. No apparent injuries to myocardium or spinal cord
E. Massive contusion and hemorrhage in rat ovaries

1014. Transient elevations of the following enzymes in serum or urine have been observed in the immediate post lithotripsy period EXCEPT:

A. Lactic dehydrogenase
B. Gamma-glutamyl transpeptidase
C. Alanine aminotransferase
D. *N*-Acetyl-beta-glucosaminidase
E. Creatine phosphokinase

1015. Which one of the following statements concerning the effect of ESWL on the kidney is *false*?

A. Gross hematuria, which occurs almost universally after ESWL, is thought to be due to parenchymal injury as opposed to urothelial damage from fragments.
B. The majority of kidneys treated with the Dornier HM-3 exhibit swelling in the immediate postoperative period.
C. Five per cent of kidneys show subcapsular bleeding or perinephric fluid collections on radiographic studies immediately following ESWL treatment.
D. In animal studies, chronic changes noted in the renal tissue along the path of the shockwave include calcifications, hyalinized scars, loss of nephrons and dilated veins.
E. Animal studies show capillary and small vein damage, intraparenchymal hemorrhage, and tubular injury in kidneys immediately after ESWL treatment.

1016. The following statement concerning imaging of calculi during ESWL is *false*:

A. The HM-3 (the most widely used lithotriptor in the world today) uses two fluoroscopes mounted in a transverse plane to the body's long axis at a 90 degree angle to one another and at a 45 degree angle to the horizon.
B. Most stones can be visualized by ultrasound if they are greater than 2–3 mm in size.
C. Low ureteral stones in the juxta- and intravesical areas may be localized and treated by ultrasound guidance.
D. To treat radiolucent stones with fluoroscopically guided lithotriptors requires stent placement or instillation of contrast through ureteral catheters or nephrostomy tubes for stone localization.
E. The latest variant in imaging for ESWL, the CT-guided lithotriptor (Litho-Cat), allows precise localization and visualization of all stone types and eliminates the need for contrast use.

1017. Concerning stone fragmentation and the focal point F2, the following statement is *false*:

A. The efficacy of fragmentation diminishes rapidly as one moves away from F2, and at 2 cm from F2, pressures are only 20 per cent of those at F2.
B. The "blast path" refers to a course which extends from F2 at a 25 degree angle to the cross hairs.
C. In general, with the HM-3 machine if body habitus places the stone greater than 13 cm from the ellipsoid, successful fragmentation is less likely.
D. Successful fragmentation can occur up to 12 cm beyond F2 if the stone lies on the "blast path."
E. In general if the energy per shockwave (kV) is increased a greater pressure gradient develops at F2 leading to faster fragmentation with larger size fragments.

1018. Preoperative preparation for ESWL includes all of the following EXCEPT:

A. Urine cultures for those with struvite stones of urinary tract infection.
B. Appropriate pre-operative antibiotic therapy for those with nephrostomy tubes, indwelling stents and catheters, and for patients with struvite stones.
C. Placement of a double-J ureteral stent when treating a stone greater than 1 cm.
D. Placement of a ureteral stent or nephrostomy tube in at least one renal unit when treating bilateral calculi at the same setting.
E. Full mechanical bowel prep to aid visualization of calculi.

1019. Contraindications to ESWL include all of the following EXCEPT:

A. Uncontrolled coagulation parameters
B. Childhood
C. Pregnancy
D. Stones whose treatment leads to placement of a calcified aortic aneurysm in the "blast path"
E. Obstruction distal to the stone

1020. The following statement concerning stone composition and ESWL monotherapy is *false*:

A. The stone-free rate for brushite stones is 53 per cent.
B. Cystine stones and calcium oxalate dihydrate stones fragment poorly.
C. Uric acid and struvite stones break up readily.
D. The stone-free rate for calcium oxalate monohydrate stones is 74 per cent.
E. The highest stone-free rates are observed with treatment of uric acid stones.

1021. Which one of the following statements concerning the treatment of renal calculi is *false*?

A. The stone free rate for solitary renal stones that average 1.2 cm in size using ESWL monotherapy is 87 per cent.
B. In the treatment of staghorn calculi with open anatrophic nephrolithotomy, the success rate is 94 per cent.
C. When ESWL monotherapy is used to manage staghorn calculi, most series show a 50 per cent stone-free rate.
D. Combined ESWL and percutaneous lithotripsy for management of staghorn calculi yields stone-free rates of 77–88 per cent.
E. Percutaneous lithotripsy as the sole therapy for staghorn stones has a success rate of 68 per cent.

1022. Which statement concerning the management of ureteral stones is *false*?

A. Treatment of upper ureteral stones in situ with the HM-3 lithotripter has a 60–85 per cent success rate.
B. Higher stone-free rates are obtained when an upper ureteral stone is treated with the "push up and smash" technique—pushing the stone into the kidney and treating with ESWL.
C. Operators often use higher kilovoltage and fewer shock waves to treat ureteral stones in situ in comparison to similar renal calculi.
D. It is necessary to treat the patient in the prone position when the stone resides in the ureter overlying the pelvic bones and one is using ESWL.
E. Ureteroscopic techniques have a higher success rate (95 per cent) and are less expensive overall than management with ESWL for distal ureteral stones.

1023. Factors which decrease the likelihood of a stone free status following ESWL include all of the following EXCEPT:

A. Increasing stone burden
B. Marked hydronephrosis
C. The presence of stone in lower pole calyces or in a calyceal diverticulum
D. Horseshoe kidney
E. Absence of a ureteral stent

1024. Which of the following statements concerning long term effects of ESWL is *false*?

A. Swelling of the kidney, perinephric fluid collections, and intranephric fluid collections seen immediately following ESWL on magnetic resonance imaging appear to resolve by 3 months.
B. A decrease in effective renal plasma flow is noted at 17 months following ESWL.
C. There is definitely a 2- to 3-fold increase in the incidence of hypertension following ESWL.
D. At 4 years post ESWL, no adverse effects are seen on renal scans with ^{131}I hippurate.
E. The majority of ESWL patients appear to suffer little long-term morbidity.

1025. All of the following are true concerning Steinstrasse EXCEPT:

A. Indications for steinstrasse intervention include: solitary kidney, pain, total obstruction, and a ureteral segment 3 cm in length full of fragments.
B. Intervention for steinstrasse is necessary in 35 per cent of cases.
C. Upper ureteral steinstrasse can sometimes be cleared by repeat ESWL to the lead fragment.
D. 75 per cent of steinstrasse cases occur in the distal ureter and 18 per cent in the proximal ureter.
E. Steinstrasse occurs in less than 5 per cent of ESWL cases.

1026. All of the following are true concerning severe complications after ESWL EXCEPT:

A. ESWL has a mortality of 0.02 per cent.
B. Iliac artery and vein thrombosis has been reported after ESWL of ureteral stones.
C. Severe pulmonary damage in infants and children may be avoided by shielding the chest with styrofoam.
D. Pancreatitis occurs in 5–10 per cent of ESWL cases.
E. Renal artery aneurysm rupture has not been reported following ESWL, although one should be concerned about this possibility.

1027. Which of the following specifications in the design of lithotriptors does *not* decrease the anesthesia requirement?

A. The use of a water cushion
B. A widened dish or ellipsoid aperture

C. A wide shock wave skin entry radius
D. A reduction in the power of the shock wave generator
E. A decreased focal zone

1028. When comparing lithotriptors, the following are true EXCEPT:

A. The "effectiveness quotient" relates the stone-free rate to the incidence of additional therapy including repeat ESWL and is calculated by: EQ = per cent stone free × 100 / (100 + per cent retreatment + per cent auxiliary procedures).
B. The retreatment rate is 30 per cent for lower power, "anesthesia-free," machines.
C. The piezoelectric lithotriptor by Wolf is truly an anesthesia-free machine.
D. Overall, the HM-3 is superior to other machines when treating stones <2 cm in size with an "effectiveness quotient" of 90 per cent.
E. The Dornier MPL 9000 has been used to treat cholelithiasis.

1029. Indications for percutaneous lithotripsy include all of the following EXCEPT:

A. Ureteropelvic junction obstruction with coexisting calculi in the collecting system
B. Caliceal diverticula containing calculi
C. Collecting system calculi in a gravid patient
D. Collecting system calculi and previous ureteroneocystostomy
E. Body habitus that excludes extracorporal shockwave lithotripsy (ESWL), such as obesity or severe scoliosis

1030. Which of the following statements concerning percutaneous management of struvite stones is *false*:

A. With percutaneous lithotripsy (PL) alone, stone free rates of 85–90 per cent can be achieved in experienced hands.
B. The combined technique of PL and ESWL consists of an initial debulking or removal of large stone volume with percutaneous lithotripsy followed by ESWL of residual stone followed by a final percutaneous endoscopic procedure to remove fragments.
C. When a given staghorn calculus requires three or more access tracts to manage percutaneously, a nephrolithotomy may be indicated.
D. The combined technique of PL and ESWL has a slightly better stone free rate than PL alone.
E. The advantage of ESWL in the combined technique is that it reduces the need for additional access tracts, and greatly simplifies the second endoscopic procedure.

1031. The stone type *least* likely to require percutaneous lithotripsy for a stone-free state is:

A. Cystine
B. Uric acid
C. Brushite
D. Calcium oxalate monohydrate
E. Struvite

1032. In general, percutaneous lithotripsy is preferred to ESWL when:

A. An upper pole renal calculus is present.
B. A renal calculus has a diameter of 3.0 cm or more.
C. A renal calculus has a diameter of 2.0 cm.
D. The stone composition is calcium oxalate dihydrate.
E. A 2.0-cm stone exists at the UPJ in a solitary kidney.

1033. The following guidelines for obtaining percutaneous access to the collecting system are true EXCEPT:

A. An excretory urogram or retrograde pyelogram should first be obtained and reviewed to select the optimum tract.
B. With caliceal or diverticular stones, access should be obtained directly into the calyx or diverticulum of interest.
C. An upper pole approach is suboptimum for work at the UPJ.
D. Enlargement of the spleen, liver, or colon may exclude the possibility of safe percutaneous access.
E. Lateral caliceal access is generally optimum.

1034. Which statement concerning percutaneous stone removal is *false*?

A. Power lithotripsy is generally required and ultrasonic lithotripsy is generally preferred.
B. Electrohydraulic lithotripsy is useful for fragmentation of hard stones.
C. The nephroscope should not be inserted for a second procedure for 3–4 postoperative days.
D. Common reasons for early termination of the procedure include bleeding which obscures vision and extravasation of irrigant.
E. A large nephrostomy tube and ureteral catheter should be placed at the completion of the procedure.

1035. The following statements concerning complications of percutaneous access are true EXCEPT:

A. Patients who have undergone intestinal bypass procedures should be suspected of having colonomegaly and may be at risk for colon injury during access.
B. Placement of a tract medial to the calyces may lead to large vessel injury or tearing of the renal parenchyma.
C. Dilators should be placed no further than the stone itself.
D. A suboptimal access point should be changed to another location prior to dilatation.
E. Pneumothorax is of little concern for approaches below the 11th rib.

1036. The following statements concerning complications of percutaneous lithotripsy (PL) are true EXCEPT:

A. Colonic perforation may be managed with percutaneous drainage through the retroperitoneum.
B. Arterial injury occurs in less than 1 per cent of PL cases.
C. Arteriography should be performed immediately if significant vessel injury is suspected, and the offending artery embolized.
D. Stone fragments extruded through the collecting system into perinephric tissue need not be removed.

E. UPJ obstruction is a common long-term complication following PL.

1037. Which of the following statements with respect to extravasation of irrigant during percutaneous lithotripsy (PL) is *false*?

A. Normal saline should be used for irrigation fluid during percutaneous lithotripsy.
B. Healthy adults can absorb 1000 ml of extravasated normal saline without complication.
C. If the nephroscope must be placed farther in to access the stone as the procedure progresses, significant retroperitoneal extravasation should be suspected.
D. As with transurethral resection of the prostate, when significant venous bleeding is observed through the nephroscope, intravascular extravasation may be significant.
E. Extravasation is more likely when the Amplatz sheath is used for PL.

1038. Which of the following statements concerning the anatomic relationships of the ureter is *false*?

A. The ureter begins at the ureteral pelvic junction and is covered by the descending duodenum on the right and the beginning portion of the jejunum on the left.
B. As the ureter descends from the renal pelvis, it lies lateral to the inferior vena cava, anterior to the psoas major muscle, and posterior to the genital femoral nerve.
C. Near the level where the ureters cross the bifurcation of the common iliac arteries, the right ureter lies directly posterior to the right colic and ileocolic blood vessels and terminal ileum, and the left ureter lies posterior to the left colic vessels and line of attachment of the sigmoid mesocolon.
D. As the ureters enter the true pelvis, they course ventral to the hypogastric arteries and medial to the obturator nerves and arteries.
E. Near the region of the ischial spine, the ureter bends medially and anteriorly to reach the bladder at the ureterovesical junction.

1039. All of the following are true concerning the histologic structure of the ureter EXCEPT:

A. The mucosal layer consists of transitional cell epithelium and lamina propria, and is thickest (six cell layers deep) in the calyces and renal pelvis.
B. The outermost layer, the tunica adventitia, is a continuous fiber structure that runs from the renal sinus along the ureter and inserts into the fibrous coat of the bladder giving rise to Waldeyer's sheath.
C. Nerve fibers, lymphatics and blood vessels are contained in the fibrous outer layer.
D. In the middle and distal ureter, the muscular layer is composed of three distinct muscle layers: inner longitudinal, middle circular, and outer longitudinal.
E. In the submucosal ureter, the muscular layer is sparse with only a semicircle of longitudinal fibers around the lateral aspect and few fibers along the medial aspect.

1040. Endoscopy of the renal collecting system and ureter may reveal all of the following EXCEPT:

A. Papilla appearing as a rounded cone with a pink, easily friable epithelium.
B. Displacement of the ureter anteriorly by psoas hypertrophy in young muscular male patients.
C. Narrowing of the ureteral lumen at the ureteral pelvic junction, the pelvic brim, and the ureteral vesical junction.
D. Respiratory movement of the renal pelvis and proximal ureter, with the renal pelvis and proximal ureter moving in a caudal direction during expiration.
E. A bend or lip of ureteral mucosa in the posterolateral ureteral lumen of the proximal ureter near the ureteral pelvic junction.

1041. Indications for ureteroscopy include all the following EXCEPT:

A. Impacted lower ureteral calculi
B. Steinstrasse
C. A large ureteral pelvic junction calculus
D. Retrieval of broken or migrated ureteral stents
E. Surveillance following segmental ureterectomy for a urothelial tumor

1042. Indications for diagnostic ureteroscopy include the following EXCEPT:

A. A radiographic filling defect of the ureter or renal pelvis
B. A tumor found near or at the ureteral orifice
C. Unilateral upper tract hematuria
D. Upper tract cytology findings suggestive of malignancy
E. Multiple bladder tumors suggestive of upper tract seeding

1043. Routine preoperative evaluation and treatment prior to ureteroscopy should include each of the following EXCEPT:

A. Administration of intravenous indigo carmine when the patient receives anesthesia.
B. Administration of broad-spectrum antibiotics to decrease the risk of sepsis following intravasation of irrigant or urine.
C. Bimanual examination.
D. Performance of retrograde pyelography when the ureter is not adequately visualized on radiographic studies.
E. A detailed history, including an inquiry regarding prior pelvic or urologic surgery, and whether pelvic radiation has been given.

1044. Which of the following statements concerning dilation of the ureteral orifice and intramural ureter is *false*?

A. Dilation to 14-15 French has no detrimental effect on the structure or function of the orifice.
B. Hydraulic dilation by pressurized pumping may be performed, but can be associated with intravasation of fluid.
C. Cone-shaped metal bougies may be passed up the ureter to the level of the pelvic brim.
D. Subacute or passive dilation is not preferred when diagnostic ureteroscopy is planned.
E. In general, dilating methods which proceed over a positioned guide wire are safer than

other methods, with fewer false passages and ureteral perforations.

1045. When performing balloon dilation of the ureteral orifice or intramural ureter, all of the following are true EXCEPT:

A. Inflation is carried out at a rate of 2 atmospheres per minute.
B. Once the balloon is fully inflated, it is kept in place for 10 minutes.
C. The balloon is inflated with a 50 per cent radiocontrast solution in order that it may be seen fluoroscopically.
D. Generally less than 10 atmospheres is needed to dilate the nondiseased orifice.
E. Reimplanted or scarred ureters may require pressures as high as 15 atmospheres to dilate the orifice.

1046. Which of the following statements concerning dilation of the supravesical ureter is *false*?

A. The ureteral orifice should always be dilated prior to supravesical ureteral balloon dilation because once the balloon is used in the supravesical ureter it may not resume its preinflation diameter.
B. A partially inflated balloon should not be moved in the ureter or ureteral mucosa may be avulsed.
C. Buckling of the guidewire may lead to ureteral perforation by the end of the balloon catheter.
D. Inflation of the balloon at rates greater than 1.5 atmospheres per minute may lead to ureteral rupture in the supravesical ureter.
E. The inability to pass the guidewire smoothly into the renal pelvis should lead one to suspect the possibility of a submucosal tunnel.

1047. All of the following techniques are useful when introducing the ureteroscope into the ureter EXCEPT:

A. Rotation of the rigid ureteroscope 90 to 180 degrees as it enters the ureter, enabling the beveled tip to "lift" the upper lip of the orifice permitting smooth insertion
B. Placement of a guide tube in the ureter over a flexible dilator, and its later use as an introducer sheath for the flexible ureteroscope
C. Use of the cystoscope sheath as a rigid sheath to guide the flexible ureteroscope to the orifice and prevent coiling of the scope in the bladder
D. Positioning of a guide wire in the ureter to visualize the orifice and ureteral lumen when introducing the ureteroscope
E. Avoiding the temptation to pass the flexible ureteroscope over a guidewire

1048. Concerning the use of ultrasonic lithotripsy through the ureteroscope, it is *not true* that:

A. Thermal urothelial injury is less likely in the distal ureter than in other locations.
B. High-frequency vibrations of a rigid metal transducer provide the energy for stone fragmentation.
C. The tip of the transducer must be in contact with the stone for fragmentation to occur.
D. Thermal injury to the urothelium may be avoided by flowing irrigation past the probe when it is in use.
E. The stone should be fixed in place with a basket to facilitate ultrasonic fragmentation when using the ureteroscope.

1049. The following statement concerning fragmentation of ureteral calculi with electrohydraulic shock wave lithotripsy (EHL) is *false*:

A. With use of EHL on nonimpacted ureteral calculi, a 10–15 per cent ureteral perforation rate is reported.
B. Impacted ureteral calculi should not be fragmented by this technique.
C. The coaxial probe must be in contact with the stone for fragmentation.
D. Normal saline may be used as an irrigant for EHL.
E. EHL is performed under direct visualization unlike ultrasonic lithotripsy which may be carried out with tactile sensation and fluoroscopic visualization.

1050. Which of the following statements concerning laser lithotripsy is *false*?

A. The light-conducting fiber must be in contact with the stone for effective fragmentation.
B. Ideally, the stone is entrapped in a basket and held in position for laser fragmentation.
C. 200 to 300 micron size quartz fiber is used to conduct light through the ureteroscope.
D. Thermal injury to ureteral mucosa is rare.
E. 50 millijoules is the upper limit of energy at which the laser should be set for work in the ureter.

1051. The following statements concerning ureteroscopic biopsy and resection or fulguration are true EXCEPT:

A. Ureteral biopsy should be performed during the initial pass of the ureteroscope to avoid avulsion and loss of the lesion.
B. Glycine should not be used as irrigant in the proximal ureter.
C. Only intraluminal tumor should be resected with the loop, no attempt should be made to take arcing bites into the ureteral wall.
D. Following resection of a luminal lesion, the base is fulgurated lightly with a loop or Bugbee electrode.
E. The neodymium-yttrium-aluminum-garnet laser is valuable for ablation of lower ureteral tumors because it avoids stimulation of the obturator nerve which may occur with use of electrocautery.

1052. Which of the following statements concerning the etiology and incidence of ureteral injuries with ureteroscopy is *false*?

A. EHL has greater potential than ultrasonic or laser lithotripsy for thermal injury to the ureteral mucosa, and is associated with the greatest incidence of ureteral injury.
B. Ureteral perforation occurs in approximately 7 per cent of ureteroscopic cases.
C. The risk of complete ureteral perforation is greater in the proximal ureter than in the distal or intramural ureter.

D. The incidence of ureteral stricture following ureteroscopy is approximately 8 per cent.
E. It is more common to have a false passage develop in the distal ureter (including the intramural region) than in other regions of the ureter.

1053. Which of the following statements concerning the prevention and management of complications due to ureteroscopic procedure is *false*?

A. The most common cause of ureteral avulsion is attempting to extract a calculus too large for the ureter.
B. Fluoroscopy is mandatory and should be used early in the procedure (when a guidewire is first placed in the ureter).
C. Following a documented ureteral perforation, urinary diversion with a nephrostomy tube or ureteral stenting is typically maintained for 1 to 2 weeks.
D. One can usually manage a ureteral perforation or false passage with an internal ureteral stent or ureteral catheter.
E. Distal ureteral avulsion may be repaired using a ureteral reimplant with a psoas hitch or Boari flap.

1054. Which of the following statements concerning the incidence and severity of complications of percutaneous access to the renal collecting system is *false*?

A. Acute bleeding necessitating nephrectomy occurs in 0.19 per cent.
B. Acute bleeding requiring transfusion occurs with an incidence <5 per cent.
C. With an intercostal approach, pleurotomy occurs in 12 per cent.
D. Septicemia occurs with an incidence of 5 per cent.
E. Delayed hemorrhage occurs with an incidence of <0.5 per cent.

1055. All of the following are useful when performing a percutaneous nephrostomy EXCEPT:

A. Resistance to passage of the needle is noted when the renal capsule is encountered but not when the calyx is punctured.
B. The lumbodorsal fascia is incised by passing a 13.5 French shovel-shaped incising needle over the guide wire twice with a 90 degree difference in rotation on the second pass.
C. When the patient is prone, the posterior calyces may be outlined by instilling 10 cc of carbon dioxide through a retrograde ureteral catheter.
D. When using C-arm fluoroscopy, the needle is advanced 5 cm on a straight path into the flank to fix its trajectory; the C-arm may then be rotated to a lateral position to view the tip of the needle.
E. When placing a tube for drainage of pyonephrosis, an infracostal path should be used and the tract dilated minimally (10 French).

1056. All of the following are true regarding the prevention and management of complications of percutaneous nephrostomy EXCEPT:

A. Hemorrhage is best managed by immediate tamponade, which can be effectively done with a Kaye catheter.
B. Delayed bleeding, after nephrostomy tube removal, often requires angiographic embolization.
C. When a retrorenal colon is perforated, it may be managed simply by placing the nephrostomy tube into the colon and diverting the urine with an external retrograde ureteral catheter.
D. Collecting system perforations require only 48-hour urinary drainage with ureteral stent or nephrostomy tube.
E. Urothorax should be managed with an intrapleural Foley catheter and leg bag until the nephropleural fistula resolves.

1057. All of the following statements concerning the etiology of hematuria from the upper urinary tract are true EXCEPT:

A. Forty-two per cent is due to renal or ureteral calculi.
B. Transitional cell carcinoma accounts for 20 per cent.
C. Renal cell carcinoma accounts for 10 per cent.
D. <1 per cent is due to renal arteriovenous fistula.
E. Nineteen per cent is due to renal disease other than malignancy.

1058. In the evaluation of radiolucent upper urinary tract filling defects with CT scan, which statement is *false*?

A. Uric acid stones are > 300 Hounsfield units.
B. Fungal balls are 20–40 Hounsfield units.
C. Transitional cell carcinoma is 30–40 Hounsfield units.
D. A sloughed papilla is 20–40 Hounsfield units.
E. Blood clots are 60–90 Hounsfield units.

1059. In the evaluation of radiolucent upper urinary tract filling defects, pertinent medical history might reveal any of the following EXCEPT:

A. Analgesic abuse
B. Gouty arthritis
C. Sarcoidosis
D. Immunosuppression
E. Diabetes mellitus

1060. All of the following statements regarding the ureteroscopic evaluation of essential hematuria which has not been diagnosed by radiographic or urine studies are ture EXCEPT:

A. Bleeding is localized to a lower pole site in 50 per cent of cases and to an upper pole site in 20 per cent of cases.
B. The most common finding is a small vascular abnormality—hemangioma or arteriovenous malformation.
C. It is extremely rare that the bleeding site is localized to the ureter.
D. Vascular abnormalities giving rise to hematuria are most commonly seen directly on a papilla.
E. Bleeding due to a renal artery aneurysm has not been observed in multiple series.

1061. All of the following statements are true regarding ureteroscopic evaluation of a collecting system filling defect EXCEPT:

A. When no lesion is seen, radiographic findings may be due to a crossing vessel.

B. A sloughed papilla appears as a freely floating object with a dull gray appearance.
C. Fungal balls have a black gelatinous appearance and are free floating.
D. Papillary transitional cell tumors appear similar to those seen in the bladder.
E. A fibroepithelial polyp appears as a smooth-walled pedunculated lesion.

1062. In the diagnosis and management of a uriniferous pseudocyst or urinoma, all of the following are true EXCEPT:

A. It is important to distinguish between pancreatic pseudocyst and urinoma prior to therapy, and this can be done by analysis of aspirate.
B. CT attenuation is usually 10–20 Hounsfield units for a urinoma which has not taken up contrast.
C. When no communication is seen between collecting system and urinoma, percutaneous drainage of the urinoma usually ceases within 72 hours.
D. Commonly a fistula persists despite percutaneous drainage, in which case ureteroscopy or antegrade nephroscopy and fulguration of the tract leading to the urinoma is successful.
E. In the largest series reported of treated urinomas, nephrectomy was required in 50 per cent.

1063. Which one of the following statements concerning the diagnosis and management of perinephric abscess is *false*?

A. If after percutaneous drain placement, drainage persists for more than 7 days, a urinary fistula should be suspected.
B. If a large cavity remains after adequate percutaneous drainage of a perinephric abscess, it may be sclerosed with 95 per cent ethanol or 50 mg/ml of tetracycline.
C. Ureteroscopic incision and drainage of the abscess into the nonobstructed collecting system has a similar success to that of percutaneous procedures.
D. The mortality rate for percutaneous management of perinephric abscess is 8 per cent.
E. Unfavorable factors for percutaneous management of a perinephric abscess include multiloculated abscess, infected hematoma, abscess material with a high viscosity, calcifications, and air-fluid levels on CT scan indicative of an enteric-retroperitoneal fistula.

1064. Which one of the following statements concerning the management of renal cysts is *false*?

A. The endoscopic approach (either ureteroscopic or percutaneous nephroscopic) to renal cyst management has a 20 per cent higher success rate than sclerotherapy.
B. For standard sclerotherapy, ethanol is injected to fill 25 per cent of the cyst volume and is left in place for 10–20 minutes before withdrawing.
C. Absolute contraindications to percutaneous sclerotherapy include a parapelvic cyst or communicating pyelovenous cyst.
D. With the direct approach, a transcystic nephrostomy tract is established, a nephroscope placed into the cyst, and the wall between cyst and pelvis excised marsupializing the cyst into the renal pelvis.
E. Simple cyst drainage cures 4 to 19 per cent of renal cysts.

1065. In the management of calyceal diverticula, all of the following statements are true EXCEPT:

A. The antegrade percutaneous approach has the best results of endosurgical methods.
B. With percutaneous approaches, the first step is to pass a retrograde ureteral catheter and occlusion balloon into the renal pelvis.
C. The indirect percutaneous approach is difficult because a nondilated collecting system must be accessed and the communication between diverticulum and collecting system may be difficult to locate.
D. The use of ureteroscopic dilation of the neck of the diverticulum and stone extraction combined with ESWL for diverticular stones has a reported stone free rate of 73 per cent.
E. After fulguration of the neck of the diverticulum, sclerosing agents such as ethanol or bismuth phosphate may be injected into the diverticulum.

1066. Which one of the following statements concerning the diagnosis of upper urinary tract obstruction is *false*?

A. Renal artery disease may give rise to false negatives with the diuretic washout renal scan.
B. With the Whitaker test, a renal pelvis/bladder pressure differential above 22 cm of water is considered positive for obstruction.
C. In the diuretic washout renogram, 50 per cent of the radionuclide tracer should drain from the kidney within 10 minutes following the administration of intravenous furosemide in a patient with two nonobstructed kidneys.
D. False negatives may result with the Whitaker test when extravasation occurs or when the renal pelvis is not completely filled prior to obtaining pressures.
E. A normal diuretic washout renal scan is a reliable indicator of a nonobstructed system.

1067. All of the following techniques are employed when performing an antegrade endopyelotomy EXCEPT:

A. A 0.035-inch guidewire is first passed into the renal pelvis in retrograde fashion.
B. Percutaneous access should be to an upper or middle posterior calyx.
C. The incision should be full thickness (exposing retroperitoneal fat), and adequacy of the incision is verified by rapid extravasation of contrast through the incised region.
D. The incision is made along the anteromedial border of the ureteropelvic junction (UPJ) and extended caudally to a point 1 cm past the obstruction.
E. A 6-mm balloon is inflated along the course of UPJ obstruction and the incision performed alongside the inflated balloon.

1068. Which one of the following statements concerning the results of endourologic surgery for UPJ obstruction is *false*?

A. With antegrade endopyelotomy, durable success rates of 72 to 87 per cent are reported in most series.

B. Poorly functioning renal units have success rates similar to renal units with good function at the time of endopyelotomy.
C. The majority of failures occur within 3 months.
D. Adult patients with chronic massive hydronephrosis who undergo endopyelotomy have a high failure rate.
E. Retrograde endopyelotomy has success rates similar to the antegrade endopyelotomy; however, it is technically more difficult and has the additional delayed complication of distal ureteral stricture.

1069. When performing endoureterotomy, all of the following points are valid EXCEPT:

A. For the endosurgical management of a complete obstruction in the distal ureter, a nephrostomy tract is not necessary.
B. Endosurgical approaches can be attempted for complete ureteral obstruction if the occlusion is <1 cm in length.
C. When incising the ureter below the iliac vessel crossing, a direct medial incision is made.
D. The goal in treating distal ureteral strictures is marsupialization of the stricture into the bladder, which can be done with a retrograde approach and a cold-knife urethrotome, or by inflating a balloon in the distal ureter and incising from the bladder onto the balloon.
E. The endosurgical technique for proximal ureteral strictures is similar to that of the antegrade endopyelotomy.

1070. Which one of the following statements concerning the results of endosurgical management of ureteral strictures is *false*?

A. Lasting overall success rates are similar for endoincision and balloon dilation, and are in the range of 50 to 60 per cent.
B. Strictures due to ischemic problems do not respond as well as those due to nonischemic factors; 40 per cent versus 58 per cent, respectively.
C. The success rate of endoureterotomy for strictures >1 cm is as low as 11 to 18 per cent.
D. Proximal and distal ureteral strictures which may be marsupialized to the bladder or renal pelvis have a much higher success rate than mid-ureteral strictures; 80 per cent versus 25 per cent respectively.
E. The duration of stricture prior to endosurgery impacts outcome; strictures >18 months having a significantly lower success than those <12 months.

1071. Which of the following statements concerning endosurgical management of upper tract transitional cell carcinoma (TCC) is *false*?

A. In patients with TCC of the renal pelvis, the 2-year recurrence and open surgical rate following endosurgical treatment is 30 per cent.
B. Reports of nephrostomy tract seeding or retroperitoneal recurrence of TCC following endosurgical resection are rare, unlike the 11 per cent retroperitoneal seeding reported following surgical pyelotomy.
C. Ureteral tumors respond less well to endosurgical management than renal pelvic tumors, having a 2-year recurrence rate of 40 per cent and a progression of 30 per cent.
D. Understaging of TCC of the renal pelvis may be as high as 60 per cent with endoscopic techniques.
E. The results of endosurgical management for upper tract TCC are remarkably similar to results of open conservative therapy.

1072. The following techniques are applicable to endosurgical management of upper tract TCC EXCEPT:

A. An antegrade percutaneous approach is preferred for resection of tumors >1 cm in the kidney or renal pelvis.
B. In the upper tract, random urothelial biopsies near the tumor site following tumor ablation or resection are *not* recommended as these traumatized areas provide excellent sites for tumor seeding.
C. With ureteroscopic resection, irrigant pressure should be less than 40 cm water to prevent vascular entry of tumor cells with renal backflow.
D. With flexible ureteroscopy, tumors may be ablated with a 400 μm Nd:YAG laser set at 25 to 30 watts.
E. Tumors located in the ureter above the iliac vessels may be resected with the rigid ureteroscope and electrocautery loop in females; however, this is not recommended in males.

1073. Which of the following statements with regard to techniques of laparoscopic urologic surgery is *false*?

A. Pressure within the abdomen is maintained in the range of 10 to 15 mm Hg.
B. To introduce the pneumoperitoneum, the Veress needle is passed into the peritoneal space through an infraumbilical midline approach.
C. During laparoscopic nephrectomy, after detachment of the kidney, it is removed through a small flank incision.
D. In the laparoscopic drainage of lymphoceles, the lymphocele is marsupialized to the intraperitoneal space by excision of overlying peritoneum.
E. In the laparoscopic varicocelectomy, the spermatic veins are divided just proximal to joining the vas and entering the internal inguinal ring.

PART XIII

URINARY LITHIASIS

CHAPTERS 58 THROUGH 62

ANSWERS

984-D *(Campbell's, pp. 2086–2134)*

Since the beginning of the 19th century, coinciding with industrial development, stones of patients in Western countries have occurred predominantly in the upper urinary tract. Pre-industrialized countries still have a high incidence of bladder calculi, often in children and often formed of ammonium acid urate. Dietary changes in industrialized countries are thought to explain the differences in clinical patterns of stone disease.

985-C *(Campbell's, pp. 2087–2088)*

Blacks appear to have a hereditary protection against stone disease, possibly because of the forces of natural selection in the hot climate of Africa.

986-D *(Campbell's, p. 2089)*

The "stone belt" in the United States, where the incidence of stone disease is highest, is the Southeast. Reasons for this remain unclear.

987-D *(Campbell's, p. 2094)*

Spontaneous nucleation of crystals occurs at concentrations above the formation product. The metastable zone refers to concentrations of crystallizable substances between the solubility product and the formation product. Spontaneous nucleation does not occur in the metastable zone, even though the solution is supersaturated.

988-E *(Campbell's, p. 2096)*

Epitaxy may be clinically important in the case of uric acid and calcium oxalate. The presence of uric acid crystals may promote formation of calcium oxalate stones. Since calcium oxalate and uric acid have similar crystal lattices, the presence of uric acid crystals may promote the formation of calcium oxalate stones. In contrast, cystine crystals rarely deposit on the surface of previously formed uric acid or calcium oxalate crystals, since the mismatch in surface lattices is too great.

989-B *(Campbell's, pp. 2096–2097)*

The smallest diameter calculus that can cause ureteral obstruction is 2 mm.

This is based on the clinical observation that the majority of urinary calculi causing symptoms are greater than 2 mm in diameter.

990-A *(Campbell's, pp. 2098–2099)*

Substance A is a mucoprotein found in urine that has been suggested to be a promoter of stone formation. Citrate, magnesium, pyrophosphate, and zinc have all been suggested to be inhibitors. The existence of stone promoters and inhibitors has been postulated because of the observation that stone formation seems to depend on factors other than the saturation levels of crystallizable substances.

991-D *(Campbell's, p. 2092)*

"Moving irritation" is typical of renal colic; that is, patients are not able to obtain relief in any position. This is in contrast to conditions causing intraperitoneal inflammation, such as appendicitis, where certain positions may sometimes result in pain relief.

992-A *(Campbell's, p. 2103)*

Ten per cent of patients with urinary lithiasis may not have gross or microscopic hematuria, particularly when the calculus has created complete obstruction. Moderate pyuria may occur with uninfected urinary lithiasis. On occasion, urine crystals of the same type that are creating the calculus will be observed in the urine.

993-D *(Campbell's, pp. 2103–2104, 2111)*

Of the common urinary calculi, only uric acid stones, which make up approximately 10 per cent of the total, are not sufficiently radiodense to be visualized on a plain film.

994-D *(Campbell's, pp. 2103–2104, 2134–2135)*

Cystine stones, contrary to relatively common misconception, are not radiolucent, but have a radiodensity that often results in a ground glass appearance. Cystine stones are approximately 0.45 times as radiopaque as calcium oxalate calculi. With the exception of uric acid, all of the other radiolucent stones are very rare.

995-B *(Campbell's, p. 2109)*

Complete ureteral obstruction, without infection, will cause at least some irreversible loss of renal function by 2 weeks, although obstruction lasting 6 weeks or longer is necessary to completely destroy renal function.

996-A *(Campbell's, pp. 2111–2112)*

Calcium oxalate is the most common type of urinary calculus in the developed world, although many stones are mixed with smaller amounts of calcium phosphate.

997-C *(Campbell's, p. 2112)*

Hyperparathyroidism is associated with calcium phosphate stone disease, possibly because the tendency toward urine alkalinity in this metabolic disease causes increased deposition of phosphate during stone formation. Calcium phosphate stones also predominate in patients with renal tubular acidosis and medullary sponge kidney.

998-C *(Campbell's, p. 2113)*

Destruction of renal parenchyma by calculus disease and infection can lead to xanthogranulomatous pyelonephritis. *Proteus mirabilis* is the organism most often associated with this process.

999-C *(Campbell's, p. 2114)*

The pKa of uric acid is 5.75; at this pH, 50 per cent of uric acid is in the form of relatively insoluble uric acid and 50 per cent as the more soluble urate salt. With increasing acidity (i.e., pH's below 5.75), even more uric acid is in the insoluble form and stones are more likely to form.

1000-A *(Campbell's, p. 2116)*

The chronic diarrhea associated with ileostomies leads to bicarbonate loss, systemic acidosis and acidic urine, which increases the risk of uric acid stone disease.

1001-E *(Campbell's, p. 2118)*

Allergic or idiosyncratic reactions including arthralgia, rash, and nephrotic syndrome are the most important complication of D-penicillamine. This drug acts to increase solubility of cystine in urine.

1002-A *(Campbell's, pp. 2118, 2120)*

E. coli apparently does not produce urease. Bacterial production of urease, and the resultant enzymatic breakdown of urea to CO_2 and NH_3 leading to alkaline urine, is the basis pathophysiologic explanation of struvite stone disease.

1003-E *(Campbell's, pp. 2125–2126)*

Parathormone promotes renal production of 1–25-dihydroxycholecalciferol, the active form of vitamin D, as well as increasing calcium and decreasing phosphorus absorption.

1004-C *(Campbell's, p. 2130)*

Regional ileitis and ileal bypass surgery for obesity have been associated with increased intestinal absorption of oxalate leading to increased renal oxalate excretion and stone disease.

1005-E *(Campbell's, p. 2133)*

Thiazide diuretics decrease urinary calcium excretion. Because this effect can be negated by dietary salt intake and increased vascular volume, patients should restrict dietary salt.

1006-D *(Campbell's, p. 2135)*

The potassium-sparing diuretic triamterene can (rarely) precipitate in urine leading either to pure triamterene or mixed calcium and triamterene stones. This drug should be used with caution in patients with a history of stone disease.

1007-E *(Campbell's, p. 2140)*

Obstruction due to prostate enlargement, bladder neck contracture, or urethral stricture is the most important factor in formation of bladder stones. Bladder stones are much less common in women than in men.

1008-A *(Campbell's, p. 2140)*

Although struvite stones make up a larger percentage of bladder stones than they do of renal stones, calcium oxalate is the most common type of bladder stone.

1009-B *(Campbell's, pp. 2142–2143)*

Most prostatic stones are of calcium phosphate; calcium carbonate may be found as a secondary constituent. These stones are relatively common in men over age 50, and are observed during transurethral resection of the prostate in the plane between the adenoma and the surgical capsule. Specific treatment is usually not necessary.

1010-D *(Campbell's, pp. 2159–2160)*

When the shock wave strikes the stone surface nearest the source, the wave is split into a proceeding compressive wave and a reflected tensile wave giving rise to a high pressure gradient at the stone surface. This gives rise to a tensile force at the surface which overcomes forces holding the stone intact and leads to disintegration at the surface nearest the source. A similar phenomenon occurs at the distal surface when the proceeding compressive wave is again split into opposing components and a high pressure gradient develops at the distal surface. The mechanism is depicted in Fig. 59–5 of *Campbell's Urology.*

1011-E *(Campbell's, pp. 2158–2159)*

A spark plug which discharges in a liquid medium is used to generate shock waves by the spark gap generator. These waves are then reflected by a hemiellipsoid shell toward the object to be fragmented. The discharge of the spark plug must occur during the refractory period of the heart or arrhythmias may develop. In the piezoelectric lithotriptors, the shock wave is generated by ceramic elements which are excited by high frequency, high voltage pulses. This manner of generation of a shock wave does not lead to development of cardiac arrhythmias. In the electromagnetic generator, a shock wave is generated by rapid magnetic repulsion of the plate within a shock tube. These waves are then focused with an acoustic lens. In the microexplosive lithotripter, the shock waves are generated by microexplosive charges. The SZ–1 microexplosive lithotriptor by Yachiyoda Company is one such machine, which uses lead azide pellets for the explosive charge and focuses the shock waves with an ellipsoid. An acoustic lens is not used with the microexplosive lithotriptor.

1012-D *(Campbell's, p. 2161)*

The Munich team initially had performed studies of lithotriptor shock waves on tissue and cell culture. It is true that shocking whole blood at the F2 focal zone leads to an increase in free plasma hemoglobin which appears to be linearly related to the number of shocks delivered. Proximal and distal tubular cells from tissue culture do show decreased viability due to shock waves and this appears to be influenced by the number of shock waves rather than the energy per shock wave. Randazzo and colleagues treated an in vitro model of renal cell carcinoma with shock waves and found decreased viability, cell growth, and cell attachment. Other studies of tissue subjected to shock waves show that cavitation effects appear to be the cause of tissue injury. These effects are increased when the frequency or rate of delivery of shock waves increases. Finally, studies have been performed on bacterial viability and no effects have been seen by bacterial cultures subjected to shock wave lithotripsy.

REFERENCES

1. Chaussy, C.G., Schmeidt, E., Jocham, D., et al.: *In* Chaussy, C. (Ed.): Extracorporeal Shock Wave Lithotripsy. Munich, Karger Verlag, 1982.
2. Fischer, N., Muller, H.M., Gulham, A., et al.: Cavitation effects: possible cause of tissue injury during extracorporeal shock wave lithotripsy. J. Endourol., *2*: 215, 1988.
3. Delius, M.: This month in investigative urology: effect of extracorporeal shock waves on the kidney. J. Urol., *140*:390, 1988.
4. Randazzo, R.F., Chaussy, C.G., Fuchs, G.J., et al.: The in vitro and in vivo effects of extracorporeal shock waves on malignant cells. Urol Res., *16*(6):419, 1988.
5. Elbers, J., Seline, P., and Clayman, R.V.: The effects of shock wave lithotripsy on urease-positive calculogenic bacteria. *In* Lingeman, J.E. and Newman, D.M. (Eds.): Shock Wave Lithotripsy. New York, Plenum Press, 1988, p. 391.
6. McAteer, J.A., Evans, A.P., Hoak, R., et al.: Cell culture and in vitro systems to assess the bioeffects of ESWL. J. Urol., *141*:228A, 1989.
7. Clayman, R.V., Preminger, G.M., Long, S., et al.: A comparison of in vitro cellular effects of shock waves generated by electrohydraulic, electromagnetic, and piezoelectric sources. J. Urol., *141*:228A, 1989b.

1013-E *(Campbell's, pp. 2161–2163)*

It is true that a single shock wave to the thorax causes massive hemoptysis in rats. It is also true that epiphyseal growth plate abnormalities in immature rats are noted following ESWL and that 17 per cent of treated rats experienced shortened extremities. Complete devastation of chick embryos is documented after ESWL. No apparent injury is noted in the spinal cord or in myocardium in animal studies following ESWL. After treatment of rat ovaries, no adverse effects were found on the fetal morphology, numbers, or weight, or within the ovaries.

REFERENCES

1. Chaussy, C., Schmeidt, E., Jocham, D., et al.: *In* Chaussy, C. (Ed.): Extracorporeal Shock Wave Lithotripsy. Munich, Karger Verlag, 1982.
2. McCullough, D.L., Yeaman, L.D., Bo, W., et al.: Effects of shock waves on the rat ovary. J. Urol., *141*: 666, 1989.
3. Yeaman, L.D., Jerone, C.P., and McCullough, D.L.: Effect of shock waves on structure and growth of the immature rat epiphysis. J. Urol., *141*:670, 1989.
4. Moran, M.E., Sandock, D., and Drach, G.W.: Effects of high energy shock waves on chick embryo development. J. Urol., *143*:167A, 1990.

1014-C *(Campbell's, p. 2161)*

In the immediate postlithotripsy period, transient elevations of creatine phosphokinase, *N*-Acetyl-beta-glucosaminidase, beta-galactosidase, gamma-glutamyltranspeptidase, and lactic dehydrogenase are seen. No elevation in alanine aminotransferase is reported.

REFERENCES

1. Assimos, D.G., Boyce, W.H., Furr, E., et al.: Selective elevation of urinary enzyme levels after extracorporeal shock wave lithotripsy. J. Urol., *142*:687, 1989.
2. Karlin, G.S., Urivetsky, M., and Smith, A.S.: Side effects of extracorporeal shock wave lithotripsy: Assessment of urinary excretion of renal enzymes as evidence of tubular injury. *In* Lingeman, J.E., and Newman, D.M. (Eds.): Shock Wave Lithotripsy 2. New York, Plenum Press, 1989.
3. Kishimoto, T., Yamamato, K., Suginoto, T., et al.: Selective elevation of urinary enzyme levels after extracorporeal shock wave lithotripsy for upper urinary tract stones. Eur. Urol., *12*:308, 1986.

1015-C *(Campbell's, p. 2162)*

Gross hematuria universally occurs after ESWL and is thought to be due to parenchymal injury. The Dornier HM-3 machine is a higher energy machine and most kidneys treated with this do exhibit swelling in the immediate post-operative period. Of kidneys treated with ESWL, approximately 15 to 30 per cent show subcapsular bleeding, perinephric fluid collections or subcapsular hematomas. Pathologic studies of renal tissue following ESWL show fibrosis occurring up to approximately 1 per cent renal volume along the path of the shock wave. Other changes include focal calcification, loss of nephrons, dilated veins and acellular and hyalinized scars. Studies do show capillary and small vein damage, intraparenchymal hemorrhage, and tubular injury in kidneys immediately following ESWL.

REFERENCES

1. Jaegar, P., Redha, F., Uhlschmid, G., et al.: Morphologic changes in canine kidneys following extracorporeal shock wave treatment. J. Endourol., *2*:205, 1988.
2. Dyer, R.B., Karstaedt, N., McCullough, D.L., et al.: Magnetic resonance imaging evaluation of immediate and intermediate changes in kidneys treated with extracorporeal shock wave lithotripsy. J. Lithotripsy Stone Dis., *2*:302, 1990.

3. Rubin, J.I., Arger, P.H., Pollack, H.M., et al.: Kidney changes after extracorporeal shock wave lithotripsy: CT evaluation. Radiology, *162*:21, 1987.

1016-E *(Campbell's, p. 2163)*

The HM-3 Dornier lithotriptor is the most widely used lithotriptor in the world and does use two fluoroscopes mounted as noted in answer A for visualization of calculi. Low ureteral stones may be localized by ultrasound and treated. Adequate localization of a stone by ultrasound units usually requires the fragment be at least 2 to 3 mm in size. When treating uric acid calculi or lightly calcified struvite stones which may be radiolucent, the stone should be localized by instilling contrast into the collecting system or ureter when using fluoroscopy to visualize the stone. Additionally, a ureteral catheter may be placed and used for guidance if one knows in what position the stone lies along the ureteral catheter. There is no CT guided lithotriptor.

1017-D *(Campbell's, p. 2164)*

The maximum pressure gradient for disintegration of stones is achieved at the focal point F2. As one moves away from the focal point, the pressures rapidly decline and at 2 cm from F2, they are only approximately 20 per cent of the pressure at F2 and fragmentation efficacy rapidly diminishes. There is a course which is referred to as the "blast path" which does extend from the focal point at a 25 degree angle to the cross hairs on the HM-3 machine. When a stone lies outside of the focal point but is along this "blast path," it may be fragmented even up to 10 cm away from F2. Successful fragmentation has not been reported beyond this point. With the HM-3 machine, 13 cm is the distance F2 is from the ellipsoid and, therefore, if body habitus places the stone at a position greater than this, the stone will not lie within the focal zone and successful fragmentation is less likely. It is true that as one increases the energy of the shockwave, he increases the pressure gradient that develops at F2 leading to faster fragmentation; with this, larger size fragments develop.

REFERENCES

1. Hunter, P.T., Finlayson, B., and Hirkso, R.I.: Measurement of shock wave pressures used for lithotripsy. J Urol., *136*:733, 1986.

1018-E *(Campbell's, pp. 2164, 2169)*

A urine culture should be obtained prior to ESWL for any patient who may have infected urine, and this includes those patients with struvite stones. This allows the guidance of antibiotic therapy and aids in the prevention of sepsis postoperatively. Patients with collecting systems that may be colonized such as those with nephrostomy tubes, indwelling stents and catheters or patients with struvite stones should have appropriate preoperative antibiotic therapy. The author of Chapter 59 also makes the point that most urologists prefer the placement of a double J ureteral stent when treating a stone that is greater than 1 cm in size to possibly enhance passage of fragments and maintain a nonobstructed system. Transient renal failure has been reported following ESWL and may be more likely with bilateral ESWL. Therefore, it is recommended that if bilateral treatment of calculi is planned at the same setting, one or both renal units should be stented.

1019-B *(Campbell's, p. 2164)*

Pregnancy and uncontrolled coagulation parameters are absolute contraindications to ESWL. Obstruction distal to the stone which would prevent passage of fragments is a contraindication. Care should be taken to avoid having renal artery calcifications or aortic aneurysms in the "blast path" or at the focal point and are a relative contraindication. Patients with aneurysms have been treated successfully; however, one should be concerned about the possibility of rupture. Initially, childhood was felt to be a contraindication; however, children have been successfully treated with ESWL. Care should be taken to shield the lungs with styrofoam padding prior to their treatment.

1020-B *(Campbell's, p. 2165)*

Uric acid calculi and calcium oxalate dihydrate calculi fragment readily. Calcium phosphate dihydrate (also known as brushite) is difficult to fragment and tends to fragment into large pieces when treated with ESWL. The stone-free rate for brushite stones is 53 per cent when ESWL is used as the sole therapy. Calcium oxalate monohydrate stones are harder to fragment than their dihydrate counterparts and have a somewhat lower stone-free rate (74 per cent). Cystine stones are probably the hardest to fragment using ESWL and many urologists will consider percutaneous procedure for a cystine stone of 2 cm or larger. The highest stone-free rates according to Newman and colleagues as listed in Chapter 59 occur with uric acid stones (85 per cent for ESWL monotherapy). Struvite stones also readily break up; however, they have a lower stone-free rate due to reoccurrence because of their infectious nature.

1021-E *(Campbell's, pp. 2165–2166)*

With ESWL, stone-free success appears to be highly related to stone size. Stones less than or equal to 1 cm are ideal and often a 90 per cent stone-free rate is reported. For stones up to 1.2 cm, stone-free rate is noted to be 87 per cent with ESWL alone. When very large stones such as staghorn calculi are treated with ESWL monotherapy, stone-free rates may be as low as 30 per cent, and most studies report about a 50 per cent stone-free rate with multiple ESWL procedures. When anatrophic nephrolithotomy is used for the management of staghorn calculi, the success rate is 94 per cent. There does appear to be a cutoff for stones that are approximately 3 cm or larger where most urologists would prefer percutaneous lithotripsy or other therapy for treatment rather than ESWL as the sole treatment. When ESWL is combined with percutaneous lithotripsy to manage staghorn calculi, stone-free rates of 77 to 88 per cent are noted. Percutaneous lithotripsy alone as the sole therapy for staghorn stones has a similar success rate of up to 86 per cent.

REFERENCES

1. Riehle, R.A., and Naslund, E.B.: Patient management and results after ESWL. *In* Riehle, R.A., and Newman, D.M. (Eds.): Principles of Extracorporeal Shock Wave Lithotripsy. New York, Churchill Livingstone, 1987, p. 121.

2. Boyce, W.H., and Elkins, I.B.: Reconstructive renal surgery following anatrophic nephrolithotomy: followup of 100 consecutive cases. J. Urol, *111*:307, 1974.
3. Winfield, H.N., Clayman, R.V., Chaussy, C.G., et al.: Monotherapy of staghorn renal calculi: a comparative study between percutaneous nephrolithotomy and extracorporeal shock wave lithotripsy. J. Urol., *139*:895, 1988.
4. Eisenberger, F., Fuchs, G., Miller, K., et al.: Extracorporeal shock wave lithotripsy (ESWL) and endourology—an ideal combination for the treatment of kidney stones. World J. Urol., *3*:41, 1985.
5. Thomas, R., Figuera, T.W., and Macaluso, J.: Advances in management of staghorn renal calculi. *In* Lingeman, J.E. and Newman, D.M. (Eds.): Shock Wave Lithotripsy. New York, Plenum Press, 1988, p. 71.

1022-C *(Campbell's, pp. 2166–2167)*

When the HM-3 lithotriptor is used to treat upper ureteral stones, success rates of 60 to 85 per cent were initially reported. Higher stone-free rates are achieved when the stone is pushed from the ureter up into the kidney and then treated with ESWL and this is known as the "push up and smash" technique. In general, lithotriptor operators have used more shock waves and higher kilovoltage when treating ureteral stones in situ in comparison to treatment of the same size stone within the kidney. When treating a stone which overlies the pelvic bones, the patient must be positioned in the prone position to prevent the shock waves from being shielded by the pelvis. Finally, debate does exist concerning the best way to treat lower ureteral stones. Ureteroscopic techniques are reported to be 95 per cent successful and are less expensive; however, they are more invasive and have a higher complication rate.

REFERENCE

1. Blute, M.L., Segura, J.W., and Patterson, D.E.: Ureteroscopy. J. Urol., *139*:510, 1988.

1023-E *(Campbell's, p. 2168)*

Factors which lead to a persistence of residual fragments following ESWL decrease the likelihood of a stone-free status. Patients with an increased stone burden such as those with multiple stones, stones greater than 2 cm, or staghorn stones have a longer duration of persistence of fragments and have less chance of a stone-free status. Patients who have factors which lead to reduced clearance of fragments exhibit a lower stone-free rate. Reduced clearance of fragments may occur when stone is present in lower pole calyces, stone is present in a calyceal diverticulum, long-standing marked hydronephrosis occurs, or stone is present in a horseshoe kidney. Stone composition is also a factor in achieving a stone-free rate. Stones which are harder to fragment and have larger fragments which do not easily pass (such as brushite or cystine) have lower stone-free rates with ESWL. The presence or absence of a ureteral stent does not necessarily affect the stone-free rate, but may be a factor with larger stones.

1024-C *(Campbell's, pp. 2168–2169)*

Multiple studies do show swelling of the kidney as well as perinephric fluid collections and intranephric fluid collections immediately following ESWL, and this is seen with both magnetic resonance imaging and with radiographic studies. These acute changes appear to resolve in three months. However, when renal plasma flow is evaluated with nuclear studies, an immediate decrease in renal plasma flow is noted in 30 per cent of kidneys after ESWL. A decrease in effective renal plasma flow was noted to persist as long as 17 to 21 months following ESWL. One long-term study by Chaussy notes no adverse effects on renal scan at four years after ESWL. The development of hypertension as a result of ESWL has not been proven. In one study, the incidence of hypertension increased from 2 to 3.5 per cent to approximately 8 per cent after ESWL; other studies do not show this. It is apparent at this time that the majority of patients who have been treated with ESWL have little long-term morbidity.

REFERENCES

1. Baumgartner, B.R., Dickey, K.W., Ambrose, S.S., et al.: Kidney changes after extracorporeal shock wave lithotripsy: appearance on MR imaging. Radiology, *163*: 531, 1987.
2. Kaude, J.V., Williams, C.M., Millner, M.R., et al.: Renal morphology and function immediately after extracorporeal shock wave lithotripsy. AJR, *145*:305, 1985.
3. Williams, C.M., Kaude, J.V., Newman, R.L., et al.: ESWL: long-term complications. AJR, *150*:311, 1988.
4. Lingeman, J.E., Woods, J., and Toth, P.D.: Blood pressure changes following extracorporeal shock wave lithotripsy and other forms of treatment for nephrolithiasis. JAMA, *263*:1789, 1990.

1025-A *(Campbell's, pp. 2169)*

Steinstrasse refers to a condition where a series of stone fragments line up in the ureter, forming a column of stone. Often a large fragment at the bottom of this column is responsible for the jam or obstruction. This is a rare complication following ESWL, occurring in less than 5 per cent of cases and probably occurs in as low as 1 per cent of cases of ESWL. When steinstrasse does occur, intervention is indicated when there is total obstruction of the ureter, intractable pain, obstruction of a solitary kidney, evidence of renal failure, or when urosepsis develops. An additional indication may be the failure of fragments to pass over a reasonable period of time. Intervention appears to be necessary in approximately 35 per cent of cases with steinstrasse. About 75 per cent of cases with steinstrasse develop in the distal ureter while 18 per cent develop in the proximal ureter. When the lead fragment which may be responsible for the obstruction is in the upper ureter, it may successfully be fragmented with an additional ESWL treatment. Other methods of treatment include ureteroscopic extraction of stones as well as percutaneous drainage and management. Simple ureteral stenting may also be sufficient. The fact that a 3-cm length of ureter is full of fragments is not necessarily an indication for intervention when steinstrasse occurs.

REFERENCE

1. Fedullo, L.M., Pollack, H.M., Banner, M.P., et al.: The development of steinstrasse after ESWL: frequency, natural history, and radiologic management. AJR. *151*: 1145, 1988.

1026-D *(Campbell's, pp. 2169–2170)*

Severe pulmonary injury and hemoptysis are potential complications in infants and children who undergo ESWL, in particular myelodysplastic patients. This occurs when shock waves are directed at the lungs. Shielding of the chest and lungs can be successfully done with a thin piece of styrofoam. Patients who suffered pulmonary damage recovered uneventfully in one study. Cases are noted of iliac artery and vein thrombosis following ESWL of ureteral stones in the lower ureter. No reports exist of rupture of aortic or renal artery aneurysms following ESWL, although this has been an area of concern. Pancreatitis is rarely reported. The mortality of ESWL is 0.02 per cent and deaths were primarily due to pulmonary emboli, myocardial infarction and cerebrovascular accident. One death has been reported due to retroperitoneal hemorrhage and one to mesenteric thrombosis after ESWL. Additional data on complications can be found in Table 59–1 on page 2170 of *Campbell's Urology* from the American Urologic Association Lithotripsy Committee.

REFERENCES

1. Kroovand, R.L.: Extracorporeal shock wave lithotripsy in the pediatric stone patient: Problems and results. Probl. Urol., *1*(4):682, 1987.
2. Desmet, W., Baert, L., Vandeursen, H., et al.: Iliac vein thrombosis after extracorporeal shock wave lithotripsy (letter to editor). N. Engl. J. Med., *321*:907, 1989.
3. Keeler, L., McNamara, T.C., Dorey, F.O., et al.: Extracorporeal shock wave lithotripsy for lower ureteral calculi: Treatment of choice. J. Endourol., *4*:71, 1990.

1027-A *(Campbell's, pp. 2171–2172)*

Pain is generally increased when the energy of the shock waves is increased. Therefore, reducing the power of the shock wave generator will lead to a decrease in anesthesia requirement in general. Another factor which affects pain is the area of the skin through which the shock wave penetrates. A wide shock wave skin entry radius generally reduces the pain felt in this region. This can be achieved with a widened dish or ellipsoid aperture. Lastly, a smaller focal zone is also associated with lower pain.

1028-D *(Campbell's pp. 2171–2173)*

The "effectiveness quotient" was introduced by Clayman and colleagues and is used to compare the effectiveness of different lithotriptors. The "effectiveness quotient" is calculated according to the equation that is given in answer A. This quantity attempts to relate the stone-free rate to the incidence of additional therapy including both repeat ESWL and auxiliary procedures. The HM-3 machine which has been found to be superior to others for the treatment of stones smaller than 2 cm has an effectiveness quotient according to this formula of 63 per cent. In general, machines which are touted as being anesthesia free use less power and ultimately require a higher retreatment rate. This has been stated to be as high as 30 per cent retreatment. Of the lithotriptors on the market, the author of Chapter 59 feels the piezoelectric lithotriptor by Wolf is truly an anesthesia free machine in comparison with all other lithotriptors. The use of lithotriptors to treat cholelithiasis has been under investigation and the Dornier MPL 9000 is a machine that has been used in these studies.

1029-C *(Campbell's, pp. 2183–2185)*

Calculi in the collecting system coexisting with a UPJ obstruction are most appropriately managed by the percutaneous approach, which would allow removal of the calculi as well as endopyelotomy to relieve the UPJ obstruction in a single procedure. Likewise, calculi contained in caliceal diverticula are appropriately managed with PL. When such calculi are managed with extracorporeal shockwave lithotripsy (ESWL), fragments frequently remain in the diverticula. Often the diverticular opening does not allow easy passage of the fragments. The stone-free rate with ESWL of calculi contained in caliceal diverticula may be as low as 20 per cent. Scar tissue present along the course of the ureter may restrict passage of stone fragments. A ureteroneocystostomy or ureteroileal anastamosis are two such cases where a narrow scarred segment of ureter may exist. When large calculi exist in these patients, percutaneous lithotripsy may be the treatment of choice to avoid the passage of fragments down the scarred ureter. Body habitus such as obesity or severe scoliosis may prevent the use of extracorporal shockwave lithotripsy, and in these patients percutaneous lithotripsy may be indicated. Answer C is incorrect and the condition of pregnancy does not necessitate that stones be treated with percutaneous lithotripsy. The patient may simply be stented until delivery and then the stones managed appropriately.

REFERENCES

1. Psihramis, K.E., and Dretler, S.P.: Extracorporeal shock wave lithotripsy of calyceal diverticular calculi. J. Urol., *138*:707–711, 1987.
2. LeRoy, A.J., Segura, J.W., Williams, H.J., and Patterson, D.E.: Percutaneous renal calculus removal in an extracorporeal shock wave lithotripsy practice. J. Urol., *138*:703, 1987.

1030-D *(Campbell's, pp. 2184–2186)*

Successful treatment of struvite stones depends on the complete removal of the stone; otherwise persistent infection and regrowth of the stone will occur. With percutaneous lithotripsy (PL) alone, stone-free rates of 85 to 90 per cent can be achieved. When percutaneous lithotripsy is combined with extracorporeal shock wave lithotripsy (ESWL), the stone free rates are no better; however, it is felt that the combined therapy does simplify treatment. The combined technique of PL and ESWL consists of an initial debulking or removal of large stone volume by PL, followed by ESWL of residual stone. After ESWL is completed, a final percutaneous endoscopy is performed to remove the remaining fragments. The advantage of performing ESWL is that it reduces the need for additional access tracts to remove stone from difficult to reach calyces, and it greatly simplifies the second endoscopic procedure. When a staghorn struvite stone is present and three or more access tracts may be needed to manage this percutaneously, a nephrolithotomy should be considered.

REFERENCE

1. Patterson, D.E., Segura, J.W., and LeRoy, A.J.: Long-term follow-up of patients treated by percutaneous ultrasonic lithotripsy for struvite staghorn calculi. J. Endourol., *1*:777, 1987.

1031-B *(Campbell's, p. 2186)*

Struvite stones are appropriately managed percutaneously because of the need to remove all fragments of stone. Brushite stones fragment poorly after ESWL and in some cases may be managed more appropriately with percutaneous lithotripsy. Both calcium oxalate monohydrate and cystine stones are very hard, and when large calculi are present, multiple ESWL procedures may be required to break up these stones. Such cases may be more appropriately managed with a single percutaneous procedure. Of the answers, uric acid stones are the least likely to require percutaneous lithotripsy since the stones can be managed with oral therapy in addition to ESWL. However, when staghorn uric acid calculi occur, percutaneous lithotripsy may be necessary.

1032-B *(Campbell's, pp. 2184–2186)*

Presently, it is recommended that renal calculi with a diameter greater than 3.0 cm be treated with percutaneous lithotripsy because of the volume of stone material present and the number of ESWL procedures that will be required. An upper pole renal calculus is ideally treated by ESWL. No recommendations are given for stones in solitary kidneys; however, such calculi could be managed with a stent and ESWL. ESWL is commonly used to treat calcium oxalate stones prior to other methods unless there are definite indications for percutaneous lithotripsy such as stone size.

REFERENCE

1. Lingeman, J.E., Smith, L.H., Woods, J.R., and Newman, D.M.: Urinary Calculi-ESWL, Endourology, and Medical Therapy. Philadelphia, Lea & Febiger, 1989.

1033-C *(Campbell's, p. 2188)*

An excretory urogram or a retrograde pyelogram should be obtained and used to determine the optimum calyces to be accessed for management of the stone. When the calculi is in a diverticulum or calyx, access should be obtained directly into the calyx or diverticulum containing the stone. Optimum access is generally through a lateral calyx, since this allows maneuverability and enables removal of a large amount of pelvic stone material. Access through the upper pole ensures good access to the pelvis and UPJ; therefore, answer C is incorrect. However, upper pole access often has increased risks of pleural injury. Finally, prior to obtaining percutaneous access, one must consider whether there is any enlargement of the spleen, liver, or colon, any of which may exclude the possibility of safe percutaneous access.

1034-C *(Campbell's, pp. 2188–2189)*

Generally, use of the ultrasonic lithotripter is preferred when power lithotripsy is required. However, the time required to fragment very hard stones may be excessive, and in these cases, the electrohydraulic probe may be more useful. Extravasation of irrigant either into the retroperitoneum or into the intravascular space may limit the time of the operation. Likewise, bleeding which obscures vision may necessitate an early termination of the procedure. When the procedure is terminated early, usually one can repeat nephroscopy in 48 hours and proceed with removal of remaining stone fragments. Therefore, answer C is incorrect. At the termination of the procedure, a large Foley catheter or nephrostomy tube and a ureteral catheter are left in place.

1035-E *(Campbell's, pp. 2189–2191)*

Colonomegaly should be suspected in patients who have undergone intestinal bypass procedures. This may occur because of increased volumes passing through the colon. Since colonomegaly may be a contraindication to percutaneous access, if colonomegaly is suspected, a flat plate of the abdomen should be obtained prior to attempting percutaneous access. Optimum access traverses the bulk of the kidney entering the collecting system through one of the calyces and then traverses the infundibulum into the renal pelvis. When the tract is placed medial or lateral to the calyx, a parenchymal tear or injuries to large vessels may occur. If suboptimal access is obtained, the tract should not be dilated. A new access point should be obtained prior to dilatation. Dilators should be placed no further than the stone itself because aggressive dilatation can produce perforation of the collecting system. Finally, one should be concerned of the possibility of pneumothorax anytime the approach is above the 12th rib; therefore, answer E is incorrect.

1036-E *(Campbell's, pp. 2190–2192)*

Colonic perforation is indeed rare following percutaneous access. Such perforations of the colon have been managed with percutaneous drainage of the colonic perforation through the retroperitoneum and internal drainage of the kidney with a double J stent. Significant arterial injury occurs in less than 1 per cent of percutaneous lithotripsy cases. Injury should readily be indentifiable through the nephroscope by the loss of visibility even with good irrigation and the lack of response to tamponade. In this case, arteriography should be performed immediately and the offending vessel embolized. Often, a pseudoaneurysm is observed on arteriography. Stone fragments extruded through the collecting system into the perinephric tissues need not be removed. Answer E is incorrect, since long-term complications following percutaneous lithotripsy are rare.

REFERENCES

1. Patterson, D.E., Segura, J.W., LeRoy, A.J., et al.: The etiology and treatment of delayed bleeding following percutaneous lithotripsy. J. Urol., *133*:447, 1985.
2. Marberger, M., Stackl, W., Hruby, W., et al.: Late sequelae of ultrasonic lithotripsy of renal calculi. J. Urol., *133*:170, 1984.

1037-E *(Campbell's, pp. 2191–2192)*

Because of the possibility of significant extravasation, normal saline should be used for irrigation fluid to prevent hyponatremia. It is true that healthy adults can absorb 1 liter of normal saline from extravasation without complications. Significant venous bleeding during the procedure can be identified by bleeding which resolves when irrigant is turned on, and in such cases one must be concerned with significant intravascular absorption of the irrigant. This is similar to the absorption of the irrigating fluid through the sinuses during transurethral resection of the prostate. The Amplatz sheath allows irrigating fluid to be removed through the sheath and therefore leads to a lower pressure system, and with this extravasation is less likely. Therefore, answer E is incorrect. As the procedure progresses, if it is noted that the nephroscope must be placed further and further into the kidney to access the stone, one must be concerned that the retroperitoneal space is expanding due to retroperitoneal extravasation.

1038-B *(Campbell's, p. 2196)*

At the ureteral pelvic junction, the abdominal portion of the ureter begins and is covered by the descending duodenum on the right and the beginning portion of the jejunum on the left. As the ureter descends from the renal pelvis, it lies lateral to the inferior vena cava and anterior to both the psoas major muscle and genital femoral nerve. Statement B is, therefore, false. The ureter then takes a slightly medial course crossing transverse processes of the third to fifth lumbar vertebral bodies along their ventral surface. Near the level where the ureters cross the bifurcation of the common iliac arteries, the right ureter lies directly posterior to the right colic and ileocolic blood vessels and the terminal ileum, and the left ureter lies posterior to the left colic vessels and line of attachment of the sigmoid mesocolon. As the ureters enter the true pelvis, they course ventral to the hypogastric arteries and medial to the obturator nerves and arteries. Near the region of the ischial spine, the ureter bends medially and anteriorly to reach the bladder at the ureteral vesical junction.

1039-A *(Campbell's, pp. 2196–2197)*

The ureter is composed of three layers which are fibrous, muscular, and mucosal. The outermost layer, the tunica adventitia, is a continuous fiber structure that runs from the renal sinus along the ureter and inserts into the fibrous coat of the bladder giving rise to Waldeyer's sheath. The middle muscular layer consists of a inner circular and outer longitudinal muscular layer in the proximal ureter. In the middle and distal ureter, the muscular layer has three layers consisting of inner longitudinal, middle circular and outer longitudinal fibers. The muscular layer diminishes in the intramural ureter with the number of longitudinal muscle fibers decreasing as the ureteral orifice is approached. There is only a semi-circle of longitudinal muscle fibers around the lateral aspect of the intramural ureter with few fibers along the medial aspect. The mucosal layer of the ureter consists of transitional cell epithelium and lamina propria. The transitional cell layer is thickest in the distal ureter where it is approximately 6 cell layers deep and is thinnest in the proximal ureter where it is approximately 2 cell layers thick.

1040-D *(Campbell's, pp. 2197–2198)*

With endoscopy of the renal collecting system and ureter, the renal papillae appear as rounded cones with a pink, easily friable epithelium. As one moves up the ureter, in the proximal ureter, just below the ureteral pelvic junction, a bend or lip of ureteral mucosa is seen in the posterolateral ureteral lumen. This is an indicator that one is just about to enter the renal pelvis. Also seen in the region of the proximal ureter and in the renal pelvis is movement secondary to respiration. With inspiration, the diaphragm pushes downward on the kidney causing a simultaneous caudal movement of the renal pelvis and proximal ureter. Narrow sites of the ureteral lumen seen on ureteroscopy include the ureteral pelvic junction, the pelvic brim, and the ureteral vesical junction. In young muscular male patients, psoas hypertrophy leads to the displacement of the ureter anteriorly making its course more difficult to traverse with the rigid ureteroscope. A lateral view of the ureter in Figure 61–1 on page 2196 of *Campbell's Urology* gives some appreciation for the difficulty anterior displacement of the ureter may cause with rigid ureteroscopy.

1041-C *(Campbell's, pp. 2198–2205)*

Indications for ureteroscopy are summarized in Table 61–1 on page 2198 of *Campbell's Urology*. These include removal of lower ureteral calculi as well as management of post ESWL steinstrasse. In some cases, upper ureteral calculi and renal calculi may be managed with the ureteroscope; however, the treatment of choice for a large ureteral pelvic junction calculus would be ESWL. Ureteroscopy is also indicated for the evaluation of filling defects (both in the renal pelvis and in the ureter), and for the surveillance of the ureter following removal of a ureteral tumor, such as after segmental ureterectomy for urothelial tumor. Other therapeutic indications for ureteroscopy include passage of a ureteral catheter for obstruction or fistula, dilation or incision of strictures and retrieval of foreign bodies (including broken and migrated ureteral stents).

1042-E *(Campbell's, p. 2202)*

Indications for diagnostic ureteroscopy include the following: radiographic filling defect or obstruction; tumor found cystoscopically near or at the ureteral orifice; unilateral upper tract hematuria; and upper tract urinary cytology findings which indicate malignancy. The presence of multiple bladder tumors is not an indication for ureteroscopy without other evidence for upper urinary tract tumor such as suspicious cytologies from ureteral samples.

REFERENCES

1. Gittes, R.F., and Varaday, S.: Nephroscopy in chronic unilateral hematuria. J. Urol., *126*:2297, 1981.
2. Huffman, J.L., Bagley, D.H. and Lyon, E.S.: Ureteral catheterization, retrograde ureteropyelography and self-retaining ureteral stents. *In* Bagley, D.H., Huffman, J.L., and Lyons, E.S. (Eds.): Urologic Endoscopy: A Manual and Atlas. Boston, MA, Little, Brown and Co., 1985, pp. 163–176.

1043-A *(Campbell's, p. 2206)*

Preoperative evaluation for ureteroscopy begins with a detailed history and examination when the patient presents. The history should include pelvic and urologic surgery and whether the patient has received pelvic radiation. A bimanual exam is essential and allows evaluation of the mobility of the urethra, bladder, and lower ureter. If these structures are frozen, rigid ureteroscopy may not be possible and flexible ureteroscopy may be significantly more difficult. At the time of surgery, sterile urine is essential because of the possibility of intravasation of urine and irrigant which may lead to sepsis. Therefore, preoperative antibiotics are recommended and a broad spectrum antibiotic should be chosen. Radiographic studies should be available at the time of surgery and if the lower ureter is not well visualized, a retrograde pyelogram should be performed prior to initiating ureteroscopy. The administration of intravenous indigo carmine (which might be useful in the identification of the ureteral orifices) is not routinely recommended in the preoperative treatment for ureteroscopy.

1044-C *(Campbell's, p. 2208)*

Clinical evidence suggests that dilation of the ureteral orifice to sizes of 14–15 French has no detrimental effect on the structure or function of the orifice. Dilation to these sizes allows sufficient passage of operating instruments for ureteroscopy. Passive or subacute dilation of the ureteral orifice is accomplished by placing a ureteral stent 1 to 3 days prior to performing the ureteroscopic procedure. The stent accomplishes the dilation of the ureteral orifice. This form of dilation is not recommended when diagnostic ureteroscopy is planned because it may give rise to inflammation and confuse the findings of diagnostic ureteroscopy. Acute methods of dilation of the ureter include the passage of progressively larger ureteral catheters at the time of ureteroscopy or the use of cone-shaped metal bougies. Acute dilation is also accomplished through methods performed over a guidewire which includes use of graduated fascial dilators or balloon dilating catheters. Hydraulic dilation of the ureter by pressurized pumping may also be performed but this method may be associated with intravasation of fluid. In general, dilating methods which proceed over a positioned guidewire are safer than other methods, with fewer false passages and ureteral perforations. When the cone-shaped metal bougies are used, they should be passed to the level of the detrusor hiatus and not further.

REFERENCES

1. Greene, L.F.: The renal and ureteral changes induced by dilating the ureter. An experimental study. J. Urol., *52*:505–521, 1944.
2. Ford, T.F., Parkinson, M.C., and Wickham, J.E.A.: Clinical and experimental evaluation of ureteric dilation. Br. J. Urol., *56*:460–463, 1984.
3. Huffman, J.L., and Bagley, D.H.: Balloon dilation of the ureter for ureteroscopy. J. Urol., *140*:954–956, 1988.
4. Perez-Castro, E.: Ureteromat: method to facilitate ureterorenoscopy and avoid dilatation. Urol. Clin. North Am., *15*:315, 1988.

1045-B *(Campbell's, pp. 2212–2214)*

When performing balloon dilation of the ureteral orifice, a guidewire is first placed in the ureter. The positioning is monitored with fluoroscopy, and fluoroscopy is used throughout the dilation process. The balloon catheter is then passed over the wire and positioned across the intramural ureteral tunnel and orifice with the proximal end of the balloon visualized in the bladder with the cystoscope. Once the balloon is positioned, it is inflated with 50 per cent radiocontrast solution at a rate of 2 atmospheres per minute using a screw-type inflation syringe. When the balloon is fully inflated and all "waisting" of the balloon is removed, dilation is complete and the balloon is deflated. Generally, the ureteral orifice can be dilated with pressures less than 10 atmospheres; however, in the case of reimplanted or scarred ureters, pressures as high as 15 atmospheres may be required.

1046-D *(Campbell's, pp. 2214–2215)*

When performing dilation of the supravesical ureter, the ureteral orifice should be first dilated. An uninflated balloon may pass through the ureteral orifice, but once it has been inflated and deflated it may not resume its preinflation diameter and, therefore, it may not be able to pass back through the ureteral orifice unless the orifice has been dilated. Guidewire placement in the ureter is critical and if the guidewire does not pass smoothly and easily into the renal pelvis, one must be concerned with the possibility that a submucosal tunnel has been formed. Dilation of such a tunnel by passing the balloon over the guidewire could have disastrous results. When the balloon is inflated in the ureter, care should be taken not to move it because movement of even a partially inflated balloon may cause avulsion of ureter mucosal. Additionally, buckling of the guidewire with the balloon in place may lead to perforation of the ureter at the end of the balloon catheter. When performing dilation of the supravesical ureter, the actual technique of dilating is similar to that described for the ureteral orifice in question 1045. The rate of inflation of the balloon may be 2 atmospheres per minute.

1047-E *(Campbell's, p. 2215)*

To facilitate introduction of the ureteroscope into the ureteral orifice, a guidewire is left in place in the ureter to help with identification of the orifice and alignment with it. When the rigid ureteroscope is passed into the orifice, it is helpful to rotate the instrument 90 to 180 degrees as it enters the ureter. This action allows the beveled tip to "lift" the upper lip of the orifice permitting a smooth insertion. The flexible ureteroscope may be advanced into the ureter directly over a guidewire which has been passed through a working channel. Answer E is, therefore, incorrect. The flexible ureteroscope can also be inserted directly under vision without aid of any other instruments. When buckling or coiling in the bladder is a problem with the flexible ureteroscope, it may be passed through the rigid cystoscope sheath and the sheath employed to prevent buckling and coiling by bringing it right to the ureteral orifice. Another way of introducing the flexible ureteroscope involves the placement of a flexible dilator with a guidetube outer sheath into the ureter. After removal of the dilator the guidetube sheath is in place and may be used as a conduit from the bladder into the ureter for the flexible scope to be passed.

REFERENCE

1. Bagley, D.H.: Ureteropyeloscopy with flexible fiberoptic instruments. *In* Huffman, J., Bagley, D., and

Lyon, E. (Eds.): Ureteroscopy. Philadelphia, W.B. Saunders Co., 1988, pp. 131–155.

1048-A *(Campbell's, p. 2217)*

With the ultrasonic lithotriptor, high frequency vibrations of the rigid metal transducer generate the energy for stone fragmentation. The tip of the transducer must be in contact with the stone for fragmentation to occur. The energy may fragment the stone or carve a path through the calculus. To facilitate fragmentation with this technique, the stone should be fixed in place with a basket, and the probe introduced into the basket against the stone. Ultrasonic transducers do generate heat during operation and the probe must be cooled throughout its use to avoid thermal injury to the ureteral mucosa. This can be done with irrigation solution. Additionally, it is advisable to negotiate the stone and basket into the more proximal ureter where the ureter is of larger diameter. In this region, heat may be better dissipated in the spacious ureter where fluid can surround the basket. Thermal urothelial injury is less likely in the proximal ureter than other locations.

REFERENCES

1. Huffman, J.L., Bagley, D.H., Schoenberg, H.W., and Lyon, E.S.: Transurethral removal of large ureteral and renal pelvic calculi using ureteroscopic ultrasonic lithotripsy. J. Urol., *130*:31–34, 1983.
2. Howards, S.S., Merrill, E., Harris, S., and Cohn, J.: Ultrasonic lithotripsy. Invest. Urol., *2*:273–277, 1974.

1049-C *(Campbell's, pp. 2218–2221)*

With the electrohydraulic lithotriptor, an electrohydraulic shockwave generator and a coaxial probe are used to produce a shock wave that causes fragmentation when directed toward a stone. When EHL is used in the ureter, the calculus is approached with the ureteroscope and the coaxial probe is advanced toward the stone but it is not placed in contact with the stone. After fragmentation is complete, fragments are removed with the basket which is inserted after the EHL probe is removed. EHL is performed under direct visualization whereas ultrasonic lithotripsy may be carried out with tactile sensation and fluoroscopic visualization. There is a 10 to 15 per cent rate of ureteral perforation when EHL is used on non-impacted ureteral calculi. This technique should not be used on impacted ureteral calculi.

REFERENCES

1. Goodfriend, R.: Ultrasonic and electrohydraulic lithotripsy of ureteral calculi. Urology, *23*:5–8, 1984.
2. Green, D.F., and Lytton, B.: Early experience with electrohydraulic lithotripsy of ureteral calculi using direct vision ureteroscopy. J. Urol., *133*:767, 1985.
3. Willscher, M.K., Conway, J.F., Babayan, R.K., et al.: Safety and efficacy of electrohydraulic lithotripsy by ureteroscopy. J. Urol., *140*:957–958, 1988.
4. Denstedt, J.D., and Clayman, R.V.: Electrohydraulic lithotripsy of renal and ureteral calculi. J. Urol., *143*: 13, 1990.

1050-E *(Campbell's, pp. 2221–2223)*

Laser lithotripsy employs a pulsed-dye laser which produces light of 504 nanometers wavelength. This is conducted through a quartz fiber approximately 200 to 320 μm in size. When this is performed in the ureter, the fiber is passed through the working channel of the ureteroscope until it makes contact with the stone. Preferably, the stone is held in place with a basket. The fiber must remain in contact with the stone for effective fragmentation since the laser energy rapidly dissipates. The energy setting for the laser is generally 60 to 80 millijoules. Temperature increases do occur at the stone's surface, but thermal injury occurring to the surrounding mucosa is rare.

REFERENCES

1. Watson, G.M., and Wickham, J.E.A.: Initial experience with a pulsed-dye laser for ureteric calculi. Lancet, *1*:1357, 1986.
2. Dretler, S.P.: An evaluation of ureteral laser lithotripsy: 225 consecutive patients. J. Urol., *143*:267–273, 1990.

1051-B *(Campbell's, pp. 2223–2224)*

When performing ureteral biopsy, this should be done with the initial pass of the ureteroscope in order to avoid avulsion of the suspicious lesion and loss of it. With ureteroscopic resection or fulguration, basic principles apply as with electrosurgery transurethrally. Irrigants should consist of either glycine or water. When resecting an intraluminal tumor, no attempt should be made to take arcing bites into the ureteral wall. Only the intraluminal portion of the tumor is resected. After resection is complete, the base of the luminal lesion is then fulgurated lightly with either the loop or a Bugbee electrode. This technique minimizes ureteral perforation. When working in the distal ureter, electrosurgical techniques may cause stimulation of the obturator nerve with disastrous consequences. A neodymium-yttrium-aluminum-garnet or KTP laser may be used to ablate lower ureteral tumors without stimulating the obturator nerve.

1052-D *(Campbell's, pp. 2225–2226)*

The incidence of ureteral injuries with ureteroscopy is shown in Table 61–6 on page 2226 of *Campbell's Urology*. Ureteral perforation has been noted in approximately 7 per cent of cases. Ureteral stricture occurs in approximately 1.4 per cent of cases. Ultrasonic lithotripsy, EHL, and laser lithotripsy all have the potential for thermal injury to the ureteral mucosa; however, EHL has greatest potential for thermal injury. The proximal ureter has a thinner mucosal layer as well as a thinner muscular layer and is therefore at greater risk for complete perforation than the distal or intramural ureter. The muscular layers are much greater in the distal and intramural ureter and the potential for false passage development in these regions is greater.

REFERENCE

1. Huffman, J.L.: Injuries to the upper urinary tract. Urol. Clin. North Am., *16*:249–254, 1989.

1053-C *(Campbell's, pp. 2226–2227)*

Fluoroscopy should be mandatory for ureteroscopy and is definitely advantageous for the prevention of complications. It should be used even with the initial placement of a guidewire in the ureter at the start of the procedure. Ureteral avulsion is most commonly caused when one attempts to extract a calculus too large for the ureter. Lithotripsy techniques should be available at the time of ureteroscopy and one should not hesitate to use intraureteral lithotripsy for larger calculi. The majority of ureteral injuries following ureteroscopy can be managed conservatively without open surgery. Ureteral perforation or false passage development can usually be managed with an internal ureteral stent or a ureteral catheter. When a documented ureteral perforation is found and urinary diversion with a nephrostomy tube or ureteral stenting is performed, diversion or stenting is usually maintained for 6 weeks. A contrast study is then done to document healing prior to removal of the catheter or nephrostomy tube. When distal ureteral avulsion occurs and an open procedure is necessary, ureteral repair may be done using ureteral reimplant with a psoas hitch or Boari flap.

REFERENCES

1. Benjamin, J.C., Donaldson, P.J., and Hill, J.T.: Ureteric perforation after ureteroscopy: Conservative management. Urology, *29*:623–624, 1987.

1054-D *(Campbell's, p. 2236)*

The incidence and severity of complications of percutaneous access to the renal collecting system are as follows. Acute bleeding requiring transfusion occurs in less than 5 per cent. Of those with acute bleeding, less than 0.5 per cent require emergent embolization and nephrectomy may be required in up to 0.19 per cent. Delayed hemorrhage is seen in less than 0.5 per cent. Septicemia occurs in less than 1 per cent. Injury to the bowel or spleen occurs in less than 1 per cent. With the intercostal approach, pleurotomy and possible pleural effusion occurs in 12 per cent.

REFERENCE

1. Picus, D.D., Weyman, P.J., Clayman, R.V., et al.: Intercostal-space nephrostomy for percutaneous stone removal. Am. J. Rad., *147*:393, 1986.

1055-A *(Campbell's, pp. 2236–2241)*

For patients undergoing diagnostic or therapeutic nephrostomy, it is helpful to initially pass a retrograde ureteral catheter. Through this catheter, the collecting system may be opacified. In general, approaches to the collecting system are going to be through posterior calyces. When the patient is positioned prone, 10-cc of carbon dioxide may be instilled through the retrograde ureteral catheter and the posterior calyces will be outlined by the carbon dioxide. If contrast is injected in the prone position, the anterior calyces are filled first because the contrast is denser than urine. With fluoroscopy guidance, the desired calyx of entry is identified and the needle is advanced in a straight path toward this calyx for approximately 5 cm into the flank. At this point, the entire needle appears only as a radiodense dot overlying the calyx. Once the needle's trajectory is fixed, the C-arm may be rotated to a lateral position to view the needle and shaft in relation to the calyx. When only a fixed fluoroscopy unit is available, the physician must rely on the feel of the needle as it passes through various layers. Resistance to passage of the needle is noted when the renal capsule is encountered and when the calyx is punctured. Once the collecting system is entered, a guidewire is passed through the needle into the collecting system. The lumbodorsal fascia may be incised by passing a 13.5 French shovel shaped incising needle over the guidewire twice with a 90 degree difference on rotation on the second pass. The tract is then dilated to the desired size and the nephrostomy tube placed. When a nephrostomy tract is desired for drainage of pyonephrosis an infracostal path should be used and the tract should be minimally dilated (10–12 French).

1056-E *(Campbell's, pp. 2244–2245)*

The best management of hemorrhage at the time of percutaneous nephrostomy is immediate tamponade with a Kaye catheter. Rarely, arterial embolization or open surgical therapy is necessary. On the contrary, when delayed hemorrhage occurs, usually after nephrostomy tube removal, angiographic embolization is often required. This complication, however, develops in less than 0.5 per cent. Collecting system perforations typically resolve within 48 hours given proper drainage of the collecting system. These are simply managed with a ureteral stent or nephrostomy tube. Between 2 to 10 per cent of patients may have a retrorenal colon when prone; however, perforation of the colon is indeed rare. When this occurs, it can be managed by placing a nephrostomy tube into the colon to drain the perforated site and by maintaining urinary tract drainage with an external retrograde ureteral catheter. A colostomy is only indicated when peritonitis develops. With the supracostal approach for percutaneous nephrostomy, pleurotomy may occur in 12 per cent of cases which may then be associated with a hydro- or pneumothorax. Appropriate treatment would involve placement of a chest tube. The occurrence of chronic nephropleural fistula is rare.

REFERENCES

1. Clayman, R.V., Surya, V., Hunter, D., et al.: Renal vascular complications associated with percutaneous removal of renal calculi. J. Urol., *132*:228, 1984.
2. Winfield, H.W., and Clayman, R.V.: Complications of percutaneous removal of renal and ureteral calculi. Part I. World Urology Update Series, Vol. 2, Lesson 37, 1985.
3. Young, A.T., Hunter, D.W., Castaneda-Zuniga, W.R., et al.: Percutaneous extraction of urinary calculi: Use of the intercostal approach. Radiology, *154*:633, 1985.
4. Hopper, K.D., Sherman, J.L., Luethke, J.M., et al.: The retrorenal colon in the supine and prone patient. Radiology, *162*:443, 1987.

1057-B *(Campbell's, p. 2249)*

Approximately 10 per cent of macro- or microscopic hematuria has a source localized to the upper urinary tract. When bleeding is due to an upper urinary tract etiology, 42 per cent of cases are found to be due to renal or ureteral calculi, 19 per cent are due to medical renal disease, 10 per cent are due to renal cell carcinoma, 7 per cent are due to transitional cell carcinoma and less than 1 per cent are due to arteriovenous fistula.

REFERENCE

1. Mariani, A.J., Mariani, M.C., Macchioni, C., et al.: The significance of adult hematuria: 1000 hematuria evaluations including a risk-benefit and cost-effectiveness analysis. J. Urol., *141*:350, 1989.

1058-E *(Campbell's, p. 2253)*

In the evaluation of upper urinary tract filling defects on CT scan, the following attenuations are seen: uric acid stones greater than 300 Hounsfield units, fungal balls 20 to 40 Hounsfield units, a sloughed papilla 20 to 40 Hounsfield units, transitional cell tumor 30 to 40 Hounsfield units, and blood clot 30 to 55 Hounsfield units.

REFERENCE

1. Pollack, H.M., Arger, P.H., Banner, M.P., et al.: Computed tomography of renal pelvic filling defects. Radiology, *138*:645, 1981.

1059-C *(Campbell's, pp. 2249–2251)*

The differential diagnosis of radiolucent upper urinary tract filling defects includes: tumor, uric acid urolithiasis, sloughed papilla, blood clots, fungal infection with fungal ball, foreign bodies, and iatrogenic air from recent genitourinary tract manipulation. Gouty arthritis may be associated with uric acid urolithiasis, and is important information from the medical history. Analgesic abuse and diabetes mellitus are both predisposing factors in papillary necrosis (and the possibility of a sloughed papilla) and are, therefore, important points to note in the medical history. Finally, patients that are immunosuppressed are predisposed to fungal infection and may develop fungal ball in the renal pelvis. Sarcoidosis is not necessarily associated with radiolucent upper urinary tract filling defects.

1060-A *(Campbell's, p. 2249)*

By the time ureteroscopy is performed on patients with essential hematuria, radiographic and urine studies have usually eliminated the diagnosis of urolithiasis or tumor. Although 42 per cent of upper tract hematuria is due to ureteral calculus, in this select group the most common lesion found on ureteroscopy is a discreet, small vascular abnormality such as a hemangioma or arteriovenous malformation. It is extremely rare in this select group of patients that the bleeding site is found in the ureter. When a small vascular abnormality is found, it is most often seen directly on a papilla. In multiple series, bleeding due to renal artery aneurysm has not been reported. Presently, bleeding sites localized to the lower pole are not reported to have a higher incidence than other sites.

REFERENCES

1. Bagley, D.H., and Allen, J.: Flexible ureteropyeloscopy in the diagnosis of benign essential hematuria. J. Urol., *143*:549, 1990.
2. Gittes, R.F., and Varady, S.: Nephroscopy in chronic unilateral hematuria. J. Urol., *126*:297, 1981.
3. Kumon, H., Tsugawa, M., Matsumura, Y., et al.: Endoscopic diagnosis and treatment of chronic unilateral hematuria of uncertain etiology. J. Urol., *143*:554, 1990.
4. Patterson, D.E., Segura, J.W., Benson, R.C., Jr., et al.: Endoscopic evaluation and treatment of patients with idiopathic gross hematuria. J. Urol., *132*:1199, 1984.

1061-C *(Campbell's, p. 2254)*

When ureteroscopy is performed in the evaluation of a collecting system filling defect, the following may be seen. Sloughed papillae have a dull, gray appearance and are free-floating. A fungal ball appears as a white gelatinous free-floating object. Fibroepithelial polyps appear as smooth-walled pedunculated lesions. Papillary transitional cell tumors are similar in appearance to those seen in the bladder. When no lesion is identified on ureteroscopy, the radiographic finding may be due to a crossing vessel. If this is thought to be the case, the collecting system can be slowly filled with contrast and on fluoroscopy the filling defect should appear initially if it is due to a crossing vessel; however, as the pelvis is distended the defect should disappear.

1062-D *(Campbell's, p. 2256)*

A uriniferous pseudocyst or urinoma of the retroperitoneum may be due to renal trauma, ureteral obstruction with calyceal forniceal rupture or a complication following endosurgical procedures. If a urinoma is suspected, it is important to determine whether ureteral obstruction exists, extravasation from the collecting system is occurring, and whether the kidney is functioning. Appropriate radiographic studies include an IVP or antegrade nephrostogram, a retrograde ureterogram, or a CT scan. On CT scan, the attenuation of a urinoma which has not taken up contrast is 10 to 20 Hounsfield units. It is important to distinguish between a urinoma and pancreatic pseudocyst prior to therapy because of the different therapies required. Fluid should be analyzed for the presence of creatinine and amylase. When no communication exists between the collecting system and urinoma, percutaneous drainage is often successful and urinoma drainage will cease within 48 to 72 hours. If a fistulous tract is present, it may be necessary to place a retrograde ureteral catheter or percutaneous nephrostomy to divert the urine from the fistulous tract. It is rare that a fistula will not respond to diversion of the urine; however, when this occurs, antegrade nephroscopy or ureteroscopy may be performed with fulguration of the fistulous tract. The experience with this is rare. It is true that in the largest series of treated urinomas, half of the patients required nephrectomy.

REFERENCES

1. Lang, E.K., and Glorioso, L.W., III: Management of urinomas by percutaneous drainage procedures. Radiol. Clin. North Am., *24*:551, 1986.
2. Thompson, I.M., Ross, G. Jr., Habib, E.H., et al.: Experiences with 16 cases of pararenal pseudocyst. J. Urol., *116*:289, 1976.

1063-C *(Campbell's, pp. 2257–2258)*

A perinephric abscess is a life-threatening illness. Without drainage, the mortality rate approaches 80 per cent; however, with surgical therapy the mortality is often 11 to 22 per cent. With less invasive percutaneous procedures, a mortality rate of 8 per cent is reported. Factors which decrease the likelihood of successful percutaneous drainage include the occurrence of a multiloculated abscess, infected hematoma, high viscosity abscess material, calcifications present in the abscess, and air fluid levels on CT scan indicative of enteric-retroperitoneal fistula. When percutaneous drainage of the abscess is employed, drainage usually ceases within 5 to 7 days unless a urinary fistula is present. After adequate drainage of the abscess cavity, a large cavity may persist and this can be effectively sclerosed using 95 per cent ethanol or tetracycline 50 mg/ml. Ureteroscopic incision of the abscess into the collecting system is not reported as appropriate therapy.

REFERENCES

1. Altemeyer, W.A., and Alexander, J.: Retroperitoneal abscess. Arch. Surg., *83*:512, 1961.
2. Thorley, J.D., Jones, S.R., and Sanford, J.P.: Perinephric abscess. Medicine, *53*:441, 1974.
3. Haaga, J.R.: Imaging intra-abdominal abscesses and nonoperative drainage procedures. World J. Surg., *14*: 204, 1990.
4. Caldamone, A.A., and Frank, I.N.: Percutaneous aspiration in the treatment of renal abscess. J. Urol., *123*: 92, 1980.

1064-A *(Campbell's, pp. 2259–2261)*

Simple drainage of renal cysts cures only 4 to 19 per cent. Sclerotherapy after cyst aspiration, however, has a very high success rate with a 100 per cent success in some series. Endosurgical management of renal cysts is also reported to have a 93 per cent success rate but it is no more effective than sclerotherapy and is more invasive. With standard sclerotherapy, after aspiration of the cysts ethanol is injected into the cyst to fill 25 per cent of the volume and is left in place 10 to 20 minutes and then withdrawn. Alternative sclerotherapy can be performed using 5 to 10 ml of bismuth phosphate which may be left in the cyst. Contraindications to sclerotherapy include a communication between cyst and renal pelvis or any component of the collecting system. With the direct endosurgical approach, a transcystic nephrostomy tract is established, a nephroscope is placed in the cyst and the wall between the cyst, and renal pelvis excised, marsupializing the cyst into the renal pelvis.

REFERENCES

1. Holmberg, G., and Hietala, S.O.: Treatment of simple renal cysts by percutaneous puncture and instillation of bismuth phosphate. Scand. J. Urol. Nephrol., *23*: 207, 1989.
2. Ozgun, S., Cetin, S., and Ilken, Y.: Percutaneous renal cyst aspiration and treatment with alcohol. Int. Urol. Nephrol., *20*:481, 1988.
3. Hubner, W., Pfab, R., et al.: Renal cysts: Percutaneous resection with standard urologic instruments. J. Endourol., *4*:61, 1990.

1065-E *(Campbell's, pp. 2262–2265)*

For management of calyceal diverticula, the antegrade percutaneous approach indeed has the best results of endosurgical methods, with successful removal of calculi in approximately 100 per cent and obliteration of the diverticulum in up to 85 per cent. Results of ESWL for diverticular calculi are discouraging. However, when ureteroscopy and dilation of the calyceal neck is performed with ESWL, a stone-free rate of up to 73 per cent has been reported. With percutaneous approaches, the first step is to pass a retrograde ureteral catheter and occlusion balloon into the renal pelvis. In the direct antegrade percutaneous approach, the nephrostomy tube is placed directly into the calyceal diverticulum and the neck of the diverticulum may be identified by injecting dye through the ureteral catheter with the balloon inflated to occlude the pelvis. In the indirect antegrade percutaneous approach, the nephrostomy tract is placed into the collecting system. This technique is more difficult than the direct technique because a nondilated collecting system must be accessed and then the neck of the diverticulum must be identified, which may be difficult. The walls of the diverticulum are fulgurated to cause scarring and hasten collapse of the diverticulum. The use of sclerosing agents is not reported.

REFERENCES

1. Eshghi, M., Tuong, W., Fernandez, R., et al.: Percutaneous (endo) infundibulotomy. J. Endourol., *1*:107, 1987.
2. Hulbert, J.C., Hernandez, J., Hunter, D.W., et al.: Current concepts in the management of pyelocaliceal diverticula. J. Endourol., *2*:11, 1988.
3. Fuchs, G.J., and David, R.D.: Flexible ureterorenoscopy, dilation of narrow caliceal neck, and ESWL: A new, minimally invasive approach to stones in caliceal diverticula. J. Endourol., *3*:255, 1989.

1066-A *(Campbell's, pp. 2269–2270)*

Two tests are available which can diagnosis functional obstruction and these are the diuretic wash-out renogram and the Whitaker renal pelvic/bladder differential pressure study. With the diuresis renogram, ^{131}I Hippuran or DTPA is given and renal images taken through 30 minutes. If the curve appears to demonstrate obstruction, a diuretic such as furosemide is given intravenously at 30 minutes. In the non-obstructive situation, 50 per cent of the radionuclide tracer should drain from the kidney within 10 minutes. When 50 per cent drainage requires between 10 to 20 minutes, the study is considered equivocal; drainage times longer than 20 minutes are associated with obstruction. Medical renal disease or renal artery disease may confuse the results of this test by affecting the excretion of radionuclide, and massive hydronephrosis by its diluting effect may also confuse the result of this study. These disease processes lead to false-positive results. In general, a normal diuretic washout renal scan is a reliable indicator of a non-obstructive system. Renal artery disease may give rise to a false-positive rather than false-negative diuretic wash-out renal scan.

The Whitaker test is an invasive study which involves placing a small nephrostomy tube into the renal collecting system and a urethral catheter into the bladder. The collecting system is then fully distended and perfused percutaneously at a rate of 10 ml/min. Pressure readings are then recorded both in the renal pelvis and in the bladder. A pressure differential between renal pelvis and bladder of 15 cm of water or less is considered unobstructed. The differential in the range of 15 to 22 cm is equivocal and a pressure differential above 22 cm is considered to indicate obstruction. False-negative results may occur with the Whitaker test when extravasation occurs from the renal pelvis or when the renal pelvis is not fully distended when the pressures are recorded.

REFERENCES

1. Talner, L.B.: Obstructive uropathy. *In* Pollack, H.M. (Ed.): Nuclear Medicine Techniques in Clinical Urography. Philadelphia, W.B. Saunders Co., 1990, p. 1570.
2. Whitaker, R.H.: An evaluation of 170 diagnostic pressure flow studies of the upper urinary tract. J. Urol., *121*:602, 1979.

1067-D *(Campbell's, pp. 2274–2275)*

When performing an antegrade endopyelotomy, a 0.035-in. guidewire is first passed into the renal pelvis in a retrograde fashion. A standard percutaneous nephrostomy is then placed and access should be to an upper or middle posterior calyx. This allows your point of access to be in line with the ureteral pelvic junction. A 6 mm balloon is inflated along the course of the UPJ obstruction, placing the UPJ tissue under tension. The balloon is maintained and the incision is made alongside the balloon. The incision should be made full-thickness (exposing retroperitoneal fat) and adequacy of the incision is verified by rapid extravasation of contrast through the incised region. The incision should be made along the posterolateral border of the UPJ and carried caudally for approximately 1 cm beyond the point of UPJ obstruction.

REFERENCE

1. Karlin, G.S., and Smith, A.D.: Endopyelotomy. Urol. Clin. North Am., *15*:433, 1988.

1068-B *(Campbell's, pp. 2277–2280)*

Antegrade endopyelotomy has lasting success rates reported in the range of 72 to 87 per cent. When failure occurs, it is usually seen within 3 months of the procedure. Similar success has been found with the retrograde endopyelotomy; however, it is considerably more difficult technically. In addition, the occurrence of ureteral strictures following a retrograde endopyelotomy has been reported as high as 20 per cent. Chronic massive hydronephrosis is an unfavorable condition for endopyelotomy and adults with this condition who undergo endopyelotomy have a higher failure rate. This is thought to be due to the inability to tailor the renal pelvis for proper drainage as can be done with an open surgical procedure. When poor renal function is present, endopyelotomy also has a poor success rate because the UPJ has a tendency to scar. Evaluation of renal function is recommended prior to the endopyelotomy with a renal scan and if the kidney poorly functions, obstruction should be relieved with a nephrostomy tract. If compromise of function persists endopyelotomy has a greater tendency to fail. Answer B is therefore incorrect.

REFERENCES

1. Brannen, G.E., Bush, W.H., and Lewis, G.P.: Endopyelotomy for primary repair of ureteropelvic junction obstruction. J. Urol., *139*:29, 1988.
2. Karlin, G.S., Badlani, G.H., and Smith, A.D.: Endopyelotomy versus open pyeloplasty: Comparison in 88 patients. J. Urol., *140*:476, 1988.
3. Motola, J.A., Badlani, G.H., and Smith, A.D.: Endopyelotomy: Long-term follow-up of 156 cases. J. Endourol., *4*:S139, 1990.
4. Badlani, G., Karlin, G., and Smith, A.D.: Complications of endopyelotomy: Analysis in series of 64. J. Urol., *140*:473, 1988.
5. Clayman, R.V., Basler, J.W., Kavoussi, L., et al.: Ureteronephroscopic endopyelotomy. J. Urol., *144*:246, 1990.

1069-A *(Campbell's, pp. 2280–2286)*

The endosurgical management of proximal ureteral strictures is similar to that of antegrade endopyelotomy with a similar technique. The incision in the upper ureter is again made in the posterolateral region of the ureter. If the stricture directly overlies the iliac vessels, the incision is made anteriorly, and below the iliac vessels the incision is made medial to avoid branches of the internal iliac vessels. As with the endopyelotomy, the incision should be full thickness and periureteral fat should be seen. In the management of distal ureteral strictures, marsupialization of the stricture into the bladder is the goal. This can be done with a retrograde approach and a cold knife urethrotome or by inflating a balloon in the distal ureter and incising from the bladder onto the balloon. Complete obstruction may be successfully managed with endosurgical techniques when the ureteral obstruction is less than 1 cm in length. Typically, an approach from both the proximal and distal ureter will be required and therefore a nephrostomy tract will be necessary.

1070-E *(Campbell's, pp. 2287–2288)*

Durable overall success rates are similar for endoincision and balloon dilation of ureteral strictures and are in the range of 50 to 60 per cent. Ureteral strictures greater than 1 cm in length respond poorly to endoureterotomy, which has a success rate of only 11 to 18 per cent in these cases. Strictures which are due to ischemic problems do not respond as well as those due to non-ischemic factors when endosurgical techniques are used, and a 40 per cent success rate is reported for ischemic strictures versus a 58 per cent success rate for those which are non-ischemic in origin. Strictures which may be marsupialized into either the bladder or pelvis have a much higher success rate than midureteral strictures which may not be marsupialized. An 80 per cent success rate is reported for proximal and distal ureteral strictures which can be marsupialized versus a 25 per cent success rate for midureteral strictures. Presently, there is no evidence that duration of stricture prior to endosurgery impacts the outcome.

REFERENCES

1. Gothlin, J.H., Gadeholt, G., Farsund, T., et al.: Percutaneous antegrade dilatation of distal ureteral strictures and obstruction. Eur. J. Radiol., *8*:217, 1988.

2. Johnson, D.C., Oke, E.J., Dunnick, R.N., et al.: Percutaneous balloon dilation of ureteral strictures. Am. J. Roentgenol., *148*:181, 1987.
3. Lang, E.K., and Glorioso, L.W., III: Antegrade transluminal dilation of benign ureteral strictures: Long-term results. Am. J. Roentgen., *150*:131, 1988.
4. O'Brien, W.M., Maxted, W.C., and Pahira, J.J.: Ureteral stricture: Experience with 31 cases. J. Urol., *140*: 737, 1988.
5. Chang, R., Marshall, F.F., and Mitchell, S.: Percutaneous management of benign ureteral strictures and fistulas. J. Urol., *137*:1126, 1987.
6. Netto, N.R., Jr., Ferreira, U., Lemos, G.C., et al.: Endourological management of ureteral strictures. J. Urol., *144*:631, 1990.
7. Meretyk, S., Clayman, R.V., Kavoussi, L.R., et al.: Endoureterotomy for treatment of ureteral strictures. J. Urol., 1991.

1071-C *(Campbell's, pp. 2298–2302)*

When endosurgical techniques are employed to evaluate transitional cell tumors of the renal pelvis, understaging may occur in as many as 60 per cent of cases. This may, in part, be due to fear of perforating the renal pelvis or ureter or in part to missing urothelial changes which may be consistent with CIS or dysplasia during endoscopic techniques of the renal pelvis. When endosurgical resection is employed in the ureter, the recurrence rate at approximately 2 years is 15 per cent and progression to open ablative surgery occurs in approximately 13 per cent. With endosurgical management of transitional cell tumors of the renal pelvis, results are poorer than the ureter and recurrence or open surgery rates at 2 years are approximately 30 per cent. When endosurgical management of upper tract transitional cell carcinoma is compared to open conservative therapy, results are similar. However, one must keep in mind that endoscopic therapy is primarily reserved for low-grade solitary lesions. Following surgical pyelotomy, an 11 per cent retroperitoneal seeding rate was reported; however, reports of nephrostomy tract seeding following endosurgical techniques are exceedingly rare. Additionally, reports of retroperitoneal recurrence following endosurgical resection are also rare.

REFERENCES

1. Blute, M.L., Segura, J.W., Patterson, D.E., et al.: Impact of endourology on diagnosis and management of upper urinary tract urothelial cancer. J. Urol., *141*: 1298, 1989.
2. Huffman, J.L.: Endoscopic management of upper urinary tract urothelial cancer. J. Endourol., *4*:S–141, 1990.
3. Huffman, J.L., Bagley, D.H., Lyon, E.S., et al.: Endoscopic diagnosis and treatment of upper tract urothelial tumors. A preliminary report. Cancer, *55*:1422, 1985.
4. Nurse, D.E., Woodhouse, C.R.J., Kellett, M.J., et al.: Percutaneous removal of upper tract tumors. World J. Urol., *7*:131, 1989.
5. Orihuela, E., and Smith, A.D.: Percutaneous treatment of transitional cell carcinoma of the upper urinary tract. Urol. Clin. North Am., *15*:425, 1988.

1072-B *(Campbell's, pp. 2300–2301)*

In general, tumors that are greater than 1 cm in diameter in the renal pelvis are difficult to ablate or resect with the ureteroscope, and an antegrade percutaneous approach is preferred. Both approaches have the risk of perforation of the renal pelvis with retroperitoneal seeding but, in addition, the percutaneous procedure has the risk of seeding of the access tract; however, this has not been found to be a problem. With the percutaneous approach, a standard resectoscope may be used or the tumor alternatively can be ablated with a laser or fulgurated. However, with ureteroscopy, one is generally limited to the use of laser or fulguration if it is a tumor in the proximal ureter or renal pelvis. In females, the rigid ureteroscope may be passed to a level above the iliac vessels and resection of tumor carried out with an electrocautery loop through the rigid ureteroscope. This, however, is not recommended in males. When performing endoscopic resection of the upper tract, care should be taken to ensure that irrigant pressure is not above 40 cm of water. Higher pressures may lead to renal back-flow and may have the risk of entry of tumor cells into the vascular system. When performing laser ablation of the tumor, a 400 μm Nd:YAG laser probe is used and the energy is set at 25 to 30 watts. When tumor is either completely resected or ablated with the laser, random biopsies should be performed of the urothelium around the tumor site.

1073-C *(Campbell's, pp. 2303–2304)*

Within the realm of urologic surgery, laparoscopy has been employed to perform pelvic node dissection, varicocelectomy, nephrectomy, lymphocele drainage, removal of ureteral calculi, and in the evaluation of the non-palpable testes. Standard techniques in all laparoscopic procedures include the induction of pneumoperitoneum (which is done with carbon dioxide gas) as well as the placement of trocars and sheaths into the intraperitoneal space. The pneumoperitoneum is first induced, and this is done by passing a Veress needle into the abdominal cavity through a infraumbilical midline approach and insufflating with carbon dioxide. The pressure in the abdomen is brought to the range of 10 to 15 mm of Mercury and maintained there. In the laparoscopic varicocelectomy, the spermatic veins are observed immediately superior to the internal inguinal ring and seen to join the vas in this region. They are ligated and divided just proximal to joining the vas. With the laparoscopic drainage of a lymphocele, the peritoneum overlying the lymphocele is resected or incised and the lymphocele is marsupialized to the intraperitoneal space. A piece of omentum may be placed into the lymphocele to maintain patency of the orifice between the lymphocele and peritoneal cavity. With the laparoscopic nephrectomy, after detachment of the kidney, it is entrapped in a surgical sack that is passed into the abdomen and drawn up to the under surface of the abdominal wall. The kidney is then morcellated in the sack and the contents aspirated. The kidney is not removed through a flank incision.

REFERENCES

1. Semm, K.: Endoscopic Abdominal Surgery. Chicago, Year Book Medical Publishers, 1987, p. 499.
2. Winfield, H.N., and Ryan, K.G.: Experimental laparoscopic surgery: Potential clinical applications in urology. J. Endourol., *4*:37, 1990.
3. Clayman, R.V., Kavoussi, L.R., Soper, N.J., et al.: Laparoscopic nephrectomy: Initial case report. J. Urol., *146*:1, 1991.

PART XIV

UROLOGIC SURGERY

CHAPTERS 63 THROUGH 87

DIRECTIONS: Each question below contains suggested responses. Select the ONE BEST response to each question.

1074. The two strongest predictors of perioperative cardiac morbidity are recent myocardial infarction and:

A. Rhythm other than sinus or sinus with premature atrial contractions
B. Age over 70 years
C. Poor general medical status
D. Congestive heart failure
E. Emergency operation

1075. The indications for preoperative administration of digitalis include all of the following EXCEPT:

A. Prior history of congestive heart failure
B. Cardiac dysfunction with evidence of impaired ventricular performance
C. Nocturnal angina
D. Atrial fibrillation or flutter with a rapid ventricular response
E. Advanced age

1076. What percentage of perioperative myocardial infarction are silent?

A. 10 per cent
B. 30 per cent
C. 50 per cent
D. 70 per cent
E. 90 per cent

1077. Supraventricular tachycardia occurs postoperatively in what percentage of surgical patients?

A. Less than 5 per cent
B. 10 per cent
C. 15 per cent
D. 20 per cent
E. 25 per cent

1078. All of the following statements are true about hypertension EXCEPT:

A. Patients with a diastolic blood pressure less than 120 mm Hg do not have an increased risk of cardiac complications.
B. Patients whose normal systolic pressure drops by one third for 10 minutes have an increased incidence of cardiovascular complications.
C. Abrupt cessation of clonidine may precipitate severe hypertension.
D. Beta-adrenergics should be withdrawn prior to surgery.
E. Patients receiving diuretics should be evaluated for hypokalemia.

1079. Which one of the following statements about myocardial depression and anesthetic agents is *true*?

A. Morphine produces a relatively large amount of myocardial depression.
B. Meperidine produces a relatively large amount of myocardial depression.
C. Halothane produces little myocardial depression.
D. Barbiturates have a marked depressant effect even in small doses.
E. Nitrous oxide produces marked myocardial depression.

1080. All of the following are indications for direct blood pressure monitoring EXCEPT:

A. Age over 70 years
B. Rapid change in blood pressure due to cardiac disease
C. Expectation of large volumes of blood loss
D. Sudden changes in blood pressure due to nature of the surgery
E. Need for postoperative vasodilator or vasopressor therapy

1081. All of the following are associated with increased postoperative pulmonary morbidity EXCEPT:

A. Cigarette smoking
B. Upper abdominal incision
C. Procedure over 3 hours
D. Mild obesity
E. Protein-depleted nutritional status

1082. Which of the following statements about mechanical ventilation is *false*?

A. Cardiac output may be decreased due to increased intrathoracic pressure.
B. Oxygen toxicity becomes a concern when FIO_2 is greater than 50 per cent.
C. Ventilation-perfusion imbalance results from the larger influence of disease and positioning on perfusion than on ventilation.
D. Barotrauma can be a major complication.
E. Respiratory alkalosis is related to hyperventilation.

1083. All of the following statements are true regarding regional vs. general anesthesia EXCEPT:

A. Regional anesthesia carries a lower perioperative mortality in hip surgery.
B. Regional anesthesia is *not* associated with a de-

creased morbidity in high-risk patients within 3 months of myocardial infarction.
C. Evidence suggests that FRC (functional residual capacity) is better preserved with regional anesthesia.
D. Regional anesthesia is associated with a 35 per cent lower blood loss in retropubic prostatectomy.
E. There is a significant decrease in thromboembolic events utilizing regional anesthesia in surgery below the umbilicus.

1084. What percentage of deep venous thromboses (DVTs) are clinically silent?

A. 10 per cent
B. 20 per cent
C. 30 per cent
D. 40 per cent
E. 50 per cent

1085. Risk factors for deep venous thrombosis (DVT) include all of the following EXCEPT:

A. Anesthesia duration greater than 1 hour
B. Age greater than 60 years
C. Presence of malignant disease
D. Use of estrogens
E. Race

1086. All of the following statements are true regarding the prevention and treatment of DVT EXCEPT:

A. Early ambulation has been shown to decrease the incidence of DVT in patients after myocardial infarction.
B. Regional anesthesia reduces the incidence of DVT.
C. Antiplatelet therapy, specifically aspirin derivatives, has been shown to prevent DVT.
D. Low-dose heparin is effective in the prevention of DVT and is not associated with an increased risk of bleeding.
E. Pneumatic compression devices are effective in prevention of DVT through mechanisms other than the direct mechanical compression.

1087. Which one of the following statements about patients with renal insufficiency is *true*?

A. Under normal conditions patients are able to maintain potassium balance only until GFR (glomerular filtration rate) falls below 50 ml/min.
B. Metabolic alkalosis is rarely encountered postoperatively.
C. Diabetics with renal insufficiency (creatinine >1.7 mg/dl) have a 10 per cent risk of mild nephropathy after receiving contrast compared to a 2 per cent risk in patients not receiving contrast.
D. Hypocalcemia and hypophosphatemia are rarely seen.
E. The best test to assess their increased risk of hemorrhage is the prothrombin time.

1088. The most common cause of anemia is:

A. Vitamin B_{12} deficiency
B. Iron deficiency
C. Folic acid deficiency
D. Hemolytic anemia
E. Chronic renal insufficiency

1089. All of the following statements are true about hemostatic competence EXCEPT:

A. Patients with sickle cell trait experience no increased surgical risk.
B. von Willebrand's disease is related to a deficiency in factor VII complex.
C. Platelet function is measured by bleeding time.
D. Prothrombin time assesses the extrinsic pathway.
E. Patients with vitamin K deficiency have prolongation of prothrombin and partial thromboplastin time.

1090. Blood glucose should be maintained in what range perioperatively to decrease the incidence of wound infection?

A. Less than 100 mg/dl
B. 80 to 125 mg/dl
C. 125 to 250 mg/dl
D. Less than 300 mg/dl

1091. All of the following statements are true about supplemental steroid therapy perioperatively EXCEPT:

A. Markedly impaired cortisol secretion during surgery is unlikely if a normal response to adrenocorticotropic hormone is demonstrated preoperatively.
B. No supplemental therapy is needed for patients receiving topical therapy.
C. Patients receiving systemic steroids for greater than 1 week in the previous 6 months should receive supplemental therapy.
D. Patients with anticipated bilateral adrenalectomy should receive supplemental therapy.
E. Patients with anticipated unilateral adrenalectomy for a cortisol-producing tumor should receive supplemental therapy.

1092. What percentage of catheterized patients will have urinary tract infection after 10 days?

A. 50 per cent
B. 60 per cent
C. 70 per cent
D. 80 per cent
E. 90 per cent

1093. All of the following statements are true about urologic surgery in pregnancy EXCEPT:

A. Radiographic evaluation of the urinary tract should be limited to emergency situations.
B. Endoscopic extraction of distal ureteral calculi is possible during any phase of pregnancy.
C. Percutaneous nephrostomy drainage may be safely employed during pregnancy.
D. The dose of radiation associated with fetal harm is in excess of 50 rad (cGy), a dose over 50 times that associated with the usual intravenous pyelogram.
E. The incidence of renal calculus in pregnancy is approximately 2.5 times that of nonpregnant women.

1094. The right adrenal vein drains into the:

A. Right renal vein
B. Inferior phrenic vein
C. Inferior vena cava
D. Right gonadal vein
E. Lumbar vein

1095. The adrenal medulla develops from the:

A. Endoderm
B. Mesoderm
C. Mesonephric duct
D. Paramesonephric duct
E. Neuroectoderm

1096. The only source of aldosterone production is the:

A. Zona glomerulosa
B. Zona fasciculata
C. Zona reticularis
D. Adrenal medulla
E. Macula densa

1097. Adrenocorticotropic hormone (ACTH) shares a common precursor protein with all of the following EXCEPT:

A. β-Lipotropin (β-LPH)
B. α-Melanocyte stimulating hormone (α-MSH)
C. β-Melanocyte stimulating hormone (β-MSH)
D. Thyroid-stimulating hormone (TSH)
E. β-Endorphin

1098. The production of which adrenal hormone is not primarily influenced by ACTH:

A. Cortisol
B. Aldosterone
C. Dehydroepiandrosterone
D. 17-Hydroxyprogesterone
E. 11-Deoxycortisol

1099. All of the following statements regarding adrenal cortical hormones are true EXCEPT:

A. They exert their effects primarily in the nucleus of cells.
B. Glucocorticoids are essential for life.
C. Aldosterone stimulates sodium reabsorption and increased secretion of potassium and hydrogen.
D. Adrenal androgens are only weakly active compared to testosterone.
E. Glucocorticoids stimulate glycogenolysis and enhanced peripheral glucose utilization.

1100. The predominant hormone produced by the adrenal medulla is:

A. Cortisol
B. Aldosterone
C. Epinephrine
D. Norepinephrine
E. Topamine

1101. The primary metabolite of adrenal catecholamines found in the urine is:

A. Metanephrine
B. Vanillyl mandelic acid (VMA)
C. Normetanephrine
D. Epinephrine
E. Homovanillic acid

1102. Cushing's syndrome is caused by excess circulating:

A. Aldosterone
B. Glucocorticoids
C. Dehydroepiandrosterone
D. Epinephrine
E. Norepinephrine

1103. The most common cause of Cushing's syndrome is:

A. Pituitary adenoma
B. Adrenal adenoma
C. Adrenal carcinoma
D. Exogenous ingestion of steroids
E. Ectopic ACTH production by tumors

1104. All of the following are found in patients with Cushing's syndrome EXCEPT:

A. Loss of diurnal variation in cortisol levels
B. Suppression of cortisol release with low-dose dexamethasone
C. Elevated serum cortisol levels
D. Elevated levels of urinary free cortisol

1105. Treatment with which of the following agents impairs aldosterone production?

A. Metyrapone
B. Ketoconazole
C. Bromocriptine
D. Pituitary irradiation
E. Aminoglutethimide

1106. A 40-year-old white female undergoes a CT scan of the abdomen for intermittent epigastric discomfort and is found to have a 4-cm solid right adrenal mass. Biochemical evaluation is without evidence of a functioning tumor. The tumor/liver intensity on MRI is less than 2. The appropriate next step in management is:

A. Exploration and right adrenalectomy
B. Fine needle aspiration of the lesion under CT guidance
C. Treatment with aminoglutethimide
D. Follow-up CT scans at 6-month intervals for at least 18 months
E. No further work-up

1107. The hallmark of Cushing's syndrome secondary to adrenal carcinoma is:

A. Purple striae
B. Virilization
C. Temporal hair loss
D. Hypertension
E. Thin skin

1108. All of the following statements regarding adrenocortical carcinoma are true EXCEPT:

A. The most common site of metastasis is the lung.
B. Five-year survival approaches 70 per cent.
C. These tumors often extend into adjacent structures, especially the kidney.
D. Most of these tumors are hormonally active.
E. Hormone levels can be used as markers for tumor recurrence after surgical removal.

1109. The most successful adrenolytic agent used in metastatic adrenal carcinoma is:

A. o, p′-DDD
B. Aminoglutethimide
C. Ketoconazole
D. Metyrapone
E. Suramin

1110. A 53-year-old white male with history of tuberculosis in the past undergoes right radical nephrectomy for renal cell carcinoma. Postoperatively, the patient is noted to be febrile (101°) and to have hypotension, which responds to saline boluses. Laboratory abnormalties include Na, 124; K, 5.4; glucose, 300; Hb, 13; Hct, 38. The treatment of choice is:

A. Broad-spectrum antibiotics
B. Alpha-adrenergic agonist
C. 3 per cent saline fluid administration
D. Transfusion of packed red blood cells
E. Glucocorticoids

1111. All of the following are characteristics of hyperaldosteronism EXCEPT:

A. Hypertension
B. Metabolic alkalosis
C. Elevated aldosterone levels despite sodium loading
D. Hyperkalemia
E. Low plasma renin activity despite sodium restriction

1112. All of the following statements regarding pheochromocytoma are true EXCEPT:

A. It has been associated with both sustained hypertension and paroxysmal hypertension.
B. It has been associated with multiple endocrine adenoma I (MEA I).
C. Metaiodobenzylguanidine (MIBG) scans can be used to localize the tumor.
D. Preoperative alpha-adrenergic block is recommended.
E. Intraoperative arrhythmias can be managed with either lidocaine or propanolol.

1113. A 25-year-old male undergoes surgery to remove a right pheochromocytoma. Upon ligation of the adrenal vein, a precipitous fall in blood pressure is noted. The first step in management should be:

A. Remove the ligature from the adrenal vein, then slowly clamp the vein before ligating it
B. A saline infusion
C. Low-dose norepinephrine
D. Beta blockade
E. Cross-clamp the patient's aorta

1114. In a patient suspected of having a left adrenal pheochromocytoma, the incision of choice is a:

A. Posterior approach
B. Modified posterior approach
C. 12th rib flank incision
D. Transabdominal chevron
E. Thoracoabdominal approach

1115. The incision of choice for bilateral adrenal ablation is the:

A. Bilateral posterior approach
B. 11th rib approach (flank)
C. Modified posterior approach
D. Transabdominal chevron
E. Thoracoabdominal approach

1116. All of the following are constant vascular segments of the kidney EXCEPT:

A. Apical
B. Anterior
C. Posterior
D. Lateral
E. Basilar

1117. In patients with impaired respiratory function, the preferred approach to remove a renal mass is:

A. Flank
B. Anterior
C. Dorsal
D. Thoracoabdominal
E. Laparoscopic

1118. All of the following conditions of a patient following unilateral nephrectomy with a normal contralateral kidney are true EXCEPT:

A. Stable overall renal function
B. Normal life expectancy
C. Increased risk of hypertension
D. No increased risk of proteinuria
E. Glomerular filtrating rate ultimately maintained at up to 75 per cent of the normal valve when compensatory hypertrophy occurs

1119. The maximum tolerable period of warm ischemia (renal arterial occlusion) before permanent renal damage is sustained is:

A. 10 minutes
B. 20 minutes
C. 30 minutes
D. 60 minutes
E. 90 minutes

1120. All of the following have been shown to increase the risk of damage by renal ischemia EXCEPT:

A. Intermittent clamping of the renal artery, as opposed to continuous arterial occlusion
B. Intravenous administration of mannitol *prior* to arterial occlusion
C. Manual renal compression to control hemorrhage, as opposed to simple arterial occlusion
D. Continuous occlusion of both the renal vein and artery, as opposed to the artery clamp
E. Lack of use of renal hypothermia

1121. When performing a flank incision, one can expect to find the intercostal neurovascular bundle:

A. Superficial to the external oblique aponeurosis
B. Between the external oblique and internal oblique muscles
C. Between the internal oblique and transversus abdominis muscles
D. Between the transversus abdominis muscles and the transversalis fascia
E. Deep to the transversalis fascia

1122. The principal advantage of the abdominal approach for renal surgery is:

A. Low incidence of postoperative ileus
B. Lower risk of bowel obstruction
C. Ease of access to upper pole masses
D. Excellent exposure of the renal pedicle
E. Lower incidence of splenic trauma

1123. All of the following are indications for simple nephrectomy EXCEPT:

A. Nonfunctioning kidney that is chronically infected
B. Pyelocutaneous fistula and normal contralateral kidney in a patient whose general condition is too poor to permit a reconstructive operation

C. Renovascular hypertension due to uncorrectable renal artery disease
D. Multicystic dysplastic kidney impeding alimentation or respiration
E. 4-cm renal cell carcinoma with a normal contralateral kidney

1124. During radical nephrectomy, vena caval hemorrhage is frequently caused by laceration or avulsion of all the following veins EXCEPT:

A. Inferior mesenteric vein
B. Lumbar veins
C. Right gonadal vein
D. Right adrenal vein
E. Renal veins

1125. The mortality rate for radical nephrectomy is approximately:

A. <4 per cent
B. 6 per cent
C. 8 per cent
D. 10 per cent
E. 12 per cent

1126. All of the following are indications for partial nephrectomy in patients with renal malignancy EXCEPT:

A. Bilateral renal cell carcinoma
B. Localized unilateral renal cell carcinoma in a patient with renal insufficiency
C. Localized renal cell carcinoma and a contralateral kidney involved with renal calculi
D. Localized renal cell carcinoma and a normal opposite kidney
E. Renal cell carcinoma in a solitary kidney

1127. A 56-year-old white male undergoes a left lower pole partial nephrectomy for localized renal cell carcinoma. Three days postoperatively, his serum hematocrit drops from 34 to 27 per cent over 24 hours. He is afebrile, neither tachycardic nor hypotensive, and clinically he appears well. Initial management should be:

A. Hematology consult
B. Bed rest, serial hematocrit determinations, and blood transfusions as needed
C. Angiography and embolization of bleeding sites
D. Reoperation and suture ligation of bleeding sites
E. Reoperation and nephrectomy

1128. After an anatrophic nephrolithotomy for a calcium oxalate staghorn calculus, a patient is found to have a residual 1.5-cm fragment in a mid-pole calyx on postoperative KUB. Renal scan reveals good function bilaterally without evidence of obstruction. The next step in management should be:

A. Renacidin irrigation
B. Extracorporeal shock wave lithotripsy (ESWL) in 4–6 weeks
C. Extended pyelolithotomy
D. Reexploration and anatrophic nephrolithotomy
E. Nephrectomy

1129. All of the following are indications for surgical repair of ureteropelvic function obstruction EXCEPT:

A. Symptoms of obstruction
B. Impaired renal function
C. Bilateral involvement with normal renal function in an asymptomatic patient
D. Development of calculi in the involved system
E. Recurrent pyelonephritis on the involved side

1130. The procedure of choice to best manage a 38-year-old white male with recurrent episodes of left flank pain and a work-up consistent with left ureteropelvic function obstruction in a functioning kidney is:

A. Observation with follow-up renal scans
B. Ureteral stent placement
C. Ureteropelvic junction balloon dilatation
D. Open pyeloplasty
E. Nephrectomy

1131. All of the following regarding techniques of pyeloplasty are true EXCEPT:

A. The Foley Y-V plasty was specifically designed for reconstruction of UPJ obstruction associated with a lower ureteral insertion.
B. Only a dismembered pyeloplasty allows complete excision of the abnormal ureteropelvic junction.
C. The Culp-DeWeerd spiral flap is very helpful in UPJ obstruction associated with a long upper ureteral stricture.
D. To preserve vascular integrity in flap pyeloplasties, the ratio of flap length to width should not exceed 3 to 1.
E. The Scardino-Prince vertical flap has largely been supplanted by the standard dismembered pyeloplasty.

1132. A 57-year-old white male is referred with persistent urinary drainage following an open pyelolithotomy and pyeloplasty. Antegrade nephrostogram and retrograde pyelogram showed an intrarenal pelvis with a 3-cm strictured area between the renal pelvis and the patient's ureter. Renal scan revealed good renal function. The procedure of choice to repair the problem is:

A. Endopyelotomy
B. Dismembered pyeloplasty
C. Scardino vertical flap
D. Ureterocalycostomy
E. Nephrectomy

1133. Open renal biopsy is generally preferred over percutaneous needle biopsy in all of the following situations EXCEPT:

A. Solitary kidney
B. Transplant kidney
C. Coagulopathy
D. Atypical anatomy
E. Infants and children

1134. The preferred surgical approach to repair a ureteropelvic junction obstruction in a horseshoe kidney is:

A. Flank
B. Dorsal lumbotomy
C. Anterior subcostal extraperitoneal
D. Midline transabdominal
E. Thoracoabdominal

1135. Concerning the percentage of end-stage renal disease (ESRD) due to different disease states, which of the following is *false*?

A. 30 per cent is due to diabetes mellitus
B. 14 per cent is due to glomerulonephritis
C. 12 per cent is due to cystic kidney disease
D. 26 per cent is due to hypertension
E. 6 per cent is due to other urologic diseases

1136. Pretransplant urologic evaluation includes all of the following EXCEPT:

A. Upper tract evaluation usually by sonography
B. Urine or bladder wash culture
C. Retrograde contrast study of existing urinary diversion to assess suitability for urinary tract reconstruction
D. Voiding cystourethrography
E. Cystoscopy and bladder biopsy in patients who have contracted bladders after multiple lower urinary tract operations

1137. The following urologic interventions are appropriate prior to renal transplantation EXCEPT:

A. Transurethral prostatectomy in men with obstructing prostates
B. Bilateral orchiectomy in a 72-year-old patient with slowly rising PSA
C. The use of semirigid penile prosthesis if the prosthesis is placed prior to transplantation
D. Pretransplant bilateral nephrectomy for hypertension refractory to dialysis and medications
E. Suprapubic cystostomy with bladder outlet procedures, such as TURP, to allow instillation of sterile water and voiding in the oliguric patient

1138. In the evaluation of potential kidney donors, serologic screening should be performed for all of the following EXCEPT:

A. Hepatitis
B. Varicella-zoster virus
C. Cytomegalovirus
D. Syphilis
E. Human immunodeficiency virus

1139. The evaluation of potential living kidney donors should include each of the following studies EXCEPT:

A. Intravenous pyelography
B. Chest x-ray
C. Aortography or digital subtraction arteriography of the renal vessels in potential donors who have satisfied all other requirements
D. Serial serum creatinine levels
E. Abdominal computed tomography scan with contrast

1140. Which of the following is *not* recommended when performing a living-donor nephrectomy?

A. The patient is fully heparinized prior to clamping the renal vasculature and removing the kidney.
B. Diuresis is confirmed by transecting the ureter and observing urine flow before interrupting renal circulation.
C. 25 grams of mannitol is given intravenously over 1 hour beginning with the skin incision.
D. After removal of the kidney, it is immediately flushed with Ringer's lactate, Euro-Collins solution, or UW solution at 4°C.
E. Living-donor nephrectomy is performed through a flank incision.

1141. Which of the following consequences of donor nephrectomy is *false*?

A. Endogenous creatinine clearance rapidly approaches 70 to 80 per cent of the preoperative level following donor nephrectomy.
B. The risk of developing late hypertension following donor nephrectomy is nearly the same as that of the general population.
C. Mild anemia develops in 5 per cent of patients following donor nephrectomy.
D. Acceptable levels of endogenous creatinine clearance are sustained for more than 10 years following donor nephrectomy.
E. The long-term risks of donor nephrectomy are low enough such that it is an acceptable procedure when patients are fully informed.

1142. Which of the following statements concerning cadaveric donors and grafts is *false*?

A. Eighteen months is generally accepted as the lower age limit for cadaveric kidneys.
B. In adult recipients graft, survival is significantly lower when the donor is below age 6 as compared to above age 6.
C. Fifty-five years has been used as the upper age limit for the cadaveric pool.
D. Age-matching of donor and recipient improves graft survival.
E. The 1-year graft survival for grafts from donors between ages 55 and 60 is 12 per cent lower than that for grafts from donors between ages 16 and 30.

1143. All of the following malignancies are contraindications for cadaveric kidney donation EXCEPT:

A. Bronchioalveolar carcinoma
B. Astrocytoma
C. Colorectal adenocarcinoma
D. Infiltrating duct carcinoma
E. Malignant melanoma

1144. All of the following steps are recommended for renal preservation in the brain-dead cadaver EXCEPT:

A. Maintenance of blood pressure and urinary output with a fluid challenge
B. Use of furosemide or a mannitol infusion if vasopressors and intravascular volume expansion do not maintain a urine output of 0.5 ml/kg/hr
C. Administration of Pitressin for unmanageable diabetes insipidus
D. Infusion of dopamine, dobutamine, or isoproterenol when central venous pressure is greater than 15 cm H_2O and urine output is below 0.5 ml/kg/hr
E. Papaverine infusion to the renal arteries when other measures fail to maintain urine output

1145. All of the following statements concerning warm ischemic injury to the kidney are true EXCEPT:

A. Depletion of ATP leads to impairment of the cellular sodium-potassium pump, which leads

in turn to cellular swelling when sodium ion and water passively diffuse into the cell.
B. During reperfusion, hypoxanthine from ATP degradation is oxidized, giving rise to the formation of free radicals, which cause additional cell damage.
C. Increasing intracellular magnesium levels lead to poisoning of mitochondrial enzymes and complete arrest of oxidative phosphorylation.
D. Anaerobic glycolysis lowers intracellular pH and leads to lysosomal enzyme activation with resultant cell membrane damage.
E. Influx of calcium into the cell through damaged cell membrane leads to cell death.

1146. University of Wisconsin (UW) solution contains all of the following EXCEPT:
A. ATP-$MgCl_2$
B. Allopurinol
C. Glutathione
D. Potassium lactobionate
E. Adenosine

1147. Which of the following statements concerning renal preservation is *false*?
A. The use of UW solution results in a significantly more rapid reduction in postoperative serum creatinine level following renal transplantation than the use of Euro-Collins solution.
B. UW solution may be used to preserve other abdominal organs.
C. UW solution contains dexamethasone as a membrane-stabilizing agent.
D. The function of the calcium channel blocker in Euro-Collins solution is to reduce cellular damage by inhibiting intracellular calcium influx.
E. Euro-Collins solution contains glucose and sodium bicarbonate, unlike UW solution.

1148. Which of the following statements concerning the standard technique for renal transplantation is *false*?
A. In adults and large children, the kidney is placed extraperitoneally in the iliac fossa contralateral to the donor nephrectomy site.
B. Mannitol infusion should begin when the vascular anastomosis is started.
C. An antireflux ureteroneocystostomy is commonly performed from an extravesical approach.
D. In men, the spermatic cord should be preserved by mobilizing and retracting it medially during the procedure.
E. Placement of a double-J ureteral stent is the rule.

1149. Following renal transplantation, early postoperative management includes all of the following EXCEPT:
A. Monitoring of serum electrolyte levels every 4 to 8 hours.
B. Continuous bladder irrigation with antibiotic solution until the Foley catheter is removed.
C. Intravenous fluid replacement with 0.45 per cent saline at a rate of hourly urine output plus insensible losses until diuresis slows and oral intake is established.
D. Catheter urinary drainage until a retrograde cystogram documents the absence of extravasation.
E. Radioisotope renogram and ultrasonogram of the transplant 24 to 48 hours after the procedure.

1150. Which of the following statements concerning renal allograft rejection is *false*?
A. Graft losses due to acute rejection usually occur within 3 months of transplantation.
B. Hyperacute rejection occurs immediately following revascularization and is due to circulating host cytotoxic antibodies.
C. Accelerated rejection occurs within weeks to months and is mediated by humoral and cellular components of the immune response.
D. Typical histologic findings for acute rejection consist of mononuclear cellular infiltration and vasculitis.
E. Signs of acute rejection include pain over the graft, decreased urinary output, fluid retention, and decreased glomerular filtration and tubular function on nuclear renal scan.

1151. Which of the following statements concerning histocompatibility is *false*?
A. Histocompatibility of HLA class I antigens is of greater importance than ABO compatibility.
B. Major histocompatibility class I antigens are present on all nucleated cells and are detected by serotyping T-lymphocytes.
C. Major histocompatibility class II antigens HLA-DR, HLA-DQ, and HLA-DP are present on B-lymphocytes, monocytes, macrophages, dendritic cells, activated T-lymphocytes, and on some endothelial cells.
D. Major histocompatibility antigens are encoded by major histocompatibility complex autosomal genes on the short arm of chromosome 6.
E. There is a .25 probability of HLA identity between sibling and patient.

1152. Which of the following statements concerning the immune response of the host toward graft tissue is *false*?
A. Class I and II major histocompatibility (MHC) antigens on donor dendritic cells stimulate recipient T-lymphocytes and initiate rejection.
B. Host macrophages process MHC antigens and present class II antigens to host CD4+ helper T-cells, and class I antigens to CD8+ precursor cytotoxic T-cells.
C. Class I antigen activated B lymphocytes are transformed by IL-4, IL-5, and IL-6 into plasma cells that produce cytotoxic antibodies against the graft class I MHC molecules.
D. Gamma interferon secreted by antigen-activated T-helper cells induces the expression of MHC class II antigens on kidney graft cells.
E. Activated cytotoxic cells secrete IL-1 which causes recruitment and activation of macrophages and monocytes.

1153. Which of the following statements concerning the mechanism of action of immunosuppressive agents is *false*?
A. Glucocorticoids block T-cell proliferation by blocking the production of IL-1 and IL-6.

B. Cyclosporine stops production and release of IL-2, and inhibits IL-2 receptor expression on helper and cytotoxic T-lymphocytes.
C. Azathioprine is an antimetabolite that is structurally similar to purine, and inhibits DNA synthesis and thus T-cell proliferation.
D. FK 506 is structurally similar to the macrolide antibiotics and similarly inhibits T-lymphocyte protein synthesis.
E. Monoclonal antibodies anti-Tac and 33B3.1 bind to the IL-2 receptor and prevent T-cell clonal expansion.

1154. Of the drugs below, the one that does *not* increase serum cyclosporine levels is:

A. Diltiazem
B. Phenytoin
C. Ketoconazole
D. Metoclopramide
E. Danazol

1155. In addition to nephrotoxicity, side effects of cyclosporine include the following EXCEPT:

A. Hirsutism
B. Gingival hypertrophy
C. Pruritus
D. Hypertension
E. Breast fibroadenomas

1156. All of the following facts are useful in distinguishing cyclosporine nephrotoxicity from acute rejection EXCEPT:

A. Graft blood flow is normal with cyclosporine toxicity but is reduced during acute rejection.
B. Serum creatinine usually rises rapidly when acute rejection is present in contrast to a slow rise with cyclosporine nephrotoxicity.
C. Fever may develop with acute rejection.
D. Urinary output may be maintained with cyclosporine nephrotoxicity but usually decreases with acute rejection.
E. Ultrasonography shows increased graft size with cyclosporine nephrotoxicity, but an unchanged graft size with acute rejection.

1157. In the management of pelvic fluid collections following renal transplantation, all of the following statements are true EXCEPT:

A. Large, uninfected lymphoceles may be marsupialized to the bladder.
B. Uninfected lymphoceles can be aspirated and sclerosed with iodine.
C. Small urinary leaks may be managed with simple bladder catheter drainage with or without percutaneous nephrostomy.
D. If extensive urinary tract repair is required for leakage, an omental wrap may be beneficial.
E. Excretory urography or percutaneous antegrade pyelography may be necessary to define the site of urinary extravasation when a retrograde cystogram fails.

1158. The incidence of renovascular hypertension among 60 million hypertensive patients in the United States is:

A. <1 per cent
B. 1–5 per cent
C. 5–10 per cent
D. 10–15 per cent
E. 15–25 per cent

1159. Which of the following statements concerning atherosclerotic renal artery lesions is *false*?

A. Atherosclerotic lesions make up two thirds of pathologic renal artery lesions.
B. Unilateral lesions more frequently involve the right renal artery.
C. Lesions may consist of a circumferential atheroma containing lipid with focal calcification.
D. Lesions may consist of an eccentric fibrous plaque composed of lipid deposits and collagen.
E. Lesions develop at or near the origin of the main renal arteries.

1160. The following are true concerning the renal mural dysplasias EXCEPT:

A. Multiple microaneurysms are seen with medial fibroplasia.
B. With subadventitial fibroplasia severe stenotic lesions develop, with dense collagen deposition in the outer portion of the media.
C. With true fibromuscular hyperplasia, segmental stenotic lesions develop unassociated with dissecting aneurysms.
D. For most renal mural dysplasias, the natural history involves progressive occlusion with dissection or development of aneurysms.
E. At the time of presentation, the mean age of patients is 35.

1161. Which of the following statements concerning renal artery aneurysms is *false*?

A. Saccular and fusiform aneurysms are associated with a high risk of spontaneous rupture.
B. Saccular aneurysms usually develop at the bifurcation of the main renal artery or a branch of the main renal artery.
C. Fusiform aneurysms typically lack calcifications and occur in young hypertensive patients with fibrous mural dysplasia.
D. Surgical intervention is not required for well-calcified aneurysms less than 2 cm when the patient is normotensive and asymptomatic.
E. Dissecting aneurysms are typically associated with atherosclerosis, intimal fibroplasia, and perimedial fibroplasia.

1162. Renal artery aneurysms are associated with each of the following diseases EXCEPT:

A. Takayasu's arteritis
B. Neurofibromatosis
C. Trauma
D. Scleroderma
E. Atherosclerosis

1163. Indications for corrective surgery in patients with renovascular disease include each of the following EXCEPT:

A. Poor compliance
B. Uncontrollable hypertension despite aggressive medical therapy
C. Deteriorating renal function
D. Failure of percutaneous angioplasty
E. Bilateral renal artery disease

1164. The following principles are applicable in the treatment of renovascular disease EXCEPT:

A. Percutaneous balloon angioplasty is an excellent method for treating renal artery stenosis due to atherosclerosis.
B. Medial fibroplasia should be treated with antihypertensives until hypertension can no longer be controlled.
C. In general lesions due to mural dysplasias respond well to balloon angioplasty, with an overall success rate of up to 85 per cent.
D. Complications such as renal artery intimal dissection or rupture following percutaneous balloon angioplasty usually are limited to patients who undergo multiple such dilations.
E. Failure or recurrence after a single trial of balloon angioplasty warrants surgical intervention in the case of renal artery lesions due to mural dysplasia.

1165. Perioperative monitoring and therapy during renovascular surgery include the following EXCEPT:

A. Swan-Ganz catheter monitoring
B. Systemic anticoagulation 30 minutes prior to cross-clamping the renal vessels
C. Electroencephalographic monitoring in patients with significant carotid artery disease
D. Mannitol and Lasix 1 to 2 hours before clamping of the renal vessels
E. Renal dose dopamine infusion

1166. Which of the following concerning approaches to the renal vasculature is *false*?

A. A supracostal 11th rib incision is adequate when repairing left renal artery stenosis.
B. A transverse upper abdominal incision from the lateral border of the contralateral rectus extending to the ipsilateral flank between the 11th and 12th ribs provides excellent access to high-lying aortorenal junctions.
C. The best exposure of the renal vessels comes through reflecting the colon.
D. To mobilize the colon for exposure of the right hilum and aorta, the peritoneum is incised from the cecum up to the hepatic flexure.
E. During the reflection of the distal transverse and descending colon, the spleen is protected by dividing the gastrocolic ligament and extending the incision laterally, finally dividing the splenocolic ligaments.

1167. Indications for nephrectomy in patients with renovascular disease include each of the following EXCEPT:

A. Extensive unilateral disease of the segmental vessels in high-risk or elderly patients
B. Total renal artery occlusion with back-bleeding found distal to the occlusion when the renal arteriotomy is made
C. Complete graft occlusion following failure of arterial reconstruction
D. Total renal artery occlusion with no evidence of perihilar or capsular collaterals on arteriogram
E. Severe unilateral parenchymal disease

1168. In performing a polar nephrectomy, all of the following are true EXCEPT:

A. After identifying the diseased polar vessel, it is ligated and injected distally with dilute methylene blue dye in order to define the avascular region.
B. The main renal artery need not be occluded during the procedure.
C. The collecting system is closed separately with 5.0 prolene suture.
D. The capsule over the pole to be resected is preserved for closure over the exposed parenchyma.
E. A Penrose drain is left adjacent to the site of partial nephrectomy.

1169. Which of the following is *inappropriate* therapy for a lesion occurring in a segmental artery that produces segmental ischemia, localized overproduction of renin, and hypertension?

A. Arterial bypass, when the segmental branch is large enough
B. Polar nephrectomy
C. Arteriotomy and dilation in the pediatric population
D. Midpolar partial nephrectomy
E. Angiography and complete embolization of the diseased segmental artery

1170. In performing a midpolar partial nephrectomy, all of the following statements are true EXCEPT:

A. A coronal semicircular incision is made in the capsule over the midpolar region, and the capsule peeled back on each side to expose a wedge of parenchyma which should show demarcation from injected dye.
B. The renal hilum is exposed, arterial branches meticulously identified, and diseased branches controlled with Silastic loops.
C. Diseased arterial branches are injected with a dilute solution of indigo carmine or methylene blue to demarcate the parenchyma supplied by these branches.
D. After closure of the collecting system, it is checked for leaks by injecting dilute methylene blue solution into the renal pelvis.
E. For closure, exposed parenchymal areas of each pole are covered with capsule initially peeled toward the pole, and then each pole is pexed to surrounding fascia to prevent its torsion.

1171. Disadvantages of renal endarterectomy include all of the following EXCEPT:

A. Complete cross-clamping of the aorta is required.
B. Vein patch angioplasty is often necessary to close the thin-walled renal artery without causing stenosis.
C. A substantial incidence of recurrent stenosis exists.
D. Thrombosis due to distal intimal flap is not uncommon.
E. Achieving adequate exposure for the aortic portion of the endarterectomy is difficult.

1172. All of the following describe appropriate techniques in transaortic endarterectomy EXCEPT:

A. The aorta is mobilized from the superior mesenteric artery to the iliac bifurcation.
B. A vertical aortotomy is made from the level of the inferior mesenteric artery cephalad to a

point above and to the left of the superior mesenteric artery.
C. Removal of the plaque begins circumferentially in the distal aorta and proceeds cephalad, and with traction on the plaque development of the plane in the proximal renal arteries proceeds.
D. A Fogarty catheter is routinely passed down the renal vessels to remove separated fragments of plaque.
E. The distal intima within the aorta is transfixed to the outer aortic wall with 4-5 mattress sutures using 6-0 polypropylene to prevent dissection.

1173. In the selection of a graft for aortorenal bypass graft surgery, which of the following is *false*?

A. In children with renal artery disease, Gor-Tex is the material of choice because of the small size of the saphenous vein.
B. Autogenous hypogastric artery has excellent long-term patency rates; however, in adults this vessel is often diseased.
C. Saphenous vein is the conduit of choice for aortorenal bypass.
D. Dacron has a high rate of early thrombosis.
E. When saphenous vein is not available in adults, cephalic vein is preferred over Gor-Tex.

1174. The following statements are true concerning saphenous vein aortorenal bypass grafting EXCEPT:

A. An end-to-end anastomosis between vein and renal artery is preferred because it permits the best laminar flow.
B. The graft is positioned anterior to the vena cava when performing a right renal artery bypass.
C. The vein graft is spatulated and anastomosed to the aorta with continuous 4-0 silk suture.
D. The single most important factor for long-term patency is a wide renal artery anastomosis.
E. An interrupted suture line is preferred for the renal artery anastomosis in children to prevent a purse-string effect with growth.

1175. Which of the following statements concerning splenorenal arterial bypass is *false*?

A. Splenorenal bypass should not be performed when the flow through the splenic artery is less than 125 ml/min.
B. If splenic artery length is insufficient, a saphenous vein interposition graft should be used to allow a tension-free anastomosis.
C. The splenic artery may be mobilized by a purely retroperitoneal approach.
D. After mobilization of the splenic artery, it is covered with papaverine-soaked sponges to cause dilation of the vessel.
E. The splenic artery is divided just proximal to its bifurcation in the hilum of the spleen, and a standard splenectomy is then performed.

1176. Which of the following statements concerning renal bypass grafting when extensive atherosclerosis or previous aortic surgery precludes the use of the aorta is *false*?

A. Liver function is not compromised, and renal-hepatic steal has not been demonstrated following hepatic-to-renal artery bypass graft.
B. For hepatorenal bypass, a reverse autogenous saphenous vein graft is used with an end-to-end anastomosis to the right hepatic artery.
C. Hepatic-to-renal artery saphenous vein bypass or gastroduodenal-to-renal artery bypass are preferred for the treatment of right renal artery stenosis.
D. The gastroduodenal artery is divided and anastomosed directly to the right renal artery in end-to-end fashion in the gastroduodenal-to-renal artery bypass.
E. The superior mesenteric-to-renal artery saphenous vein bypass may be used as a "bailout procedure" for both right or left renal artery lesions.

1177. Which of the following statements concerning the complications of renal revascularization is *false*?

A. Renal artery thrombosis is the most prevalent postoperative complication.
B. When severe unexplained hypertension persists following revascularization, digital subtraction angiography is indicated early to determine graft patency.
C. Coincidental splenectomy during renal bypass does not increase the incidence of postoperative complications.
D. Late studies show the development of aneurysmal dilation of saphenous vein grafts; however, no rupture of such grafts is reported.
E. When embolization of aortic plaque to the lower extremity occurs, systemic heparinization, papaverine, and fasciotomy may be of help.

1178. In the surgical management of renovascular disease, the following results are noted EXCEPT:

A. The National Cooperative Study Group showed a 66 per cent cure and improvement rate with an overall operative mortality of 8 per cent.
B. Due to an increase in surgical management of high-risk patients (those with bilateral renal artery disease), cure rates have declined to 44 per cent.
C. When revascularization is performed primarily to preserve renal function, successful outcomes are seen in 85 per cent.
D. A graft occlusion rate of 6.5 per cent is reported with a mean follow-up of more than 2 years.
E. Graft patency rates are significantly higher for visceral artery bypass procedures in comparison to aortorenal bypass.

1179. Following transection of the ureter, ureteral smooth muscle is usually completely healed by:

A. 48–72 hours
B. 1 week
C. 3 weeks
D. 6 weeks
E. 6 months

1180. All of the following are indications for proximal urinary diversion in ureteral surgery EXCEPT:

A. Uncomplicated repair of through and through ureteral incision
B. Infection with abscess

C. Contaminated wound
D. Impaired renal function
E. Difficult anastomosis in a solitary kidney

1181. All of the following factors regarding ureteral anastomosis should be adhered to in order to ensure successful healing EXCEPT:

A. Tension-free mucosa-to-mucosa anastomosis
B. Spatulated ureteral ends
C. Monofilament non-absorbable suture
D. Internal stents
E. Drainage of the periureteral area

1182. The most important factor in deciding the incision and approach to the ureter is:

A. Surgeon's preference
B. Segment of ureter to be operated on
C. Extent of disease
D. Patient's body habitus
E. Type of disease necessitating surgery

1183. A 52-year-old white male with idiopathic retroperitoneal fibrosis and right hydroureteronephrosis above the pelvic brim is initially managed with cystoscopy and right ureteral stent placement. The best approach to definitively manage this patient's problem is:

A. Observation
B. Balloon dilation of the right ureter
C. Right flank approach with ureterolysis
D. Gibson incision with biopsy of lesion and ureterolysis and lateralization of right ureter
E. Midline transabdominal approach, biopsy of mass, ureterolysis, and either intraperitonealization or lateralization of both ureters

1184. In performing ureterectomy for tumor, the major disadvantage of bladder cuff excision without vesicotomy is:

A. Increased risk of tumor spillage
B. Inability to identify and prevent injury to the contralateral ureteral orifice
C. Increased risk of injury to the ipsilateral superior vesicle pedicle
D. Inability to adequately resect the entire ureteral orifice
E. Increased risk of iatrogenic bladder diverticulum

1185. All of the following are options for surgical approaches in a 40-year-old female with a distal right ureteral calculus requiring ureterolithotomy EXCEPT:

A. Extraperitoneal flank
B. Lower midline
C. Pfannenstiel
D. Gibson
E. Transvaginal

1186. When performing ureterolithotomy, the incision in the ureter which best allows removal of the stone with the least chance of disrupting ureteral blood supply is:

A. Removal of a vertical ellipse of tissue
B. Transverse incision
C. Ureteral transection above the stone with subsequent reanastomosis
D. Oblique incision

1187. The most common complication of ureterolithotomy is:

A. Wound infection
B. Prolonged urinary leakage
C. Ureteral stricture
D. Urinoma
E. Sepsis

1188. All of the following statements regarding transvaginal approaches to the ureter in stone surgery are true EXCEPT:

A. Ureteroscopy has made this operation virtually unnecessary.
B. Recovery period is short.
C. Postoperative ureterovaginal fistula rate is high.
D. A major disadvantage is the extensive tissue dissection involved.
E. It is best not to attempt unless the stone can be palpated.

1189. The primary contraindication to ureteroureterostomy is:

A. Presence of abscess, hematoma, or urinoma
B. Vascular compromise of the ureter
C. Inadequate length to ensure a tension-free anastomosis.
D. Previous ureteral injury
E. Previous radiation therapy

1190. All of the following are contraindications to transureteroureterostomy EXCEPT:

A. Previous radiation therapy
B. Recurrent calculi
C. Defects in middle or lower third of the ureter
D. Uroepithelial tumors
E. Retroperitoneal fibrosis

1191. In transureteroureterostomy, the donor ureter is tunneled beneath the sigmoid mesenteric and preferentially:

A. Above the inferior mesenteric artery
B. Below the inferior mesenteric artery
C. With a sweep as acute as possible
D. Spatulated on its mesenteric border
E. Anastomosed to the recipient ureter as proximally as possible

1192. When performing a psoas hitch to repair a distal ureteral injury, the surgeon is unable to find the psoas tendon. The next step should be:

A. Downward renal mobilization and ureteroneocystostomy despite anastomotic tension
B. Creation of a Boari flap
C. Use of an intestinal interposition graft
D. Perform a psoas hitch by ensuring that large bites of muscle are taken with the sutures
E. Perform transureteroureterostomy

1193. When performing a Boari flap, the width of the base of the flap should be at least:

A. 1 cm
B. 2 cm
C. 3 cm
D. 4 cm
E. 5 cm

1194. All of the following statements regarding cutaneous ureterostomy are true EXCEPT:

A. It is often simple to perform with minimal exposure and trauma.
B. Due to vast ureteral blood supply, distal ureteral slough and stomal stricture are rare.
C. Both ureters should be brought to the skin to a simple stoma.
D. Preoperative irradiated skin or ureters increase the risk of stomal stenosis.
E. Conversion of cutaneous ureterostomy to intestinal conduit has been required in up to 50 per cent of patients.

1195. All of the following are contraindications for ileoureteral substitution EXCEPT:

A. Bilateral ureteral disease
B. Bladder outlet obstruction
C. Compromised renal function with serum creatinase of 2.0
D. Diffuse retroperitoneal malignancy
E. Crohn's disease

1196. Which of the following has the *lowest* priority in the management of the trauma patient with genitourinary tract injury?

A. Obtaining a computed tomography scan of the abdomen and pelvis
B. Establishment of an adequate airway
C. Establishment of vascular access, and subsequent fluid resuscitation
D. Gastric decompression in the unconscious patient
E. Control of hemorrhaging points

1197. Which of the following statements concerning the use of computed tomography (CT) in the evaluation of the genitourinary tract is *false*?

A. Minimal urinary extravasation not seen on intravenous pyelography may be discerned by CT scan with intravenous contrast.
B. CT scan accurately rules out a major renal vessel injury.
C. CT scan is the best study for identification of ectopic kidneys or congenital absence of a kidney.
D. Renal lesions, including infarction, as small as 1.5 cm can be diagnosed with CT scan.
E. On CT scan, the cortical rim sign is an indication of collateral arterial flow to a kidney.

1198. In the traumatized patient the following statement concerning the evaluation of the upper urinary tract is *false*:

A. If a nephrogram shows on IVP, there is a 95 per cent chance that no surgically correctable renal artery injury is present.
B. CT scan is the study of choice for evaluation of upper urinary tract trauma.
C. There is no place for the use of radionuclide studies in the early evaluation of blunt upper urinary tract trauma.
D. When a CT scan indicates possible main renal vessel injury, selective renal arteriography should be performed before deciding on nonoperative management.
E. When access to CT scanning is not available, the use of IVP and renal sonography is an acceptable alternative in the evaluation of blunt trauma to the upper urinary tract.

1199. In the traumatized patient, the need for retrograde urethrography prior to urethral catheterization is suggested by all of the following EXCEPT:

A. The patient is known to have sustained a straddle injury.
B. Blood is noted at the meatus on initial examination.
C. A Malgaigne fracture is present.
D. A scrotal laceration is found on examination.
E. Ecchymosis of the perineum is noted on examination.

1200. Concerning trauma to the adrenal gland, which of the following statements is *false*?

A. Isolated adrenal injuries among the population of blunt and penetrating trauma patients are exceedingly rare.
B. The adrenal medulla is very susceptible to hemorrhage from trauma, usually iatrogenic in nature.
C. Bilateral adrenal trauma during breech extraction occurs rarely.
D. Adrenal medulla hemorrhage is occasionally observed following harvest of the adrenal gland, for transplantation.
E. Immediately following blunt trauma to the adrenal gland, patients should be treated with 5 mg of phentolamine intravenously.

1201. All of the following are accepted indications for radiographic evaluation of the upper urinary tract in the trauma patient EXCEPT:

A. Gross hematuria
B. Microhematuria defined as less than 500 RBC/high power field
C. Microhematuria and a history of systolic BP less than 80 mm Hg
D. Penetrating abdominal trauma
E. Normal urinalysis and history indicating a fall from great height

1202. Which of the following is classified as a *major* renal injury?

A. A contained subcapsular hematoma
B. A nonexpanding perirenal hematoma with laceration of parenchyma extending 1 cm into the cortex
C. Microhematuria and a small parenchymal laceration noted to have perirenal extravasation on CT scan
D. A renal contusion measuring 2 cm on CT scan
E. Gross hematuria with a small renal contusion on CT scan

1203. Which of the following statements concerning renal pedicle injuries is *false*?

A. Pedicle injuries are associated with rapid deceleration from a high velocity.
B. Pedicle injuries include UPJ disruption and/or renal arterial intimal tear.
C. In children, greater spinal mobility is thought to be a factor in UPJ disruption.
D. Greater than 20 per cent of pedicle injuries are bilateral.

E. A significant mortality rate has been observed in trauma patients with renal pedicle injuries.

1204. The following surgical techniques are used when gaining exposure to the traumatized kidney EXCEPT:

A. A midline incision from xiphoid to pubis in multisystem trauma patients
B. Incision of the posterior peritoneum parallel to the inferior mesenteric vein and cephalad retraction of the left renal vein to expose the right and left renal arteries
C. Incision around the cecum and through the root of the mesentery, sacrificing both the inferior mesenteric artery and vein
D. The Kocher maneuver in exposing the right renal hilum
E. The dorsal lumbotomy incision when isolated renal trauma from a penetrating flank injury occurs in the adult

1205. When repairing a renal polar rupture or laceration, all of the following steps are advisable EXCEPT:

A. A devascularized pole should be excised.
B. The capsule should always be reflected from the segment removed and then used to cover remaining bare areas of parenchyma.
C. When repairing a lower pole injury, the lower pole should be positioned away from the UPJ region and fat interposed between the healing kidney and the UPJ region to prevent UPJ obstruction.
D. 3.0 silk may be used to close the collecting system following partial nephrectomy.
E. Nephropexy of the kidney to muscle fascia after partial nephrectomy may prevent Dietl's crisis and postoperative torsion of the pedicle.

1206. The following are true concerning ureteral injuries EXCEPT:

A. A direct ureteral injury from penetrating trauma is a rare event.
B. The occurrence of hematuria is a reliable indicator of ureteral injury.
C. With iatrogenic ureteral injuries, the ureter is most commonly injured at the pelvic brim.
D. A high-velocity missile (>2200 ft/s) may cause extensive coagulation necrosis of the ureter.
E. Unrecognized iatrogenic ureteral injuries usually manifest themselves between postoperative days 4 and 9 with flank pain and fever.

1207. Concerning the management of ureteral injuries, the following are true EXCEPT:

A. For injuries to the upper and middle third of the ureter, ureteroureterostomy with spatulation and ureteral stenting is the preferred method of management.
B. In elderly patients who require vascular graft placement at the time of ureteral injury or who have existing vascular grafts, nephrectomy may be preferable to ureterostomy and ureteral ligation followed by delayed ureteral repair.
C. Mobilization of both kidney and bladder is not required for ureteral repair unless 15 cm or more of ureter is destroyed.
D. When ureteral injury presents with urinoma and abscess formation, management should be in two stages, with initial drainage and diversion followed by definitive repair.
E. A psoas-bladder hitch and reimplantation or Boari bladder flap are useful when small lengths of distal ureter are destroyed.

1208. Which of the following statements concerning the etiology and diagnosis of the ruptured urinary bladder is *false*?

A. Intraperitoneal rupture of the bladder is indicated by poorly localized abdominal tenderness, hematuria, and intermittent inability to void.
B. To establish the diagnosis on cystogram, the bladder should be distended to a minimum of 250 ml with sterile contrast.
C. Both intraperitoneal and extraperitoneal ruptures may be associated with pelvic fractures without lacerations of the bladder due to bone fragments.
D. Extraperitoneal rupture often occurs when blunt external force is applied to the lower abdomen and the bladder is full.
E. Rupture of the bladder is found in approximately 5 per cent of patients suffering a pelvic fracture.

1209. Concerning the management of the ruptured urinary bladder the following are true EXCEPT:

A. Exploration of the peritoneal cavity should be performed if bloody fluid is observed there at the time of suprapubic cystostomy or if an intraperitoneal bladder rupture occurs.
B. The bladder wall is closed in three layers with chromic catgut or Vicryl suture, and typically a 20 French suprapubic tube is brought out through a separate stab wound in the bladder.
C. In the trauma patient with a ruptured bladder and a complete spinal cord injury, urinary diversion with conduit or vesicostomy should be considered at the time of repair of the perforation.
D. Extraperitoneal drainage is advantageous.
E. Typically, the suprapubic tube remains in place only 10 to 14 days unless the patient is immobilized due to other injuries.

1210. Concerning urinary trauma and pregnancy, the following statement is *false*:

A. Angioinfarction should be considered for branch lesions of the renal artery.
B. Radiation exposure should be minimized early in pregnancy, and ultrasonography may be used to assess renal injuries as well as evaluate the fetus and locate the placenta.
C. Cesarean section is indicated for gravid trauma patients when fetal distress is noted and gestational age is beyond 26 weeks.
D. Exploration for major renal injuries, nephrectomy, and/or urinary drainage should be performed for the "usual" indications regardless of pregnancy.
E. Penetrating trauma to the uterus and bladder must be managed with immediate C section followed by bladder repair.

1211. The following statement concerning the diagnosis of posterior urethral rupture is *false*:

A. On radiographic studies, the bladder silhouette is seen floating above the symphysis.

B. "Pie in the sky" refers to a radiographic view showing an intact vesicle neck and a bladder distended with contrast above the sacroiliac joint.
C. Extraperitoneal vesicle rupture can be confused with posterior urethral rupture when contrast material is seen in a deformed bladder and descends to the symphysis in teardrop fashion.
D. Urethrography with water-soluble contrast confirms the diagnosis.
E. Frequently the prostate is difficult to examine due to superior displacement—a finding first reported by Vermooten.

1212. The following are true concerning posterior urethral disruptions EXCEPT:

A. Major complications associated with posterior urethral injury include stricture, urinary incontinence, and impotence.
B. Complications associated with posterior urethral rupture may be minimized when delayed urethral repair is performed.
C. A vesicostomy is an acceptable alternative to suprapubic cystostomy in the infant with posterior urethral rupture.
D. More than 90 per cent of posterior urethral disruptions are complete and stricture of the disrupted region is the rule.
E. Complete epithelial apposition is not required for a good result during repair of the disrupted urethra.

1213. The following statement concerning rupture of the anterior urethra is *false*:

A. In Texas, a common cause of a blow to the perineum is from the toe of a boot, and this may lead to injury of the anterior urethra.
B. If Buck's fascia remains intact following anterior urethral rupture, extravasation will follow the shaft of the penis.
C. If Buck's fascia is violated, extravasation of urine and blood may proceed to the level of the clavicle.
D. Anterior urethral injuries are less common than posterior urethral injuries and most commonly occur as a result of straddle injuries.
E. Retrograde urethrography confirms the diagnosis of a ruptured anterior urethra.

1214. All of the following statements concerning the management of anterior urethral injuries are true EXCEPT:

A. If there is any doubt as to the integrity of the urethra, suprapubic cystostomy and delayed reconstruction of the urethra is recommended.
B. Severance of the urethra by a stab wound or blunt trauma to the perineum may be treated with exploration through a perineal incision at the time of injury, and oblique spatulated reanastomosis of the urethra.
C. The proximal urethra should be fixed to the underlying fascia during repair to minimize postoperative urethral stricture.
D. When evaluating anterior urethral injuries that occur with penetrating perineal trauma, proctoscopy must be included as part of the workup.
E. The urethra should be stented a minimum of 3 weeks following anterior urethral repair.

1215. All of the following statements regarding the management of penile injuries are true EXCEPT:

A. Split thickness skin grafts to the penis need to be 0.10 mm thick to allow for expansion during erection.
B. When rupture of the corporal fascia has occurred, immediate repair minimizes the development of scar tissue causing Peyronie's-like symptoms.
C. Objects that are placed around the penis circumferentially and give rise to strangulation may be removed by reducing the distal penile diameter with a tightly circumferentially wound string starting at the meatus.
D. When repairing penile amputation, survival of the distal part depends simply on reestablishment of venous drainage and approximation of the corpora.
E. Icing down the dismembered portion as soon as possible following penile amputation is the most important factor for subsequent survival after reattachment.

1216. In the management of scrotal injuries, the following statements are true EXCEPT:

A. Placement of the testis following scrotal loss in the superficial thigh is preferable to a subcutaneous abdominal placement.
B. Perineal skin may provide a useful flap to supplement lost scrotal tissue.
C. Following debridement of a testicle suffering a penetrating injury, a drain should be left beneath the tunica albuginea.
D. In patients with massive scrotal injury, the testicles may be left exposed if repeated debridements are contemplated, but should be treated with application of warm saline.
E. Broad-spectrum antibiotics are indicated when testicular parenchyma is exposed to foreign materials in the trauma setting.

1217. When using the stomach for reconstructive urologic surgery, which blood vessel(s) is (are) used to mobilize a pedicle of stomach to the pelvis?

A. Left gastric artery
B. Gastroepiploic arteries
C. Short gastric arteries
D. Right gastric artery
E. Gastroduodenal artery

1218. Unique properties of the ileum that allow distinction from the jejunum intraoperatively include all of the following EXCEPT:

A. The ileum has a small diameter.
B. The ileum has multiple arterial arcades.
C. The mesentery of the jejunum is thicker than the ileal mesentery.
D. The vessels composing the jejunal arcades are larger in diameter.
E. The ileum is more distal in location.

1219. The stomach has all of the following advantages over other intestinal segments EXCEPT:

A. It is less permeable to urinary solutes.
B. It acidifies the urine.

C. The incidence of bacteriuria is lower.
D. It produces less mucus.
E. The incidence of postoperative bowel obstruction is less than that seen with colonic segments.

1220. Mechanical bowel preparation via whole-gut lavage is contraindicated in all of the following conditions EXCEPT:

A. Unstable cardiovascular disease
B. Cirrhosis
C. Severe renal disease
D. Insulin-dependent diabetes mellitus
E. Congestive heart failure

1221. Preoperative antibiotic bowel preparation:

A. Is effective in patients with bowel obstruction
B. Reduces the risk of pseudomembranous enterocolitis
C. May allow the tenuous anastomosis to survive
D. Reduces postoperative thrush and stomatitis
E. Reduces postoperative diarrhea

1222. All of following techniques should be followed when anastomosing bowel EXCEPT:

A. Drains should be placed on or near the anastomoses.
B. The mesentery of the two segments of bowel must be realigned.
C. Irradiated bowel should be avoided if possible.
D. There should be accurate apposition of serosa to serosa.
E. Sutures should not be tied tightly, only enough to approximate tissue.

1223. What advantage do hand-sewn bowel anastomoses have over stapled anastomoses in urologic surgery?

A. Reduced tissue manipulation
B. A lower incidence of stone formation when exposed to urine
C. A better blood supply to the healing tissue
D. A wider lumen
E. Reduced length of postoperative paralytic ileus

1224. In an otherwise healthy patient who has no complications following intestinal surgery, colonic activity usually returns in:

A. Hours after the operative event
B. 24 hours
C. 2–4 days
D. 5–7 days
E. 7–8 days

1225. Urinary fistulas generally occur during what time frame following urinary intestinal diversion?

A. 7–10 days
B. >10 years
C. 1–3 days
D. 3–4 months
E. 8–10 months

1226. The most common cause of bowel obstruction following urinary intestinal diversion is:

A. Recurrent cancer
B. Volvulus
C. Internal hernia
D. Adhesions
E. Ogilvie's syndrome

1227. The causes of ureterointestinal anastomotic stricture include all of the following EXCEPT:

A. Ischemia
B. Urine leak
C. Radiation
D. Infection
E. Use of Silastic stents

1228. All of the following are nonrefluxing ureterointestinal anastomoses EXCEPT:

A. Bricker technique
B. Split nipple technique
C. Stickler technique
D. Leadbetter and Clarke technique
E. Goodwin technique

1229. The most successful technique for treating uretero-intestinal stricture is:

A. Antegrade incision of the stricture
B. Balloon dilatation of the stricture
C. Open surgical correction—resection and reimplantation
D. Retrograde incision of the stricture

1230. What type of urinary intestinal diversion has the highest incidence of sepsis and renal failure?

A. Ileal conduit
B. Ureterosigmoidostomy
C. Continent ileal cecal diversion
D. Gastric conduit
E. Jejunal conduit

1231. The electrolyte disorders of hyponatremia, hypochloremia, and hyperkalemia are most commonly seen with what type of urinary diversion?

A. Gastric conduit
B. Ileal conduit
C. Ileal cecal conduit
D. Jejunal conduit
E. Colonic conduit

1232. The appropriate treatment for the electrolyte disorders in question 1231 is:

A. Rehydration with sodium chloride
B. Furosemide
C. Intravenous calcium gluconate
D. Chlorpromazine
E. Kayexalate

1233. In a patient who is status-postileal conduit and has severe congestive heart failure, the best treatment for his (her) persistent hyperchloremic metabolic acidosis would be:

A. Sodium bicarbonate
B. Bicitra (sodium citrate and citric acid)
C. Furosemide
D. Polycitra (potassium citrate, sodium citrate, citric acid)
E. Nicotinic acid

1234. A patient who is status-postureterosigmoidostomy is undergoing treatment of severe hyperchloremic metabolic acidosis with sodium bicarbonate. During the course of treatment, he develops total paralysis. The most likely metabolic cause is:

A. Hypocalcemia
B. Body potassium depletion
C. Hyponatremia

D. Ammonia toxicity
E. Hypermagnesemia

1235. Patients who have had urinary intestinal diversions frequently have bacteriuria. Asymptomatic patients with relatively pure cultures of which of the following organisms require treatment?

A. *E. coli*
B. *Proteus*
C. *Klebsiella*
D. *Staphylococcus*
E. *Serratia*

1236. All of the following vitamin deficiencies may be directly attributed to resection of the ileocecal valve EXCEPT:

A. Vitamin B_{12}
B. Vitamin A
C. Vitamin D
D. Vitamin C
E. Vitamin K

1237. The development of which technique was one of the most important advances toward making lower urinary tract reconstruction possible?

A. Clean intermittent catheterization
B. Augmentation cystoplasty
C. Antirefluxing ureteral reimplantation
D. Artificial genitourinary sphincter
E. Continent urinary diversion

1238. Use of all of the following bowel segments in urinary tract reconstruction will cause a metabolic acidosis EXCEPT:

A. Ileum
B. Cecum
C. Sigmoid
D. Stomach
E. Rectum

1239. The major determinant of success in lower urinary tract reconstruction is:

A. Preoperative renal function
B. Adequate bladder volume
C. A low-pressure, compliant bladder
D. A leak point pressure >40 cm H_2O
E. Patient attitude and support systems

1240. Continence can be restored in what percentage of patients with dysfunctional lower urinary tracts?

A. 20 per cent
B. 50 per cent
C. 67 per cent
D. 90 per cent
E. 100 per cent

1241. Which of the following tissues should *not* be used to augment the bladder?

A. Ureter
B. Stomach
C. Colon
D. Ileum
E. All of the above can be used

1242. Which of the following techniques does not incorporate cecum?

A. Indiana pouch
B. MAINZ pouch
C. Hemi-Kock pouch
D. "Le Bag"
E. Penn pouch

1243. All of the following are advantages of using stomach segments for bladder augmentation or substitution EXCEPT:

A. Ease of ureteral reimplantation
B. Less cystitis than with other bowel segments
C. Gastric tissue is rarely exposed to radiation
D. Does not cause metabolic acidosis
E. Less mucus production

1244. Complications of cystoplasty include all of the following EXCEPT:

A. Vesicoureteral reflux
B. Stone formation
C. Development of malignancy
D. Acidosis
E. Spontaneous perforations

1245. All of the following would be good choices to increase outlet resistance in a patient with "normal voiding" EXCEPT:

A. Alpha agonists
B. Beta antagonists
C. Kropp procedure
D. Young-Dees-Leadbetter procedure
E. Artificial urinary sphincter

1246. The primary objective in patients having surgery for incontinence is:

A. Daytime continence
B. Total continence
C. Protection of the upper tracts
D. A compliant bladder
E. Prevention of UTIs

1247. If the bladder is entered during the placement of an artificial urinary sphincter, proper management is to:

A. Continue with the procedure
B. Close with two layers, place a suprapubic tube, and abandon placement of the sphincter
C. Administer triple antibiotics
D. Heavily irrigate with antibiotics
E. Place the sphincter through a perineal approach

1248. An artificial GU sphincter should not be placed in the bulbar urethra in which of the following circumstances?

A. Prepubertal males
B. Postmenopausal women
C. After radical prostatectomy
D. After TURP
E. After epispadias repair

1249. New onset of incontinence in a previously dry patient after placing an artificial urinary sphincter is usually due to:

A. Sphincter malfunction
B. Cuff leak
C. Cuff erosion
D. A change in bladder dynamics
E. Urinary tract infection

1250. Which of the following complication rates relating to artificial urinary sphincters is inaccurate?

A. A failure rate of 5 per cent

B. Technical problems in 20 to 35 per cent
C. Erosion or infection of the sphincter in 8 to 13 per cent of children
D. The need for revision in 25 to 50 per cent
E. Secondary bladder augmentation in 30 per cent of patients with neurogenic bladder

1251. Important principles for stoma creation include all of the following EXCEPT:

A. The stoma should be placed away from fat creases.
B. The stoma should be close to prior incisional sears.
C. The stoma should traverse the rectus muscle.
D. The stoma should be as far lateral as possible.
E. The stoma should be placed in the right or left lower abdomen.

1252. When cutaneous ureterostomies are to be performed and one of the ureters is dilated, the best procedure to perform is:

A. To bring them both out the abdominal wall as a double-barreled ureterostomy
B. To bring them out separately to the skin
C. Perform a proximal TUU with the normal ureter and bring the dilated ureter to the skin
D. Perform a proximal TUU with the dilated ureter and bring the normal ureter to the skin
E. To manage it with an intestinal diversion

1253. The optimal management of stomal stenosis with cutaneous ureterostomy consists of:

A. Conversion to an intestinal conduit
B. Local revisions with skin V-flaps
C. Resection of stenosis and pulling normal ureter up for a new stoma
D. Bringing the ureter through to a new skin site
E. Ureterosigmoidostomy

1254. The best segment of bowel to use for conduit diversion in a patient who has had extensive pelvic radiation is:

A. Ileum
B. Jejunum or transverse colon
C. Rectum
D. Sigmoid colon
E. Stomach

1255. When both ureters are spatulated and sewn together prior to anastomosis to the ileum, this is called the:

A. Deaver technique
B. Turnbull technique
C. Bricker technique
D. Wallace technique
E. Leadbetter-Politano technique

1256. Extravasation of urine at the ureteroileal anastamosis is less common today due to the use of:

A. Perioperative antibiotics
B. Nonabsorbable sutures
C. The Bricker anastomosis
D. The Wallace anastomosis
E. Stents

1257. Ureterointestinal anastomotic strictures:

A. Usually occur early postoperatively
B. Are more common on the left
C. Always require surgical revision
D. Are successfully managed with dilation and stenting 90 per cent of the time
E. Are rarely due to recurrence of malignancy

1258. The most common complication of a jejunal conduit is:

A. A hyponatremic, hypochloremic acidosis
B. A hyperchloremic metabolic acidosis
C. A ureterointestinal anastomosis stricture
D. Stomal stenosis
E. Radiation enteritis

1259. When comparing ileal and colon conduits, all of the following are true EXCEPT:

A. A tunneled nonrefluxing ureteral anastomosis can be created in colon conduits.
B. The stoma location is in the left lower quadrant for colon conduits.
C. There is a lower incidence of ureterointestinal stenosis with colon conduits.
D. There is a higher incidence of parastomal hernias with colon conduits.
E. There is a lower incidence of stomal stenosis with colon conduits.

1260. Preoperative evaluation prior to ureterosigmoidostomy should include all the following EXCEPT:

A. Sigmoid biopsy
B. Evaluation of renal function
C. Evaluation of hepatic function
D. Studies for bowel disease
E. Testing for adequate sphincter integrity

1261. In the patient with a rectal bladder, acidosis not corrected by oral medication is best managed by:

A. Antibiotic suppression
B. Increasing fluid intake
C. Conversion to a continent diversion
D. Daily cleansing enemas
E. Nighttime drainage with a rectal tube

1262. Rectal bladder formation with a posterior perineal sigmoidostomy is called the:

A. Mauclaire technique
B. Heitz-Boyer Hovelacque technique
C. Augmented valved rectum technique
D. Duhamel technique
E. Gersuny technique

1263. The principal rationale behind the augmented valved rectum is to:

A. Prevent reflux
B. Decrease infection
C. Confine urinary absorption to a smaller colon segment
D. Be able to anastamose dilated ureters
E. Decrease diarrhea

1264. Nocturnal enuresis is common with orthotopic diversions due to:

A. Small capacity pouches
B. Loss of the spinal reflex arc recruiting external sphincter contraction
C. No voluntary sphincter control while asleep
D. Injury to the external sphincter
E. Injury to the neurovascular bundle

1265. The risk of urethral cancer recurrence after orthotopic diversion is:

A. 0 per cent
B. 5 per cent
C. 15 per cent
D. 25 per cent
E. 50 per cent

1266. The orthotopic diversion with the lowest continence rate is the:

A. "Le Bag"
B. Sigmoid pouch
C. Camey II
D. Ileal Neobladder
E. Hemi-Kock pouch

1267. The harmful effects of reflux are lessened in the Studer pouch (low-pressure bladder substitute) by:

A. A nonrefluxing ureteroileal anastomosis
B. A proximal nipple value
C. An intact proximal 25-cm segment of ileum
D. A completely detubularized bowel segment
E. Utilizing the ileocecal value

1268. The continence mechanism which is easiest to catheterize in an orthotopic location is the:

A. Mitrofanoff principle
B. Nipple valve
C. Benchekroun nipple
D. Flap valve
E. Imbricated and tapered ileal segment

1269. The biggest disadvantage of the nipple valve continence mechanism is:

A. The time required to construct it
B. Its propensity for stone formation
C. Incontinence rate
D. Nipple value failure/instability
E. Difficult catheterization

1270. Concerning the nipple valve continence mechanism, the minimal intussuscepted nipple length required for continence is:

A. 0.5–2 cm
B. 2.5–3 cm
C. 3.5–5 cm
D. 5–7.5 cm
E. 7.5–8 cm

1271. Which of the following pouches does not utilize cecum and terminal ileum?

A. Hemi-Kock pouch
B. MAINZ pouch
C. Duke pouch
D. Indiana pouch
E. Penn pouch

1272. Which of the following pouches does not use a nipple valve for the continence mechanism?

A. Hemi-Kock pouch
B. MAINZ pouch
C. UCLA pouch
D. "Le Bag"
E. Indiana pouch

1273. All the following techniques help prevent failure of the nipple valve EXCEPT:

A. Removing mesenteric attachments from the bowel segment to be intussuscepted
B. Stapling the nipple valve to itself
C. Complete detubularization of bowel
D. Stapling the nipple valve to the reservoir
E. Placing absorbable mesh collar around the base of the nipple valve

1274. The Miami and the Florida pouches are most similar to which of the following pouches?

A. Indiana pouch
B. Hemi-Kock pouch
C. Penn pouch
D. MAINZ pouch
E. "Le Bag"

1275. Which development has had the greatest impact in making undiversion possible?

A. New surgical techniques using bowel segments
B. Nonrefluxing ureteral reimplantation
C. Intermittent catheterization
D. Stapling devices
E. Modern-day antibiotics

1276. Which of the following is a contraindication to urinary undiversion?

A. Age >30
B. Prior diversion performed >20 years ago
C. Renal insufficiency
D. Negative psychosocial factors
E. Previous pelvic radiation therapy

1277. The best method to predict how well a defunctionalized bladder will work is:

A. Urodynamic studies
B. Bladder cycling
C. VCUG
D. Videourodynamics with EMG studies
E. Measuring preoperative bladder capacity and post-void residual

1278. Proper management of urethral valves in a patient whose bladder has been diverted is:

A. Fulguration 2 weeks prior to undiversion
B. Balloon dilatation of valves
C. Leaving the patient diverted as long as renal function is stable
D. Open excision of valves followed by urethrourethrostomy
E. Fulguration only if cycling or diversion are to be performed immediately

1279. In mobilization of the ureter, the gonadal vessels should:

A. Be divided distally if necessary to preserve collaterals to ureter
B. Never be divided or testicular atrophy will ensue
C. Be separated from the ureter
D. Be divided proximally as they place tension on the ureteral anastomosis
E. Be temporarily clamped to see if they provide any blood supply to the ureter prior to dividing

1280. A reimplanted ureter or bowel segment should have a tunnel-length to ureter-diameter ratio of:

A. 1:1
B. 2:1
C. 3:1
D. 5:1
E. 10:1

1281. A transureteroureterostomy should be performed:

A. Always, if possible
B. Only if no other options exist
C. When there is not enough room for two reimplants in the bladder or one ureter is short
D. In patients with prior stone disease
E. Only when one or both ureters are dilated

1282. The best way to manage the old ileal conduit during undiversion is to:

A. Discard it
B. Utilize it as distal ureter after tapering it and reimplant it into the bladder
C. Utilize it as a bowel patch for augmentation
D. Intussuscept the distal end to create a nonrefluxing situation for the ureters
E. Leave it disconnected as dissection to remove it may compromise ureteral blood supply

1283. Important steps to follow when reimplanting a bowel segment include all the following EXCEPT:

A. Removing a strip of bowel one third the circumference of bowel to taper it
B. Creating a long tunnel with 5:1 length-to-width ratio
C. Employing a psoas hitch
D. Only a refluxing anastomosis may be made
E. Assuring lifelong follow-up

1284. The most common complication of the use of staples in urinary tract undiversion is:

A. Infection
B. Stone formation
C. Fistula formation
D. Ischemia of intussuscepted segment
E. Nipple valve failure

1285. The best choice of bowel segment in a patient with very poor renal function would be the:

A. Stomach
B. Jejunum
C. Ileum
D. Cecum
E. Sigmoid colon

1286. All of the following regarding open bladder surgery are true EXCEPT:

A. The majority of the blood supply to the bladder can be interrupted without major untoward effects.
B. Nonabsorbable suture should never be used in the bladder.
C. Suprapubic tube drainage should be avoided in bladder cancer.
D. Preoperative irradiation in patients with bladder cancer has been proven to result in longer survival than cystectomy alone.
E. The most common open bladder surgery performed is radical cystectomy.

1287. The first posterior branch of the internal iliac artery is the:

A. Superior vesical artery
B. Superior gluteal artery
C. Inferior vesical artery
D. Inferior gluteal artery
E. Inferior epigastric artery

1288. During radical cystectomy, ligation of the internal iliac artery above its first posterior branch may result in:

A. Impotence
B. Lower leg weakness
C. Gluteal claudication
D. Sigmoid colon ischemia
E. Incontinence

1289. Most blood loss during radical cystectomy usually occurs during which maneuver?

A. Pelvic lymphadenectomy
B. Control of lateral pedicles
C. Incision of endopelvic fascia
D. Ligation of dorsal vein complex
E. Urethral mobilization

1290. The mortality rate for radical cystectomy should be approximately:

A. 2 per cent
B. 5 per cent
C. 10 per cent
D. 15 per cent
E. 20 per cent

1291. A 67-year-old white male is admitted in preparation for radical cystectomy for clinical stage B, transitional cell carcinoma of the bladder. On the morning of the operation, he develops anterior chest pain. Despite the completion of a full bowel preparation, the operation is canceled and a cardiology evaluation is performed, which reveals no significant abnormality. The patient is readmitted 2 weeks later for radical cystectomy. Which one of the following is contraindicated in preoperative preparation?

A. Intravenous hydration before surgery
B. Mechanical bowel preparation
C. Oral antibiotic bowel preparation
D. Preoperative oral antifungal agents
E. Prophylactic intravenous antibiotics on call to surgery

1292. During radical cystectomy in a female patient, the first structure encountered during incision of the lateral peritoneal reflection is the:

A. Hypogastric artery
B. Broad ligament
C. Uterine artery
D. Obturator nerve
E. Round ligament

1293. Which of the following is most useful in dissecting and finding the vaginal vault and in preventing rectal and bladder injury during radical cystectomy in a female?

A. A Foley balloon in the bladder
B. A sponge on a forceps placed in the vagina
C. A finger in the rectum
D. An Allis forceps used for traction in the uterus
E. Dissection in the plane between the uterus and the bladder

1294. A 57-year-old female who underwent radical cystectomy and ileal loop diversion for muscle invasive bladder carcinoma approximately 6 months ago complains of dyspareunia. Work-up reveals vaginal contracture. The initial treatment of choice is:

A. Topical estrogen cream
B. Lidocaine jelly before intercourse
C. Vaginal dilation
D. Reconstruction with skin flaps
E. Reconstruction using bowel segments

1295. Which of the following is a contraindication to partial cystectomy in most patients?

A. Carcinoma in situ found on random biopsy samples
B. Solitary bladder tumor in the dome in an elderly patient who poses a significant surgical risk
C. Superficial transitional cell carcinoma in a bladder diverticulum
D. Persistent Hunner's ulcers despite transurethral resection
E. Invasion of bladder wall by colon cancer

1296. The major complication of bladder diverticulectomy is:

A. Bleeding
B. Urine leak
C. Rectal injury
D. Ureteral injury
E. Recurrent diverticulum

1297. The most common cause of enterovesical fistulas is:

A. Colon cancer
B. Crohn's disease
C. Diverticular disease
D. Trauma
E. Bladder cancer

1298. The most common presentation in patients with enterovesical fistulas is:

A. Urinary tract infection
B. Pneumaturia
C. Fecaluria
D. Urine per rectum
E. Tenesmus

1299. Which of the following is most accurate to diagnose a colovesical fistula?

A. Intravenous urogram
B. Cystogram
C. Barium enema
D. Sigmoidoscopy
E. Cystoscopy

1300. The most compelling indication for simultaneous urethrectomy in radical cystectomy is:

A. Solitary bladder tumor at bladder neck
B. Multifocal bladder tumors
C. Carcinoma in situ on bladder biopsy
D. Stage B2 transitional cell carcinoma of the bladder
E. Prostatic urethral involvement

1301. After radical cystectomy, the segment of urethra most likely to be involved with recurrent tumor is:

A. Bulbomembranous
B. Distal bulbar
C. Penile
D. Fossa navicularis
E. External meatus

1302. The external sphincter in the female is formed by fibers of the:

A. Pubococcygeus muscle
B. Bulbocavernosus muscle
C. Iliococcygeus muscle
D. Ischiococcygeus muscle
E. Transverse perineal muscle

1303. Normal continence in females results from all of the following EXCEPT:

A. Coaptation of urethral mucosal surface
B. Critical functional and anatomic urethral length
C. Increased urethral pressure by reflex pelvic contraction at time of stress
D. Proper anatomic location of the sphincteric unit
E. Urethral hypermobility

1304. Major support for the bladder neck and proximal urethra is provided by the:

A. Pubourethral ligaments
B. Urethropelvic ligaments
C. Pubocervical fascia
D. Cardinal ligaments
E. Periurethral fascia

1305. Which one statement regarding the intrinsic urethral mechanism is *false*?

A. Urethral pressure profilometry provides the best means to evaluate this continence mechanism.
B. Hormonal influences are intimately involved in this continence mechanism.
C. Coaptation is provided by the urethral mucosa.
D. The surrounding urethral smooth muscle coat exerts a constant tonus and directs submucosal expansile pressures inward toward the mucosa to maintain this mechanism.
E. The submucosa, which consists of smooth muscle bundles, loosely woven connective tissue, and an elaborate vascular plexus, creates the "washer effect" for the continence mechanism.

1306. Which statement concerning the classification of female urinary incontinence is *true*?

A. The majority of incontinent females are classified with pure stress urinary incontinence.
B. Type III incontinence in the McGuire and Blaivas classifications corresponds to the anatomic type stress incontinence in the Raz classification.
C. The Raz classification divides stress incontinence into anatomic incontinence or intrinsic sphincter dysfunction incontinence based on malposition of an intact sphincter unit versus malfunction of the sphincter with or without urethral hypermobility.
D. In the McGuire classification, types I and II stress incontinence are associated with a urethral closure pressure less than 20 cm H_2O.
E. In the Blaivas classification, type I stress incontinence occurs when the bladder neck and urethra open and descend more than 2 cm during stress with cystocele.

1307. Medical therapy for stress urinary incontinence includes intervention with all of the following EXCEPT:

A. Biofeedback
B. Estrogen supplementation
C. Tricyclic antidepressants
D. Alpha sympathomimetics
E. Kegel exercise

1308. The Q-tip test, which grossly defines the degree of urethral mobility, indicates urethral hypermobility when the Q-tip angle changes more than ____ with straining:

A. 0°
B. 5°
C. 15°
D. 25°
E. 35°

1309. Which one of the following statements regarding the use of a cystogram in the assessment of stress incontinence is *true*?

A. Funneling of the bladder neck on a cystogram is pathognomonic for stress incontinence.
B. In a patient with anatomic stress urinary incontinence, a cystogram reveals a fixed and open bladder neck.
C. A urethrotrigonal angle greater than 120° signifies bladder neck funneling on a true lateral cystogram.
D. An angle of inclination of the urethra to the vertical axis in an erect female greater than 35° indicates urethral hypermobility.
E. In the normal continent female, the bladder base lies above the inferior pubic ramus and does not descend more than 2 cm with straining during cystographic evaluation.

1310. Anatomic stress urinary incontinence can be surgically corrected by all of the following EXCEPT:

A. Raz needle suspension
B. Stamey needle suspension
C. Periurethral collagen injection
D. Burch colposuspension
E. Marshall-Marchetti-Krantz procedure

1311. All of the following statements concerning the Marshall-Marchetti-Krantz procedure are true EXCEPT:

A. Postoperative urethral obstruction occurs secondary to the close proximity of sutures to the urethra.
B. Absorbable sutures are used to anchor the perivaginal fascia and vaginal wall to Cooper's ligament.
C. A concomitant cystocele cannot be simultaneously corrected.
D. Success rates vary from 57 to 95 per cent.
E. Osteitis pubis is a potential complication of the procedure.

1312. Which surgical procedure corrects both urethral hypermobility and cystocele?

A. Kelly plication
B. Marshall-Marchetti-Krantz procedure
C. Stamey needle suspension
D. Gittes needle suspension
E. Burch colposuspension

1313. Which one of the following statements concerning the Raz transvaginal needle bladder neck suspension is *false*?

A. The suspension sutures incorporate the urethropelvic ligament, pubocervical fascia, and anterior vaginal wall and are anchored to the rectus fascia.
B. Cystourethroscopy is performed during the procedure to rule out bladder and/or ureteral injury.
C. Appropriate candidates for this procedure include patients with anatomic stress incontinence with mild to no cystocele.
D. Absorbable suture, such as chromic, is recommended for use as the suspending suture.
E. The procedure requires an incision in the anterior vaginal wall and detachment of the urethropelvic ligament from its lateral pelvic wall attachment to allow entrance into the retropubic space.

1314. Intrinsic sphincter dysfunction incontinence can be treated by all of the following EXCEPT:

A. Four-corner bladder and bladder neck suspension
B. Periurethral collagen injection
C. Pubovaginal sling
D. Vaginal wall sling
E. Artificial urinary sphincter

1315. Which statement concerning the complications of female urologic vaginal surgery is *false*?

A. Excessive bleeding during vaginal surgery can be controlled by overinflation of a Foley catheter intravaginally.
B. Urinary tract infections are the most common infections associated with vaginal surgery.
C. Partial ureteral tears are best treated by reimplantation.
D. Vaginal stenosis is best prevented by avoiding excessive excision of the vaginal wall.
E. Urinary retention can occur secondary to transient postoperative edema of the bladder neck and urethra, denervation, or misplaced suture.

1316. Which of the following is *not* characteristic of rectocele and perineal repair for posterior vaginal wall prolapse?

A. Preoperative preparation with enemas is recommended, since rectal injury is a potential complication.
B. The rectocele is repaired with a single running layer of absorbable suture incorporating the vaginal epithelium, prerectal fascia, and pararectal fascia.
C. The pubococcygeus muscle is excluded from the suture reapproximating the posterior vaginal wall.
D. Rectal injuries are avoided intraoperatively by retracting the rectal wall downward with a Deaver or Heaney retractor.
E. Perineorrhaphy corrects perineal laxity by reapproximating superficial and deep transverse perineal muscles, bulbocavernosus muscle, and levator ani complex in the midline.

1317. All of the following are used in the diagnosis of a urethral diverticulum EXCEPT:

A. Positive pressure urethrography
B. Urethroscopy
C. Intravenous urography
D. VCUG
E. Cystometrography

1318. Which statement concerning female urethral diverticulum is *true*?

A. Blacks and whites are equally affected.
B. The majority of urethral diverticula are acquired secondary to infection, parturition, or iatrogenic injury.
C. The incidence in adult females is approximately 10 per cent.
D. The majority of urethral diverticula open into the proximal urethra.
E. Hematuria is the most common presenting complaint in patients with urethral diverticula.

1319. Urethral diverticula are treated by all of the following EXCEPT:

A. Transvaginal excision
B. Spence marsupialization
C. Endoscopic urethrotomy
D. Suprapubic catheter drainage

1320. The most common cause of vesicovaginal fistulas is:

A. Gynecologic surgery
B. Obstetric trauma
C. Radiation therapy
D. Urologic surgery
E. Gastrointestinal surgery

1321. Which one of the following statements regarding vesicovaginal fistulas is *true*?

A. A Martius flap, peritoneal flap, or gracilis muscle flap can be used to reinforce the closure of a vesicovaginal fistula.
B. A 3-month waiting period is recommended prior to surgically repairing a radiation therapy induced vesicovaginal fistula.
C. Estrogen replacement therapy has a minimal role in the management of vesicovaginal fistulas.
D. Intermittent episodes of incontinence are characteristic of vesicovaginal fistula.
E. A single layer closure is usually adequate to repair the fistula.

1322. The most common cause of involuntary loss of urine in women is:

A. Cystitis
B. Uninhibited contractions
C. Stress urinary incontinence
D. Neurogenic bladder
E. Congenital anomalies

1323. All of the following are true concerning stress urinary incontinence EXCEPT:

A. One third to two thirds of patients with surgically curable incontinence also have urgency incontinence.
B. Postoperatively, urgency incontinence immediately improves in half the patients.
C. Most urgency incontinence postoperatively will resolve by 6 months.
D. Urgency incontinence often requires long-term anticholinergics.
E. Postoperative urgency incontinence is seen more often in women over 65 who had preoperative urgency incontinence.

1324. The best evidence for surgically correctable incontinence is:

A. An open bladder neck at cystoscopy
B. Demonstration of incontinence directly related to coughing
C. An open bladder neck on a lateral VCUG
D. A positive Q-tip test
E. A positive Bonney test

1325. In incontinent females, trigonitis is associated with:

A. Long-standing cystocele
B. Bladder stones
C. Cystitis
D. Early dysplasia
E. There is no such definable pathologic condition.

1326. A normal lateral straining cystogram will show all the following EXCEPT:

A. A flat and posteriorly directed base of bladder
B. A posterior urethrovesical angle of 90°
C. A proximal urethra directed posteriorly
D. A high position of urethrovesical junction behind the symphysis pubis
E. Complete emptying

1327. How much is the urethrovesical junction elevated by the Kelly anterior colporrhaphy?

A. Not at all
B. 1 cm
C. 2.5 cm
D. 4 cm
E. 5.5 cm

1328. The Stamey endoscopic vesical neck suspension is contraindicated in:

A. Stress urinary incontinence
B. Pure urgency incontinence
C. Stress urinary incontinence with a component of urgency incontinence
D. Patients with an acontractile bladder
E. Patients with an incompetent urethra

1329. Which of the following statements is *false*?

A. Patients with nonstress urinary incontinence have higher maximal detrusor pressures during voiding than stress urinary incontinence patients.
B. Maximal urethral closure pressures are much lower in women with stress urinary incontinence than in healthy continent controls.
C. Stress incontinence patients have equal closure pressures in the anterior and posterior urethra.
D. Vesical neck suspension doubles the urethral closure pressure in the posterior urethra.
E. Urethral closure pressures decline dramatically with age.

1330. The fascial layer which forms the bulk of the urethral suspension tissue is the:

A. Pubocervical fascia
B. Periurethral fascia
C. Cardinal ligament
D. Anterior vaginal wall
E. Denonvillier's fascia

1331. The correct place to pass the Stamey needles is:

A. Submucosally
B. In the mid-urethra
C. Just proximal to the urethrovesical junction
D. Exactly at the urethrovesical junction
E. Just distal to the urethrovesical junction

1332. The suprapubic suspending sutures should be tied:

A. Firmly to prevent the suspension from slipping
B. When the bladder neck is seen to be narrowed cystoscopically
C. Before closing the vaginal mucosa
D. Under no tension
E. When the vesical neck has been elevated 5.5 cm

1333. Which one of the following statements regarding the Stamey vesical neck suspension is *true*?

A. Most patients can void on the second or third postoperative day.
B. One suture must be removed due to pain or infection in 1 to 2 per cent.
C. The Dacron buttress should be left in place when the suture is removed for infection.
D. Success rate is around 70 per cent.
E. It cannot be repeated in the same patient.

1334. Which of the following is a contraindication for an open prostatectomy?

A. A gland that has previously been resected
B. Renal failure
C. A gland smaller than 50 grams
D. A large bladder diverticulum
E. Ankylosis of the hips

1335. The preoperative preparation for a patient undergoing open prostatectomy should include all of the following EXCEPT:

A. Cystoscopy
B. Transrectal ultrasound
C. Upper urinary tract imaging
D. Banking of autologous blood
E. An enema on the night prior to surgery

1336. Which of the following is true regarding suprapubic prostatectomy?

A. The procedure involves total removal of the prostate.
B. Vasectomy should be performed in all patients.
C. Traction should be applied to the urethral Foley catheter postoperatively.
D. The 5 and 7 o'clock vessels should be ligated even if there is no active bleeding.
E. Following incision of the mucosa, the adenoma should be excised by blunt dissection only.

1337. Which of the following is true regarding the complications of suprapubic prostatectomy?

A. Delayed bleeding is more common than following TURP.
B. Urethral stricture is more common than following TURP.
C. Bladder neck contracture is more common than following TURP.
D. Excessive blood loss is the most common immediate complication.
E. Retrograde ejaculation is uncommon.

1338. Which of the following statements regarding the comparison of suprapubic and retropubic prostatectomies for BPH is *false*?

A. The suprapubic approach is preferred when a simultaneous bladder diverticulectomy is needed.
B. The suprapubic approach has a lower incidence of incontinence.
C. The suprapubic approach is preferred when the prostatic enlargement involves mainly the median lobe.
D. The retropubic approach allows for easier detection of residual adenoma.
E. The retropubic approach allows for easier detection of bleeding points.

1339. Which of the following is *not* a recommended step in a simple retropubic prostatectomy?

A. Ligation of the lateral pedicles
B. Ligation of the dorsal vein complex
C. A longitudinal incision of the prostatic capsule
D. Division of the puboprostatic ligaments
E. Sharp dissection between the anterior adenoma and prostatic capsule

1340. The most common complication of simple retropubic prostatectomy is:

A. Retrograde ejaculation
B. Excessive postoperative bleeding
C. Epididymitis
D. Impotence
E. Bladder neck contracture

1341. The major arterial supply to the prostate is from the:

A. External iliac
B. Superior vesical
C. Inferior vesicle
D. Obturator
E. Inferior epigastric

1342. The pelvic plexus, which gives rise to the cavernous nerves, is located:

A. 20 cm above the anal verge
B. At the dome of the bladder
C. At the level of the tip of the seminal vesicle
D. Posterior to the bifurcation of the aorta
E. Lateral to the rectum adjacent to the apex of the prostate

1343. All of the following are true EXCEPT:

A. Ligation of the lateral prostatic pedicle in its midportion transects the nerve supply to the corpora.
B. The prostate receives its blood supply and autonomic innervation through the leaves of the lateral pelvic fascia.
C. The striated urethral sphincter is a vertically oriented tubular sheath rather than a pair of transverse muscles.

D. When dissecting the prostate off the rectum, separating the anterior and posterior layers of Denonvillier's fascia decreases the risk of rectal injury.
E. The venous drainage of the prostate is into Santorini's plexus.

1344. After transurethral resecting of the prostate, radical prostatectomy for adenocarcinoma should be deferred for:

A. 1 week
B. 2 weeks
C. 3 weeks
D. 6 weeks
E. 12 weeks

1345. All of the following regarding pelvic lymphadenectomy in radical prostatectomy are true EXCEPT:

A. Spinal or epidural anesthesia has been associated with less blood loss.
B. Transection of the vas deferens is recommended to more adequately mobilize the peritoneum.
C. Lymphadenectomy is a staging procedure (not therapeutic).
D. The lymphatics overlying the external iliac artery are preserved.
E. The distal margin of dissection is the node of Cloquet at the femoral canal.

1346. Incision of the endopelvic fascia too close to the bladder or prostate increased the risk of:

A. Residual tumor
B. Impotence
C. Lymphocele
D. Urinoma
E. Severe blood loss

1347. Excessive traction on the urethra prior to urethral transection in radical prostatectomy can increase the risk of:

A. Delayed return of urinary control
B. Impotence
C. Anastomotic stricture
D. Anastomotic leak
E. Rectal injury

1348. After urethral division in radical prostatectomy, with traction on the catheter, one can visualize a complex of skeletal muscle and fibrous tissue tethering the apex of the prostate to the pelvic floor. This complex is best identified as:

A. Rectourethralis muscle
B. Anterior rectal wall
C. Striated urethral sphincter
D. Levator in muscle fibers
E. Urogenital diaphragm

1349. All of the following are contraindications to a nerve-sparing procedure in radical prostatectomy EXCEPT:

A. Preoperative impotence
B. Induration involving the lateral sulcus found on preoperative physical examination
C. Induration in the lateral pelvic fascia found intraoperatively after incising the endopelvic fascia
D. Age over 70
E. Adherence of the neurovascular bundle to the prostate after incising the lateral pelvic fascia

1350. The most common intraoperative complication of radical retropubic prostatectomy is:

A. Hemorrhage
B. Rectal injury
C. Ureteral injury
D. Obturator nerve injury
E. Pneumothorax during placement of central lines

1351. In a previously healthy patient, rectal injury during radical retropubic prostatectomy is best managed by:

A. Aborting the prostatectomy, performing diverting colostomy, and delaying definitive completion of the operation 6 weeks to 6 months
B. Completing the prostatectomy and vesicourethral ovostomosis and observing the patient on broad-spectrum antibiotics
C. Completing prostatectomy, closing the rectum in 2 layers, dilating the anal sphincter, performing the vesicourethral anastomosis, and broad-spectrum antibiotics
D. Completing the prostatectomy, closing the rectum in 2 layers, completing the vesicourethral anastomosis, and performing temporary diverting colostomy
E. Aborting the prostatectomy, closing the rectum in 2 layers, dilating the anal sphincter, and delaying definitive completion of the operation 6 weeks to 6 months

1352. The risk of pulmonary embolus in radical retropubic prostatectomy is approximately:

A. 1 per cent
B. 5 per cent
C. 15 per cent
D. 20 per cent
E. 30 per cent

1353. On the second postoperative day after radical retropubic prostatectomy, the patient's Foley catheter is mistakenly removed. The most appropriate management is:

A. Observation while allowing the patient to void spontaneously
B. Percutaneous suprapubic cystostomy tube placement
C. One attempt at gentle passage of a small-caliber Foley catheter, and if this is without success, cystoscopy with catheter placement under direct vision
D. Filiform and followers with placement of a council-hipped catheter over a filiform placed in the bladder
E. Reexploration with revision of the vesicourethral anastomosis after direct Foley catheter placement

1354. Mucosal advancement in reconstruction of the bladder neck reduces the risk of:

A. Impotence
B. Incontinence
C. Bladder neck bleeding
D. Bladder neck contracture

E. Disruption of the anastomosis during the postoperative period

1355. The most important factor in determining continence after radical retropubic prostatectomy is:

A. Prior transurethral resection of the prostate
B. Preservation of the anterior component of the striated urethral sphincter
C. Pathologic stage of the tumor
D. Preservation of the neurovascular bundle
E. Age of the patient

1356. All of the following affect postoperative potency in patients undergoing radical prostatectomy EXCEPT:

A. Capsular penetration
B. Grade of tumor
C. Age of patient
D. Seminal vesicle invasion
E. Preservation or excision of the neurovascular bundle

1357. All of the following are advantages of the perineal approach over the retropubic approach in radical prostatectomy EXCEPT:

A. Provision of a relatively avascular field
B. Better exposure for vesicourethral anastomosis
C. Dependent postoperative drainage
D. Easier preservation of the neurovascular bundle
E. Less compromise of postoperative pulmonary function in elderly patients

1358. All of the following statements regarding the preparation for perineal prostatectomy are true EXCEPT:

A. Transrectal ultrasound offers no greater advantage over digital rectal examination for clinical staging.
B. Patients with extension of disease beyond the prostatic capsule are not candidates for this surgery.
C. Preoperative cystoscopy is recommended if the patient has had a prior transurethral resection.
D. Sterilization of the bowel with oral antibiotics is recommended in case of rectal injury.
E. The appropriate placement of the patient for surgery is the exaggerated lithotomy position.

1359. After division of the central tendon, the important landmark to aid in developing the path to the prostate and prostatic apex is (are) the:

A. Anterior rectal fascia
B. Rectourethoalis muscle
C. Levator ani
D. Seminal vesicles
E. Bulbocavernosus muscles

1360. During dissection of the prostatic apex in perineal prostatectomy, vigorous venous bleeding is encountered. The appropriate management is:

A. Stop the dissection and control the venous bleeding with suture ligatures.
B. Control the bleeding with pressure behind a curved narrow Deaver retractor and continue dissecting out the prostate from the bladder neck.
C. Place the patient in the supine position and get control of the dorsal vein via a retropubic approach.
D. Abort the procedure, place a large Foley catheter on traction, and treat the patient with external beam radiation therapy in 6 weeks.
E. Abort the procedure, pack the wound until bleeding stops, and reattempt the procedure in 3 to 5 days.

1361. During perineal prostatectomy, a large median lobe prevents separation of the prostate from the posterior bladder neck and the lobe cannot be delivered through the bladder neck into the operative field. The next step should be:

A. Abort the procedure, close the wound, perform transurethral resection of the median lobe in 6 weeks and radical retropubic prostatectomy 6 weeks after the TURP.
B. Dissect the posterior bladder wall off the rectum and enter the bladder posteriorly above the level of the obstructing median lobe.
C. Sharply amputate the median lobe at its neck and repair it following completion of the prostatectomy.
D. Abort the procedure, close the wound, and treat the patient with external beam radiation therapy.
E. Use intraoperative laser to shrink the median lobe.

1362. Following radical perineal prostatectomy, prolonged drainage from the perineal incision after Foley catheter removal is initially best managed by:

A. Opening the incision and draining the wound
B. Replacing the Foley catheter for several days
C. Suprapubic cystotomy tube drainage
D. Open revision of the ureterovesical anastomosis
E. Adjunctive external beam radiation therapy to sclerose off the area of leakage

1363. The incidence of urinary incontinence after radical perineal prostatectomy is:

A. <2 per cent
B. 4 per cent
C. 8 per cent
D. 16 per cent
E. 32 per cent

1364. After perineal prostatectomy, the best site for placement of an artificial sphincter in those patients with persistent incontinence is around the:

A. Membranous urethra
B. Ureterovesical anastomosis
C. Bulb of the urethra
D. Proximal penile urethra
E. Distal penile urethra

1365. The following statements are true regarding transurethral resection of the prostate EXCEPT:

A. The chance of a 40-year-old man having a prostatectomy in his lifetime is between 10 and 30 per cent.
B. The incidence of prostatectomy in the United States is double that of England.
C. The development of acute retention is predict-

able based on the severity of a patient's symptoms.
D. Following TURP, over 80 per cent of patients experience improved urinary flow rates.
E. The most common reason for TURP are symptoms of prostatism.

1366. The most common cause of death following TURP is:

A. Sepsis
B. Myocardial infarction
C. Hemorrhage
D. Pulmonary complications
E. Renal failure

1367. In a patient with BPH, the irritative symptoms of urinary urgency, frequency, and nocturia usually result from:

A. Bladder calculi
B. Bladder (detrusor) hyperreflexia
C. Prostatic calculi
D. External sphincter dyssynergia
E. Detrusor areflexia

1368. The following are true regarding anesthesia during TURP EXCEPT:

A. TURP may be performed with general, spinal, epidural, or local anesthesia.
B. There is no significant difference in blood loss between epidural and general anesthesia.
C. Postoperative morbidity rates are not significantly different between spinal and general anesthesia.
D. There is no higher incidence of cardiac arrhythmias with general anesthesia.
E. Postoperative mortality rates are not significantly different between spinal and general anesthesia.

1369. All of the following are true regarding technical aspects of TURP EXCEPT:

A. The bladder should be moderately distended before proximal resection near the vesical neck is begun.
B. If the bladder is filled during resection of the apex, the prostatic fossa is distended, making resection more difficult.
C. Proximal resection with the bladder nondistended carries the danger of resecting the walls of the bladder adjacent to the prostate, with possible perforation.
D. The proximal resection should be carried deep to the circular fibromuscular fibers of the vesical neck.
E. The TURP should begin with urethral calibration.

1370. Which of the following statements regarding TURP is *true*?

A. The prostatic capsule is easily recognized by its granular appearance.
B. Sterile water should be used as the irrigating solution.
C. The posterior aspect of the vesical neck should be resected deeply.
D. In cases of meatal postnavicular stenosis, a generous ventral meatotomy should be performed.
E. The most common area of damage to the external sphincter is at the 12 o'clock position.

1371. The following statements are true regarding hemostasis during TURP EXCEPT:

A. Arterial bleeding generally is easily controlled by electrocoagulation.
B. The surgeon should be persistent in attempting to control venous sinus bleeding by electrocoagulation.
C. Arterial bleeding should be controlled in one stage before moving to the next stage of the resection.
D. Pressure in the venous sinuses is approximately 10–12 mm Hg, which is lower than the pressure of the irrigant leading to intravasation of the fluid.
E. The bleeding venous sinus can usually be controlled by proper placement of the urethral catheter at completion of the procedure.

1372. Which of the following statements regarding TURP is *false*?

A. The mortality rate is less than 1 per cent.
B. Intraoperative bleeding is related to the size of the prostate and the length of surgery.
C. TUR syndrome is characterized by mental confusion, nausea, vomiting, hypertension, bradycardia, and visual disturbances.
D. Penile erections during surgery have been successfully managed with ketamine and/or intracorporal epinephrine.
E. The incidence of TUR syndrome is not related to gland size nor length of surgery.

1373. The metabolic abnormality observed in TUR syndrome is:

A. Hyponatremia
B. Hypokalemia
C. Hyperkalemia
D. Elevated serum osmolality
E. Hypernatremia

1374. The most immediate postoperative complication after TURP is:

A. Bleeding requiring transfusion
B. Infection
C. Failure to void
D. Clot retention
E. Myocardial infarction

1375. A patient is 5-week status post-TURP and initially had a good urinary stream; however, he now presents with a marked reduction in his stream. The most likely diagnosis is:

A. Urethral stricture
B. Vesical neck contracture
C. Residual adenoma
D. Infection
E. Clot formation

1376. A 72-year-old male presents with severe obstructive symptoms, no obvious prostate enlargement, but with uroflow values suggesting outlet obstruction. He would probably be best managed with:

A. Open prostatectomy
B. TURP
C. TUIP (transurethral incision of the prostate)

D. Observation
E. Pharmacotherapy

1377. A 68-year-old male with an 80-g prostate and a 3 × 5-cm bladder calculus would be best managed by which of the following procedures:

A. Mechanical litholapaxy
B. Electrohydraulic lithotripsy (EHL) and TURP
C. TURP and mechanical litholapaxy
D. Open prostatectomy and vesicolithotomy
E. Electrohydraulic lithotripsy

1378. In tissues exposed to 40°C, which of the following effects are noted?

A. Protein coagulation
B. Loss of structural integrity
C. Vaporization
D. Cell death
E. No irreversible cellular damage

1379. The direct cause of stone disruption in laser lithotripsy is:

A. Thermal energy
B. Vaporization
C. Plasma expansion
D. Spark gap
E. Photosensitization

1380. The wavelength of the emitted light in laser surgery is determined by the:

A. Power of the laser
B. Energy density
C. Diameter of the fiber used
D. Distance between the fiber tip and the tissue surface
E. Active medium

1381. Tissue penetration of the argon laser is approximately:

A. 0.5 mm
B. 1 mm
C. 2 mm
D. 5 mm
E. 10 mm

1382. The laser associated with the most coagulation effect on tissues is:

A. CO_2
B. Neodymium:YAG
C. KTP-532
D. Pulsed-dye
E. Argon-dye

1383. All of the following statements regarding laser treatment of penile condyloma acuminata are true EXCEPT:

A. When using the CO_2 laser, a power output of 3–5 watts will usually suffice.
B. When using the neodymium:YAG laser, a power output of 15–20 watts will usually suffice.
C. Recurrence rates are high in patients with microscopic subclinical lesions.
D. Laser therapy of aceto-white microscopic condyloma can decrease recurrence rates.
E. The KTP-532 laser may be preferred in black patients due to its affinity for melanin.

1384. The preferred laser for tumor ablation in CIS of the penis is:

A. CO_2
B. Neodymium:YAG
C. Argon
D. KTP-532
E. Pulsed-dye

1385. All of the following regarding laser treatment of urethral stricture disease are true EXCEPT:

A. CO_2 laser energy is rapidly extinguished by water, limiting its feasibility with endoscopy.
B. Suprapubic venting does not decrease the risk of air embolus with the CO_2 laser.
C. Laser therapy has been proven to have a lower recurrence rate than internal urethrotomy.
D. After neodymium:YAG laser treatment of urethral strictures, dilation of the stricture is usually necessary to provide immediate symptomatic relief.
E. Contact tips increase the energy density and cutting effect of a neodymium:YAG laser.

1386. The treatment of choice for bladder hemangioma is:

A. Transurethral resection
B. Partial cystectomy
C. Neodymium:YAG laser
D. Photodynamic therapy
E. Intravesical BCG

1387. Which of the following is a contraindication to neodymium:YAG laser treatment of superficial bladder cancer?

A. Previous history of superficial transitional cell carcinoma
B. Low-grade malignant cells on voided cytology examination
C. Tumors overlying the ureteral orifice
D. Lesions greater than 3.0 cm in diameter
E. Inability to tolerate general or regional anesthesia

1388. Two days after neodymium:YAG laser treatment for superficial transitional cell carcinoma of the bladder, a patient complains of abdominal pain and nausea. Physical examination reveals a temperature of 102°F and a rigid abdomen with rebound tenderness. The most likely diagnosis is:

A. Urinary tract infection due to endoscopic procedure
B. Bladder perforation
C. Small bowel perforation
D. Severe inflammatory reaction due to necrosing tumor
E. Meningitis from spinal anesthesia

1389. All of the following regarding photodynamic therapy are true EXCEPT:

A. Hemotoporphyrin derivative is the photosensitizer of choice.
B. The KTP-532 laser is the laser of choice.
C. The mechanism of cellular death is uncertain.
D. Phototoxicity precludes exposure to direct sunlight for at least 6 weeks.
E. The optimal time for the delivery of the laser energy after drip administration is unknown.

1390. The greatest risk of ureteral injury in the laser treatment of ureteral calculi is associated with:

A. Ureteroscopy itself
B. Use of power greater than 20 millijoules
C. Thermal injury
D. Discharge frequencies greater than 5 Hz
E. Inadvertent firing of the probe while it is in contact with the ureteral mucosa

1391. The calculus most easily fragmented by laser lithotripsy is:

A. Calcium oxalate monohydrate
B. Calcium oxalate dihydrate
C. Uric acid
D. Calcium phosphate
E. Cystine

1392. The theoretical advantages of laser assistance in vasovasostomy include all of the following EXCEPT:

A. Increased patency
B. Decreased incidence of sperm granuloma
C. Ability to perform the laser weld rapidly
D. Minimal local tissue reaction
E. Improved pregnancy rates

1393. Which statement concerning the embryology and development of the seminal vesicles is *false*?

A. The seminal vesicle begins with the development of a dorsolateral bulbous swelling of the distal mesonephric duct around 13 fetal weeks.
B. The seminal vesicle has no female homologue.
C. 30 per cent of ectopic ureters are found to drain into the seminal vesicles.
D. Absence of the vas deferens confirms absence of the ipsilateral seminal vesicle.
E. The seminal vesical is commonly absent in patients with cystic fibrosis.

1394. Which statement concerning the anatomy of the seminal vesicles is *false*?

A. The normal adult seminal vesicle is 5 to 10 cm in length, 3 to 5 cm in diameter, and has a volume capacity of 13 ml on average.
B. The seminal vesicle is innervated by adrenergic fibers from the hypogastric nerve.
C. Primary blood supply to the seminal vesicles is derived from the umbilical artery through a branch known as the vesiculodeferential artery.
D. The middle rectal artery provides a communicating vessel supplying the seminal vesicles.
E. The right seminal vesicle is slightly larger than the left in one third of men and the size of both glands will decrease with age.

1395. Components of seminal vesicle secretions include:

A. D-Fructose, prostaglandin A, prostaglandin E, coagulation factor
B. IgA, D-fructose, prostaglandin A, prostaglandin F
C. D-Fructose, D-sorbitol, prostaglandin E, prostaglandin F
D. α-Tocopherol, D-fructose, prostaglandin F, coagulation factor
E. Carbohydrates, IgA, prostaglandin E, α-tocopherol

1396. On semen analysis, all of the following indicate absence of the seminal vesicles EXCEPT:

A. Lack of fructose
B. Liquefaction of semen
C. Low sperm count
D. Low semen volume
E. Lack of carbohydrate

1397. Which statement concerning imaging of the seminal vesicles is *true*?

A. Vasography accurately demonstrates pathology of the seminal vesicles in patients with vesiculitis, tumors, and cysts.
B. TRUS can distinguish between seminal vesical inflammation and prostatodynia or chronic prostatourethritis.
C. CT scan adequately distinguishes primary from secondary tumors.
D. On MRI, hemorrhagic cysts are readily identified because of high-intensity T1- and T2-weighted images.
E. MRI may be used to distinguish benign seminal vesicle tumors from primary malignancies.

1398. Which statement concerning infections of the seminal vesicles is *false*?

A. Tuberculosis and schistosomiasis remain common causes of seminal vesicle masses and calcifications in the third world today.
B. In the United States, infection of the seminal vesicles is rare.
C. Bacterial infections are thought to be secondary to bacterial prostatitis, and typically pathogens are colonic flora.
D. Recurrent septicemia secondary to seminal vesiculitis should be treated by excision of the infected seminal vesicle.
E. Transrectal needle aspiration followed by antibiotic therapy is the treatment of choice for seminal vesiculitis with apparent glandular congestion on radiographic imaging.

1399. Characteristics of primary adenocarcinoma of the seminal vesicle include each of the following EXCEPT:

A. Elevated serum CEA levels
B. Normal serum PSA and PAP levels
C. A pathologic analysis showing a mucin-producing papillary carcinoma or anaplastic carcinoma that may contain lipofuscin
D. Hematospermia as the primary presenting complaint
E. Rare occurrence before age 50

1400. Benign and malignant tumors of the seminal vesicles include the following EXCEPT:

A. Fibroma
B. Papillary adenocarcinoma
C. Cystic teratoma
D. Leiomyosarcoma
E. Cystadenoma

1401. Metastatic malignancies, which have been reported to involve the seminal vesicles, include each of the following EXCEPT:

A. Adenocarcinoma of the vas deferens
B. Colorectal adenocarcinoma
C. Transitional cell carcinoma

D. Lymphoma
E. Adenocarcinoma of the prostate

1402. Which of the following statements concerning treatment for symptomatic seminal vesicle cyst is *incorrect*?

A. Initial therapy should be transperineal or transrectal ultrasound-guided aspiration.
B. Large recurring cysts may be marsupialized to the bladder via the transvesical approach.
C. Reaspiration with injection of a sclerosing agent may be performed for recurrent cysts.
D. When aspiration fails, proximal seminal vesical cysts adjacent to the prostate may be unroofed with deep transurethral resection at the 5 or 7 o'clock position.
E. Transperineal excision may be performed for small recurrent symptomatic cysts.

1403. Preoperative preparation for open seminal vesicle procedures includes all of the following EXCEPT:

A. Mechanical bowel preparation the evening prior to surgery
B. A standard oral antibiotic regimen, including neomycin/erythromycin for bowel preparation
C. A prophylactic systemic antibiotic of choice administered immediately preoperatively
D. Type and cross for 2 units of packed cells for perineal or transcoccygeal approaches and 3 units for anterior approaches
E. Preoperative heparinization

1404. Concerning the transperineal approach to the seminal vesicles, all of the following statements are true EXCEPT:

A. The seminal vesicle containing pathology should be completely dissected out prior to ligating its entry into the prostate.
B. A vertical incision is made through Denonvilliers' fascia at the level of the base of the seminal vesicles on the prostate when attempting to preserve potency.
C. Dissection near the base of the seminal vesicles is enhanced by posterior traction on a Lowsley tractor placed through the urethra.
D. The vascular pedicle is encountered approximately 1 cm from the distal end of the vesicle.
E. A Penrose drain should be left in the bed of the resected seminal vesicle.

1405. Concerning the transvesical approach to seminal vesiculectomy, all of the following statements are true EXCEPT:

A. It is preferable to place ureteral catheters prior to dissection through the trigone to help avoid ureteral injury.
B. The best exposure to the seminal vesicles is obtained by making a transverse incision through the posterior trigone approximately 5 cm in length.
C. Rectal laceration is much less likely than with alternative approaches.
D. Suprapubic cystostomy is not necessary.
E. Once the trigone is opened, the seminal vesicles are found just lateral to the ampullae at the base of the prostate.

1406. Which of the following statements concerning the paravesical approach to seminal vesicle surgery is *true*?

A. This approach is ideal for treatment of a small unilateral seminal vesicle cyst.
B. Placing a catheter in the bladder and distending the bladder helps to develop the plane between cyst and bladder.
C. This approach is useful in children with a large unilateral seminal vesicle cyst who may also require a nephroureterectomy.
D. The ipsilateral superior and inferior vesicle arteries may not be sacrificed when exposing the seminal vesicle.
E. Care must be taken when dissecting medially to the affected seminal vesicle to maintain potency.

1407. Concerning the retrovesical approach to seminal vesicle surgery, the following statement is *true*:

A. A suprapubic incision is made and the space of Retzius is opened.
B. A catheter is placed and the bladder filled to facilitate development of the plane between seminal vesicle cyst and bladder.
C. The prostatic urethra is transected at the bladder neck, and the bladder elevated off the seminal vesicles.
D. This approach is ideal for excision of large seminal vesicle tumors.
E. The reflection of the peritoneum over the rectum at the posterior bladder wall is incised transversely to gain access to the seminal vesicles.

1408. Which of the following concerning seminal vesicle surgery via the transcoccygeal approach is *false*?

A. The patient is positioned prone on the table in a relative jackknife position.
B. An L-shaped incision is made from the midsacral region, angled at the tip of the coccyx.
C. The lateral wall of the rectum on the affected side is dissected medially from the levator ani muscle and surrounding tissue until the prostate is exposed.
D. Dissection inferior to the base of the prostate reveals the ampulla and seminal vesicle lateral to this.
E. Use of an O'Connor sheath and finger in the anus helps in the development of the correct plane.

1409. All of the following are true statements concerning skin grafts EXCEPT:

A. Graft "take" involves two stages: (1) imbibition—absorbing nutrients ($\cong$ 48°) and (2) inosculation—reestablishing anastomosis of graft vessels to those in the host bed ($\cong$ 4 days).
B. Split thickness skin grafts are advantageous because the removal of the reticular dermis exposes the papillary dermis with its abundant blood supply and thinness allowing rapid inosculation and imbibition.
C. The disadvantage of the full-thickness skin graft is that it revascularizes more slowly and, because the dermis is left, it is more prone to contraction than is split-thickness skin graft.

D. A meshed skin graft has the advantages of being able to cover an area 1.5 to 2 times the site of the harvested graft and it is better suited to suboptimal graft sites or when infection may be present.

1410. Which one of the following statements concerning penile anatomy is *false*?

A. Buck's fascia closely surrounds the cavernosal bodies and splits to surround the corpus spongiosum.
B. The arterial supply consists of the paired bulbourethral, dorsal, and cavernosal arteries.
C. The three-level venous drainage of the penis consists of superficial dorsal veins, which usually drain into the left saphenous vein; deep dorsal and circumflex veins, which drain into Santorini's plexus; and the caval/cavernosal veins, which empty into internal pudendal veins and ultimately the internal iliac veins.
D. The lymphatics of the penis drain primarily into the superficial inguinal and internal iliac lymph nodes.
E. Cowper's glands lie within the urogenital diaphragm and empty into the urethra at the bulb.

1411. Which one of the following statements concerning hypospadias is *false*?

A. The urethral meatus may be on the ventral glans, shaft of the penis, scrotum, or perineum.
B. There is typically a ventral hooded prepuce.
C. The mesenchyme of the corpus spongiosum may be dysgenetic, forming ventral bands, which may result in ventral bending or chordee.
D. Incomplete development of the phallus is caused by deficient androgen effects.

1412. Adequate correction of a penoscrotal hypospadias includes/requires all of the following EXCEPT:

A. Excision/release of all dysgenetic tissue for correction of chordee
B. Artificial erection to confirm a straight phallus
C. Full-thickness tubularized vascularized skin graft with spatulated anastomosis to a spatulated distal urethra
D. Temporary suprapubic tube urinary diversion for 3 to 4 weeks while healing takes place
E. An inverting urethral closure of the tubularized graft with a second layer of 6-0 absorbable suture to bury the urethral closure

1413. All of the following are true concerning urethral fistula EXCEPT:

A. Meatal stenosis or stricture may be an associated and potentially causative co-feature in fistula after hypospadias repairs.
B. The urethra should be closed with 6 or 7-0 absorbable suture with everting of all mucosal edges.
C. A fistula is a tract from the urethra to the skin lined with epithelium.
D. Postsurgical fistula repair should be delayed 3 to 6 months, for resolution of all inflammation.
E. A small fistula may be closed primarily while larger fistula may require a flap or patch urethroplasty.

1414. All of the following are true concerning urethral diverticulum EXCEPT:

A. The diagnosis is most reliably made with voiding cystourethrogram.
B. Males may have a congenital posterior urethral diverticulum, which may be a large müllerian remnant or enlarged utricle which usually requires no therapy.
C. Large posterior urethral diverticula in males may require transsacral access, whereas small ones may be approached transvesically though the center of the trigone.
D. Patients may present with urethral symptoms, recurrent UTIs, post-void dribbling due to urine draining from diverticulum or a tender periurethral mass.
E. Females may have diverticula from dilated periurethral glands.

1415. The goals of reconstructive penile surgery in male patients with exstrophy include all of the following EXCEPT:

A. Obtaining a penis with adequate length for sexual function that dangles naturally by releasing the proximal corporal bodies from the widespread pubic rami
B. Avoiding injury to the dorsolaterally located vessels and nerves while the corporal bodies are mobilized
C. Correction of chordee by release of dysgenetic tissue, inward corporal rotation and Nesbit tucks or dermal graft patching to correct any residual curvature
D. Staged (later) or simultaneous bladder neck reconstruction for incontinence
E. Urethral reconstruction with full thickness skin graft to bring the urethra to a ventral position on the glans penis

1416. All of the following are correct statements concerning penile/genital trauma EXCEPT:

A. With fracture or suspected fracture of the penis (disrupted tunica albuginea) immediate exploration and surgical repair should be undertaken.
B. An amputated penis should be reimplanted with microvascular reanastomosis. If the distal phallus is not suitable, a staged radial forearm flap is the mainstay for distal penile reconstruction.
C. With severe genital burn injuries a urethral catheter should be used early to prevent urinary retention due to penile edema. Aggressive debridement of questionably viable tissue as always with burns is the rule.
D. With degloving injuries of the penis and scrotum, the penis should be covered with a split-thickness skin graft and the testes pexed in their anatomic position and covered with a meshed split-thickness skin graft.

1417. Which one of the following statements concerning urethral strictures is *false*?

A. Strictures may be caused by infection (gonorrhea- or catheter-associated) or due to trauma to the urethra (instrumentation, catheter, transurethral surgery).

B. Chlamydia and ureaplasma are becoming more common as causes of urethral stricture.
C. Symptoms are predominantly obstructive, but patients may have dysuria or a history of recurrent prostatitis.
D. The urethra proximal to the stricture is usually dilated due to increased pressures during active voiding.
E. If the urethra proximal to the stricture is not dilated but rather narrows, it should be suspected of being diseased as well and included in any area of repair.

1418. Which of the following is appropriate therapy for a 1.0-cm stricture of the bulbar urethra with full thickness fibrosis of the spongiosum?

A. Island flap urethroplasty
B. Urethral dilatation
C. Open excision and primary spatulated reanastomosis
D. Visual internal urethrotomy
E. Open split-thickness skin graft urethroplasty

1419. The most important factor in the evaluation of a patient with erectile dysfunction is:

A. History
B. Nocturnal penile tumescence monitoring
C. Response to papaverine
D. Dynamic cavernosometry
E. Visual sexual stimulation testing

1420. The systemic medical disorder most often associated with impotence is:

A. Multiple sclerosis
B. Hypothyroidism
C. Cirrhosis
D. Diabetes mellitus
E. Pituitary insufficiency

1421. The class of drugs most often associated with erectile dysfunction is:

A. Antidepressant medications
B. Histamine receptor antagonists
C. Antihypertensives
D. Antianxiety medications
E. Cardiac glycosides

1422. Nocturnal penile tumescence testing is most useful in:

A. Distinguishing endocrine from vascular impotence
B. Distinguishing arterial insufficiency from inadequate venous occlusion
C. Determining adequacy of erectile sustainability
D. Assessing adequacy of erectile rigidity
E. Distinguishing psychogenic from organic impotence

1423. Visual sexual stimulation testing (VSS) has been used during evaluation of men with sexual dysfunction in place of:

A. History
B. Physical examination
C. Duplex ultrasound
D. Nocturnal penile testing
E. Pharmacologic injection

1424. A methodology for testing neurologic function in patients with erectile dysfunction that is practical for routine use is:

A. Biothesiometry
B. Waveform analysis of corporal smooth muscle electrical activity
C. Measurement of dorsal nerve conduction velocity
D. Dorsal nerve somatosensory evoked response testing
E. Bulbocavernosus reflex latency testing

1425. Hypogonadotropic hypogonadism can be distinguished from hypergonadotropic hypogonadism by:

A. Measurement of serum testosterone
B. Measurement of LH
C. Measurement of prolactin
D. Measurement of FSH
E. A brain CT

1426. Of the following statements, which is the most accurate description of serum testosterone levels?

A. Serum testosterone levels remain constant.
B. Serum testosterone varies diurnally with peak levels in the morning.
C. Serum testosterone varies diurnally with peak levels in the evening.
D. Serum testosterone varies on a monthly cycle.
E. There is no consistent pattern of serum testosterone.

1427. Hyperprolactinemia is thought to cause impotence by:

A. Decreasing serum testosterone
B. Increasing serum estrogen
C. Interfering with peripheral action of testosterone
D. Increasing serum FSH
E. Both decreasing serum testosterone and interfering with its peripheral action

1428. The major disadvantage of the penile brachial index in evaluating possible arterial insufficiency in men with erectile dysfunction is the:

A. Expense of the study
B. Complexity of the study
C. Discomfort of the study
D. Inability to specifically measure cavernous artery pressure
E. Inability to specifically measure dorsal artery pressure

1429. The major disadvantage of duplex ultrasonography for evaluation of possible arterial insufficiency in men with erectile dysfunction is the:

A. Operator dependence of the results
B. Discomfort of the study
C. Inability to specifically assess cavernous arteries
D. Inability to specifically assess dorsal arteries
E. Inability to specifically assess pudendal arteries

1430. A normal cavernosal artery occlusion pressure is:

A. Greater than systolic blood pressure
B. Greater than diastolic blood pressure
C. Not more than 35 mm Hg less than systolic pressure

D. Not more than 35 mm Hg greater than systolic pressure
E. Equal to systolic pressure

1431. The major potential difficulty in accurately identifying patients with corporal veno-occlusive dysfunction is:

A. Radiographically identifying venous leaking
B. Distinguishing arterial insufficiency from venous leaking
C. Producing a full pharmacologic-induced erection
D. Overcoming anxiety-induced smooth muscle contraction that prevents full activation of the veno-occlusive mechanism
E. Accurately measuring intracavernous pressure

1432. Normal findings during gravity pharmacocavernosometry would be an:

A. Intracavernosal pressure similar to pressure of infused saline and low volume infused
B. Intracavernosal pressure similar to pressure of infused saline and high volume infused
C. Intracavernosal pressure less than pressure of infused saline and low volume infused
D. Intracavernosal pressure less than pressure of infused saline and high volume infused
E. Intracavernosal pressure greater than pressure of infused saline and high volumes infused

1433. The primary goal of psychologic therapy for men with erectile dysfunction is to:

A. Increase self-esteem
B. Uncover repressed conflicts from early childhood
C. Overcome performance anxiety
D. Achieve psychoanalytic insight
E. Overcome inhibitions regarding sexuality

1434. Testosterone as therapy for sexual dysfunction is indicated:

A. In all impotent men, as a therapeutic trial
B. In men with hyperprolactinemia
C. Following a blood test that demonstrates low testosterone
D. Following several blood tests demonstrating consistently low testosterone
E. For men with decreased libido

1435. Hyperprolactinemia as a cause of sexual dysfunction is treated medically with:

A. Testosterone
B. LH-RH agonists
C. L-Dopa
D. Trazodone
E. Bromocriptine

1436. All of the following are potential difficulties associated with the use of the vacuum constrictor device for erectile dysfunction EXCEPT:

A. Inadequate penile diameter during erection
B. Ecchymoses
C. Pivoting of the penis at its base
D. Penile edema and cyanosis
E. Difficulty with ejaculation

1437. Intracavernosal injection of pharmacologic agents can be expected to be successful for treatment of erectile dysfunction due to all of the following EXCEPT:

A. Diabetes mellitus
B. Multiple sclerosis
C. Corporal veno-occlusive dysfunction
D. Psychologic impotence
E. Arteriosclerotic vascular disease

1438. A man treated for erectile dysfunction with a penile prosthesis complains of persistent penile pain without fever or purulent discharge. A major consideration in the differential diagnosis should be:

A. Erosion of prosthesis
B. Inappropriately sized prosthesis
C. Infection
D. SST deformity
E. Injury to the neurovascular bundle

1439. In men with a penile prosthesis, which of the following underlying diseases is most often associated with prosthesis erosion in the long term?

A. Arteriosclerotic vascular insufficiency
B. Priapism
C. Peyronie's disease
D. Paraplegia
E. Impotence postradical prostatectomy

1440. Vascular reconstruction for treatment of erectile dysfunction has been most successful for men with:

A. Aortoiliac occlusive disease
B. Internal iliac occlusive disease
C. Diffuse arteriosclerotic vascular disease
D. Vascular disease associated with diabetes mellitus
E. Traumatic lesions involving the pudendal or penile arteries

1441. The Virag procedure for erectile dysfunction refers to:

A. Ligation of the deep dorsal vein
B. Anastomosis of inferior epigastric artery to deep dorsal vein
C. Anastomosis of inferior epigastric artery to dorsal artery of penis
D. Anastomosis of inferior epigastric artery to tunica albuginea of corpus cavernosum
E. Anastomosis of inferior epigastric artery to cavernosa artery

1442. Which of the following class of patients with corporal veno-occlusive dysfunction would not be good candidates for venous surgery?

A. Patients with coexisting arterial disease
B. Patients in whom perineal compression reduces venous leakage
C. Patients with spongiosal leaking
D. Patients with leakage through dorsal vein
E. Patients with leakage through crural veins

1443. A proximal corpus spongiosum shunt for treatment of priapism is indicated when:

A. The patient is uncircumcised
B. Cosmetic concerns are important
C. Priapism is of only short duration
D. Priapism is recurrent
E. Severe tissue changes are present distally

1444. In females, lymphatic drainage of the distal urethra goes primarily to the:

A. Superficial inguinal nodes
B. Deep inguinal nodes
C. External iliac nodes
D. Internal iliac nodes
E. Presacral nodes

1445. All of the following regarding the histology of urethral carcinomas are true EXCEPT:

A. It significantly influences tumor progression and management.
B. Secondary transitional cell carcinomas generally involves the urethra as a manifestation of bladder carcinomas.
C. Adenocarcinoma usually arises in the distal urethra.
D. Distal squamous cell carcinoma tends to remain localized for a relatively long period of time.
E. Total en block urethrectomy is routinely included as part of a radical cystectomy in the female.

1446. All of the following regarding radiotherapy for penile cancer are true EXCEPT:

A. Palpable inguinal adenopathy is more appropriately managed with surgery.
B. External beam is associated with better local control than interstitial techniques.
C. Pretreatment circumcision and meatotomy are mandatory.
D. After treatment, appearance of new lesions is more commonly due to new tumor formation rather than tumor persistence.
E. Therapy is more morbid if there is associated infection.

1447. The desired extent of tumor margin that affords excellent local control in partial penectomy for penile carcinoma is:

A. 0.5 cm
B. 1.0 cm
C. 2.0 cm
D. 3.0 cm
E. 4.0 cm

1448. The major factor in deciding between partial and total penectomy in the treatment of penile cancer is:

A. Patient's preference
B. Residual penile length sufficient to permit directable micturition after partial penectomy
C. Grade of the tumor
D. Presence of inguinal metastases
E. Presence of urethral stricture disease

1449. When performing partial penectomy, the urethra is:

A. Transected at the same level as the corporeal bodies
B. Transected 1 cm proximal to the transected corporeal bodies
C. Transected 1 cm distal to the transected corporeal bodies
D. Spatulated ventrally only
E. Anastomosed to penile skin using nonabsorbable suture

1450. The most cephalad extent of the deep inguinal nodes is:

A. Sentinel lymph node
B. Node of Cloquet
C. Virchow's node
D. Lateral to the femoral nerve just below the inguinal ligament
E. Within Camper's fascia just above the inguinal ligament

1451. The femoral nerve supplies motor function to all of the following muscles EXCEPT:

A. Pectineus
B. Vastus medialis
C. Sartorius
D. Biceps femoris
E. Vastus lateralis

1452. The lateral margin of the femoral triangle is:

A. Femoral nerve
B. Femoral artery
C. Sartorius muscle
D. Tensor fascia lata
E. Pectineus muscle

1453. The percentage of patients with penile carcinoma presenting with palpable inguinal lymphadenopathy is:

A. 5–10
B. 15–25
C. 30–60
D. 60–70
E. 75–90

1454. A 56-year-old black male who had a partial penectomy for T1: grade II squamous cell carcinoma of the penis undergoes right inguinal mode dissection for persistently palpable adenopathy despite antibiotics, and his is found to have evidence of metastatic disease on frozen section. The risk of contralateral metastases in this patient is approximately:

A. <5 per cent
B. 10 per cent
C. 20 per cent
D. 40 per cent
E. 60 per cent

1455. The sentinel lymph node is located:

A. Between the superficial external pudendal and superficial epigastric veins
B. Lateral to the saphenofemoral junction
C. Two fingerbreadths inferomedial to the pubic tubercle
D. Just inferomedial to the superficial external pudendal vein
E. Just below the saphenofemoral junction anterior to the femoral vein

1456. The muscle used to cover the femoral vessels after inguinal lymph node dissection should be:

A. Pectineus
B. Adductor longus
C. Adductor brevis
D. Gracilis
E. Sartorius

1457. At inguinal lymph node dissection, when attempting to close the skin incision, it is noted that the margins are slightly ischemic and some tension exists along the closure when placing the sutures. The best approach to management is:

A. Close the wound as is despite tension.
B. Debride the ischemic areas and close the wound primarily despite tension.
C. Debride the ischemic areas, leave the wound open and perform delayed closure in 4 days.
D. Debride the ischemic areas and close with the aid of myocutaneous flaps.
E. Debride the ischemic area and cover the skin defect with split-thickness skin grafts.

1458. Modified groin lymphadenectomy differs from the standard dissection in all of the following ways EXCEPT:

A. Skin incision is shorter.
B. Lateral margin is the femoral nerve.
C. Saphenous vein is preserved.
D. Sartorius muscle is not transposed.
E. Inferior margin excludes regions caudal to the fossa ovules.

1459. A 65-year-old white male is diagnosed with an invasive proximal bulbomembranous squamous cell carcinoma of the urethra. Metastatic work-up is negative. The treatment of choice for the primary lesion is:

A. Transurethral resection
B. Neodymium:YAG laser fulguration
C. Total penectomy
D. Extended excision (cystectomy, urethrectomy, and excision of the pubic arch)
E. Radiation therapy

1460. In urethral carcinoma, palpable inguinal adenopathy is most commonly due to:

A. Inflammation
B. Infection
C. Nodal metastasis
D. Lymphatic obstruction from radiation therapy
E. Lymphatic obstruction from chemotherapy

1461. The incidence of subsequent severe epithelial atypia or frank in-situ urethral carcinoma in male patients in whom urethrectomy in not performed prophylactically during cystectomy of bladder cancer is estimated to be approximately:

A. 10–12 per cent
B. 25 per cent
C. 50 per cent
D. 75 per cent
E. 90 per cent

1462. During urethrectomy, the urethral branches of the internal pudendal arteries are ligated and divided as they enter the bulb:

A. At 12 and 6 o'clock
B. At 4 and 8 o'clock
C. Superior to the perineal membrane
D. After passing through the corpora cavernosa
E. Superior to the bulbocavernosus muscle

1463. Therapy of urethral carcinoma in the female is based primarily on:

A. Stage
B. Grade
C. Size
D. Histologic type
E. Patient age

1464. A 50-year-old white female is diagnosed with invasive well-differentiated squamous cell carcinoma of the urethral meatus. Metastatic work-up is negative. The recommended management should be:

A. Radiation therapy
B. Transurethral resection
C. Circumferential local excision of the distal urethra only
D. Circumferential local excision of the distal urethra and adjacent portion of anterior vaginal wall
E. Anterior pelvic exenteration

1465. All of the following regarding the management of a primary testicular tumor are true EXCEPT:

A. In patients with an unequivocal testicular mass on physical examination, ultrasound is unnecessary.
B. Early control of the cord vessels must always be achieved to prevent potential tumor spread.
C. The scrotal approach offers the best chance for surgical resection of tumor, especially in large masses.
D. The vas should be ligated separately from the rest of the cord structures.
E. The internal ring should be obliterated with a suture before closing the external oblique fascia.

1466. A 35-year-old man is referred after a right scrotal orchiectomy for a T2 seminoma. Metastatic work-up including B-HCG, AFP, CXR, and CT scan of abdomen and pelvis are without evidence of metastatic disease. The next step in management should be:

A. Observation
B. Hemiscrotectomy and ipsilateral inguinal lymph node dissection
C. Radiation therapy to the retroperitoneum, right hemiscrotum, and ipsilateral inguinal lymph nodes
D. Radiation therapy to the retroperitoneum and ipsilateral inguinal lymph nodes after hemiscrotectomy
E. 3 cycles of platinum-based chemotherapy

1467. A 25-year-old white male is referred after a left scrotal orchiectomy reveals T3 embryonal cell carcinoma. Metastatic work-up, including B-HCG, AFP, CXR, and CT scan of abdomen and pelvis, is without evidence of metastatic disease. The treatment of choice is:

A. Observation
B. Modified retroperitoneal lymph node dissection only
C. Modified retroperitoneal lymph node dissection and excision of the prior scrotal incision and residual stump of the spermatic cord
D. Modified retroperitoneal lymph node dissection and radiation therapy to the left hemiscrotum
E. 3 cycles of platinum-based chemotherapy

1468. A 30-year-old white male is found to have an abdominal mass on CT scan for abdominal pain. CXR is without lesions. B-HCG is 40 MIU/ml and

AFP is 80 mg/ml. Physical examination and scrotal ultrasound reveal normal testes. Retroperitoneal lymph node dissection reveals a 4-cm mass anterior to the aorta just below the left renal vein, and pathologic examination reveals teratocarcinoma. Throughout his course of chemotherapy, physical examination and follow-up ultrasound fail to reveal any evidence of testicular lesions. The next step in management is:

A. Observation with physical examination, tumor markers, and serrated ultrasounds
B. Bilateral testicular biopsies inguinal approaches
C. Bilateral orchiectomy
D. Left orchiectomy and right testicular biopsy
E. Radiation therapy to the scrotum

1469. A 35-year-old white male with a left testicular mass and a B-HCG of 250 MIU/ml and AFP of zero undergoes left radical orchiectomy. Pathologic examination reveals stage T3 pure seminoma. CT scan reveals no obvious masses. The treatment of choice is:

A. Observation every 6 months
B. Radiation therapy
C. Platinum-based combination with chemotherapy
D. Radiation therapy and platinum-based chemotherapy
E. Modified retroperitoneal lymph node dissection

1470. All of the following are associated with higher risk of metastatic spread in patients with nonseminomatous germ cell tumors EXCEPT:

A. Embryonal cell type
B. Vascular invasion
C. Lymphatic invasion
D. Yolk sac elements
E. Epididymal involvement

1471. Which of the following is not recommended as part of the staging work-up of testicular tumors:

A. Serum B-HCG
B. Serum AFP
C. Serum LDH
D. Chest radiograph
E. CT scan of chest

1472. Clinical surveillance of patients with low stage nonseminoma:

A. Is better with MRI than with CT scan
B. Is associated with the development of metastatic disease in 25 to 35 per cent of patients
C. Is more accurate with the addition of lymphangiogram
D. Results in similar retroperitoneal recurrence rates as compared with retroperitoneal lymph node dissection
E. Is most commonly associated with the development of lung metastases

1473. The incidence of retroperitoneal recurrence following thorough lymph node dissection is:

A. <1 per cent
B. 5 per cent
C. 10 per cent
D. 20 per cent
E. 50 per cent

1474. When performing a limited retroperitoneal lymph node dissection, the most important area to preserve is:

A. Anterior to the aorta above the origin of the inferior mesenteric artery
B. Overlying the aorta and sacrum below the origin of the inferior mesenteric artery
C. Overlying the common iliac arteries
D. Overlying the sacrum below the aortic bifurcation
E. Interaortacaval area below the superior mesenteric artery

1475. After modified nerve-sparing RPLND, ejaculation can be preserved in approximately what percentage of patients:

A. 30 per cent
B. 50 per cent
C. 60 per cent
D. 80 per cent
E. 100 per cent

1476. A patient with clinical stage A teratocarcinoma undergoes nerve-sparing retroperitoneal lymph node dissection. At exploration, he is found to have gross adenopathy and a 3-cm mass anterior to the aorta just below the left renal vein. Appropriate management should be:

A. Continue with limited nerve-sparing RPLND
B. Limited nerve-sparing RPLND and postoperative adjunctive chemotherapy
C. Full bilateral RPLND with suprahilar dissection
D. Full bilateral RPLND with postoperative adjunctive chemotherapy
E. Limited nerve-sparing RPLND and postoperative radiation therapy

1477. The risk of tumor recurrence with surgical therapy alone (RPLND) in low volume pathologic stage II disease is:

A. 5–10 per cent
B. 10–30 per cent
C. 30–50 per cent
D. 55–70 per cent
E. 70–90 per cent

1478. The advantages of the transabdominal approach over the thoracoabdominal approach of RPLND include all of the following EXCEPT:

A. Shorter operation time due to faster opening and closure of the incision
B. Easier access to the suprahilar area
C. More familiar to most surgeons
D. Lower risk of atelectasis
E. Lower risk of pulmonary injury

1479. When performing a thoracoabdominal approach for RPLND, the skin incision is usually made:

A. Over the bed of the sixth rib
B. Over the bed of the seventh rib
C. Over the bed of the eighth or ninth rib
D. Over the bed of the 10th rib
E. Between ribs 7 and 8

1480. The lateral margin of dissection in a full bilateral RPLND should be:

A. Medial aspect of the gonadal vessels

B. Medial aspect of the ureters
C. Lateral aspect of the psoas muscle
D. Lateral border of the quadrators lumbering muscle
E. Iliohypogastric nerve

1481. The most common intraoperative complication in RPLND is:

A. Colonic injury
B. Duodenal injury
C. Vascular injury
D. Bladder injury
E. Hepatic injury

1482. During RPLND, it is noted that during mobilization of the adipose tissue around the renal hilum, the superior segmental branch of the right renal artery was ligated and transected. The next step in management should be:

A. Completion of the procedure and observation
B. Primary reanastomosis
C. Use of Gor-Tex interposition graft between the two transected ends of the vessel
D. Aortic to superior segmental artery revascularization using a Gor-Tex graft
E. Right upper pole nephrectomy

1483. The most common long-term complication of full RPLND is:

A. Hypertension
B. Bowel obstruction
C. Impotence
D. Anejaculation
E. Incisional hernia

1484. During RPLND, division of the inferior mesenteric vein facilitates:

A. Mobilization of the pancreas
B. Mobilization of the mesenteric of the left colon
C. Mobilization of the right colon
D. Access to ligament of Treitz
E. Access to the infrahilar interaortocoval tissue

1485. Nerve-sparing RPLND attempts to isolate which of the following structures?

A. Sympathetic chain
B. Preganglionic sympathetic fibers T8-T10
C. Postganglionic sympathetic fibers emanating from the lumbar ganglia L1 to L4
D. Hypogastric plexus
E. Pelvic nerves

1486. In adults, which of the following cell types requires RPLND regardless of results with chemotherapy?

A. Seminoma
B. Choriocarcinoma
C. Embryonal cell
D. Yolk sac
E. Teratoma

1487. After 3 cycles of platinum-based chemotherapy for stage III embryonal cell carcinoma, a patient is found to have a 4-cm residual retroperitoneal mass on CT scan but no other evidence of disease. The most appropriate management is:

A. Observation with repeat CT scan and tumor markers in 3 months
B. Full RPLND
C. Salvage chemotherapy
D. CT-guided needle biopsy of the mass
E. Radiation therapy

1488. A major risk factor for increased morbidity in patients undergoing RPLND is:

A. Obesity
B. Immunologic status
C. Hormonal dysfunction
D. Preoperative chemotherapy
E. Prior abdominal surgery

1489. The major factor related to pulmonary complications in RPLND after bleomycin chemotherapy is:

A. Use of colloids for hydration
B. Increased inspired oxygen concentrations
C. Thoracoabdominal incision
D. Atelectasis
E. Suprahilar dissection

1490. During RPLND for abdominal disease after primary chemotherapy the ipsilateral ureter cannot be separated from the tumor. The patient has a normal contralateral kidney. The procedure of choice is:

A. Leave behind tumor around the ureter and treat the patient with adjuvant chemotherapy.
B. Resect the ureter and perform permanent nephrotomy tube placement.
C. Resect the ureter and perform ileal interposition graft.
D. Leave behind the tumor around the ureter, place ureteral stent, and treat with adinguinal radiation therapy and chemotherapy.
E. Perform ipsilateral nephrectomy with the dissection.

1491. Which of the following is an indication for testicular biopsy?

A. Unexplained oligospermia
B. Azoospermia with small, firm testes and elevated FSH
C. Azoospermia with testes of normal size and consistency, palpable vasa deferentia and normal FSH
D. Absent vasa deferentia
E. Oligospermia with >10 WBCs per high-power field

1492. All of the following are true regarding vasography EXCEPT:

A. The vas should be explored through an inguinal incision if prior inguinal surgery has occurred.
B. If no fluid is found in the cut vas lumen, epididymal obstruction is confirmed.
C. The vas should be opened at the junction of the straight and convoluted portions to perform the vasogram.
D. Water-soluble contrast should be used.
E. Vasography should be injected toward the testis when epididymal obstruction is suspected.

1493. If vasal fluid contains sperm and the vasogram is normal, which of the following may be responsible?

A. Retrograde ejaculation
B. Lack of emission
C. Vas aperistalsis

D. All of the above
E. None of the above

1494. Which of the following is *not* an advantage of the no-scalpel vasectomy technique?

A. Lower failure rate
B. Less hematomas
C. Less infection
D. Less pain
E. Takes less time

1495. All of the following decrease the failure rate of vasectomy EXCEPT:

A. Removal of long segments of vas
B. Tight suture ligature of both ends
C. Hemoclips applied to both ends
D. Intraluminal occlusion with needle electrocautery
E. Interposition of fascia between the cut ends

1496. Complication rates of vasectomy are most affected by the:

A. Completeness of the shave and prep
B. Size of incision created
C. Use of electrocautery for hemostasis
D. Method of vasal occlusion
E. Experience of the surgeon

1497. When thick white fluid without sperm is found after the vas is transected, the best management strategy would be to:

A. Recut the vas closer to the epididymis
B. Treat with antibiotics postoperatively
C. Perform vasovasostomy if there is no evidence of more proximal obstruction
D. Perform vasoepididymostomy
E. Use a two-layered vasovasostomy anastomosis

1498. All the following are true regarding vasovasostomy EXCEPT:

A. The testicular side lumen of the vas is usually equal in size to the abdominal side.
B. Extravasated sperm negatively affects the success of the repair.
C. A one-layer anastomosis may be satisfactory.
D. Crossed vasovasostomy should be performed with unilateral vasal obstruction or aplasia of the inguinal vas or ejaculatory duct and contralateral epididymal obstruction.
E. One good anastomosis is better than two mediocre ones.

1499. Pregnancy rates following vasovasostomy when sperm were identified on at least one cut vas are:

A. 10–15 per cent
B. 25–33 per cent
C. 50–60 per cent
D. 70–80 per cent
E. 90–98 per cent

1500. Anatomic considerations of importance for epididymal surgery include all the following EXCEPT:

A. Short epididymal lengths will not allow for sperm to acquire motility and fertilizing capacity.
B. The distal epididymis is preferred for anastomosis.
C. Spermatic cord vessels enter medial to the epididymis at the junction of the middle and upper thirds of the testis.
D. Efferent ducts are located superior to the vascular pedicle of the testis.
E. The epididymis has a rich blood supply.

1501. The most common solid epididymal mass is a(n):

A. Spermatocele
B. Sperm granuloma
C. Rhabdomyosarcoma
D. Adenomatoid tumor
E. Leiomyoma

1502. End-to-end vasoepididymostomy is indicated when:

A. Epididymal tubules are dilated
B. Adequate vasal length is present
C. Congenital epididymal obstruction is present
D. Proximal obstruction of the epididymis is present
E. Obstruction occurs near the vasoepididymal junction

1503. Pregnancy rates after vasoepididymostomy are:

A. <5 per cent
B. 15–30 per cent
C. 50–60 per cent
D. The lower, the more distal the anastomosis
E. Equal to vasovasostomy rates

1504. Ejaculatory duct obstruction is characterized by all the following EXCEPT:

A. Elevated FSH
B. Low semen volume
C. Low fructose level in semen
D. Normal spermatogenesis on testis biopsy
E. Palpable vas deferens

1505. In obstructed systems, sperm motility is:

A. Best in the distal epididymis
B. Best in the proximal epididymis
C. Absent
D. Best after washing
E. Best when mixed with blood

1506. Venous drainage of the testis after microsurgical varicocelectomy is through the:

A. Cremasteric vein
B. Inguinal and retroperitoneal collaterals
C. Vasal vein
D. Gubernacular collaterals
E. External spermatic veins

1507. Postoperative hydroceles after varicocelectomy:

A. Are due to poor venous drainage
B. Are secondary to postoperative inflammatory changes
C. Do not occur after a retroperitoneal approach
D. Are due to ligated lymphatics
E. Never become symptomatic so as to require treatment

1508. Varicocele recurrence is lowest with:

A. Retroperitoneal repairs
B. Repairs in adolescents
C. Microsurgical high inguinal repairs
D. Radiographic occlusion techniques
E. Laparoscopic approaches

1509. Which of the following statements regarding varicocelectomy is *false*?

A. Varicocelectomy produces significant improvement in semen parameters in 33 per cent of cases.
B. Average pregnancy rate after varicocele repair is 35 per cent.
C. Varicoceles are found in 35 per cent of men with primary infertility and 85 per cent of cases of secondary infertility.
D. Varicoceles are seen in 15 per cent of normal men.
E. Better results are seen after repair in adolescents and of large varicoceles.

1510. The most common complication of a hydrocelectomy is:

A. Infection
B. Recurrence
C. Testicular artery injury
D. Hematoma formation
E. Epididymal injury

PART XIV

UROLOGIC SURGERY

CHAPTERS 63 THROUGH 87

ANSWERS

1074-D *(Campbell's, p. 2315)*

Congestive heart failure and recent myocardial infarction (within 6 months) remain the two strongest predictors of perioperative cardiac morbidity.

REFERENCES

1. Goldman, L., Calders, D.L., Nussbaum, S.R., et al.: Multifactorial index of cardiac risk in noncardiac surgical procedures. N. Engl. J. Med., *297*:345, 1977.
2. Detsky, A.S., Abrams, H.B., Forbath, N., et al.: Cardiac assessment for patients undergoing noncardiac surgery. A multifactorial clinical risk index. Arch. Intern. Med., *146*:2131, 1986.

1075-E *(Campbell's, p. 2317)*

The indications for preoperative administration of digitalis include: (1) a prior history of congestive heart failure; (2) cardiac dysfunction with evidence of impaired ventricular performance; (3) nocturnal angina; (4) atrial fibrillation or flutter with a rapid ventricular response; and (5) frequent episodes of paroxysmal atrial or junctional tachycardia. Digitalis is not recommended on the basis of either advanced age or thc presence of coronary artery disease alone. Digitalis should be started several days before surgery so that adequate therapeutic level can be achieved.

REFERENCE

1. Mason, D.T.: Cardiovascular management. *In* Mason, D.T. (Ed.): Essays in Medicine, New York, Medcom Publishers, 1974.

1076-C *(Campbell's, p. 2317)*

Perioperative myocardial infarction usually occurs in the first postoperative week and is silent in about 50 per cent of patients. The mortality from an initial myocardial infarction is about 20 to 30 per cent, whereas the mortality from a recurrent myocardial infarction is between 50 and 80 per cent. Patients who undergo surgery within 3 months after a myocardial infarction have up to a 37 per cent incidence of reinfarction. The overall reinfarction rate has been reduced to less than 6 per cent within 3 months of a previous infarction if aggressive intraoperative monitoring and extended stay in an intensive care unit are utilized.

REFERENCES

1. von-Knorring, J.: Postoperative myocardial infarction: A prospective study in a risk group of surgical patients. Surgery, *90*:55, 1981.
2. Rao, T.K., Jacobs, K.H., El-Etr., A.A.: Reinfarction following anesthesia in patients with myocardial infarction. Anesthesiology. *59*:499, 1983.

1077-A *(Campbell's, p. 2318)*

Supraventricular tachycardia occurs in about 4 per cent of surgical patients postoperatively. Atrial fibrillation is the most common supraventricular tachyarrhythmia and accounts for about half of the cases. Preoperative factors that are associated with the development of postoperative arrhythmias include age greater than 70 years, major thoracic abdominal or vascular operations, and the presence of pulmonary rales.

REFERENCE

1. Goldman, L., Calders, D.L., Southwick, F.S., et al.: Cardiac risk factors and complications in noncardiac surgery. Medicine, *57*:537, 1978.

1078-D *(Campbell's, p. 2319)*

All of the statements are true except D. Patients with a diastolic blood pressure less than 120 mm Hg do not have an increased risk of cardiac complications. Patients with a diastolic blood pressure above 120 mm Hg do have an increased risk of complications. Patients whose normal systolic pressure drops by one third for as little as 10 minutes have an increased incidence of cardiovascular complications. Abrupt cessation of clonidine may precipitate severe hypertension. This medication deserves special attention in patients who will be unable to resume oral medications immediately postoperatively and should be withdrawn and replaced with another medication several weeks prior to surgery. Beta-adrenergics should not be withdrawn prior to surgery. Patients receiving diuretics should be evaluated for hypokalemia and hypovolemia.

REFERENCES

1. Goldman, L., and Calders, D.: Risks of general anesthesia and elective operation in the hypertensive patient. Anesthesiology, *50*:285, 1979.

2. Blaschke, T.F., and Melmon, R.L.: Antihypertensive agents and the drug therapy of hypertension. *In* Goodman, A.G., Goodman, L.S., and Gilman, A. (Eds.): Goodman and Gilman's Pharmacological Basis of Therapeutics. 6th ed. New York, Macmillan Publishing Co., 1980.

1079-B *(Campbell's, p. 2319)*

Meperidine produces a relatively large amount of myocardial depression as does halothane. Morphine and nitrous oxide, on the other hand, produce relatively little myocardial depression, and barbiturates do not have a marked myocardial depressant effect in smaller doses.

1080-A *(Campbell's, pp. 2319–2320)*

All of the statements are true except A. The indications for direct blood pressure monitoring include expected rapid changes in blood pressure as a result of underlying cardiac disease, expected sudden changes in blood pressure because of the nature of the surgical procedure, the expectation of postoperative instability requiring intravenous infusions of vasopressor or vasodilating therapy, and the expectation of large volumes of blood loss. The patient's age is not an indication for direct blood pressure monitoring.

REFERENCE

1. Merritt, W.T.: Monitoring modalities. *In* Breskow, M.J., Miller, C.F., and Rogers, M.C. (Eds.): Perioperative Management. St. Louis, C.V. Mosby Co., 1990, p. 64.

1081-D *(Campbell's, p. 2322)*

Cigarette smokers and patients with chronic obstructive pulmonary disease have a 2- to 3-fold increased risk for postoperative pulmonary morbidity and a 7- to 10-fold higher mortality rate. In one study, 25 per cent of patients who had upper abdominal incisions developed pulmonary complications. Anesthesia time in excess of 3 hours is associated with increased pulmonary complications. Protein-depleted patients demonstrated significant reduction in respiratory muscle strength, vital capacity, and peak expiratory flow rate. The risk of developing pneumonia is significantly higher in protein-depleted patients. *Severe* obesity is associated with a greatly increased risk of pulmonary complications.

REFERENCES

1. Ray, S., et al.: Effects of obesity on respiratory function. Am. Rev. Respir. Dis., *128*:501, 1983.
2. Winser, J.A., and Hill, G.L.: Risk factors for postoperative pneumonia. Am. Surg., *208*:209, 1988.
3. Roukema, J.A., Carol, E.J., and Prins, J.G.: The prevention of pulmonary complications after upper abdominal surgery in patients with noncompromised pulmonary status. Arch. Surg., *123*:30, 1988.
4. Forthman, H.J., and Shepard, A.: Postoperative pulmonary complications. South. Med. J., *62*:1198, 1969.
5. Fowkes, F.G.R., et al.: Epidemiology in anesthesia, III. Mortality risk in patients with coexisting physical disease. Br. J. Anesth., *34*:819, 1982.

1082-C *(Campbell's, pp. 2324–2325)*

All of the statements are true except C. During mechanical ventilation, cardiac output may be decreased due to increased intrathoracic pressure. Oxygen toxicity becomes a concern when FIO_2 is greater than 50 per cent. Barotrauma can be a major complication, as can respiratory alkalosis, which is related to hyperventilation and may be physiologic, iatrogenic, or reflex. Ventilation perfusion imbalance results from the influence of disease and positioning, causing decreased ventilation with little effect on the perfusion.

REFERENCES

1. Gillmour, I.J.: Preoperative respiratory care. Urol. Clin. North Am., *10*:65, 1983.
2. Douglas, W.W., Rehder, K., Beyman, F.M., et al.: Improved oxygenation in patients with acute respiratory failure. The prone position. Am. Rev. Respir. Dis., *115*:559, 1977.
3. Colgan, F.J., Barrow, R.E., and Fanning, G.L.: Continuous positive pressure breathing and cardiorespiratory function. Anesthesiology, *34*:145, 1979.

1083-B *(Campbell's, p. 2326)*

All of the statements are true except B. Regional anesthesia is associated with a decreased morbidity in high-risk patients within 3 months of myocardial infarction. It also carries a lower perioperative mortality in hip surgery. Although it has not been proved, evidence suggests that regional anesthesia is better than general anesthesia in preserving FRC (functional residual capacity) postoperatively. It is associated with significantly reduced bleeding in patients undergoing hysterectomy, lower and vascular surgery, and hip replacement, and results in a 35 per cent reduction in blood loss during retropubic prostatectomy. Multiple studies have demonstrated that significant decrease in both deep venous thrombophlebitis and pulmonary embolism for operations below the embolic is performed under regional anesthesia. However, no benefit has been observed for upper abdominal surgery.

REFERENCES

1. Valentin, N., Lomholt, B., Jensen, J.S., et al.: Spinal or general anesthesia for surgery of the fractured hip. Br. J. Anesth., *58*:284, 1986.
2. Reiz, S., Balfors, E., Sorrensen, M.B., et al.: Risk of complications during intravenous heparin therapy. West. J. Med., *136*:189, 1982.
3. Catley, D.M., Thornton, C., Jordan, C., et al.: Pronounced episodic desaturation in the postoperative period. Its association with ventilatory pattern and analgesic regime. Anesthesiology, *65*:20, 1985.
4. David, F.M., McDermott, E., Hickson, C., et al.: Influence of spinal and general anesthesia on hemostasis during total hip arthroplasty. Br. J. Anesth., *59*:561, 1987.
5. Hendolin, H., Mattila, M.A.K., and Poikolainen, E.: The effect of lumbar epidural analgesia on the development of deep venous thrombosis of the legs after open prostatectomy. Acta Chir. Scand., *147*:425, 1981.

6. MacKenzie, P.J., Wishart, H.Y., Gray, J., et al.: Effect of anesthetic technique on deep vein thrombosis. Br. J. Anesth., *57*:853, 1985.

1084-E *(Campbell's, pp. 2327–2328)*

Nearly all clinically significant pulmonary emboli originate in the deep veins of the leg. It is difficult to estimate the incidence of deep venous thrombosis by physical examination because at least 50 per cent of venous thrombi in the leg are clinically silent. By utilizing radioactive iodine-labeled fibrinogen scanning or venography, the incidence of DVT in patients undergoing urologic surgery has been found to be between 30 and 60 per cent.

REFERENCES

1. Hovig, O.: Source of pulmonary emboli. Acta Chir. Scand. Suppl., *478*:42, 1977.
2. Moser, K.M., Brach, B., and Dolan, G.F.: Clinically suspected deep venous thrombosis of the lower extremities. JAMA, *237*:2195, 1977.
3. Kutnowski, M., Vandendris, M., Steinberger, R., et al.: Prevention of postoperative deep-vein thrombosis by low-dose heparin in urological surgery. A double blind randomized study. Urol. Res., *5*:123, 1977.

1085-E *(Campbell's, p. 2328)*

All of the statements are true except E. The duration of anesthesia is a major risk factor contributing to thromboembolic disease, and incidence of DVT increases markedly when anesthesia time is greater than 1 hour. Other risk factors for thromboembolic disease include age greater than 60 years, the presence of malignant disease, the use of estrogens, and the period and degree of immobility after surgery.

REFERENCES

1. Kakkar, V.V.: Prophylaxis of venous thromboembolism. Proc. R. Soc. Med., *68*:263, 1975.
2. Moser, K.M.: Thromboembolic disease in the patient undergoing urologic surgery. Urol. Clin. North Am., *10*:101, 1983.

1086-C *(Campbell's, pp. 2328–2330)*

All of the statements are true except C. Antiplatelet therapy, specifically aspirin derivatives, is of value in prophylaxis of certain arterial occlusive diseases such as transient ischemic attacks and myocardial infarction; however, it has not been shown to be effective in the prevention of venous thromboembolic disease. Early ambulation has been shown to decrease venous thrombosis after myocardial infarction, although its efficacy for surgical patients has not been established. Regional anesthesia also reduces the incidences of DVT. Pneumatic compression devices are effective in the prevention of DVT through mechanisms other than a direct mechanical compression as shown by measurement of euglobulin lysis time. Further, the devices have been shown to result in an increased venous capacitance and outflow when applied only unilaterally. Low-dose heparin effectively reduces both DVT and pulmonary embolism and has not been shown to be associated with an increased risk of bleeding or a significant blood loss when compared to untreated patients. The incidence of wound hematoma is significantly more frequent with heparin treated patients but no significant morbidity is associated with this.

REFERENCES

1. Clagett, G.P., and Reisch, J.S.: Prevention of venous thromboembolism in general surgical patients. Ann. Surg., *208*:227, 1988.
2. Kiil, J., Axelsen, F., et al.: Prophylaxis against postoperative pulmonary embolism and deep-vein thrombosis by low-dose heparin. Lancet, *1*:1115, 1978.
3. Caprini, J.A., and Natonson, R.A.: Postoperative deep vein thrombosis: Current clinical consideration. Semin. Thromb. Hemost., *15*:244, 1989.
4. Inada, K., Koike, S., Shirai, N., et al.: Effects of intermittent pneumatic leg compression for prevention of postoperative deep venous thrombosis with special reference to fibrinolytic activity. Am. J. Surg., *155*:602, 1988.
5. Blackshear, W.M., Prescott, C., LePain, F., et al.: Influence of sequential pneumatic compression on postoperative venous function. J. Vasc. Surg., *5*:432, 1987.
6. Miller, R.R., Lies, J.E., and Caretta, R.F.: Prevention of lower extremity venous thrombosis by early mobilization. Ann. Intern. Med., *84*:700, 1976.

1087-C *(Campbell's, pp. 2331–2334)*

In all patients, GFR decreases intraoperatively and immediately postoperatively. In patients with preexisting renal insufficiency, this can be a devastating occurrence. Under normal conditions, patients are able to maintain a potassium balance until GFR falls to 10 ml/min; however, during the perioperative period an increased endogenous and exogenous potassium load may precipitate problems. Thus hyperkalemia is a potentially major problem in patients with renal insufficiency who are undergoing surgery. Hypocalcemia and hypophosphatemia occur commonly in patients with renal insufficiency and are generally well tolerated. Patients with renal insufficiency frequently have metabolic acidosis because of an inability to excrete a normal acid load and to regenerate bicarbonate. Although metabolic alkalosis is seldom of renal origin, it occurs commonly in the postoperative period because of gastrointestinal losses. Metabolic alkalosis is usually corrected by the kidneys, and patients with renal insufficiency may be unable to compensate adequately. Patients with moderate or severe renal insufficiency are also at risk for increased perioperative hemorrhage, primarily from abnormal platelet function. The best laboratory test to assess the risk is the bleeding time. The prothrombin time, partial thromboplastin time, and platelet count are usually normal.

REFERENCES

1. Kasiske, B.L., Kjellstrand, C.M.: Perioperative management of patients with chronic renal failure and postoperative acute renal failure. Urol. Clin. North Am., *10*:35, 1983.
2. Burke, G.R., and Gulyassy, P.E.: Surgery on the patient with renal disease and related electrolyte disorders. Med. Clin. North Am., *63*:1191, 1979.

3. Kono, K., Philbin, D.M., Coggins, C.H., et al.: Renal function and stress response during halothane and fentanyl anesthesia. Anesth. Analog., *50*:552, 1981.
4. Parfrey, P.S., Griffiths, S.M., Barrett, B.J., et al.: Contrast material-induced renal failure in patients with diabetes mellitus, renal insufficiency, or both. N. Engl. J. Med., *320*:143, 1989.

1088-B *(Campbell's, pp. 2336–2337)*

Mild to moderate degrees of anemia do not increase the risk of elective surgery but should be evaluated to determine the etiology. Iron deficiency anemia is the most common cause of anemia. In this condition, both the mean corpusculaı volume and mean corpuscular hemoglobin content are decreased, resulting in a microcytic, hypochromic peripheral smear. The reticulocyte percentage index is less than 1 per cent.

1089-B *(Campbell's, pp. 2339–2341)*

All of the statements are true about hemostatic competence except B. von Willebrand's disease is related to deficiency of a part of the factor VIII complex. It is caused by a deficiency of the high-molecular-weight protein. Patients with sickle cell trait experience no increased surgical risk. Platelet function is measured by bleeding time. Patients with vitamin K deficiency have prolongation of prothrombin (time the measure of the extrinsic pathway) and partial thromboplastin time (the measure of the intrinsic pathways).

REFERENCES

1. Sears, D.A.: The morbidity of sickle cell trait: A review of the literature. Am. J. Med., *64*:1021, 1978.
2. Owen, C.A., Jr.: Factor VIII terminology. Letter. Lancet, *2*:359, 1981.
3. Owen, C.A., Jr., and Walter Bowie, E.J.: Disorders of coagulation. Urol. Clin. North Am., *10*:77, 1983.

1090-C *(Campbell's, p. 2341)*

Blood glucose levels should be maintained between 125 and 250 mg/dl during the perioperative period to decrease the incidence of infections and to facilitate wound healing.

REFERENCES

1. Bagdade, J.D.: Phagocytic and microbial function in diabetes mellitus. J. Endocrinol. (Suppl.), *83*:27, 1976.
2. Goodsen, W.H., and Hunt, T.K.: Studies on wound healing in experimental diabetes mellitus. J. Surg. Res., *22*:221, 1977.

1091-B *(Campbell's, p. 2343)*

Markedly impaired cortisol secretion during surgery is unlikely if a normal adrenal response to adrenocorticotropic hormone is demonstrated preoperatively. The indications for supplemental perioperative steroid therapy are as follows: (1) chronic adrenal insufficiency; (2) continuous treatment with topical steroids for greater than 1 month in the previous 6 months; (3) treatment with systemic steroids for greater than 1 week in the past 6 months; (4) current steroid therapy; (5) anticipated bilateral adrenalectomy; and (6) anticipated unilateral adrenalectomy for cortisol-producing tumor.

REFERENCES

1. Kehlet, H., and Binder, C.: Value of an ACTH test in assessing hypothalamic-pituitary-adrenocortical function in glucocorticoid-treated patients. Br. Med. J., *2*: 147, 1973.
2. Rabinowitz, I.N., Watson, W., and Farber, E.M.: Topical steroid depression of the hypothalamic-pituitary-adrenal axis in psoriasis vulgaris. Dermatologica., *154*: 321, 1977.
3. Gran, L., and Pahle, J.A.: Rational substitution therapy for steroid-treated patients. Anesthesia, *33*:59, 1978.
4. Baesl, T.J., and Buckley, J.J.: Preoperative assessment, preparation for operation, and routine postoperative care. Urol. Clin. North Am., *10*:3, 1983.

1092-A *(Campbell's, p. 2347)*

The risk of infection increases with the duration indwelling urethral catheter. Even with careful management, about 50 per cent of patients will have urinary tract infections after 10 days of catheterization.

REFERENCE

1. Nickel, J.C., Feero, P., Costerton, J.W., et al.: Incidence and importance of bacteriuria in postoperative, short-term urinary catheterization. Can. J. Surg., *32*:131, 1989.

1093-E *(Campbell's, pp. 2351–2352)*

All of the statements about urologic surgery during pregnancy are true except E. Radiographic evaluation of the urinary tracts should be limited to emergency situations. The evidence suggests that harmful radiation effects of the fetus are associated with radiation exposure in excess of 50 cGy. This dose is far in excess of that associated with the usual intravenous pyelogram, which has a radiation dosage of less than 1 cGy. In patients with demonstrated calculi it has been found that endoscopic extraction of distal ureteral calculi is possible during any phase of pregnancy and percutaneous nephrostomy drainage may be safely employed during pregnancy also. The incidence of calculus disease is no greater during pregnancy, but the symptoms are often attributed to another cause, and the diagnosis is frequently not made until after delivery.

REFERENCES

1. Coe, F.L., Parks, J.H., and Lindheimer, M.D.: Nephrolithiasis during pregnancy. N. Engl. J. Med., *298*:324, 1978.
2. Swartz, H.M., and Reichling, B.A.: Hazards of radiation exposure for pregnant women. JAMA, *239*:1907, 1978.

1094-C, 1095-E *(Campbell's, pp. 2360–2362)*

The adrenal glands are paired retroperitoneal organs that lie within perinephric fat at the anterosuperior and medial aspects of the kidney. The adrenals have a delicate and rich blood supply without a dominant single artery. The inferior phrenic artery is the main blood supply with additional branches from the aorta and the renal artery. The venous drainage is usually a common vein on the right exiting the apex of the gland and entering the posterior surface of the IVC. The left adrenal vein empties directly into the left renal vein often opposite to the gonadal vein.

Microscopically, the mature adrenal cortex constitutes 90 per cent of the gland and is divided into three zones: zona glomerulosa, zona fasciculata, and zona reticularis. The adrenal cortex develops from mesoderm and the medulla from neuroectoderm (i.e., cells of the neural crest that migrate at the seventh week to form collections which enter the fetal cortex leaving nodules of neuroblasts scattered throught the cortex). Neuroblastic cortical nodules regress as the medulla forms.

REFERENCES

1. Johnston, F.R.: The suprarenal veins. Am. J. Surg., *94*: 615, 1957.
2. Crowder, R.E.: The development of the adrenal gland in man. Carnegie Contrib. Embryol., *36*:193, 1957.

1096-A *(Campbell's, p. 2364)*

The steroid hormones produced by the adrenal cortex have an array of actions, including salt retention, metabolic homeostasis, and adrenergic development. The zona glomerulosa is the only source of the major mineralocorticoid aldosterone, which regulates sodium resorption in the kidney, gut, and salivary and sweat glands. The other zones produce and secrete cortisol and the principal androgens dehydroepiandrosterone (DHEA), dehydroepiandrosterone sulfate (DHEAS), and androstenedione. The rate-limiting step for the formation of all these hormones is the production of pregnenolone from cholesterol.

REFERENCE

1. Carey, R.M., and Sen, S.: Recent progress in the control of aldosterone secretion. Rec. Prog. Horm. Res., *42*:251, 1986.

1097-D, 1098-B *(Campbell's, pp. 2365–2366)*

The regulation of cortical steroid release involves a complex interaction of the hypothalamus, pituitary gland, and adrenal gland. ACTH is a 39 amino acid polypeptide that exerts a major influence on the adrenal cortex, and it is produced from a large protein termed propiomelanocortin (POMC). Other POMC-derived peptides include β-lipotropin (β-LPH), α-melanocyte stimulating hormone (α-MSH), β-melanocyte stimulating hormone (β-MSH), β-endorphin, and methionine enkephalin. ACTH secretion is characterized by an inherent diurnal rhythm leading to parallel changes in cortisol, and is reciprocally related to the circulating cortisol level. Adrenal androgen production in the zona reticulosa and fasciculata is also under the influence of ACTH.

In contrast to glucocorticoids and adrenal androgens, the primary physiologic control of aldosterone secretion is angiotensin II. ACTH control is secondary. The critical sensor of the renin-angiotensin-aldosterone system (RAAS) resides in the juxtaglomerular apparatus within the kidney. Thus, in situations of decreased renal perfusion, there is renin release, angiotensin II formation, and subsequent aldosterone secretion resulting in sodium and water retention in an attempt to restore renal perfusion. A second, less potent stimulus for aldosterone release is hyperkalemia.

REFERENCES

1. Tepperman, J., and Tepperman, H.: Metabolic and Endocrine Physiology, 5th ed. Chicago, Year Book Medical Publishers, 1987.
2. Parker, L., and Odell, W.: Control of adrenal androgen secretion. Endocr. Rev., *1*:392, 1980.
3. Laragh, J.H., and Sealey, J.E.: The renin-angiotensin-aldosterone system and the renal regulation of sodium, potassium and blood pressure homeostasis. *In* Windhager, E.E. (Ed.): Handbook of Physiology. New York, Oxford University Press, 1991.

1099-E *(Campbell's, pp. 2366–2367)*

All steroid hormones diffuse passively into cells where they bind to a protein receptor in the cytosol before migrating into the nucleus. In the nucleus, these hormones result in the stimulation of transcription, which is regulated by interaction with a specific group of steroid-regulated genes, resulting in new RNA and specific protein synthesis.

Glucocorticoids are essential for life, even following mineralocorticoid replacement. Their effects include accumulation of glycogen in the liver and muscle, enhanced gluconeogenesis, impaired peripheral glucose utilization, muscle wasting, and osteoporosis (see Table 64–1).

Aldosterone stimulates sodium reabsorption and increased secretion of potassium and hydrogen via Na^+, K^+-ATPase activity. Adrenal androgens are only weakly active compared to testosterone and appear to be relevant only in pathologic states in which there may be excess production (e.g., congenital adrenal hyperplasia).

1100-C, 1101-B *(Campbell's, p. 2368)*

The adrenal medulla is composed of large chromaffin cells, which primarily secrete epinephrine but also secrete norepinephrine and dopamine. The enzyme phenylethanolamine-*N*-methyltransferase (PNMT), which catalyzes the methylation of norepinephrine to form epinephrine, is almost solely localized to the adrenal medulla. Thus, if there is excessive production of both norepinephrine and epinephrine, the offending lesion is almost always within the adrenal and not other sites of chromaffin tissue.

Catecholamines are rapidly removed from the circulation with a plasma half-life less than 20 seconds. Catecholamines are degraded by the action of both catechol-O-methytransferase (DMT) and by monamine oxidase (MAO), with either enzyme beginning the degradative process. The primary metabolite in the urine is vanillylmandelic acid (VMA) with metanepines, normetanephrine, and their derivatives contributing to total metabolic products.

REFERENCE

1. Axelrod, J.: Purification and properties of phenylethanolamine-*N*-methyltransferase. J. Biol. Chem., *237*: 1657, 1962.

1102-B, 1103-D, 1104-B *(Campbell's, pp. 2639–2374)*

Cushing's syndrome is the term used to describe the symptom complex caused by excess circulating glococorticoids. It includes patients with pituitary hypersecretion of ACTH, Cushing's disease, which accounts for 75 to 85 per cent of patients with endogenous Cushing's syndrome, patients with adrenal adenomas or carcinomas, and patients with ectopic secretion of ACTH. An exogenous source of Cushing's syndrome should always be excluded first, since therapeutic steroids are the most common cause. The manifestations of the disease are due to the actions of glucocorticoids. Some of the more common clinical manifestations include truncal obesity, hypertension, diabetes mellitus, weakness, muscle atrophy, hirsutism, purple striae, moon facies, osteoporosis, acne, hyperpigmentation, headache, and poor healing.

In patients suspected of having Cushing's syndrome, attempts should be made to determine the presence or absence of the normal circadian rhythm in plasma cortisol by obtaining ambulatory A.M. and P.M. serum cortisol levels. Patients with Cushing's syndrome usually lose the diurnal variation. An alternative first line screening test would be the measurement of 24-hour urinary free cortisol levels which tend to be elevated in patients with Cushing's syndrome. The next and most valuable test is the low-dose dexamethasone suppression test. All patients with Cushing's syndrome show resistance to suppression of cortisol release to low-dose dexamethasone. Once the diagnosis of Cushing's syndrome is made, serum ACTH levels can distinguish adrenal adenomas or carcinomas (low ACTH levels) from Cushing's disease and ectopic ACTH production (elevated ACTH levels). High-dose dexamethasone can then be used to distinguish Cushing's disease from ectopic ACTH production. In patients with Cushing's disease, there should be a 50 per cent or greater suppression of cortisol release; however, most patients with ectopic ACTH fail to suppress.

In general, CT scan has become the initial imaging procedure to search for adrenal masses in patients with Cushing's syndrome. In cases of suspected adrenal carcinoma, MRI may be useful.

REFERENCES

1. Scott, H.W. Jr.: *In* Scott, H.W. (Ed.): Surgery of the Adrenal Glands. Philadelphia, J.B. Lippincott Co., 1990.
2. Carpenter, P.C.: Cushing syndrome: Update of diagnosis and management. Mayo Clin. Proc., *61*:49, 1986.

1105-E *(Campbell's, pp. 2374–2376)*

In patients with Cushing's syndrome due to ectopic production of ACTH, treatment is directed to the primary tumor. Reduction of secretion of functional steroids by utilization of blocking agents can further ameliorate symptoms. Agents utilized include aminoglutethimide, which blocks the conversion of cholesterol to pregnenolone (the rate-limiting step in adrenal androgen synthesis); metyrapone, which blocks the conversion of 11-deoycortisol to cortisol; and ketoconazole, an antifungal agent that blocks cytochrome P450-mediated side chain cleavage and hydroxylation in steroid biosynthesis. Patients given aminoglutethimide must be observed for adrenocortical insufficiency because aldosterone production is also impaired.

Patients with pituitary disease (Cushing's disease) are best treated by transsphenoidal hypophysial microsurgical resection of the pituitary adenoma, with cure rates of 85 to 95 per cent.

Adrenal adenomas causing Cushing's syndrome are treated by surgical removal.

REFERENCES

1. Scott, H.W. Jr., and Orth, D.N.: Hypercortisolism (Cushing's syndrome). *In* Scott, H.W. (Ed.): Surgery of the Adrenal Glands. Philadelphia, J.B. Lippincott Co., 1990.
2. Wilson, C.B.: A decade of pituitary microsurgery, J. Neurosurg., *61*:814, 1984.

1106-D *(Campbell's, pp. 2376–2377)*

The increased utilization of abdominal ultrasound and CT scanning has led to the frequent findings of unexpected adrenal masses. All patients with solid adrenal massed should undergo biochemical assessment. Since most adrenal malignancies are usually larger than 6 cm and since CT scan or MRI may underestimate the size of an adrenal lesion, it is recommended that lesions larger than 5 cm on CT scan or MRI be explored. In nonfunctioning adrenal masses less than 5 cm, frequent follow-up with CT scan or MRI every 6 months for at least 18 months is recommended to evaluate any change in the size of the lesion which would necessitate exploration. An additional test that may prove helpful is the tumor/liver intensity ratio on T2 images of MRI. A high tumor/liver intensity (>2) on T2 images suggests that the lesion is not a benign adenoma (see Table 64–6).

REFERENCES

1. Ross, N.S., and Aron, D.C.: Hormonal evaluation of the patient with an incidentally discovered adrenal mass. N. Engl. J. Med., *323*:1401, 1990.
2. Reinig, J.W., Doppelman, J.L., Dwyer, A.J., et al.: Adrenal masses differentiated by MR. Radiology, *158*:81, 1986.

1107-B, 1108-B, 1109-A *(Campbell's, pp. 2376–2381)*

Adrenal carcinoma is a rare disease with an incidence of approximately 2 cases per million, and a poor prognosis. Adrenal malignancies are usually larger than 6 cm in size at diagnosis, and approximately 80 per cent of these tumors are functional. Adrenal carcinoma is one of the causes of corticosteroid excess. Virilization is the hallmark of Cushing's syndrome secondary to adrenal carcinomas. Also, virilization without evidence of cortisol excess is indicative of carcinoma except in children. From a metabolic standpoint, 17-ketosteroids and DHEAS levels are often high in patients with carcinomas. Adrenal carcinomas can less commonly secrete testosterone, estrogen, or aldosterone. The radiographic study of choice is CT or MRI.

Except for testosterone-secreting tumors, adrenocortical carcinomas are highly malignant with both local and hematogenous spread and a 5-year survival rate of less than 30 per cent. The most common sites of metastasis in decreasing order of frequency are lungs (60 per cent), liver (50 per cent), lymph nodes (48 per cent), bone (24 per cent), and pleura and heart (10 per cent). In addition, these tumors often extend directly into adjacent structures, especially the kidney.

The treatment of choice for adrenal carcinoma is radical adrenalectomy via a thoracoabdominal approach. Following surgical resection of functioning adrenal tumor, the patient can be followed with appropriate hormone levels as markers for tumor recurrence.

Despite advances in diagnostic techniques, many patients present with metastatic disease. Most patients with locally resectable disease eventually succumb to recurrent local or distant disease. The search for effective chemotherapy has been frustrating and radiation therapy is only effective for palliation. The most success reported in relieving symptoms has been with mitotane (*o.p'*-DDD), which has been shown to induce tumor response in 34 per cent, although survival time has not been prolonged.

REFERENCE

1. Luton, J.P., Cerdas, S., Billaud, L. et al.: Clinical features of adrenocortical carcinoma, prognostic factors, and the effect of mitotane therapy. N. Engl. J. Med., *322*:1195, 1990.

1110-E *(Campbell's, pp. 2381–2384)*

Adrenal insufficiency (Addison's disease) is a rare condition most commonly caused by either tuberculosis or adrenal atrophy. Other causes include malignant infiltration, sarcoidosis, or fungal infections involving the adrenal. The most common symptoms and signs of chronic adrenal insufficiency are hyponatremia and hyperkalemia. Other abnormalities include hypotension, weakness, fatigue, gastrointestinal complaints, and weight loss (see Table 64–7).

The symptoms of acute adrenal insufficiency "crisis," usually due to withdrawal of exogenous steroids, sepsis, or postadrenalectomy, are similar to those of chronic adrenal insufficiency, except that in acute cases fever can occur in up to 70 per cent of patients.

The treatment of acute or chronic adrenal insufficiency is the acute administration of glucocorticoids. In acute adrenal crisis, stress level dexamethasone (8 to 12 mg/day) is given along with replacement saline and a simultaneous ACTH stimulation test to confirm the diagnosis. The treatment of chronic Addison's disease is maintenance therapy with hydrocortisone (30 mg/day) plus fluorocortisone (0.05 tp 0.1 mg/day), or a synthetic steroid.

REFERENCES

1. Nerup, J.: Addison's disease-clinical studies. A report of 108 cases. Acta Endocrinol., *76*:127, 1974.
2. Liu, L., Haskin, M.E., Rase, L.A., and Beemus, C.E.: Diagnosis of bilateral adrenal cortical hemorrhage by computerized tomography. Ann. Intern. Med., *97*:720, 1982.
3. Smith, M.G., and Byrne, A.J.: An Addisonian crisis complicating anesthesia. Anesthesia, *36*:681, 1981.

1111-D *(Campbell's, pp. 2384–2388)*

The term hyperaldosteronism was initially used to describe the clinical syndrome characterized by hypertension, hypokalemia, hypernatremia, alkalosis, and periodic paralysis due to an aldosterone-secreting adenoma. Aldosterone hypersecretion due to adrenal adenoma of hyperplasia is characterized by hypertension, hypokalemic alkalosis, suppressed plasma renin activity (PRA) and high urinary and plasma aldosterone levels. Aldosteronomas are usually less than 3 cm, occur between the ages of 30 and 60, and are more common in women than men (2:1).

Diagnostic studies for hyperaldosteronism are designed to accomplish two goals: to screen the large hypertensive population for primary hyperaldosteronism (which makes up less than 1 per cent of all cases of hypertension) and to distinguish patients with adrenal adenoma form those with bilateral hyperplasia. Major screening criteria for diagnosis inlcude: (1) hypertension; (2) hypokalemia; (3) high serum and urinary aldosterone levels in the setting of high sodium intake (negative saline load test); and (4) suppressed plasma renin levels that fail to rise under conditions of restricted sodium intake (negative Lasix stimulation test).

CT scan has become the most accurate anatomic test for localizing adrenal disease. Adrenal vein sampling for aldosterone can help in equivocal cases. Small adrenal lesions are often not well visualized with adrenal MRI. Iodocholesterol scanning has limited accuracy.

Patients with an aldosterone-producing adenoma should be managed with excision of the adrenal gland containing the adenoma (tumors are found three times more often in the left adrenal), whereas patients with idiopathic hyperaldosteronism (bilateral adrenal hyperplasia) should be managed with medical therapy—usually spironolactone.

REFERENCE

1. Vaughan, E.D. Jr., Atlas, S., and Carey, R.M.: Hyperaldosteronism. *In* Vaughan, E.D. Jr., and Carey, R.M. (Eds): Adrenal Disorders. New York, Thieme Medical Publishers Inc., 1989.

1112-B, 1113-B *(Campbell's, pp. 2389–2398)*

Pheochromocytomas are rare, usually benign tumors arising from chromaffin cells and accounting for hypertension in less than 1 per cent of the hypertensive population. Clinical manifestations are due to the hypersecretion of the amines produced by the lesion, most comonly norepinephrine and epinephrine. Pheochromocytomas usually present in adults with either sustained hypertension, paroxysmal hypertension, or most commonly sustained hypertension with superimposed paroxysms. Other common symptoms include diaphoresis, headaches, and palpitations (see Table 64–12). Approximately 5 to 10 per cent of these tumors are associated with familial syndromes such as multiple endocrine adenoma (MEA) type II, neurofibromatosis, Von Hippel-Lindau disease, and tuberous sclerosis.

The confirmation of the clinical diagnosis of pheochromocytoma involves both biochemical and radiologic studies. Biochemical studies are used to demonstrate elevated levels of catecholamines in the blood or urine, which occur in 95 to 99 per cent of patients with pheochromocytoma. MRI appears to be the imaging study of choice for suspected pheochromocytoma. CT scan may be used with an accuracy of over 90 per cent; however, the use of contrast has been known to cause the release of catecholamines, thus necessitating treatment of these patients with alpha-blockers prior to radiographic contrast studies. The metaiodobenzylguanidine (MIBG) scan, which images medullary tissue, can be used if CT or MRI findings are equivocal or to search for extra-adrenal deposits of pheochromocytomas.

Surgical extirpation is the only effective treatment for pheochromocytoma. In the pregnant patient with pheochromocytoma, oral alpha-adrenergic blockade should be used until the fetus has reached maturity. At this point, cesarean section with tumor excision in one operation should be carried out.

Preoperative alpha-blockade is recommended for patients with pheochromocytoma in an attempt to stabilize the patient's hemodynamic status, thus facilitating the procedure for both the surgeon and the anesthesiologist as well as increasing the safety to the patient. Beta-blockers can also be used preoperatively to decrease the risk of arrhythmias. Intraoperative arrhythmias can be managed with either lidocaine for ventricular arrhythmias, or propranolol to control sinus tachycardia.

When the blood supply of the tumor has been curtailed, a fall in circulatory catecholamine levels may result in hypotension. Volume replacement is the initial treatment of choice, with careful cardiovascular monitoring. Vasopressors are rarely needed, and can usually be discontinued once the vascular volume approaches normal.

REFERENCE

1. Manger, W.M., and Gifford, R.W., Jr.: Pheochromocytoma. *In* Laragh, J.H., and Brenner, B.M. (Eds.): Hypertension Pathophysiology Diagnosis and Management. New York, Raven Press, 1990.

1114-D, 1115-A *(Campbell's, pp. 2398–2406)*

The proper approach to the adrenal gland depends on the underlying cause of the adrenal pathology, the size of the adrenal, the side of the lesion, the habitus of the patient, and the experience and preference of the surgeon.

The transabdominal approach is commonly chosen for patients with pheochromocytoma to allow complete abdominal exploration to identify multiple pheochromocytomas. Small adrenal adenomas can be treated through either a posterior or an 11th rib approach. The bilateral posterior approach is primarily utilized for ablative total adrenalectomy. Adrenal carcinomas are best approached through a thoracoabdominal incision (see Table 64–16).

REFERENCE

1. Vaughn, E.D. Jr.: Adrenal surgery. *In* Marshall, F.F. (Ed.): Atlas of Urologic Surgery. Philadelphia, W.B. Saunders Co., 1991.

1116-D *(Campbell's, pp. 2413–2414)*

The kidney has four constant vascular segments that are termed apical, anterior, posterior, and basilar. Each vascular segment is supplied by one or more major arterial branches. All segmental arteries are endarteries with no collateral circulation; therefore, during renal surgery, failure to preserve one of these branches will lead to devitalization of functioning renal tissue. Multiple main renal arteries occur in 10 to 20 per cent of the population.

The renal venous drainage system differs significantly from the arterial blood supply in that the intrarenal venous branches intercommunicate freely between the various renal segments.

REFERENCES

1. Boyce, W.H., and Smith, M.G.V.: Anatrophic nephrotomy and plastic calyorrhaphy. Tran. Am. Assoc. Genitourin. Surg., *59*:18,1967.
2. Graves, F.T.: The anatomy of the intrarenal arteries and its application to segmental resection of the kidney. Br. J. Surg., *42*:132, 1954.

1117-B *(Campbell's, pp. 2414–2415)*

The flank position with lateral flexion of the spine is known to cause embarrassment of ventilatory capacity. The venous return may also be significantly diminished in this position, resulting in hypotension. Therefore, alternatives to the flank approach should be used whenever possible in the patient with a decreased pulmonary reserve. If preoperative evaluation reveals impaired respiratory function, an anterior surgical approach with the patient in the supine position is preferred.

1118-C *(Campbell's, p. 2416)*

Patients are often concerned about how removal of a kidney will affect remaining renal function. Following nephrectomy for unilateral renal disease, the opposite kidney usually undergoes compensatory hypertrophy so that the glomerular filtration rate is ultimately maintained at 75 per cent of the normal value. Following unilateral nephrectomy with a normal contralateral kidney, several long-term studies have shown no increase in hypertension or proteinuria, stable overall renal function, and a normal life expectancy.

REFERENCES

1. Robitalle, P., Mongeau, J.G., Lortie, L., and Sinnassamy, P.: Long-term follow-up of patients who underwent unilateral nephrectomy in childhood. Lancet, *1*: 197, 1985.
2. Anderson, B., Hansen, J.B., and Jorgensen, S.J.: Survival after nephrectomy. Scand. J. Urol. Nephrol., *2*: 91, 1968.

1119-C, 1120-B *(Campbell's, pp. 2417–2418)*

The extent of renal damage following normothermic arterial occlusion depends on the duration of the ischemic insult. In general, 30 minutes is the maximum tolerable period of arterial occlusion before permanent damage is sustained.

The method to achieve vascular control may also determine the amount of renal ischemic damage. Continuous occlusion of both renal artery and vein causes more functional impairment than continuous occlusion of the renal artery alone for an equivalent time period because it prevents retrograde perfusion of the kidney through the renal vein. Intermittent clamping of the renal artery with short periods of recirculation is also more damaging than continuous arterial occlusion, possibly because of the release and trapping of damaging vasoconstrictor agents within the kidney. Animal studies have further demonstrated that renal compression to control intraoperative hemorrhage is more deleterious than simple arterial occlusion.

Several general measures should be employed in all patients who are undergoing operations that involve a period of temporary renal arterial occlusion. These include generous preoperative and intraoperative hydration, prevention of hypotension during the period of anesthesia, avoidance of unnecessary manipulation of the renal artery, and intraoperative administration of mannitol. Mannitol is most effective when given 5 to 15 minutes prior to arterial occlusion.

When the anticipated period of intraoperative renal ischemia is longer than 30 minutes, additional specific protective measures are indicated to prevent permanent damage to the kidney. Local hypothermia is the most efficacious and commonly employed method for protecting the kidney from ischemic damage. The optimum temperature for hypothermia in renal preservation is 15°C, but 20 to 25°C is more practical, simpler to maintain, and still allows renal preservation for up to 3 hours of arterial occlusion.

REFERENCES

1. Neely, W.A., and Turner, M.D.: The effect of arterial, venous, and arteriovenous occlusion on renal blood flow. Surg. Gynecol. Obstet., *108*:669, 1959.
2. Collins, G.M., Green, R.D., Boyer, D., et al.: Protection of kidneys from warm ischemic injury: Dosage and timing of mannitol administration. Transplantation, *20*:83, 1980.
3. Novick, A.C.: Renal hypothermia: In vivo and ex vivo. Urol. Clin. North Am., *10*:637, 1983.

1121-C *(Campbell's, pp. 2418–2422)*

The flank approach provids good access to the renal parenchyma and collective system. It is an extraperitoneal approach which involves minimal disturbance to other viscera and avoids contamination of the peritoneal cavity. This approach is particularly useful in the obese patient. Its principal disadvantages are that (1) exposure in the area of the renal pedicle is not as good as in the anterior transperitoneal approach and (2) it may prove unsuitable for the patient with scoliosis or cardiorespiratory problems.

The most commonly chosen flank approach to the kidney is through the bed of the 11th or 12th rib. The appropriate level of the incision is determined by drawing a horizontal line on the urogram from the hilum of the kidney to the most lateral rib that it intersects. When access to the upper renal pole is required, the rib above is selected.

The intercostal neurovascular bundle courses forward and downward between the internal oblique and transversus abdominis muscles. Every effort should be made to avoid injury to the intercostal nerves, which may cause persistent postoperative pain or bulging in the flank due to paresis of the denervated muscle.

REFERENCE

1. Woodruff, L.M.: Eleventh rib, extrapleural approach to the kidney. J. Urol., *73*:183, 1955.

1122-D *(Campbell's, pp. 2423–2427)*

The principal advantage of the abdominal approach is that exposure in the area of the renal pedicle is excellent. The principal disadvantage is the somewhat longer period of postoperative ileus and the possible long-term complication of intra-abdominal adhesions, leading to bowel obstruction. It is also associated with a higher risk of visceral injury than the flank approach. The choice between a vertical or transverse type of abdominal incision is determined by the patient's anatomy and the disease entity.

The thoracoabdominal approach is desirable for performing radical nephrectomy in patients with large tumors involving the upper portion of the kidney. It is particularly useful in the right side, where the liver and its venous drainage into the upper vena cava can limit exposure and impair vascular control as the tumor mass is being removed. Less need exists for a thoracoabdominal incision on the left side because the spleen and pancreas can usually be readily elevated away from the tumor mass.

REFERENCES

1. Chute, R., Baron, J.A., Jr., and Olsson, C.A.: The transverse upper abdominal "chevron" incision in urological surgery. J. Urol., *99*:258, 1968.
2. Chute, R., and Kerr, W.: The value of thoracoabdominal incision in the removal of kidney tumors. N. Engl. J. Med., *241*:951, 1956.

1123-E *(Campbell's, pp. 2428–2435)*

Simple nephrectomy is indicated in the patient with an irreversibly damaged kidney due to symptomatic chronic infection, obstruction, calculus disease, or severe traumatic injury. It is occasionally appropriate to remove a functioning kidney involved with one of these condition's when the patient's age or general condition is too poor to permit a reconstructive operation, provided that the opposite kidney is normal. Nephrectomy may also be indicated to treat renovascular hypertension due to uncorrectable renal artery disease or to severe unilateral parenchymal damage due to nephrosclerosis, pyelonephritis, reflex, or congenital dysplasia. Simple nephrectomy can be performed through a variety of incisions including the flank and the anterior transperitoneal approaches.

The treatment of choice for patients with localized renal cell carcinoma is radical nephrectomy.

1124-A *(Campbell's, pp. 2435–2441)*

As stated above, radical nephrectomy is the treatment of choice for patients with localized renal cell carcinoma. It involves preliminary ligation of the renal artery and vein followed by the en bloc removal of the kidney, Gerota's fascia, and adrenal glands. Perhaps the most important aspect of radical nephrectomy is removal of the kidney in the tissue plane outside Gerota's fascia, because capsular invasion with perinephric fat involvement occurs in 25 per cent of patients. The operation is usually performed through a transperitoneal incision to allow abdominal exploration for metastatic disease and early access to the renal vessels. A thoracoabdominal incision is usually chosen for patients with large upper pole tumors.

During performance of radical nephrectomy, intraoperative hemorrhage can occur from the inferior vena cava or its tributaries. Undue traction on the cava can result in avulsion of lumbar veins which enter the posterolateral aspect of the vena cava. A second predictable bleeding site is the entry of the right gonadal vein into the anterolateral surface of the cava. Another common site of bleeding lies at the level of the renal veins. The right adrenal vein, which enters the inferior vena cava posterolaterally, is a fourth potential site of bleeding.

Excessive hemorrhage can usually be prevented by careful dissection in proper tissue planes above the vena cava. One should follow the general principle of isolating a relatively normal area of vena cava and working upward or downward from the area to expose the diseased portion.

If inadvertent lacerations of vena cava or avulsions of entering vena occur, direct pressure on the site of bleeding gives immediate control until additional exposure can be gained. When the laceration involves the anterior or lateral caval wall, it can be readily controlled by applying Allis clamps over the edges of the laceration, then oversewing the edges of the laceration with running 5-0 vascular suture.

If avulsion of an entering lumbar vein is the cause of bleeding, the vena cava should be rolled medially with digital compressing above and below the site of the bleeding to expose the entry site of the avulsed vein. Allis clamps can then be used in similar fashion to obtain approximation of the edges of the laceration before oversewing the edges. Bleeding from the stump of the lumbar vein, which often retracts into the psoas muscle can be controlled by inserting a figure-of-eight 2-0 silk suture through the muscle overlying the vein.

The inferior mesenteric vein is part of the portal system and drains into the portal vein not the inferior vena cava.

REFERENCE

1. Skinner, D.G., Colvin, R.B., Vermillion, C.D., et al.: Diagnosis and management of renal cell carcinoma: A clinical and pathological study of 309 cases. Cancer, *28*:1165, 1971.

1125-A *(Campbell's, pp. 2445–2448)*

Following radical nephrectomy, postoperative complications occur in approximately 2 per cent of patients, and the operative mortality rate is approximately 2 per cent. Some of the complications include myocardial infarction, cerebrovascular accident, congestive heart failure, pulmonary embolus, atelectasis, pneumonia, intraoperative gastrointestinal injury, splenic injury, liver injury, pancreatic injury, prolonged ileus, hemorrhage, pneumothorax, infection, renal insufficiency or failure, flank bulge or hernia, and prolonged postoperative pain.

REFERENCE

1. Swanson, D.A., and Borges, P.M.: Complications of transabdominal radical nephrectomy for renal cell carcinoma. J. Urol., *129*:704, 1983.

1126-D *(Campbell's, pp. 2448–2455)*

Although radical nephrectomy remains the treatment of choice for the patient with localized renal cell carcinoma and a normal opposite kidney, partial nephrectomy is the treatment of choice when localized renal cell carcinoma is present bilaterally or in a solitary functioning kidney. Indications for partial nephrectomy in the presence of renal malignancy also include the patient with localized renal cell carcinoma and a functioning opposite kidney, when that kidney is involved with a disorder (e.g., calculi, diabetes mellitus, pyelonephritis, nephrosclerosis) that might cause progressive renal functional impairment in the future; and patients with renal pelvic transitional cell carcinoma or Wilms' tumor, when preservation of functioning renal parenchyma is a clinically relevant consideration.

A variety of surgical techniques are available for performing partial nephrectomy including simple enucleation, polar segmental nephrectomy with preliminary ligation of the appropriate renal arterial branch, wedge resection, major transverse resection, and extracorporeal partial nephrectomy with renal autotransplantation. In the majority of cases, it is possible to perform partial nephrectomy in situ by choosing an operative approach that optimizes exposure of the kidney and by combining meticulous surgical technique with an understanding of the renal vascular anatomy.

Patients who are undergoing partial nephrectomy for malignancy should be studied preoperatively with renal arteriography to delineate the main renal artery and its branches.

Partial nephrectomy is also indicated in selected patients with localized benign pathology of the kidney. The preoperative considerations, operative techniques, and complications are similar to those described for partial nephrectomy for malignant renal disease.

REFERENCES

1. Novick, A.C., Streem, S., Montie, J.E., et al.: Conservative surgery for renal cell carcinoma: A single-center experience with 100 cases. J. Urol., *141*:835, 1989.
2. Leach, G.E., and Kieber, M.M.: Partial nephrectomy: Mayo Clinic experience 1957–1977. Urology, *15*:219, 1980.

1127-B *(Campbell's, p. 2455)*

Complications of partial nephrectomy include hemorrhage, urinary fistula formation, ureteral obstruction, renal insufficiency, and infection. Early control and ready access to the renal artery is essential to decreasing the risk of intraoperative bleeding. The initial management of postoperative hemorrhage is expectant with bed rest, serial hemoglobin and hematocrit determinations, frequent noniterins of vital signs, and blood transfusions as needed. Angiography and selective angioinfarction of segmental renal arteries may be useful in some cases with persistent bleeding. Severe, intractable hemorrhage may require reexploration with early control of the renal vessels and ligation of the active bleeding points. Persistent drainage after partial nephrectomy suggests the development of a urinary cutaneous fistula which can be confirmed by determination of the creatinine levels of the drainage fluid. An intravenous urogram or retrograde pyelogram should be obtained to rule out obstruction of the involved collecting system. In the event of hydronephrosis or persistent urinary leakage, an internal stent or if this is not possible, a percutaneous nephrostomy will lead to resolution of the fistula in the majority of the cases (although this may take several weeks). A second operation to close the urinary fistula is rarely necessary.

1128-B *(Campbell's, pp. 2457–2475)*

The indications for open stone surgery have decreased dramatically since the introduction of percutaneous technology and extracorporeal shock wave lithotripsy (ESWL). As a result, only approximately 5 to 10 per cent of patients with renal stones will require open surgery. The indications for open operative interventions in renal calculous disease include an associated anatomic abnormality requiring open operative intervention; a stone so large and extensive that in the judgment of an experienced urologic surgeon, a single open procedure will more likely render the patient stone-free with less risk than would multiple percutaneous and ESWL procedures; and failure of, or contraindication to, both ESWL and percutaneous nephrolithotomy.

Retained calculi is a discouraging complication that occurs in up to 20 per cent of patients. Stones associated with obstruction, pain, or chronic infection or active stone growth require further intervention. Currently, all residual calculi may be managed with percutaneous techniques or extracorporeal shock wave lithotripsy. Whenever possible, such treatment should be delayed for at least 4 to 6 weeks following the initial operative intervention. Calcium oxalate stones are resistant to irrigation techniques for dissolution.

REFERENCE

1. Assimos, D.G., Boyce, W.H., Harrison, L.H., et al.: The role of open stone surgery since extracorporeal shock wave lithotripsy. J. Urol., *142*:263, 1989.

1129-C *(Campbell's, pp. 2478–2480)*

Indications for the open surgical repair of ureteropelvic junction obstruction include the presence of symptoms from the obstruction, impairment of renal function, or the development of stones or infection. In general, such intervention should be a reconstructive procedure aimed at restoring nonobstructed urinary flow. Occasionally, if the patient is asymptomatic and the physiologic significance of the obstruction is undetermined, careful observation with serial follow-up studies may be appropriate.

REFERENCES

1. Bejjani, B., and Belman, A.B.: Ureteropelvic junction obstruction in newborns and infants. J. Urol., *128*: 770, 1982.
2. Jacobs, J.A., Berger, B.W., Goldman, S.M., et al.: Ureteropelvic obstruction in adults with previously normal pyelograms. A report of five cases. J. Urol., *121*: 242, 1979.

1130-D, 1131-A, 1132-D *(Campbell's, pp. 2480–2489)*

When intervention for ureteropelvic junction obstruction is indicated, the procedure of choice is generally an "open" repair of the ureteropelvic junction, that is, a pyeloplasty. Percutaneous endopyelotomy may also have a role, although long-term follow-up is still unknown. Nephrectomy may be indicated in patients with non-function of the involved renal unit with no hope for salvage based on radiographic and radionuclide studies; in patients with extensive stone disease with chronic infection, significant loss of renal function in the presence of normal contralateral kidney; or in patients in whom repeated attempts at repair have failed and in whom further intervention would be extremely complicated (only when the contralateral kidney is normal).

The recommended approach for most patients undergoing primary surgical repair is an extraperitoneal flank incision. Most urologists rely on a variation of a dismembered pyeloplasty, as this procedure is almost universally applicable for repair of the ureteropelvic junction. In contrast to all flap techniques, only a dismembered pyeloplasty allows complete excision of the anatomically or functionally abnormal ureteropelvic junction. A dismembered pyeloplasty is, however, poorly suited to obstruction associated with lengthy proximal ureteral structures or ureteropelvic junction obstruction associated with a small inaccessible intrarenal pelvis.

Several other techniques for reconstruction of the ureteropelvic junction have been described. The Foley Y-V plasty was originally designed for reconstruction of a ureteropelvic junction obstruction associated with a high ureteral insertion. It is specifically contraindicated when the transposition of lower pole vessels is required, and is of little value when significant reduction of renal pelvic size is required. The Culp-DeWeerd spiral flap is best suited to large, readily accessible extrarenal pelvis in which the ureteral insertion is already in a dependent position. The spiral flap may be of particular value when the ureteropelvic junction obstruction is associated with a relatively long segment of proximal ureteral narrowing or stricture. To preserve vascular integrity of the flap, the ratio of flap length to width should not exceed 3 to 1. The Scardino-Prince vertical flap may be used when a dependent ureteropelvic junction is situated at the medial margin of a large, square extrarenal pelvis, but is has been supplanted by the standard dismembered pyeloplasty.

Management of the "failed pyeloplasty" is a challenging problem. Anastomosis of the proximal ureter directly to the lower calyceal system has become a well-accepted salvage technique. It may also be used as a primary reconstructive procedure in ureteropelvic junction obstruction associated with a small intrarenal pelvis. Two important technical points to be emphasized are (1) the proximal ureter is spatulated laterally before the anastomosis is performed over an internal stent, and (2) the renal parenchyma overlying the lower pole calyx must be resected, rather than simply incised, to prevent secondary stricture.

REFERENCES

1. Nguyen, D.H., Aliabadi, H., Ercole, C.J., and Gonzalez, R.: Non-intubated Anderson-Hynes repair of ureteropelvic junction obstruction in 60 patients. J. Urol., *142*:704, 1989.
2. Ross, J.H., Streem, S.B., Novick, A.C., et al.: Ureterocalicostomy for reconstruction of complicated pelviureteric junction obstruction. Br. J. Urol., *65*:322, 1990.

1133-B *(Campbell's, pp. 2489–2491)*

Open renal biopsy may be necessary to establish a tissue diagnosis in patients with renal disease, to assess the severity of such disease, or to evaluate the potential for salvageable renal function in patients with known correctable disorder. Open biopsy is usually preferred over a percutaneous biopsy technique in a patient with solitary kidney, coagulopathy, atypical anatomy, or other factors that may increase the risk of a closed biopsy (eg, infants and children, uncontrolled hypertension). An open biopsy also provides more tissue for study and minimizes the potential for complications, such as arteriovenous fistula, perirenal hematoma, and gross hematuria. The percutaneous biopsy technique has been used successfully, and relatively safely, in the evaluation of the postrenal transplant patient.

1134-C *(Campbell's, p. 2495)*

Horseshoe kidney occurs in about one in 700 individuals and is frequently associated with other urologic anomalies. Ureteral obstruction with hydronephrosis, stone formation, or infection is the most common associated problem in this condition and may require surgical treatment. In patients with ureteral or ureteropelvic junction obstruction division of the isthmus alone is insufficient.

When performing surgery on a horseshoe kidney, an anterior subcostal extraperitoneal approach is preferred. This provides good access to the isthmus as well as to the pelvis and ureter which are rotated anteriorly.

REFERENCE

1. Culp, O.S., and Winterringen, J.R.: Surgical treatment of horseshoe kidney: Comparison of results after various types of operations. J. Urol., *73*:747, 1955.

1135-C *(Campbell's, p. 2501)*

The causes of end-stage renal disease in the United States are listed in Table 66–1 on page 2501 of *Campbell's Urology*. Approximately 30 per cent of end stage renal disease is due to diabetes mellitus; glomerulonephritis accounts for 14.4 per cent, hypertension accounts for 26 per cent, cystic kidney disease accounts for 3.6 per cent, and other urologic diseases account for approximately 6 per cent.

1136-D *(Campbell's, p. 2503)*

The pretransplant urologic evaluation includes determination of a history of urologic disease, physical examination, urinalysis, urine or bladder wash culture, and imaging of the upper urinary tract, usually with sonography. Voiding cystourethrography is probably unnecessary in a patient with no history of urologic abnormalities; however, it may be indicated based on history. In patients who have had multiple lower urinary tract operations and have developed a contracted bladder, it is wise to perform cystoscopy and obtain bladder biopsies prior to transplantation.

1137-B *(Campbell's, p. 2503)*

In older men with obstructing prostates, a pretransplant transurethral prostatectomy or transurethral incision of the bladder neck and prostate should be performed. If such patients requiring bladder outlet procedures are oliguric, a suprapubic cystostomy done at the time of bladder outlet surgery will enable the patients to instill sterile water and void until the operative site has healed. This prevents scarring and obliteration of the prostatic fossa. An alternative to suprapubic cystostomy in such patients would be daily bladder instillation through intermittent self-catheterization followed by voiding. Indications for pretransplant nephrectomy include hypertension which is not controlled by dialysis or medications, persistent renal infection, renal calculi, severe proteinuria, infected polycystic kidneys, severe bleeding and massively enlarged kidneys. The pretransplant nephrectomy is usually performed six weeks prior to transplantation. In patients who desire a penile prosthesis for impotence prior to renal transplantation, one should avoid using devices where a reservoir is placed in the prevesical space since these may interfere with urinary tract reconstruction. In these cases, a semirigid device is recommended. Patients with malignancy are not generally candidates for transplantation.

REFERENCE

1. Orandi, A.: Transurethral incision of prostate compared with transurethral resection of prostate in 132 matching cases. J. Urol., *138*:810, 1987.

1138-B *(Campbell's, p. 2505)*

Serologic screening in potential living donors should include screening for human immunodeficiency virus, human T-cell lymphotrophic virus type I, hepatitis, cytomegalovirus and syphilis. Screening for varicella-zoster virus is not routinely done.

1139-E *(Campbell's, p. 2505)*

In potential living donors in which serologic screening, blood group compatibility, and tissue typing criteria have all been satisfied, the following studies should be performed: chest x-ray, electrocardiogram, intravenous pyelography, and serial serum creatinine levels. In patients who have satisfied all of these criteria, the last study would be aortography or digital subtraction arteriography of the renal vessels in preparation for the donor nephrectomy. Abdominal CT scan is not part of the routine evaluation of potential living donor patients.

1140-A *(Campbell's, p. 2505)*

When performing a living-donor nephrectomy, a flank incision with a rib-resecting or supracostal approach is usually employed. Then 25 grams of mannitol is given in a one hour infusion beginning at the time of the skin incision. Once dissection of the kidney and ureter has been completed, the ureter is transected and urine flow from the transected ureter observed. Adequate urine flow is desired before interrupting renal circulation. After removal of the donor kidney, it is placed in a pan of ice-cold solution and flushed with either Ringer's lactate, Euro-Collins or University of Wisconsin solution at 4°C. It is not necessary to administer heparin to the living related donor.

1141-C *(Campbell's, p. 2505)*

Complications of the donor nephrectomy include those of a standard flank nephrectomy. Studies show that endogenous creatinine clearance rapidly approaches 70 to 80 per cent of the preoperative level and that this is maintained for more than 10 years. The risk of developing late hypertension following nephrectomy is nearly the same as that for the general population. Long-term risks of the living donor nephrectomy are felt to be low, and it is considered an acceptable procedure when patients are fully informed. Anemia following donor nephrectomy has not been reported to be a problem.

REFERENCES

1. Vincenti, F., Amend, W.J.C., Jr., and Kaysen, G.: Long-term renal function in kidney donors: Sustained compensatory hyperfiltration with no adverse effects. Transplantation, *36*:626, 1983.
2. Weiland, D., Sutherland, D.E.R., Chavers, B., et al.: Information on 628 living-related kidney donors at a single institution with long-term follow-up in 472 cases. Transplant. Proc., *16*:5, 1984.

1142-D *(Campbell's, pp. 2505–2506)*

Typical criteria for cadaveric donors include: age 18 months to 55 years; no hypertension requiring treatment; no diabetes mellitus; and no malignancies other than primary brain tumors or treated skin cancer. The lower age limit of 18 months is due to the size of the kidney and the risk of technical problems; however, younger donors have been harvested providing functioning grafts. Graft survival in adult recipients has been found to be significantly lower when the donor is below age 6 as compared to above age 6. The one year graft survival for grafts from donors between ages 55 and 60 has been found to be 12 per cent lower than that for grafts for donors between ages 16 and 30. Age-matching of donor and recipient is not reported to improve graft survival.

REFERENCE

1. Terasaki, P.I., Cecka, J.M., Takemoto, S., et al.: Overview. *In* Terasaki, P.I. (Ed.): Clinical Transplants, 1988. Los Angeles, UCLA Tissue Typing Laboratory, 1988, pp. 409–434.

1143-B *(Campbell's, p. 2505)*

The only malignancies that are not contraindications for cadaveric kidney donation are primary brain tumors, which would include astrocytoma, and treated skin cancer. Certainly, the other malignancies listed in this question—bronchioalveolar carcinoma, colorectal adenocarcinoma, infiltrating duct carcinoma of the breast and malignant melanoma—all have significant potential for metastasis and are, therefore, contraindications to organ donation.

1144-E *(Campbell's, p. 2506)*

For the preservation of renal function, monitoring in the brain-dead cadaveric donor should include CVP monitoring and serum electrolyte levels every 2 to 4 hours. When urine output drops, initial therapy should consist of a fluid challenge. If blood pressure and urine output cannot be maintained by fluid challenge and the central venous pressure is greater than 15 cm, vasopressors such as dopamine, dobutamine or isoproterenol can be infused. If urine output remains low after the use of vasopressors and intravascular volume expansion, loop diuretics or mannitol should be administered in an attempt to cause diuresis. When brain death results in unmanageable diuresis due to diabetes insipidus, vasopressin or Pitressin should be administered. Papaverine infusion into the renal arteries is not recommended as standard therapy to maintain renal function in the cadaveric donor.

1145-C *(Campbell's, p. 2506)*

With warm ischemia, cellular levels of ATP are depleted and the sodium-potassium pump becomes impaired due to lack of ATP. Sodium ion then accumulates in the cell from passive diffusion and water follows causing cellular swelling. Anaerobic glycolysis occurs in an attempt to meet the energy needs of the cell and results in a lowering of the pH. Lysosomal enzymes are then activated at the low pH and cause cell membrane damage. The effect of damage to the membranes is to allow the influx of calcium into the cell. Calcium then poisons mitochondrial enzymes completely arresting oxidative phosphorylation. When reperfusion of the ischemic tissue occurs, ATP degradation leads to hypoxanthine formation, which may be oxidized and give rise to free radicals. This in turn leads to additional cell membrane damage. Additionally, calcium influx increases with reperfusion again leading to the poisoning of the mitochondria. Magnesium is an intracellular ion and with ischemia is lost from the cell. Magnesium is not reported to cause mitochondrial enzyme poisoning.

REFERENCE

1. Belzer, F.O., and Southard, J.H.: Principles of solid-organ preservation by cold storage. Transplantation, *45*:673, 1988.

1146-A *(Campbell's, p. 2508)*

The University of Wisconsin solution minimizes cellular swelling with the following impermeable solutes: potassium lactobionate, raffinose, and hydroxyethyl starch. Allopurinol is a component of University of Wisconsin solution and its function is to inhibit xanthine oxidase which leads to the generation of free radicals on reperfusion. Additionally, glutathione, a free radical scavenger, is a component of the UW solution. Dexamethasone and magnesium are also components and their function is reported to be membrane stabilization. ATP magnesium chloride is not a component of UW solution; however, adenosine is added to aid ATP synthesis during reperfusion.

REFERENCE

1. Belzer, F.O., and Southard, J.H.: Principles of solid-organ preservation by cold storage. Transplantation, *45*:673, 1988.

1147-D *(Campbell's, p. 2508)*

Components of University of Wisconsin solution, Euro-Collins solution, and Collins 2 solution are found in Table 66–2 on page 2508 of *Campbell's Urology*. Collins solution contains glucose and sodium bicarbonate which are not contained in the UW solution. No calcium channel blocker is contained in Euro-Collins solution, although it has been theorized that the addition of calcium channel blockers may reduce reperfusion injury. University of Wisconsin solution contains dexamethasone as a membrane-stabilizing agent. In a prospectively randomized study, University of Wisconsin solution resulted in a significantly more rapid reduction in post-operative serum creatinine levels following transplantation in comparison to Euro-Collins solution. The University of Wisconsin solution has been found to be a preservation solution for all intra-abdominal organs.

REFERENCE

1. Ploeg, R.J.: Kidney preservation with the UW and Euro-Collins solutions. Transplantation, *49*:281, 1990.

1148-E *(Campbell's, pp. 2509–2511)*

In transplantation of adults and large children, the operation proceeds with a Gibson incision followed by placement of the kidney graft in the contralateral iliac fossa extraperitoneally. In women, the round ligament is divided. In men, the spermatic cord is mobilized, preserved and medially retracted during the procedure. Mannitol infusion is started at the time of revascularization of the graft. Implantation of ureter into the bladder proceeds with an antireflux ureteroneocystostomy from an extravesical approach. The transvesical approach may also be used. A ureteral stent may be placed when there is a concern about urinary leakage or obstruction related to a thickened bladder or to edema. However, placement of a double J ureteral stent is not the rule.

1149-B *(Campbell's, pp. 2511–2512)*

In the early postoperative care of a renal transplant, intravenous fluid replacement should consist of half-normal saline with 0 to 5 per cent dextrose solution given at a rate of insensible losses plus the previous hour's urinary output. In cases of extreme diuresis, the dextrose concentration of the intravenous fluid should be lowered. Serum electrolyte levels should be monitored every 4 to 8 hours. A nuclear renal scan and ultrasound of the transplant should be performed 24 to 48 hours after the procedure to document graft bloodflow, obtain a baseline for graft function, and evaluate the iliac fossa for fluid collections. Typically, the Foley catheter is left in the bladder up to one week and most surgeons delay removal of the Foley catheter until a retrograde cystogram documents the absence of extravasation. Continuous bladder irrigation is not routinely performed in renal transplant patients. Other postoperative care such as mobilization of the patient and feeding of the patient proceeds according to standard principles.

1150-C *(Campbell's, pp. 2512–2513)*

Hyperacute rejection occurs immediately after perfusion of the graft and is due to preformed circulating cytotoxic antibodies in the host. Accelerated rejection occurs usually within days to weeks of transplantation and does not respond to antirejection therapy. It appears to be mediated by both humoral and cellular components of the immune response. Acute rejection is seen over a time period of weeks to months following transplantation. Symptoms of rejection include flu-like symptoms, pain over the graft, fever, increased blood pressure, decreased urine output, fluid retention, graft enlargement, and rising serum levels of creatinine and blood urea nitrogen. Nuclear renal scan will show a decrease in glomerular filtration and tubular function during rejection. With acute rejection, mononuclear cellular infiltration and vasculitis are seen.

1151-A *(Campbell's, pp. 2513–2514)*

Histocompatibility systems of importance in renal transplantation are the ABO blood group and the HLA system. Donor and recipient must be ABO compatible. The A and B antigens occur on endothelial cells and most individuals have antibodies to the antigens they lack. The major histocompatibility antigens are encoded for by the major histocompatibility complex autosomal genes which occur on the short arm of chromosome 6. These antigens are divided into class I and class II antigens. Major histocompatibility class I antigens are known as HLA-A, HLA-B, and HLA-C, and are present on all nucleated cells. Detection of class I antigens is by serotyping T-lymphocytes. Class II major histocompatibility antigens consist of HLA-DR, HLA-DQ and HLA-DP and these occur on the B-lymphocytes, monocytes, macrophages, dendritic cells, activated T-lymphocytes, and on some endothelial cells. Each patient is a half match or haploidentical with his or her parents due to inheritance patterns. There is a .25 probability of complete HLA identity of a patient with his sibling, a .5 probability of haploidentity with his sibling and a .25 probability of total HLA mismatch with a sibling.

1152-E *(Campbell's, pp. 2513–2514)*

Class I and II major histocompatibility antigens on donor dendritic cells stimulate recipient T-lymphocytes and initiate rejection. Host macrophages also process donor MHC antigens and present the class II antigens to CD4+ helper T-cells and present class I antigens to CD8+ precursor cytotoxic T-cells. Macrophages also secrete interleukin 1, which may activate helper T-cells. Activated CD4+ helper T-cells then secrete T-cell growth factor. T-cell growth factor or interleukin 2 further stimulates helper T-cells and leads to the release of interleukins 3-6 as well as interferon gamma. Interleukins 4-6 are necessary for the transformation of B lymphocytes activated by class I antigen into plasma cells. These plasma cells then produce cytotoxic antibodies against the graft class I MHC molecules. Gamma interferon has the effect of inducing graft cells to express MHC class II antigens which further amplifies the rejection process. Cytotoxic cells are not reported to secrete IL-1.

1153-D *(Campbell's, pp. 2515–2517)*

Azathioprine is an antimetabolite that is structurally similar to purine. It inhibits both DNA and RNA synthesis and thus inhibits lymphocyte proliferation. Glucocorticoids block production of interleukin 1 and interleukin 6 and thereby block T-cell proliferation. Cyclosporine blocks production of interleukin 2 and also inhibits interleukin 2 receptor expression on helper and cytotoxic lymphocytes. Anti-Tac and 33B3.1 are new monoclonal antibodies which bind to the interleukin 2 receptor and therefore prevent T-cell activation and clonal expansion. These antibodies are presently experimental and have not yet been shown to be adequate therapy for treatment of acute rejection. FK506 is also an experimental drug which is structurally similar to the macrolide antibiotics. Its mechanism of action is not reported to be inhibition of T-lymphocyte protein synthesis; therefore, answer D is incorrect.

REFERENCES

1. Kahan, B.D.: Cyclosporine. N. Engl. J. Med., *321:* 1725, 1989.
2. Cantarovich, D., LeMauff, B., Hourmant, M., et al.: Anti-IL2 receptor monoclonal antibody (33B3.1) in prophylaxis of early kidney rejection in humans: A randomized trial versus rabbit antithymocyte globulin. Transplant. Proc., *21*:1769, 1989.
3. Kirkman, R.L., Shapiro, M.E., Carpenter, C.B., et al.: Early experience with anti-TaC in clinical renal transplantation. Transplant. Proc., *21*:1766, 1989.

1154-B *(Campbell's, p. 2516)*

Drugs known to increase cyclosporine levels include ketoconazole, danazol, metoclopramide, glucocoticoids and diltiazem. Phenytoin may decrease cyclosporine.

1155-C *(Campbell's, p. 2516)*

The primary disadvantage of cyclosporine is its nephrotoxicity. This is a dose-related effect and is potentially reversible. The side effects of cyclosporine include hepatotoxicity, hypertension, hirsutism, breast fibroadenomas, gingival hypertrophy and immunosuppression. Pruritus is not reported to be a significant side effect of cyclosporine.

1156-E *(Campbell's, p. 2516)*

Table 66–8 on page 2516 lists characteristics that are used to differentiate cyclosporine toxicity from acute rejection. Typically with cyclosporine toxicity, the serum creatinine level undergoes a slow rise, graft size and blood flow remain stable, no fever is observed, no graft tenderness develops, and urine output is normally maintained. With acute allograft rejection, a rapid creatinine rise is observed which may be accompanied with decreased urine output. Fever may develop as well as swelling and tenderness of the graft. Graft blood flow does appear decreased and graft biopsy would show cellular infiltration and vasculitis.

1157-A *(Campbell's, p. 2517)*

Uninfected lymphoceles may be managed by aspiration with or without iodine sclerosis, or by marsupialization into the peritoneal cavity. They are not managed by marsupialization into the bladder. Urinary leaks may be managed conservatively with bladder catheter drainage or with percutaneous nephrostomy. In defining a urinary leak, often retrograde cystogram will fail and either a percutaneous antegrade study or an excretory urography will need to be performed to define the site of urinary extravasation. When extensive open repair of the urinary tract is required, stenting should be performed, as well as placement of a nephrostomy tube. An omental wrap may be beneficial with extensive repair.

REFERENCES

1. Schweizer, R.T., Cho, S., Kountz, S.L., et al.: Lymphoceles following renal transplantation. Arch. Surg., *104*: 42, 1972.
2. Gilliland, J.D., Spies, J.B., Brown, S.B., et al.: Lymphoceles: Percutaneous treatment with povidone-iodine sclerosis. Radiology, *171*:227, 1989.

1158-C *(Campbell's, p. 2521)*

The incidence of renovascular hypertension is estimated to be 5 to 10 per cent of the 60 million hypertensive patients in the United States.

REFERENCE

1. Sosa, R.E., and Vaughan, E.D. Jr.: Renovascular hypertension. *In* Gillenwater, J. (Ed.): Adult and Pediatric Urology, Vol. 1, Chicago, Year Book Medical Publishers, Inc., 1987, pp. 752–776.

1159-B *(Campbell's, pp. 2521–2522)*

Atherosclerotic lesions account for two thirds of all renal artery pathologic lesions. Atherosclerotic lesions develop near the origin of the main renal arteries and may be bilateral; however, when a unilateral lesion exists, it is more commonly in the left renal artery. Answer B is, therefore, false. Analysis of lesions shows either circumferential atheroma containing lipid and focal calcifications or eccentric fibrous plaque, which contains lipid deposits and collagen.

1160-C *(Campbell's, p. 2522)*

The mural dysplasias include intimal fibroplasia, medial fibroplasia, fibromuscular hyperplasia, and subadventitial fibroplasia. In mural dysplasias pathology within the wall of the artery is the primary cause of a stenotic lesion. The mural dysplasias are more common in women and the mean age of patients at the time of presentation is 35. Natural history of most of the mural dysplasias involves progressive occlusion of the renal artery associated with dissection and aneurysm formation. With medial fibroplasia, multiple microaneurysms are seen. With subadventitial fibroplasia, dense collagen deposits in the outer portion of the media are seen and severe stenotic lesions develop. With true fibromuscular hyperplasia, concentric segmental stenotic lesions develop that may be associated with disruption of the internal elastic membrane and dissecting aneurysms. Intimal fibroplasia has a strong association with dissecting aneurysm in addition to stenosis.

1161-A *(Campbell's, pp. 2522–2523)*

Saccular aneurysms develop at the bifurcation of renal vessels and may be associated with medial fibroplasia or atherosclerosis. They are at risk for spontaneous rupture and thrombosis. Fusiform aneurysms are found in young, hypertensive patients with fibrous mural dysplasia. They are typically not calcified, nor are they associated with a high risk of spontaneous rupture. The major complication of fusiform aneurysms is renal artery thrombosis. Dissecting aneurysms are most often due to atherosclerosis, intimal fibroplasia and perimedial fibroplasia. Intrarenal aneurysms may be due to trauma from needle biopsy as well as atherosclerosis, fibrous dysplasia and congenital vascular malformations. In general, in the management of aneurysms, a small well-calcified aneurysm in the normotensive asymptomatic patient does not require surgical intervention.

1162-D *(Campbell's, pp. 2523–2527)*

Trauma, as noted in the answer to question 1161, may give rise to renal artery aneurysms. Additionally, atherosclerosis is a common cause of renal artery aneurysms. Takayasu's arteritis affects the aorta and its primary branches and stenosis and aneurysm formation are seen in this disease. In neurofibromatosis, vascular lesions are seen which are characterized by intimal endothelial proliferation with or without aneurysm formation. Scleroderma may lead to chronic renal failure and end stage renal disease due to renal vessel involvement; however, it is not reported to be associated with renal artery aneurysms.

REFERENCE

1. Ishikawa, K.: Natural history and classification of occlusive thromboaortopathy (Takayasu's disease). Circulation, *57*:27, 1978.

1163-E *(Campbell's, p. 2527)*

Indications for corrective surgery in patients with renovascular disease include uncontrollable hypertension despite aggressive medical therapy, poor compliance, deterioration of renal function, dissection of a renal artery lesion, total occlusion of the renal artery, occlusion of a solitary kidney with anuria, and failure of percutaneous transluminal angioplasty. The presence of bilateral renal artery disease does not necessitate corrective surgery unless other indications as listed apply to the renal artery disease.

REFERENCE

1. Libertino, J.A., and Zinman, L.N.: Surgery for renovascular hypertension. *In* Libertino, J.A. (Ed.): Pediatric and Adult Reconstructive Urologic Surgery, 2nd ed. Baltimore, Williams & Wilkins Co., 1987, pp. 119–161.

1164-A *(Campbell's, pp. 2527–2528)*

Results of percutaneous transluminal angioplasty for artherosclerotic lesions are poor, and therefore this is not recommended as a therapeutic option for such lesions. However, in high risk patients who have a short mid-main renal artery plaque, angioplasty may be of benefit. With the mural dysplasias, however, percutaneous transluminal angioplasty is very successful, with a 60 to 85 per cent overall success rate. Angioplasty is, therefore, the first line of treatment for patients with mural dysplasia. In patients with medial fibroplasia, management should be with antihypertensives until hypertension can no longer be controlled. Severe complications with percutaneous balloon angioplasty are most often seen in patients undergoing their second or third angioplastic dilation. Therefore, failure or recurrence after a single trial of angioplasty warrants a surgical intervention.

REFERENCE

1. Sos, T.A., Pickering, T.G., Saddekni, S., et al.: The current role of renal angioplasty in the treatment of renovascular hypertension. Urol. Clin. North Am., *11*: 503, 1984.

1165-C *(Campbell's, p. 2528)*

Perioperative monitoring during renovascular surgery should include hemodynamic monitoring with Swan-Ganz catheter. Doppler monitoring should be available intraoperatively to evaluate pulses. Patients who have significant carotid artery disease should undergo carotid endarterectomy prior to renovascular surgery because the lowering of blood pressure following correction of the renovascular lesion may induce transient ischemic episodes or stroke. Electroencephalographic monitoring is not routinely performed because the carotid artery disease should be repaired first. To diminish the effects of renal ischemia, mannitol and Lasix should be administered approximately 2 hours before the renal vessels are clamped. Renal dose dopamine may also be given during the procedure to enhance renal blood flow. Systemic anticoagulation is beneficial in preventing thrombosis of small renal vessels once the renal vessels are clamped and additionally in preventing embolization and thrombosis in the lower extremities if the aorta is cross-clamped.

REFERENCE

1. Javid, H., Ostermiller, W.E., Hengesh, J.W., et al.: Carotid endarterectomy for asymptomatic patients. Arch. Surg., *102*:389, 1971.

1166-D *(Campbell's, pp. 2528–2529)*

A transverse upper abdominal incision allows good access to the aortorenal junction particularly if it is highlying. This incision extends from the lateral border of the contralateral rectus muscle across the midline into the ipsilateral flank between the 11th and 12th ribs. It is shown in Figure 67–16 on page 2529 of *Campbell's Urology*. The best exposure of the renal vessels is achieved by complete reflection of the colon. The retroperitoneal space is entered through an incision along the white line of Toldt in the lateral peritoneal gutter, and the peritoneum incised from the cecum to the ligament of Treitz to reflect the right colon. The hepatic peritoneal ligaments are incised to reflect the proximal transverse colon. The duodenum is then "kocherized" to expose the right renal vein. The distal transverse colon and descending colon are mobilized by again incising the peritoneal reflection along the lateral descending colon. The gastrocolic ligament is divided and the incision extended laterally through the avascular region; finally the splenocolic attachments are divided. The spleen is protected in this manner. The splenic flexure is retracted downward exposing the left renal vein. An alternative approach to the left renal vessels for left renal artery stenosis is through a supracostal 11th rib incision. Through this incision, a splenorenal bypass can be performed in a completely retroperitoneal approach.

1167-B *(Campbell's, p. 2530)*

Patients for nephrectomy include the following. High risk or elderly patients who have unilateral disease and who because of their high-risk category are not good candidates for a lengthy procedure should undergo a nephrectomy if they have adequate function in the non-diseased kidney. In the past, total occlusion of the renal artery was felt to be an indication for nephrectomy; however, when adequate collaterals exist, the parenchyma may be preserved. This may be identified on arteriogram when perihilar or capsular collaterals are seen. In this case, a totally occluded vessel may be revascularized. Additionally, at the time of surgery, if back bleeding is noted from the renal arteriotomy distal to the total occlusion, one can assume adequate collateralization may exist and an attempt to revascularize should be made. If arterial reconstruction fails, resulting in complete graft occlusion, nephrectomy should be performed. Severe unilateral parenchymal disease most likely cannot be reversed by revascularization and is also an indication for nephrectomy.

1168-C *(Campbell's, pp. 2531–2535)*

To perform a polar nephrectomy, adequate exposure of the kidney and the renal pedicle is first achieved. The polar vessel that is diseased is then identified, controlled, and ligated. One need not occlude the main renal artery during the procedure. A dilute solution of methylene blue is then injected into the ligated, diseased artery distally to define the region of parenchyma this vessel supplies. The capsule over the pole is then incised and peeled back and preserved for closure. The avascular region as determined by the dye is then excised. The collecting system is closed with 5.0 chromic catgut sutures. The collecting system should not be closed with a permanent suture such as prolene because of the risk of stone formation. The reflected capsule is then used to cover over exposed parenchyma. A Penrose drain is left adjacent to the site of partial nephrectomy.

1169-E *(Campbell's, pp. 2530–2531)*

Stenosis of a segmental artery may produce segmental ischemia as well as localized over-production of renin and can cause significant symptoms. Therapy for such a lesion includes arterial bypass grafting when the segmental branch is large enough to be grafted, polar or mid-polar partial nephrectomy depending on the location of the diseased segmental artery, and arteriotomy and dilation of the diseased segment. Arteriotomy and dilation is particularly useful in the pediatric population. Complete embolization of the diseased segmental artery is not reported as a therapy for such lesions.

1170-E *(Campbell's, pp. 2535–2536)*

The technique of midpolar partial nephrectomy is illustrated on pages 2535–2536 of *Campbell's Urology*. Again, exposure of the kidney and the renal pedicle is achieved. The renal hilum is exposed and arterial branches meticulously dissected and identified. Diseased branches are controlled with Silastic loops. Again, a dilute solution of indigo carmine or methylene blue is injected into the diseased vessels to demarcate the parenchyma supplied by these branches. A coronal semicircular incision is then made over the capsule and the capsule peeled back on each side to expose the midpole parenchyma and the area of demarcation from the injected dye should be seen. The diseased segmental arteries are ligated and secondary veins are also ligated. After excision of the diseased parenchyma, the collecting system again is closed as with the polar nephrectomy. After closure of the collecting system, methylene blue solution is injected into the renal pelvis to check for leaks. The 2 poles are then approximated with horizontal mattress sutures encompassing the capsule to cover exposed parenchymal areas. Statement E is false because the poles are not individually pexed and left separately, but are reapproximated.

1171-A *(Campbell's, p. 2536)*

Renal endarterectomy is associated with a substantial incidence of recurrent stenosis and of renal artery thrombosis due to distal intimal flap. In this procedure, the aortic wall is only partially occluded with a vascular clamp around the orifice of the renal artery. The aorta is not completely cross-clamped. To perform safe dissection to obtain a clear demarcation between the renal artery and the aortic lesion is indeed difficult. On completion of the endarterectomy, closure of the renal artery often requires a vein patch angioplasty further complicating the procedure.

REFERENCE

1. Kaufman, J.J.: Renal vascular disorders. *In* Glenn, J.F. (Ed.): Urologic Surgery, 2nd ed. Hagerstown, MD, Harper and Row, 1975, pp. 874–918.

1172-D *(Campbell's, p. 2537)*

In the transaortic endarterectomy, the aorta is mobilized from the iliac bifurcation up to the superior mesenteric artery. Lumbar vessels are controlled with bulldog clamps. The author prefers gentle Swartz microvascular clamps for control of the distal renal arteries and mesenteric arteries. The aorta is of course cross-clamped above the superior mesenteric artery and below the inferior mesenteric artery. Systemic heparinization, again, is performed prior to cross-clamping. A vertical aortotomy is made from the level of the inferior mesenteric cephalad to a point above the superior mesenteric artery and to the left of it. Removal of the plaque begins distally circumferentially and proceeds cephalad. Traction is placed on the plaque and this aids in the development of the plane at the takeoff of the renal vessels. When the endarterectomy is complete, the distal intima within the aorta is transfixed to the outer aortic wall with 4-5 mattress sutures using 6-0 polypropylene. This is done to prevent dissection of the distal aorta. Routine passage of a Fogarty catheter down the renal vessels is not reported.

1173-A *(Campbell's, p. 2539)*

Dacron has been used extensively in renal artery reconstruction and is associated with a high-rate of early thrombosis. Autogenous hypogastric artery is of appropriate diameter for renal artery bypass and has excellent long-term patency rates. However, in adults, this vessel is often diseased and may not be useful. Autogenous hypogastric artery is useful material in children with renal artery disease because of the small caliber of the saphenous vein. Saphenous vein is less thrombogenic than prosthetic material and is readily anastomosed to the delicate distal renal artery. Saphenous vein has become the conduit of choice for aortorenal bypass in adults. When saphenous vein is not available, the cephalic vein may be substituted and if this is not available, a Gor-Tex graft should be used.

REFERENCE

1. Libertino, J.A., and Zinman, L.N.: Renal revascularization using aortorenal saphenous vein bypass grafting. Surg. Clin. North Am., *60*:487, 1980.

1174-C *(Campbell's, pp. 2540–2541)*

The single most important factor for long-term patency following saphenous vein aortorenal bypass grafting is a wide renal artery anastomosis. An end-to-end anastomosis between the vein and renal artery permits the best laminar flow and this should be performed, if possible. In children, the suture line is interrupted to prevent a pursestring effect with growth of the vessels as the child grows. 6-0 Prolene suture is employed on the venous renal artery anastomosis and 5-0 Prolene suture for the anastomosis of the saphenous vein to aorta. The graft is positioned to lie anteriorly to the vena cava when performing a right renal artery bypass and to lie anteriorly to the left renal vein when performing a left renal artery bypass. Care should be taken not to leave the vein too long such that it can bend to an acute angle, and possibly thrombose.

1175-E *(Campbell's, pp. 2542–2543)*

The splenorenal arterial bypass may be performed through a supracostal 11th rib flank incision. The splenic artery may be mobilized by a purely retroperitoneal approach in this procedure. The plane between the pancreas anteriorly and Gerota's fascia posteriorly is entered and the splenic artery identified along the superior margin of the pancreas. At this point, it should be documented that the splenic artery can accommodate a flow of 125 ml/min. If it is felt to be less than this, bypass should not be performed. The splenic artery is divided just proximal to its bifurcation in the hilum of the spleen; however a splenectomy is not required because adequate flow to the spleen occurs through the short gastric arteries. After mobilization of the splenic artery, it is treated with papaverine soaked sponges to cause dilation of the vessel prior to the anastomosis. An end-to-end anastomosis is then performed between the splenic artery and the distal renal artery using 6-0 Prolene sutures. If the splenic artery length is insufficient, a saphenous vein interposition graft should be placed between the splenic and renal arteries to allow tension free anastomosis.

1176-B *(Campbell's, pp. 2543–2545)*

Aortic thrombosis, previous aortic surgery or extensive atherosclerosis may make the aortorenal bypass procedure unfeasible. In this case, multiple alternative bypass operations have been used, including gastroduodenal-to-renal artery bypass, hepatic-to-renal artery saphenous vein bypass, superior mesenteric-to-renal artery saphenous vein bypass and iliac-to-renal saphenous vein bypass graft. When the lesion exists in the right renal artery, the hepatic-to-renal artery saphenous vein bypass is preferred, although the gastroduodenal-to-renal artery bypass is also useful. The superior mesenteric-to-renal artery saphenous vein bypass can be used for both right and left renal artery lesions and has been used as a bail-out procedure when other procedures cannot be used. The iliac-to-renal saphenous vein bypass graft has also been used as an alternative; however, often the iliac arteries are diseased as is the aorta. The technique of hepatorenal bypass employs a reverse autogenous saphenous vein graft between the common hepatic artery and the right renal artery. An end-to-end anastomosis is used between the vein and the right renal artery; however, an end-to-side anastomosis is performed between the vein graft and hepatic artery. The right hepatic artery is not sacrificed for the bypass graft. Liver function has not been compromised in these patients and renal-hepatic steal syndrome has not been observed. With the gastroduodenal-to-renal artery bypass, the gastroduodenal artery is divided and anastomosed in end-to-end fashion to the right renal artery.

1177-C *(Campbell's, pp. 2547–2549)*

Of the complications specific to renal revascularization, renal artery thrombosis is the most prevalent. Other complications include bleeding from perihilar collateral vessels (which may be significant due to the past high-grade stenosis), false aneurysms of the vascular anastomosis, aortic thrombosis and distal extremity embolization, and bleeding due to aortoduodenal erosion. In the early postoperative period when severe unexplained hypertension persists, one should suspect loss of graft patency and digital subtraction angiography should be performed. When embolization of aortic plaque occurs to the lower extremities, systemic heparinization is indicated and papaverine and fasciotomy may be useful. If a coincidental splenectomy is required, the patient is at increased risk for graft or artery thrombosis due to the hypercoagulable state following splenectomy. It is true that late studies do show aneurysmal dilation of saphenous vein grafts. However, no rupture of such grafts is yet reported. Aortoduodenal erosion occurs usually following the use of prosthetic graft material. This complication can be minimized by the use of autogenous graft material and placement of omentum between the graft and duodenum.

1178-E *(Campbell's, pp. 2549–2550)*

The National Cooperative Study Group found a 66 per cent cure and improvement rate and 34 per cent failure rate with renal vascular surgery. Overall, an operative mortality of 8 per cent was reported by this group. In Libertino's initial group of 225 patients, a 72 per cent cure rate was achieved. However, with an increase in surgical management of high-risk patients (including those with bilateral renal artery disease), his cure rate is now reported at 44 per cent. When one selectively looks at the subset of patients that undergoes renal revascularization for preservation of renal function, successful outcomes are seen in 85 per cent. In this group also, the graft occlusion rate was noted to be about 6.5 per cent with a mean followup greater than 2 years. No information is available comparing graft patency rates in visceral artery bypass procedures versus aortorenal bypass procedures.

REFERENCE

1. Foster, J.H., Maxwell, M.H., Franklin, S.S., et al.: Renovascular occlusive disease: results of operative treatment. JAMA, *231*:1043, 1975.

1179-D *(Campbell's, pp. 2553–2554)*

A number of factors affect ureteral healing. The ureter can close its own defect by regenerating all of its components. Mucosal healing is completed by 3 weeks and smooth muscle bridging by 6 weeks. Urinary flow across a repair may promote a lumen and stimulate transitional cell and muscle growth; however, urinary extravasation may lead to a reactive fibrosis with subsequent stenosis and obstruction.

Significant controversy remains over the routine placement of ureteral stents in ureteral surgery. Proponents believe that the stent will (1) immobilize the ureter until healing occurs; (2) inhibit the growth of granulation tissue and allow the orderly regrowth of an intact epithelial layer; (3) prevent the leakage of urine at the anastomotic site; (4) help maintain an adequate ureteral lumen during the healing phase; and (5) minimize any tendency to angulation of the ureter.

Some investigators believe that the risk of complications from stenting catheters outweighs their possible merits. Complications of ureteral stents include encrustation resulting in obstruction, stent migration, ureteral erosion, and stent dislodgment. The surgeon must weigh the advantages of the stent against the disadvantages of this foreign body.

REFERENCES

1. Schlossberg, S.M.: Ureteral healing. Semin. Urol., *5*: 197,1987.
2. Persky, L.: Splinting vs. nonsplinting in ureteral surgery. *In* Bergman, H. (Ed.): The Ureter. New York, Harper and Row, 1967, pp. 566–575.

1180-A *(Campbell's, pp. 2554–2555)*

During the healing phase, a ureteral defect may be watertight within 24 to 48 hours. Without adequate drainage, a marked fibrous reaction and scarring may result with poor muscular organization, stricture formation, and obstruction. The type of drain is not as important as the efficiency of the drain.

Urinary diversion is of benefit to prevent the site of repair from being bathed in urine. This task can be accomplished effectively by means of an internal stent or a nephrostomy. An important decision is whether or not to divert. The guidelines for diversion are variable. Proximal urinary diversion may not be necessary in a well-performed uncomplicated ureteral repair; however, in a patient with serious infection, contaminated wound, impaired renal function, or difficult anastomosis, proximal diversion may be left to the surgeon's preference, the patient's diagnosis and condition, the type of lesion, and the type of repair.

REFERENCE

1. Persky, L, and Carlton, C.E., Jr.: Urinary diversion in ureteral repair. *In* Scott, R., Jr. (Ed.): Current Controversies in Urologic Management. Philadelphia, W.B. Saunders Co., 1972, pp. 169–175.

1181-C *(Campbell's, p. 2555)*

At the time of the surgical procedure, delicate and gentle manipulation of ureteral tissue to minimize tissue trauma is important. To prevent ureteral crushing and vascular compromise, the ureter should be handled with fingers, fine vascular forceps, or traction sutures. The least amount of ureteral mobilization required to accomplish the operation will help to prevent vascular compromise.

Several factors affect epithelialization of a ureteral defect. These include no tension on the area to be repaired, no urinary leakage, and mucosa-to-mucosa approximation of the defect. The suture material used should be absorbable, since nonabsorbable sutures may lead to fistula formation, encrustation, and calculi. The suture should approximate and not strangulate the ureteral wall.

A circumferential scar of the ureter may contract, causing stricture and hydronephrosis; therefore, spatulation of the ureter before anastomosis is advised. An adequate debridement of devitalized tissue, a mucosa-to mucosa tension-free approximation of the defect, an internal stent, and a drain from the periureteral area are helpful in the successful healing of ureteral anastomosis.

REFERENCE

1. Silber, S.J., and Thornbury, J.: The fate of nonabsorbable intra-ureteral suture. J. Urol., *110*:40, 1973.

1182-B *(Campbell's, pp. 2555–2556)*

The incision and approach to the ureter depend primarily on the segment to be operated upon. Other considerations include the type of disease that necessitates surgery and its extent.

Surgical approaches to the upper third of the ureter are, in general, the same as those for the kidney (i.e., flank approach, dorsal lumbotomy, transabdominal). For disease processes in the middle third of the ureter, a muscle-splitting incision at the appropriate level, sometimes called a Gibson incision, provides simple access to the ureter.

The lower third of the ureter can be approached through a muscle-splitting, lower quadrant, modified Gibson incision. A transverse, Pfannenstiel, lower midline, or paramedian extraperitoneal approach may allow more exposure of the lower ureter than a Gibson-type incision.

1183-E *(Campbell's, pp. 2556–2557)*

Ureterolysis as a primary procedure is indicated whenever there is ureteral entrapment with resultant obstruction and compromise of renal function. Initial management of obstruction and timing of surgical intervention are dictated by the extent of disease and renal compromise. The primary objective of therapy is relief of obstruction by the passage of an indwelling catheter or stent. If the ureter cannot be catheterized and renal insufficiency is present, temporary upper tract diversion by a percutaneous nephrostomy is mandatory to stabilize renal function before definative therapy is undertaken.

Retroperitoneal fibrosis, whatever the etiology, may manifest itself initially as unilateral disease; however, even with what appears to be a totally normal opposite system, the other ureter may be involved with the process and may require "prophylactic therapy." Thus, a midline transabdominal incision is preferable.

Initially, routine abdominal exploration is performed. Tissue for biopsy and frozen-section examination should be obtained to rule out the presence of malignancy. Ureterolysis is accomplished from the ureteropelvic junction to below the iliac vessels.

Ureterolysis alone is not adequate treatment to prevent reinvolvement by the fibrotic process. After ureterolysis, the ureters should be handled in one of three ways: (1) intraperitonealization; (2) transposition laterally and anteriorly, positioning retroperitoneal fat between the ureter and the fibrosis; and (3) covering with omental sleeves.

REFERENCES

1. Blandy, J.: The ureter. *In* Blandy, J. (Ed.): Operative Urology, 2nd ed. Oxford, Blackwell Scientific Publications, 1986, pp. 89–114.
2. Tressider, G.C., Blandy, J.P., and Single, M.: Omental sleeve to prevent retroperitoneal fibrosis around the ureter. Urol. Int., *27*:44, 1972.

1184-B *(Campbell's, pp. 2557–2558)*

Primary ureterectomy is most frequently performed in combination with nephrectomy for the treatment of neoplasms of the renal pelvis or ureter. The most important consideration, if tumor is present, is to remove all of the tissue en bloc. If tumor is suspected but not proven, the ureteral exploration should be done first. Whether to do a nephroureterectomy though one flank incision or two separate incisions depends on the patient's body habitus and the need for a ureteral cuff excision for carcinoma.

The distal ureterectomy may be performed in one of two ways: by making a separate anterior incision in the bladder and circumscribing the ureteral orifice with a 1-cm margin, or by staying completely extravesical and placing two right-angle clamps across the ureterovesical junction, with the bladder divided between the clamps.

The major disadvantage for bladder cuff excision without vesicotomy is the inability to identify and prevent an iatragenic injury to the opposite ureteral orifice.

1185-A, 1186-D, 1187-B *(Campbell's, pp. 2558–2560)*

Advances in endoscopic techniques and the development of extracorporeal shock-wave lithotripsy have dramatically changed the indications for ureterolithotomy; however, in selected cases, ureterolithotomy may be indicated with the concomitant repair of a ureteral disorder. Documentation of the exact position of the stone should be made as close as possible to the time of surgery, even on the operating table, employing abdominal radiography to help decide on the most appropriate approach for ureterolithotomy.

For upper-third calculi, the extraperitoneal flank approach is preferred. For middle-third calculi, the approach may be extraperitoneal through a subcostal incision or a modified Gibson incision. For lower-third calculi, a midline, Pfannenstiel, or Gibson incision may be utilized. A transvaginal approach may be chosen for a calculus located near the ureterovesical junction. For a stone located in the intramural ureter, the transvesical approach may be employed. Since the ureteral blood supply travels in the periureteral tissue, the chance of disrupting ureteral blood supply is less likely with longitudinal incision than with a transverse incision. The calculus is teased out of the ureter with the end of the knife blade or small forceps.

The most common complication following a ureterolithotomy is persistent urinary leakage. In general, if drainage persists for longer that 5 to 7 days, an intravenous urography or a retrograde study should be performed to rule out distal obstruction and an indwelling ureteral catheter or a stent placed for a period of 24 to 48 hours. Rare complications include injection, ureteral structure, and urinoma. A follow-up upper tract study should be obtained about 3 months after surgery.

REFERENCE

1. Cohen, J.D., and Persky, L.: Ureteral stones. Urol. Clin. North Am., *10*:699, 1983.

1188-D *(Campbell's, p. 2560)*

Transvaginal approaches to the ureter are now rarely needed. The ureteroscope has helped to make this operation virtually unnecessary. Occasionally, a female patient with a large lower ureteral stone that is impacted may be managed with transvaginal ureterolithotomy. The advantage of this procedure is that it is rapid to perform and involves a minimum of tissue dissection and trauma. It also eliminates the complications of transabdominal surgery and the hospitalization and recovery period is short. The disadvantages of this approach include the minimal ureteral exposure, the lack of control of the proximal ureter, and the risk of postoperative ureterovaginal fistula. If the stone is dislodged and migrates proximally, retrieval may be difficult. It is best not to attempt this operation unless the stone can be palpated.

1189-C *(Campbell's, pp. 2560–2562)*

Ureteroureterostomy is defined as the end-to-end anastomosis of any two ureteral segments, including ipsilateral duplicated ureters. It may be performed in the case of resection of short segments of ureter for stricture, traumatic or iatrogenic injury, radiation injury, congenital obstruction, or localized carcinoma. The primary contraindication to ureteroureterostomy is inadequate length to assure a tension-free anastomosis. Relative contraindications include the presence of abscess, hematoma, or urinoma; vascular compromise of the ureter from mobilization; and previous ureteral injury or therapeutic irradiation.

In the case of intraoperative ureteral injury, repair can usually be made through the incision at hand. In the case of upper-third injury, the best approach is via the flank or 12th rib. For middle-third exposure, a Gibson incision is appropriate, since it can be extended either superiorly or inferiorly to achieve better exposure. The lower third approach is best made through a midline infraumbilical incision. To assure a successful anastomosis, as little dissection as necessary should be done in order to maintain the best possible blood supply. The most common anastomotic technique is spatulation, with sutures of 4-0 or 5-0 absorbable material, placed at right angles of each cut end into the angle of the spatulating incision on the opposing ureteral cut end.

Stents can be a valuable aid to ureteroureterostomy in tenuous or difficult anastomosis. Drainage of the anastomotic site is necessary and can be accomplished with either a Penrose drain or Jackson-Pratt drain.

Complications are usually rare and include prolonged drainage of urine from the drain or the incision and anastomotic stricture.

REFERENCES

1. Carlton, C.E. Jr., Scott, R. Jr., and Guthrie, A.G.: The initial management of ureteral injuries: A report of 78 cases. J. Urol., *105*:335, 1971.

2. Rober, P.E., Smith, J.B., and Pierce, J.M., Jr.: Gunshot injuries of the ureter. J. Trauma, *30*:83, 1190.
3. Young, J.D., Jr.: Ureteroureterostomy and transureteroureterostomy. *In* Gleen, J.F. (Ed.): Urologic Surgery. Philadelphia, J.B. Lippincott Co., 1983, pp. 427–434.

1190-C, 1191-A *(Campbell's, pp. 2562–2563)*

Clinically, transureteroureterostomy may be applied when it is necessary to reconstruct a lower-third or, occasionally, a middle-third ureteral defect. For the operation to succeed, there must be sufficient length for the ureter to cross the midline for a tension-free anastomosis to its mate on the opposite side. A gentle sweeping path without kinking is desired. The more proximal the end of the donor ureter, the more acute the sweep and the greater the possibility of mechanical obstruction. The optimal point for crossing the midline is at the level of the bifurcation of the aorta, where the ureters are closest to one another. Contraindications to transureteroureterostomy include inadequate length to permit a tension-free anastomosis, previous ureteral mobilization, previous ureteral injury or exposure to therapeutic radiation, recurrent renal stones, uroepithelial tumors, ureteral or renal tuberculosis, retroperitoneal fibrosis, chronic pyelonephritis, or uncorrected reflux in the recipient ureterovesical unit.

Transureteroureterostomy is best performed through an anterior midline transperitoneal incision. After the donor ureter is sufficiently freed proximally to allow a gentle sweep across the retroperitoneal space, a tunnel is created bluntly beneath the sigmoid and preferably above the inferior mesenteric artery. The donor ureter is spatulated on its antimesenteric border to a length of about 1.5 cm. An incision of equal length is made on the anteromedial surface of the recipient ureter. The anastomosis is performed with interrupted 4-0 or 5-0 absorbable suture; however, continuous sutures may be used as well. Stenting the anastomosis is optional. The area should be drained extraperitoneally.

REFERENCES

1. Pearse, H.D., Barry, J.M., and Fuchs, E.F.: Intraoperative consultation for ureter. Urol. Clin. North Am., *12*:423, 1985.
2. Udall, D.A., Hodges, C.V., Pearse, H.M., and Burns, A.B.: Transureteroureterostomy: A neglected procedure. J. Urol., *109*:817, 1973.
3. Van Arsdale, K.N., and Hackler, R.H.: Transureteroureterostomy in spinal cord injury patients for persistent vesicoureteral reflux: 6- to 14-year follow up. J. Urol., *129*:1117, 1983.

1192-D *(Campbell's, pp. 2564–2565)*

The psoas hitch is indicated whenever there is a gap in the distal ureter which prevents the direct reimplantation of the ureter into the bladder. Fixation of the ureter to the bladder wall with adequate ureteral backing is essential to help prevent reflux. The technique gives the surgeon between 3 and 5 cm of additional length. The relative contraindication to this procedure is a contracted scarred bladder or previous pelvic surgery in which the blood supply to the bladder was compromised.

Ideally, the bladder is sutured to the tendon of the psoas minor muscle with several 2-0 absorbable sutures. Frequently, this tendon is absent. In this case, it is important to ensure that large bites of the muscle are taken with the suture, being careful to avoid the genitofemoral nerve.

REFERENCE

1. Middleton, R.G.: Routine use of the psoas hitch in uretral reimplantation. J. Urol., *123*:352, 1980.

1193-D *(Campbell's, pp. 2565–2566)*

The Boari flap is a bladder tube used to bridge large ureteral defects. It can be performed through a variety of incisions, selecting whichever is appropriate to approach and resect the distal and damaged ureter. The bladder should be fully mobilized, particularly on its lateral and medial-posterior aspects.

Principles of plastic surgery usually require graft length-to-width ratio of 3:2. Since the tubularized flap has no functional activity as a tube, its opening into the bladder must always be widemouthed to drain satisfactorily.

A bladder flap is created from the posterior wall with a base of at least 4 cm and an apex of approximately 3 cm. It should be based on the superior vesical artery or one of its major branches. Under most circumstances, up to 12 cm of bladder tube can be created in this manner. An antirefluxing ureteral anastomosis to the Boari flap can be performed; however, this antireflux procedure should not be established at the sacrifice of a tension-free suture line.

Stents should be left for 10 to 14 days, and adequate drainage of the anastomosis must be maintained for at least 15 days postoperatively.

REFERENCES

1. Benson, M.C., Ring, K.S., and Olsson, C.A.: Ureteral reconstruction and bypass: Experience with ileal interposition, the Boari flap-psoas hitch, and renal autotransplantation. J. Urol., *143*:20, 1990.
2. Olsson, C.A., and Norleu, L.J.: Combined Boari bladder flap-psoas hitch procedure in ureteral replacement. Scand. J. Urol. Nephrol., *20*:279, 1986.

1194-B *(Campbell's, pp. 2566–2567)*

Cutaneous ureterostomy was the common form of urinary diversion until the 1950s when it was replaced by either the more complex forms of urinary diversion employing bowel segments. Cutaneous ureterostomy should be considered whenever intraoperative problems necessitate urinary diversion on the one hand and rapid termination of the operation on the other.

The main advantage of this procedure is that it is simple to perform and requires minimal exposure and operative trauma. There are three major disadvantages to cutaneous ureterostomy. First of all, there is the problem of two stomas. To be effective, both ureters should be brought to the skin to a single stoma so that they can be fitted with a single collection device without intubation. Second, the relatively poor ureteral blood supply frequently leads to a distal ureteral slough, recession of the stoma, or stomal stricture. Finally, urinary collection can be a problem in patients with cutaneous ureterostomies.

The most significant early complication is stoma necrosis. Compromised blood supply during mobilization, tight opening in the abdominal wall, and retraction of the stoma from the skin are believed to contribute to stoma necrosis. Stomal stricture has been reported to occur in up to 64 per cent of cutaneous ureterostomies. Risk factors for this complication include: (1) ureteral diameter less than 8 mm, (2) everted stoma, and (3) preoperative ureteral or skin irradiation. The overall long-term results of patients with permanent cutaneous ureterostomies are not satisfying. More than half require conversion to intestinal conduits within 7 years of the original ureterostomy.

REFERENCES

1. MacGregor, P.S., Montie, J.E., and Straffon, R.A.: Cutaneus ureterostomy as palliative diversion in adults with malignancy. Urology, *30*:31, 1987.
2. Eckstein, H.B.: Ureteral diversion. *In* Glenn, J.F. (Ed.): Urologic Surgery, 3rd ed., Philadelphia, J.B. Lippincott Co., 1983, pp. 491–499.

1195-A *(Campbell's, pp. 2568–2569)*

The intact isolated ileal segment provides the only reliable replacement for the ureter. An ileal segment is reserved for a patient with an extensive loss of the ureter due to trauma, previous surgery, tuberculosis, urinary stone disease, ureteral carcinoma in a single kidney, or undiversion. Uncorrected bladder outlet obstruction is a relative contraindication to surgery. Patients with compromised renal functions may deteriorate to overt renal failure because of the absorption of urine across the ileal segment. This procedure is also contraindicated in patients with diffuse malignant disease or regional enteritis.

Bilateral replacement can be done using the same ileal segment by running the proximal end from one pelvis to the other and down to the bladder. Another method for bilateral replacement uses the terminal ileum on one side and the colon on the other.

REFERENCES

1. Boxer, R.J., Fritzsche, P., Skinner, D.G., et al.: Replacement of the ureter by small intestine: clinical application and results of the ileal ureter in 89 patients. J. Urol., *121*:728, 1979.
2. Benson, M.C., Ring, K.S., and Olsson, C.A.: Ureteral reconstruction and bypass: Experience with ileal interposition, the Boari flap-psoas hitch, and renal autotransplantation. J. Urol., *143*:20, 1990.

1196-A *(Campbell's, pp. 2571–2572)*

Although the urologist is concerned primarily with the evaluation and treatment of urinary tract injuries, the ABCs of trauma management should be followed for any trauma patient. Answers B-E have priority and should be completed in the emergency room prior to obtaining any radiographic studies. These again include establishment of an adequate airway followed by establishment of vascular access and fluid resuscitation, control of hemorrhage, and, in the unconscious patient, nasogastric intubation.

1197-B *(Campbell's, pp. 2572–2575)*

CT scanning is now the study of choice in the multisystem trauma patient with suspected upper urinary tract injury. CT scan defines organ injuries more precisely than excretion urography, showing minute extravasation of contrast material from the urinary tract or bowel that might be missed on IVP, and showing areas of infarction in the kidney as small as 1.5 cm. The CT scan also is the best study for identification of ectopic kidneys or congenital absence of the kidney. The cortical rim sign is seen when the primary blood flow to a kidney has been disrupted and a capsular vessel is providing collateral flow to the outer cortex. A thin rim of functioning cortex is then observed. The CT scan can predict major renal vessel injury; however, it does not accurately definitively rule out such injury and therefore, answer B is false.

1198-C *(Campbell's, pp. 2572–2575)*

CT scanning is presently the study of choice for the evaluation of upper urinary tract trauma. When CT scanning does indicate the possibility of a main renal vessel injury, one could proceed directly to the OR for revascularization; however, if nonoperative management is selected, arteriography should be performed to ensure a main renal vessel injury is not missed. When access to CT scanning is not available, use of IVP and renal sonography is an acceptable alternative in the evaluation of upper urinary tract trauma. In addition, radionuclide studies could be used to verify blood flow to the kidneys and could possibly have a place in the early evaluation of trauma when other modalities are not available. Generally when the nephrogram is seen on intravenous pyelogram, there is a 95 to 97 per cent chance that no renal artery injury which requires surgical correction is present. Nuclear studies are often used in follow-up of major injuries to assess functional recovery.

REFERENCE

1. Cass, A.S., and Luxenberg, M.: Management of renal artery injuries from external trauma. J. Urol., *138*: 1987.

1199-D *(Campbell's, p. 2571)*

Urethral injury may occur when a patient sustains a straddle injury or when a Malgaigne fracture is present, and one should consider performing retrograde urethrography on these patients to evaluate for urethral injury. The presence of blood at the meatus in a trauma patient is an absolute indication for performing retrograde urethrography. The finding of ecchymosis of the perineum also suggests a pelvic fracture and possible urethral injury and should be evaluated with retrograde urethrography. A scrotal laceration is not necessarily an indication for retrograde urethrography; however, one might consider retrograde urethrography if a deep scrotal laceration occurs in a region such as the penile scrotal junction where the urethra might be violated.

1200-E *(Campbell's, p. 2571)*

Isolated adrenal injuries among blunt and penetrating trauma patients are exceedingly rare, with no cases being observed in over 16,000 patients at Parkland Memorial Hospital over a seven year period. The adrenal medulla is, however, very susceptible to hemorrhage from trauma, which is usually iatrogenic in nature, and this can occur during organ harvest or during breech extraction for delivery. Bilateral adrenal trauma due to breech extraction is a very rare injury. Presently, no specific pharmacologic guidelines are given for the management for blunt trauma to the adrenal glands, and therefore answer E is incorrect. Phentolamine is an alpha-blocker and might be considered for use if high doses of epinephrine were released into the system; however, this is not reported to be a concern in adrenal trauma.

REFERENCES

1. Peters, P.C., and Sagalowsky, A.I.: Genitourinary trauma. *In* Walsh, P.E., Gittes, R.F., Perlmutter, A.D., and Stamey, T.A. (Eds.): Campbell's Urology, 5th ed. Philadelphia, W.B. Saunders Co., 1986, pp. 1192–1246.
2. Skinner, E.C., Boyd, S.D., and Apuzzo, M.L.J.: Technique of left adrenalectomy for autotransplantation to the caudate nucleus in Parkinson's disease. J. Urol., *144*:838, 1990.

1201-B *(Campbell's, pp. 2574–2575)*

Radiographic imaging to evaluate for upper urinary tract injuries should be performed when gross hematuria is present, there is a history of hypotension with a systolic blood pressure of less than 80 and the presence of microhematuria when there is any penetrating abdominal trauma, and when the history suggests a mechanism of injury that may lead to upper urinary tract injury. A fall from a great height or accidents in which the patient suddenly decelerates from a high velocity may give rise to renal pedicle injuries, which may present with a normal urinalysis, and these patients should be evaluated with studies to visualize the upper urinary tract. The presence of microhematuria alone is not an indication for radiographic imaging of the upper urinary tract.

1202-C *(Campbell's, p. 2574)*

Renal injuries are often classified as major or minor. Major renal injuries include pedicle injuries (including injuries to the main renal vessels or avulsion of the ureter at the UPJ), major lacerations of the parenchyma, and lacerations of the parenchyma which extend into the collecting system. Small contained subcapsular hematomas, nonexpanding perirenal hematomas with small lacerations of the parenchyma, and small renal contusions are not considered major renal injuries. Answer C is correct because the laceration extends into the collecting system giving rise to the perirenal extravasation seen on CT scan.

1203-D *(Campbell's, p. 2575)*

Injuries to the renal pedicle include: avulsion of the main renal artery or vein, an intimal tear in the main renal artery with intimal flap formation, and disruption of the UPJ with ureteral avulsion. In blunt trauma patients, these injuries are seen usually when there is rapid deceleration from a high velocity. Disruption of the UPJ usually occurs when there is hyperextension of the spine, and is associated with a greater mobility of the spine in the child. At Parkland Memorial Hospital the mortality rate was 37 per cent among trauma patients with renal pedicle injuries, and this is related to association with other severe injuries. Although one might expect that in blunt trauma patients pedicle injuries would be bilateral, this is not observed, and therefore answer D is incorrect.

1204-E *(Campbell's, p. 2577)*

The preferred approach for most general trauma patients would be a midline incision from xiphoid to pubis. This allows exploration of abdominal organs as well as quick access to the renal vessels. Access to the renal vessels requires reflecting the colon and incising the posterior peritoneum parallel to the inferior mesenteric vein, thus exposing the great vessels and revealing the left renal vein. The left renal vein is then retracted cephalad to expose the right and left renal arteries. An alternative approach to the renal vessels involves incising around the cecum and through the root of the mesentery, sacrificing both inferior mesenteric vessels. Control of the renal pedicle is essential prior to opening Gerota's fascia and exposing the kidney. The dorsal lumbotomy incision does not allow such control and is not a preferred approach. To expose the right renal hilum, the duodenum must be mobilized medially. This can be done by the Kocher maneuver.

1205-D *(Campbell's, p. 2578)*

A partial nephrectomy should be performed in the case of major renal polar injuries and the devascularized parenchyma of the affected pole should be removed. Care should be taken to preserve the capsule, which then should be used to cover all bare areas of parenchyma after the partial nephrectomy. The collecting system should be closed with absorbable suture, preferably 4.0 chromic, to prevent stone formation from long-term foreign bodies. Similar sutures should also be used to ligate parenchymal vessels. If the injury has occurred to a lower pole, one must be concerned with the ureter adhering to the resected kidney and leading to UPJ obstruction. To prevent this, fat should be interposed between the UPJ region and the resected lower pole. After partial nephrectomy has been performed, the possibility of torsion about the renal pedicle is increased and nephropexy of the kidney to muscle fascia should be performed to prevent this. Dietl's crisis consists of vomiting and abdominal pain associated with intermittent torsion of the renal pedicle. Answer D is incorrect because of the permanent nature of the 3.0 silk suture and the possibility of formation of calculi in the collecting system.

1206-B *(Campbell's, pp. 2578–2579)*

Direct ureteral injury from penetrating trauma is indeed a very rare event. Only 24 isolated injuries to the ureter were reported in the United States forces in the Second World War. Blunt trauma to the ureter is also rare, and the most common severe injury is UPJ avulsion, which occurs with acute hyperextension of the spine in blunt trauma. Iatrogenic ureteral injuries occur often during gynecologic, urologic or pelvic vascular procedures and also with laminectomies. With iatrogenic injuries, the ureter is most commonly injured at the pelvic brim. The occurrence of hematuria is not a reliable indicator of ureteral injuries, whether traumatic or iatrogenic. Iatrogenic ureteral injuries which are not recognized at the time of operation most often present between postoperative days 4 and 9 with symptoms of flank pain and fever. It is true that high velocity injuries can cause extensive coagulation necrosis and this can occur with the ureter.

REFERENCE

1. Daly, J.W., and Higgins, K.A.: Injury to the ureter during gynecologic surgical procedures. Surg. Gynecol. Obstet., *167*:19, 1988.

1207-C *(Campbell's, pp. 2578–2581)*

Ureteral injuries are classified by location with injuries grouped into the upper, middle, or lower third of the ureter. When the diagnosis is made shortly after the injury, definitive treatment is preferred if possible. For injuries in the upper and middle third of the ureter, a ureteroureterostomy is the preferred method of management. The ureter is debrided, spatulated, and then closed with ureteral stenting. For injuries in the lower third of the ureter, ureteral reimplantation is preferred for management. A psoas-bladder hitch or reimplantation of the ureter into a Boari bladder flap are useful procedures when small lengths of distal ureter need to be made up. When there has been 7 cm of destruction of the ureter, mobilization of both the kidney and bladder are usually required for reapproximation of the ureter. Answer C is therefore false. When the possibility of contamination of vascular grafts exists, one must consider ureterostomy and ureteral ligation followed by delayed repair vs. nephrectomy. In elderly patients, a single procedure involving a nephrectomy may be advantageous. When ureteral injuries present late with urinoma and abscess formation, they should be treated in two stages with initial drainage and diversion followed by definitive repair once the inflammation is resolved.

1208-D *(Campbell's, pp. 2581–2583)*

Rupture of the urinary bladder is categorized as being intraperitoneal or extraperitoneal. Either may be seen with blunt trauma. Intraperitoneal rupture often occurs when blunt external force is applied to the lower abdomen and the bladder is full. Therefore, statement D is false, making it the correct choice. Extraperitoneal rupture is commonly associated with pelvic fracture; however, both intraperitoneal and extraperitoneal rupture may be associated with pelvic fractures where the bladder has not been lacerated due to bone fragments. A review by Herzog shows rupture of the bladder is found in approximately 5 per cent of patients suffering a pelvic fracture. Intraperitoneal rupture should be suspected when poorly localized abdominal tenderness occurs and the patient is intermittently unable to void. Both ruptures may be associated with hematuria. To establish the diagnosis of ruptured urinary bladder, a cystogram is performed, distending the bladder with a minimum of 250 ml of sterile contrast. If this volume is not instilled, a small intact bladder may be observed and contraction of bladder muscle may seal off the area of perforation.

1209-C *(Campbell's, p. 2581)*

Peters and Sagalowsky recommend exploratory laparotomy at the time of suprapubic cystostomy to evaluate for other traumatic injuries. When bloody fluid is observed in the peritoneal cavity, exploration of this space should be performed. Likewise, if one is repairing an intraperitoneal rupture, the peritoneal cavity should be explored. They prefer closure of the bladder with three layers with chromic catgut or Vicryl suture and typically leave a 20 French suprapubic tube brought out through a separate stab wound in the bladder. These authors also prefer extraperitoneal drainage with a Jackson-Pratt drain. Typically, the bladder is sealed in 10 to 14 days and the suprapubic tube removed. However, in case of immobilization of the patient due to other injuries and the possibility of long-term requirement of catheter drainage, the suprapubic tube should be left in place as opposed to using a Foley catheter. Statement C is false. In the trauma patient with a spinal cord injury, one should attempt to preserve the bladder as the urinary storage reservoir. Urinary diversion should not be considered at the time of repair of traumatic injuries; however, this may be necessary in the future if upper tract deterioration occurs.

1210-E *(Campbell's, p. 2593)*

In the work-up of genitourinary injuries in the pregnant patient, radiation exposure should be minimized, particularly in the first trimester. Ultrasonography is a very valuable tool and should be used in the initial evaluation of suspected renal trauma. Ultrasonography can also be used to locate the placenta and evaluate the status of the fetus. When major renal injuries are identified in the pregnant patient, surgical management should be performed according to the usual indications regardless of the pregnancy. Generally, no problem occurs in operating on the pregnant woman if there is an injury to the kidney, collecting system or bladder. However, if fetal distress is noted and gestational age is beyond 26 weeks, cesarean section should be performed. When branch lesions of the renal artery are identified, angioinfarction may be considered following arteriography. Exploration should be performed for all penetrating wounds to the abdomen which perforate the peritoneal cavity or the uterus. When penetrating trauma to the uterus occurs, if the fetus is viable and is less than 26 weeks gestation, repair of the uterus should be performed. Statement E is false because penetrating trauma to the uterus may be managed in some cases without immediate C section regardless of the bladder injury.

REFERENCE

1. Sakala, E.P., and Kort, D.D.: Management of stab wounds to the pregnant uterus: A case report and a review of the literature. Obstet. Gynecol. Surv., *43*: 319, 1988.

1211-B *(Campbell's, p. 2583)*

With posterior urethral rupture, frequently the prostate is difficult to examine on digital rectal examination due to superior displacement of the gland. This was first reported by Vermooten who referred to this as the "high-riding" prostate. In the evaluation of urethral injuries, urethrography should be performed with water soluble contrast and this usually confirms the diagnosis of posterior urethral rupture. On other radiographic studies, the bladder full of contrast material is usually seen to be floating above the symphysis. When an intact vesicle neck and bladder distended with contrast material is well above symphysis, this has been referred to as the "pie in the sky." Statement B, however, is false because the bladder need not necessarily lie cephalad to the sacroiliac joint. Finally, posterior urethral rupture can be confused with extraperitoneal vesicle rupture when similar radiographic findings are seen, such as the finding of contrast material in a deformed bladder with descent of contrast to the symphysis in a teardrop fashion.

REFERENCES

1. Turner-Warwick, R.T.: Prevention of complications resulting from pelvic fracture urethral injuries and from their surgical management. Urol. Clin. North Am., *16*: 335, 1989.
2. Vermooten, V.: Rupture of the urethra: A new diagnostic sign. J. Urol., *56*:228, 1946.

1212-E *(Campbell's, pp. 2583–2585)*

Nearly 95 per cent of posterior urethral disruptions are complete, and stricture of the disrupted region is the rule. Other major complications associated with posterior urethral injury include urinary incontinence and impotence. Presently there is some debate about the initial management of posterior urethral disruption. It is the consensus of the authors of Chapter 69 that an initial suprapubic cystostomy at the time the patient presents followed by a urethral reconstructive procedure approximately three months later minimizes complications associated with posterior urethral rupture. This may be simply due to avoiding operating in a pelvis full of hematoma and bone fragments in the peritraumatic period. A vesicostomy is an acceptable alternative to a suprapubic cystostomy in the infant who has disruption of the posterior urethra. McRoberts and Rajde showed in the dog model that complete epithelial apposition, when accomplished by the suture technique, yielded a lower stricture rate following urethral alignment. Therefore, statement E is false.

REFERENCE

1. McRoberts, J.W., and Rajde, H.: Severed canine posterior urethra: A study of two distinct methods of repair. J. Urol., *104*:724, 1970.

1213-D *(Campbell's, pp. 2585–2588)*

Anterior urethral injuries are more common than posterior urethral injuries and usually occur as a result of straddle injuries. Statement D is, therefore, false. Direct blows to the perineum may also lead to anterior urethral injury, and a common cause of this in Texas is a blow from the toe of a boot. As with other urethral injuries, retrograde urethrography confirms the diagnosis of ruptured anterior urethra. When Buck's fascia remains intact following the urethral injury, extravasation will be contained by this fascial layer and will follow the shaft of the penis. However, if Buck's fascia is violated, extravasation of urine and blood may be observed to the level of the clavicle. When Buck's fascia has been ruptured, Colles' fascia becomes a limiting factor for containing extravasation of fluid from the urethra. This fascia joins with the fascia lata of the thigh and prevents inferior extravasation; however, its superior margin of fusion with other fascia layers is not reached until the clavicle.

1214-E *(Campbell's, pp. 2585–2589)*

As with posterior urethral disruption, if there is any doubt as to the integrity of the anterior urethra, a suprapubic cystostomy and delayed reconstruction of the urethra is recommended. If a direct blow or stab wound to the perineum occurs, giving rise to an anterior urethral injury, exploration may be made through a perineal incision shortly after the time of injury, and urethral reanastomosis performed. In this case, an oblique spatulated anastomosis using 5.0 and 6.0 catgut suture is preferred. When this is done, the proximal urethra should be fixed to the underlying fascia to immobilize the anastomotic site and minimize the occurrence of postoperative urethral stricture. The urethral stent left in at the time of repair should be kept in place at least 10 days to 2 weeks. When penetrating trauma has occurred to the perineum, which has given rise to an anterior urethral injury, one must also be concerned about the possibility of rectal injury, and proctoscopy must be included as part of the workup.

1215-A *(Campbell's, pp. 2589–2591)*

Following degloving injuries to the penis, skin grafting may be required. When split thickness skin grafting is performed, the graft should be 0.15 mm thick to allow for normal expansion of the healed penis during erection. Therefore, statement A is false. When an aneurysm or rupture of the corporal fascia has occurred, immediate repair is preferred and this does minimize the development of scar tissue which causes symptoms similar to those seen in Peyronie's disease. Strangulating lesions of the penis may occur when objects are placed about the penis circumferentially. These often require removal under general anesthesia using cutting tools to remove the object. However, one may first attempt to decrease the diameter of the penis by wrapping a string circumferentially around the distal penis beginning at the meatus and carrying it to the object. This occasionally will allow successful removal of the object. When penile amputation occurs, the dismembered portion should be placed in ice as soon as possible after injury, and this has been found to be the most important factor in subsequent survival of the amputated tissue. A tourniquet should be applied to the proximal penile part to arrest hemorrhage until repair can be performed. The repair should be done at a facility where microsurgery can be handled. The dorsal penile arteries and veins and the urethral cavernous artery should be reapproximated with 10.0 or 11.0 nonabsorbable suture. If this cannot be done, a minimum repair can be accomplished by reestablishing venous continuity and approximating the proximal corpora to the distal part. Often then the distal member will survive if venous drainage is established. The urethra should be reapproximated in interrupted fashion with 5.0 or 6.0 chromic catgut or Vicryl suture.

1216-C *(Campbell's, p. 2591)*

When there is a significant loss of scrotal tissue and skin, one may need to find an alternative location for the testicles. Positioning is preferable in the superficial thigh because it is felt that the temperature there is slightly lower than a subcutaneous abdominal placement and that this favors spermatogenesis. If only a moderate amount of skin is lost, perineal skin may be used to provide a flap to supplement tissue. If multiple debridements of the perineal area are required, the testicles may be left exposed, however, they should be treated with application of warm saline. If granulation tissue ensues following debridement, skin grafting may be sufficient rather than relocating testicles. When testicular parenchyma has been exposed from severe blunt trauma or penetrating trauma, meticulous debridement should be performed with care to remove all foreign materials. The tunica albuginea should then be closed; no drain is left below the tunica albuginea. Broad-spectrum antibiotic coverage is indicated.

REFERENCE

1. McDougal, W.S.: Scrotal reconstruction using thigh pedicle flaps. J. Urol., *129*:757, 1983.

1217-B *(Campbell's, p. 2595)*

Utilizing the gastroepiploic arteries, a pedicle of stomach may be mobilized to the pelvis. The pedicle may consist of the entire antrum/pylorus or a wedge of the fundus. The stomach is a very vascular organ that receives its blood supply primarily from the celiac axis. The right gastroepiploic artery anastomoses with the left gastroepiploic artery and both supply the greater curve of the stomach.

1218-C *(Campbell's, p. 2596)*

No definite demarcation exists between the jejunum and ileum; however, each possesses several unique properties that allow distinction of one from the other intraoperatively. The ileum being more distal in location has a smaller diameter. It has multiple arterial arcades, and the vessels in the arcades are smaller than those in the jejunum. The ileal mesentery is thicker than the jejunal mesentery. In contrast, the jejunal diameter is larger, and the arterial arcades are usually single. The vessels composing them are larger in diameter.

1219-E *(Campbell's, p. 2598)*

The incidence of postoperative bowel obstruction when using stomach is 10 per cent, whereas the use of colonic segments results in an incidence of 4 per cent. The advantage of stomach over other intestinal segments is that it is less permeable to urinary solutes, it acidifies the urine, it produces less mucus, it has a net excretion of chloride rather than a net absorption and the incidence of bacteriuria is lower. Stomach is useful in a patient with extensive renal dysfunction, and when a decreased amount of intestine will result in serious nutritional problems.

1220-D *(Campbell's, p. 2599)*

Whole-gut irrigation may be exhausting to the patient and may in fact result in a fluid gain. Whereas there is no known contraindication in diabetics, it is contraindicated in patients with unstable cardiovascular disease, cirrhosis, severe renal disease, congestive failure, or obstructed bowel.

1221-C *(Campbell's, p. 2600)*

Most authorities believe that preoperative antimicrobial bowel preparation is advantageous in reducing postoperative complications in elective colon and small bowel surgery. Antibiotics are felt to protect vulnerable bowel and may allow a tenuous anastomosis to survive. However, in the presence of bowel obstruction, oral antibiotics are of little value. The disadvantages of antibiotics include a postoperative increase in the incidence of pseudomembranous enterocolitis, and monilial overgrowth resulting in stomatitis, thrush, and diarrhea.

1222-A *(Campbell's, pp. 2601–2602)*

The factors that significantly contribute to anastomotic breakdown include poor blood supply, drains placed on an intra-abdominal anastomosis, fecal spillage, and anastomosis performed in radiated bowel. Drains placed on an anastomosis increase the likelihood of a leak, and an anastomosis performed in irradiated bowel is more likely to result in failure. Poor blood supply and local sepsis cause ischemia.

1223-B *(Campbell's, p. 2604)*

In general, hand-sewn anastomoses are preferable to stapled anastomoses in intestine through which urine traverses, because of their lower propensity to cause stone formation. The theoretical advantages of a stapled anastomosis are (1) better blood supply to the healing margin, (2) reduced tissue manipulation, (3) minimal edema with uniformity of suture placement, (4) wider lumen, (5) greater ease and less time involved in performing the anastomosis, and (6) reduced length of postoperative paralytic ileus.

1224-C *(Campbell's, p. 2606)*

Colonic activity usually returns in 2 to 4 days after intestinal surgery. Coordinated small bowel activity begins within hours after the operative event, and stomach activity may return as early as 24 hours. Clear liquids may be begun when the paralytic ileus resolves and bowel activity resumes. Hyperalimentation should be considered in patients who are nutritionally impaired prior to surgery or who have a prolonged paralytic ileus.

1225-A *(Campbell's, pp. 2607, 2618)*

Fistulas in the postoperative period are of two types: fecal and urinary. These generally occur within the first weeks after surgery, usually within the first 7 to 10 days. Fistulas frequently result in sepsis and markedly increase morbidity and mortality. The incidence of urinary intestinal leak is markedly reduced by the use of soft Silastic stents. A urinary intestinal leak may cause periureteral fibrosis and scarring, with subsequent stricture formation.

1226-D *(Campbell's, pp. 2607–2608)*

The most common cause of obstruction is adhesions followed by recurrent cancer. These two causes account for the majority of cases. The incidence of postoperative obstruction requiring treatment when colon is utilized is 4 per cent, and 10 per cent when stomach or ileum is used. The incidence of postoperative bowel obstruction may be reduced by using nonirradiated bowel, closing all apertures, reperitonealizing the isolated segment, decompressing the gastrointestinal tract for an adequate period of time, placing omentum over the anastomosis, and reconstituting the pelvic floor following exenterative surgery.

1227-E *(Campbell's, p. 2612)*

Strictures of ureterointestinal anastomoses are generally caused by ischemia, urine leak, radiation, or infection. The incidence of leak and stricture is greatly reduced when soft

Silastic stents are used. Adherence to basic surgical principles is a must if strictures are to be avoided. Only as much ureter as needed should be mobilized so that there is no redundancy or tension on the anastomosis. Mobilization should not strip the ureter of its periadventitia, and therefore its blood supply. The ureterointestinal anastomosis must be performed with fine absorbable sutures with a watertight mucosa-to-mucosa apposition.

1228-A *(Campbell's, pp. 2612–2616)*

The Bricker anastomosis is a refluxing end-to-side ureteral small bowel anastomosis that is easy to perform and has a low complication rate. Considerable controversy exists as to whether a nonrefluxing or refluxing anastomosis is desirable for urinary tract reconstruction. Upper tract deterioration is usually related to infection or stones. It appears that reflux associated with impaired ureteral peristalsis in the presence of bacteriuria and/or obstruction results in renal deterioration.

1229-C *(Campbell's, p. 2618)*

The most successful technique for treating ureterointestinal stricture is reexploration, removing the stenotic segment, and reanastomosing the ureter to the bowel. The open procedure resulted in approximately a 90 per cent success rate, whereas endourologic methods resulted in a 70 per cent success rate. The reported success rates must be balanced against the higher morbidity of open procedures, which are frequently very difficult.

1230-B *(Campbell's, p. 2619)*

The incidence of both sepsis and renal failure is greater in patients with ureterosigmoidostomy than in those with conduits. The incidence of renal deterioration following conduit urinary intestinal diversion has varied from 10 to 60 per cent. A greater degree of renal function is necessary for continent diversions than for short conduit diversions because of the reabsorption of urinary solutes.

1231-D *(Campbell's, p. 2620)*

Electrolyte disorders that occur when jejunum is utilized include hyponatremia, hypochloremia, hyperkalemia, azotemia, and acidosis. These result from an increased secretion of sodium and chloride with an increased reabsorption of potassium and hydrogen ions. These electrolyte abnormalities result in lethargy, nausea, vomiting, dehydration, muscular weakness, and elevated temperature. If allowed to persist, the patient may become moribund and finally succumb.

1232-A *(Campbell's, p. 2620)*

The treatment for the classic electrolyte disturbances of jejunal conduits is rehydration with sodium chloride and correction of acidosis with sodium bicarbonate. Chronic salt depletion is the primary pathophysiology in this syndrome due to the high permeability of jejunum.

1233-E *(Campbell's, p. 2621)*

The treatment of hyperchloremic metabolic acidosis involves administering alkalizing agents and/or blockers of chloride transport. However, in patients in whom excessive sodium loads are undesirable, nicotinic acid or chlorpromazine may be given to limit the degree of acidosis. Chlorpromazine and nicotinic acid inhibit cyclic AMP and thereby impede chloride transport.

1234-B *(Campbell's, p. 2621)*

Hypokalemia and total body potassium depletion may develop in patients who have undergone ureterosigmoidostomies and ureterocolonic diversions. This is due to gut loss through intestinal secretion and renal potassium wasting as a consequence of renal damage. When the potassium depletion is severe, the patient may develop a flaccid paralysis. If the hypokalemia is associated with severe hyperchloremic metabolic acidosis, treatment must involve replacement of potassium as well as correcting acidosis with bicarbonate.

1235-B *(Campbell's, p. 2623)*

Deterioration of the upper tracts is more likely when the culture becomes dominant for *Proteus* or *Pseudomonas*. Thus, patients with relatively pure cultures of these organisms should be treated, whereas those with mixed cultures may generally be observed provided they are not symptomatic.

1236-D *(Campbell's, p. 2623)*

Loss of the ileocecal valve may have many untoward effects that result in decreased availability of vitamin B_{12} and deficiencies of the fat-soluble vitamins. Reflux of bacteria into the small bowel may cause bacterial metabolism of vitamin B_{12} and adversely affect fat absorption and the subsequent digestion of fat-soluble vitamins.

1237-A *(Campbell's, p. 2631)*

Clean intermittent catheterization is now widely used largely due to the efforts of Lapides and colleagues in the early 1970s. This is a simple way to manage urinary retention for the long term in the majority of patients. This also enabled the development of continent urinary diversions and augmentation cystoplasty in the long term management of complicated problems of bladder dysfunction. Although all the surgical advances are also important, CIC may be the most significant development.

1238-D *(Campbell's, p. 2631)*

Any large or small bowel segments which are used in reconstruction of the urinary tract can cause a metabolic acidosis. A hyperchloremic metabolic acidosis develops primarily due to active transport of chloride in the large and small bowel. This carries along with it a cation which is commonly either hydrogen ion or ammonium. These enter the systemic circulation and account for the acidosis. Another contributing factor includes loss of bicarbonate in the intestinal secretions. Acidosis will be exacerbated if there is an accompanying renal tubular acidification defect. The stomach has an active hydrogen ion pump and therefore acidosis is not seen.

1239-E *(Campbell's, pp. 2631–2632)*

The patient's attitudes, abilities, and self-motivation are the major determinants of success in lower urinary tract reconstruction. It is also key to have adequate support systems if the patient is not able to perform certain functions.

Age is not always correlated with the psychological maturity level of the patient, and only when a patient is ready and willing to be responsible for the long-term management and follow-up involved with the surgery should it be undertaken. Renal function can also be a very important factor, as patients with renal insufficiency will have much difficulty with metabolic acidosis. Lower urine output will create more problems with thick and viscous mucous, especially if large bowel is used. A patient with a noncompliant bladder needs to have this corrected. A leak point pressure greater than 40 cm of water is usually necessary to obtain continence in most patients.

1240-D *(Campbell's, pp. 2632–2633)*

By carefully selecting patients and assuring that there is a bladder of adequate capacity with low compliance as well as adequate urethral resistance, 90 per cent of previously wet patients can be made dry.

1241-E *(Campbell's, pp. 2634–2635)*

The bladder can be augmented with a wide variety of tissues, including ureter, ileum, cecum, colon, and stomach. Other techniques such as autoaugmentation performed by excising overlying detrusor muscle have also been used.

The principles to follow with bladder augmentation are that the segment of bowel should be long enough to adequately increase the bladder capacity, reflux should be corrected if present, and tissue should be handled with care. Most surgeons advocate the use of a midline incision. Whether the bladder should be opened in a clam shell manner and the bowel patch sewn onto this, or whether the entire supratrigonal bladder should be removed is controversial.

1242-C *(Campbell's, pp. 2636–2640)*

The hemi-Kock pouch is made of an ileal segment which is fashioned into a pouch. One of the ends is intussuscepted into the pouch to create an antirefluxing segment for the ureters to be implanted into. The Indiana pouch, MAINZ pouch, "LeBag," and Penn pouch all incorporate cecum and ileum.

1243-B *(Campbell's, pp. 2641–2643)*

When stomach is used for augmentation or for bladder substitution, one advantage is that it is easy to perform ureteral reimplantation due to the thick nature of the wall. It also is rarely exposed to radiation and is sometimes the only tissue that can safely be used in irradiated patients. As previously mentioned, it does not cause metabolic acidosis. However, a hyponatremic hypochloremic metabolic alkalosis can develop. There is also less mucous production. Cystitis can develop due to acid secretion. This can be treated with medications used to block acid secretion.

1244-A *(Campbell's, pp. 2643–2645)*

When bowel is used in the urinary tract to augment bladders or to create new bladders, there is always the risk of spontaneous bladder perforation. One of the series of patients reviewed by Rink showed 16 ruptures in 231 patients. This may be a difficult diagnosis to make. Nausea and vomiting are noted in 88 per cent, although only 50 per cent of patients have abdominal pain. Cystogram often does not identify the perforation and sometimes CT scan is necessary. It is associated with patients who wait for long intervals between catheterization and with noncompliant patients. It can be life-threatening and should be taken care of immediately. Malignancies have been seen in about 14 patients thus far. Yearly cystoscopy should begin after 10 years. Stones can form in the bladder due to poor emptying, frequent infection, and mucous. An annual KUB can help screen for these. There is no association with new onset of vesicoureteral reflux secondary to bladder augmentation.

1245-C *(Campbell's, p. 2645)*

Choice of a procedure or method to improve urethral resistance depends upon whether the patient can void normally or is dependent on CIC. Alpha-agonists will increase resistance of the bladder neck and beta-antagonists can potentiate alpha adrenergic effects. These are simple measures which could be tried prior to any invasive techniques. The Young-Dees-Leadbetter procedure involves tubularization of the bladder neck and trigone; a patient can still void normally against this increased resistance. Artificial urinary sphincter assumes that there is normal voiding pattern present, although it is possible to catheterize through this if it is necessary. The Kropp procedure involves lengthening of the urethra and reimplanting it through the trigone in a flap valve, and CIC is necessary postoperatively.

1246-D *(Campbell's, p. 2647)*

When patients undergo surgical reconstruction for incontinence, the primary objective is to have a compliant bladder. Patients with poorly compliant bladders will likely continue to leak and the increased resistance will place the upper tracts at risk of deterioration. Patients with small capacity bladders or with noncompliant bladders should undergo bladder augmentation in addition to urethral resistance procedures.

1247-A *(Campbell's, p. 2648)*

Entry into the bladder can facilitate greatly the dissection around the bladder neck and also in locating the ureteral orifices. It should be entered cephalad to where the cuff is to be placed. As long as there is sterile urine, routine prophylactic antibiotics are all that will be needed. A suprapubic tube for postoperative drainage would probably then be advisable.

1248-A *(Campbell's, p. 2648)*

Prepubertal males have very thin tissue in the immature bulbar urethra and the risk of cuff erosion is extremely high. Therefore, the urinary sphincter should be placed at the bladder neck in these individuals. None of the other choices are contraindications for placement in the bulbar urethra. Women obviously do not have a bulbar urethra.

1249-D *(Campbell's, p. 2650)*

Appearance of leakage in a patient who was previously dry with a functional artificial urinary sphincter should be assumed to be due to a change in bladder dynamics. Sphincter malfunction or cuff leak could also cause this. These patients should be evaluated in a timely fashion to avoid any upper tract damage.

1250-C *(Campbell's, p. 2650)*

Continence is achieved in up to 95 per cent of adults and children after placement of an artificial urinary sphincter. Mechanical malfunctions and surgical problems occur in 20 to 35 per cent of adults. Sphincter erosion or infection occurs in 8 to 13 per cent of adults but in 13 to 25 per cent of pediatric patients. Patients with a history of prior bladder neck or urethral surgery, particularly those with exstrophy or epispadias, have a higher risk of erosion. Reimplantation of a cuff at the site of a previous erosion has a very high chance of recurrent erosion. Sphincter revision is necessary in about 25 to 50 per cent of pediatric patients as well as adults; however, it is expected that almost all pediatric patients will ultimately require revision due to inadequate size as the patient grows. A secondary bladder augmentation is necessary in 30 per cent of the patients with neurogenic bladders who were not previously augmented. Hydronephrosis occasionally can develop due to a change in bladder physiology. This needs prompt evaluation.

1251-B *(Campbell's, pp. 2657–2658)*

Important principles for stoma creation should be followed in order to avoid stomal stenosis or parastomal hernias or infarction. A site should be chosen where there are no fat creases when the patient sits or stands. It should not be close to any other scars. It is usually brought out in either the right or the left lower quadrant of the abdomen, and always comes through the rectus muscle so as to avoid higher incidence of parastomal hernias. A long midline incision is usually created skirting the umbilicus of the side opposite the stoma site. The contralateral ureter is usually brought through the retroperitoneum below the inferior mesenteric artery.

1252-C *(Campbell's, pp. 2659–2661)*

It takes a fair amount of peristaltic power to move the urine through the rectus sheath and muscle and a dilated ureter is superior in performing this function. If both of the ureters are dilated then they should be brought out together as a double-barreled stoma site on the anterior abdominal wall. If only one of the ureters is dilated, then the normal ureter should be brought into the dilated ureter proximally and the dilated ureter should be brought out to the skin.

When performing the proximal transureteroureterostomy, the length of the spatulation and the incision on the receptive ureter should be around 2.5 to 3 cm. Every attempt should be made to avoid creating two separate stoma sites. There is a significant incidence of stomal stenosis (about 50 per cent) and this can be lessened by using the flap skin inserts in ureters that are not dilated.

1253-A *(Campbell's, p. 2661)*

Stomal stenosis occurs in as many as 50 per cent of cases as a late complication. The most common early complications are necrosis of the distal ureter and leakage from a TUU anastomosis.

Local revision of the stoma is usually insufficient to solve the problem. Converting to a intestinal conduit is the preferred method of therapy as the other procedures are usually inadequate.

1254-B *(Campbell's, p. 2663)*

Patients who have had extensive pelvic radiation will commonly have bowel with poor vascularity not suitable for conduit diversion. The rectum and sigmoid colon are always in the field of pelvic radiation. The ileum is also commonly affected. The jejunum and transverse colon are less commonly affected and would be the best choice for a conduit diversion. Stomach is always out of the field and would be an excellent choice for a continent diversion or a patch to be used for bladder augmentation in patients who have had radiation therapy. However, it has not been used for conduit diversion.

1255-D *(Campbell's, p. 2667)*

The Wallace technique involves spatulating the distal ends of both ureters and sewing to one another prior to directly anastomosing this to the open end of the ileal segment. The Bricker technique involves standard ureteroileal anastomosis with both of the ureters being individually anastomosed. The Deaver technique refers to windows constructed in the mesentery when taking down the intestinal loop. The Turnbull technique is used to create the stoma at the skin site, which can help in obese patients. The Leadbetter Politano ureteral reimplantation is a nonrefluxing anastomosis, which is not necessary in ileal conduit diversion.

1256-E *(Campbell's, p. 2669)*

The incidence of ureteroileal urine extravasation is around 1 to 3 per cent today. Prior to the use of stents the incidence was much higher, with more urinomas and the subsequent development of ureteroileal stenosis.

1257-B *(Campbell's, p. 2669)*

Ureterointestinal anastomotic strictures can occur at any time in the postoperative period. They are more common on the left due to the fact that it is necessary to free up a longer portion of the ureter from the blood supply and also because it is more likely to be angulated beneath the inferior mesenteric artery. They can be successfully managed with balloon dilatation and stenting for 6 to 8 weeks in 50 per cent of the cases. They commonly result from recurrence of malignancy, and this should always be ruled out.

1258-A *(Campbell's, p. 2670)*

A jejunal conduit might be utilized in cases where pelvic radiation has occurred. It would be best to use proximal ileum if possible. The most common complication is hyponatremic hypochloremic acidosis. At least half of the patients require sodium chloride replacement in the form of salt tablets due to the physiologic derangements. The length of the segment utilized should be as short as possible. Sometimes the stoma might need to be positioned above the umbilicus. The conduit is brought through a tunnel between the superior and inferior mesenteric arteries, the ureters anastomosed, and the conduit is brought to the skin in the usual manner. The other complications are not more common than with other bowel segments.

1259-C *(Campbell's, pp. 2671–2673)*

A tunneled nonrefluxing anastomosis is possible with the colon conduit due to a thicker more muscular wall of the bowel. Tunneled anastomoses should not be performed when the ureters are dilated, as this will usually result in worsening of hydronephrosis. Sigmoid conduits should be avoided when there has been pelvic radiation. It should also be avoided after cystectomies because of the compromise in blood supply that could occur due to injury to the internal pudendal artery. Location of the stoma is usually in the left lower quadrant. Stoma site usually is larger and a rosebud technique is performed. There is a higher incidence of ureterointestinal stenosis at 13 per cent due to the tunneling technique. There is also a higher incidence of parastomal herniation or stomal prolapse at 13 per cent and a lower incidence of stomal stenosis.

1260-A *(Campbell's, p. 2675)*

Ureterosigmoidostomy was first performed back in the 1870s. Although newer continent diversions are more commonly utilized, ureterosigmoidostomy may be a desirable procedure in some patients. Renal function should be evaluated, as patients with renal impairment are poor candidates. Patients with hepatic dysfunction are also poor candidates due to the possibility of ammonia intoxication. The bowel should be evaluated preoperatively for any sign of disease. It is mandatory that patients should have an adequate test of anal sphincter integrity, which if not intact would result in disastrous fecal and urinary incontinence. If they are able to retain an enema solution of 400 to 500 ml for an hour in the upright position, they have demonstrated integrity of the sphincter. Biopsy of the bowel would not be necessary unless abnormal findings were discovered during evaluation.

1261-E *(Campbell's, p. 2678)*

Hyperchloremic metabolic acidosis occurs in almost every patient with a rectal bladder. Many physicians will initiate bicarbonate replacement at the outset. Hypokalemia also occurs with ureterosigmoidostomy and therefore potassium citrate would be the best choice for long-term management. It is advisable to drain the urine with a rectal tube at night but many patients find this very inconvenient. If acidosis cannot be managed on oral medications, then nighttime drainage with a rectal tube is mandatory.

1262-D *(Campbell's, pp. 2679–2681)*

Because the risk of malignancy is increased by contact of the bowel with both urinary and fecal streams, multiple procedures have been devised to help prevent this. The rectal bladder is one procedure where the rectum is isolated from the fecal stream and closed off and used as a urinary reservoir. Various techniques have been developed to manage the proximal fecal stream. The Mauclaire technique involves a terminal sigmoid colostomy. More commonly, the bowel is brought down to the perineum through any of three techniques. The Gersuny technique involves bringing the sigmoidostomy anterior to the rectum and through the anal sphincter. The Duhamel technique involves bringing the sigmoidostomy posterior to the rectum yet through the anal sphincter. The Heitz-Boyer Hovelaque technique involves bringing the sigmoidostomy through the posterior wall of the rectum just under the rectal mucosa.

These procedures are not commonly used in the United States. Each of these procedures, where the sigmoid is brought down to the perineum, requires a second operation a week later after some healing has taken place to prevent the common complication of sigmoid retraction.

1263-C *(Campbell's, pp. 2682–2683)*

An augmented valved rectum is created by intussuscepting the proximal portion of the sigmoid colon. The ureters are then brought through the wall of the intussuscipiens. The main reason for augmenting the rectum is to decrease the surface area of the large bowel to which the urine is exposed and thereby decrease the electrolyte manifestations of a rectal bladder. A patch of small bowel is used to augment this. A hemi-Kock pouch can be fashioned to use as the augmented piece with the ureters brought in through the intussuscepted area of small bowel to obtain the same goals. Dilated ureters can be anastomosed into this form of diversion. It would also be hoped that reflux and infection would also be decreased as well.

1264-B *(Campbell's, p. 2685)*

Orthotopic diversions have a daytime continence rate of around 95 per cent. However, nocturnal enuresis is common because the bladder has been removed and the reflex arc which normally occurs with bladder filling and results in recruitment of external sphincteric contraction is lost. Therefore, patients are not able to supply voluntary conscious control when asleep and, since this reflex external sphincteric recruitment is not present after diversion, the patient will leak during sleep. Injury to external sphincter will result in both daytime and nighttime leakage. Injury to neurovascular bundle would not affect continence but would affect potency.

1265-B *(Campbell's, p. 2685)*

All orthotopic diversions carry the risk of the recurrence of cancer in the urethra. The risk of urethral recurrence is around 5 per cent in this group of patients. Certain patients have a higher risk: those who have invasion of the cancer into the prostatic urethra or involvement of the prostatic urethra with carcinoma in situ. In these patients, a urethrectomy would be advised and, therefore, they would not be candidates for an orthotopic diversion. Patients can be followed with urine cytologies or urethroscopy after orthotopic diversion to evaluate for urethral recurrence.

1266-A *(Campbell's, pp. 2686–2697)*

The LeBag pouch has overall lower continence rates than the other orthotopic continent diversions. Early on, this was due to incomplete detubularization; but even with complete detubularization, continence rates are still lower.

A LeBag pouch is created with a single segment of ileum along with the cecum. This is a modification of the Mainz pouch (created with the cecum and two segments of ileum). A sigmoid pouch is created by completely detubularizing the sigmoid colon and then closing it in a Heineke-Mikulicz maneuver. A Camey II is formed by a long loop of ileum which is folded over in a U-shaped fashion upon itself. The ileal neobladder utilizes about 70 cm of ileum, which is then folded in a W fashion with four loops. The hemi-Kock pouch is formed utilizing a long segment of ileum folded over upon itself in a U-shaped fashion with a proximal intussuscepted segment to prevent reflux.

1267-C *(Campbell's, p. 2692)*

The Studer pouch utilizes an intact proximal 25 centimeter ileal limb for prevention of deleterious effects of reflux. This is a very simple method to accomplish this and is confirmed to be effective with urodynamic radiographic studies.

1268-E *(Campbell's, pp. 2699–2700)*

The imbricated and tapered ileal segment, such as is used with the Indiana pouch, is simplest to catheterize from an orthotopic location. The Mitrofanoff principle involves a flap valve technique and can utilize either the appendix or ureter or tapered bowel. The nipple valve techniques are associated with the highest incidence of catheterization problems and they are not particularly adaptable to orthotopic locations. The Benchekroun nipple is created by using a reversed intussusception and utilizing the hydraulic valve technique, and has not been utilized in the orthotopic location to any great degree.

1269-D *(Campbell's, p. 2700)*

The intussuscepted nipple valve continence mechanism is technically the most difficult to construct. It has undergone many modifications since its development, primarily due to the disappointing long-term stability of the nipple valve mechanism. Failure rates of 10 to 15 per cent are seen under the best of circumstances. One of the major advances of construction has been to remove the mesenteric attachments on the 6 to 8 cm of bowel utilized. Attaching the nipple valve to the reservoir itself also is helpful in preventing failure. Because of the use of staples, however, stones may form. Continence rates have been similar to other continence mechanisms. There can be difficulty in catheterizing these, although that is not their major drawback.

1270-B *(Campbell's, p. 2707)*

The minimal nipple length required to maintain continence is 2.5 to 3 cm. Shortening can occur due to prolapse of the intussuscepted segment outward or due to ischemia of the segment. The repair can sometimes be accomplished by reintussuscepting the bowel, but occasionally an entirely new 15-cm segment of ileum must be used to create a new nipple valve. This is then spatulated and sewn onto the established pouch.

1271-A *(Campbell's, pp. 2702–2715)*

The Kock pouch is created with a 70- to 80-cm segment of ileum. The two 20-cm segments are opened and folded together in the shape of a U, leaving the two terminal 15-cm segments to intussuscept upon themselves. The MAINZ pouch utilizes the cecum and a 20-cm section of terminal ileum. The terminal ileum is intussuscepted upon itself and then this intussusception is brought through the intact ileocecal valve. The Duke pouch is created with cecum, ascending colon and distal ileum with the ileum intussuscepted to the ileocecal valve and then stabilized by suture rather than stapling. The Indiana pouch utilizes the entire right colon with a 10-cm segment of terminal ileum. The ileocecal valve is imbricated and the ileum is tapered to create the continence mechanism. The Penn pouch utilizes the cecum and a similar length of terminal ileum sutured to one another in a neotubularized fashion. The appendix is then utilized for the continence mechanism.

1272-E *(Campbell's, pp. 2702–2715)*

The Indiana pouch utilizes plication and imbrication of the terminal ileum as its continence mechanism. The other pouches utilize a nipple valve. The UCLA pouch is a variation of the MAINZ pouch, utilizing a nipple valve for the continence mechanism, and the LeBag also utilizes a nipple valve.

1273-C *(Campbell's, pp. 2700–2715)*

The failure rate of nipple valves is between 10 and 15 per cent. Techniques used to help prevent the nipple valve slipping include removing the mesenteric attachments from the 6 to 8 cm segment of bowel that will be intussuscepted upon itself, stapling or suturing the nipple valve to itself and also stapling or suturing the nipple valve to the reservoir, and placing an absorble mesh collar around the base of the nipple valve. Detubularization only decreases the pressure generated inside the reservoir, thereby creating a low pressure urinary storage system.

1274-A *(Campbell's, p. 2712)*

The Miami and Florida pouches differ from the Indiana pouch only in the manner in which the ileocecal valve is fashioned and in the fact that they both utilize a larger amount of colon in the construction of the reservoir.

1275-C *(Campbell's, p. 2721)*

Intermittent catheterization was widely popularized by Lapides in the 1970s. This has been the most important event making it possible to undivert previously diverted urinary tracts. This development has allowed new innovations in continent diversions and continence mechanisms in response to the growing need for better forms of diversion. Stapling devices certainly make some of the procedures easier but all the procedures can be done in a handsewn technique.

1276-D *(Campbell's, pp. 2722–2723)*

Any patient, regardless of age, should be considered a suitable candidate for undiversion. The length of time that the diversion has been present does not change this. Patients with renal insufficiency are also candidates, and many times a continent diversion can improve the quality of their life greatly. Oftentimes the urinary tract can be kept sterile and therefore urinary tract infections prevented, making them better candidates for transplantation. Previous pelvic radiation therapy would make the procedure more difficult and would limit the potential bowel segments utilized, but undiversion can still be performed in these cases. Negative psychosocial factors including immaturity, poor motivation, or inability to catheterize are very important in selecting candidates for undiversion, and any negative factors of this sort would be good reason to not undivert these patients.

1277-B *(Campbell's, p. 2724)*

There is no sure method available to predict how well a defunctionalized bladder will perform once it is incorporated back into the urinary tract. However, bladder cycling is the best method available. Bladder cycling is performed by serially increasing the amount of saline placed into the bladder as much as possible every day. Sometimes only a few days are needed, sometimes up to a month, depending on the response of the bladder and the cooperation of the patient. The bladder should not be overfilled as reportedly cases of rupture have occurred. Urodynamic studies are also crucial but have not been able to predict subsequent bladder function well. Cystoscopy and cystography can also yield helpful information.

1278-E *(Campbell's, p. 2724)*

When the patient has posterior urethral valves, they must be fulgurated to undivert him. If they are fulgurated prior to performing the undiversion and a dry urethra is present, then a dense stricture may develop in the urethra in the area where the valves were fulgurated. Therefore, it is important to have the patient using the urethra either by having him cycle the bladder after fulguration of the valves or to fulgurate the valves at the time of the undiversion.

1279-A *(Campbell's, pp. 2724–2725)*

When the ureter is mobilized, one should try to preserve all of the periureteral tissue including the gonadal vessels as they provide much needed collateral blood supply. They can be divided distally; it is rare to have a testis or ovary atrophy because of this. Ureteral blood supply is of paramount importance to ensure success of the ureteral anastomosis.

1280-D *(Campbell's, p. 2725)*

When reimplanting a ureter or tapered bowel segment, the tunnel length to ureter diameter ratio should be 5:1. This may make a very long tunnel necessary when a dilated ureter is present or when a bowel segment is reimplanted. A helpful technique to enable such a long tunnel would be to perform a psoas hitch. Tunnels up to 10 cm long can sometimes be created in this manner. A psoas hitch also prevents the ureter from angulating when the bladder is full. Nonabsorbable suture should be utilized to hitch the bladder to the psoas. Reimplantation should be performed prior to the psoas hitch.

1281-C *(Campbell's, p. 2725)*

Transureteroureterostomy or even transureteropyelostomy are very useful techniques when the bladder is not large enough to incorporate two long ureteral reimplants or when one of the ureters is short. It is often difficult to put two ureters into a bladder that has had multiple procedures performed on it and often these patients have diseased ureters, which may not be long enough to reach the bladder. If possible, both ureters should be reimplanted separately. Some of these patients may have had prior stone disease but there may be no other options to safely reconstruct their upper tracts. The better ureter is usually implanted and the diseased ureter should be brought over and anastomosed proximally into the better ureter over a 2- to 2.5-cm length.

1282-A *(Campbell's, p. 2729)*

When an ileal loop diversion has been performed previously, it is best to discard the bowel loop and not utilize it in the reconstruction. Reimplanting one or both ureters into the bladder is preferred. It is occasionally necessary to utilize it as a tapered segment as an extension of the ureters. Occasionally, it must be swung up near the renal pelvis and act as an ileal ureter.

1283-D *(Campbell's, pp. 2729–2731)*

When it is necessary to use the bowel segment as a substitute ureter, there are many important details which must be followed for a successful operation. The ileal loop must be mobilized very carefully from the abdominal wall. This can be facilitated by distending the loop with saline. It is sometimes necessary to incise the mesentery to straighten out the loop. A strip of bowel not more than one-third the circumference should be removed to taper the segment. An inverting closure should be performed. It is very important to create a non-refluxing anastomosis and this is possible even with bowel. A long tunnel sometimes is necessary as the diameters are often 1 to $1^1/_2$ cm. The anastomosis should lie posteriorly to help avoid fistula formation. A psoas hitch is essential to immobilize the hiatus of the bladder wall. This prevents the ileal ureter from angulating when the bladder fills. Late stricture is always a possibility with bowel used in the urinary tract. Therefore lifelong follow-up is very important with these patients.

1284-B *(Campbell's, pp. 2734–2736)*

Staples are commonly used to keep the intussuscepted segment of a nipple valve in position and also to fixate it to the wall of the diversion. Most of the time these will be covered up by mucosa; however, if they are still exposed, stones will form on them. These can become very large and difficult to remove. It is recommended that endoscopy be performed several months postoperatively and any exposed staples removed with alligator forceps. By removing some of the staples in the distal aspect of the intussuscepted nipple, this will ensure that the staples which are present will be mostly in a fold of the mucosa and therefore less likely to form stones.

1285-A *(Campbell's, pp. 2746–2747)*

In patients with very poor renal function, the electrolyte disturbances and metabolic derangements, which are associated with certain bowel segments, must be taken into consideration. Gastric mucosa secretes chloride and does not resorb any electrolytes to any significant degree. Because the pH of the urine is generally lower after stomach augmentation, there seem to be fewer urinary tract infections. Ureters are also easily implanted into the gastric wall. The stomach is very compliant as well. Sometimes patients may develop some cystitis due to the acidic nature of the secretions and this can be treated with H2 blockers.

1286-D *(Campbell's, p. 2750)*

Open bladder operations account for approximately 15 per cent of all urologic surgery. The most common is radical cystectomy for the treatment of invasive bladder cancer. Its rich blood supply allows the urinary bladder to be extensively mobilized and have the majority of that blood supply interrupted without major untoward effects on function or capacity.

Similar to elsewhere in the urinary tract, nonabsorbable suture material should never be used in the bladder because of the increased risk of stone formation or infection. Suprapubic tube drainage should be avoided in bladder cancer to prevent tumor implantation along the tube tract.

Recent cystectomy series report better survival results than the combined approach using radiation therapy followed by radical surgery. It appears that the survival benefit derived from preoperative irradiation is due to improvements in cystectomy techniques rather than to the combination of radiation and radical cystectomy.

REFERENCE

1. Freiha, F.S.: Treatment options for patients with invasive bladder cancer. Monogr. Urol., *11*:34–47, 1990.

1287-B, 1288-C *(Campbell's, p. 2755)*

During radical cystectomy, the internal iliac artery is identified beyond the common iliac bifurcation and followed toward the bladder. The first anterior branch is usually the superior vesical artery, which can be cross-clamped and tied at its origin. The obturator and other smaller arteries may arise from the internal iliac or from the superior vesical artery at this site. They can be cross-clamped and tied. The continuation of the internal iliac becomes the inferior vesical, which can be cross-clamped and tied beyond the origin of the superior vesical artery. Care must be taken to avoid tying the superior gluteal artery, which arises from the internal iliac close to the origin of the superior vesical and dips posterolaterally. Tying the superior gluteal may cause gluteal claudication.

REFERENCE

1. Skinner, D.G.: Cystectomy for bladder cancer. *In* Crawford, E.D., and Das, S. (Eds.): Current Genitourinary Cancer Surgery. Philadelphia, Lea & Febiger, 1990, pp. 235–246.

1289-D *(Campbell's, pp. 2757–2759)*

Control of the dorsal vein complex is the most critical step in radical cystectomy because the volume of lost blood is usually determined during this maneuver. Occasionally, while attempting to ligate the dorsal vein complex, excessive bleeding is encountered. A suture ligature of O chromic on a 5/8 needle placed as far distally as possible usually controls the bleeding. However, if bleeding continues, it is recommended to use blunt finger dissection to separate the membranous urethra from the anterior rectal wall, after which the dorsal vein complex and urethra are transected just distal to the apex of the prostate. The prostatic apex is then lifted superiorly, and a 24 French Foley catheter with a 30 ml balloon is inserted per urethra into the pelvic cavity; the balloon is inflated to 30 to 60 ml, and traction on the catheter is applied. Once the bladder and prostate are removed, better visualization of and access to the pelvis is possible.

1290-A *(Campbell's, pp. 2761–2762)*

Modern day anesthesia, complete and careful preoperative preparation, good surgical technique, and intensive postoperative care have significantly reduced the morbidity and mortality from radical cystectomy. Two major intraoperative complications are excessive blood loss and rectal injury. Autotransfusion and cell savers have reduced the need for donor blood. Rectal injuries are rare, and most are small and can be corrected with a two-layer closure followed by dilation of the anal sphincter. In patients with a history of radiation therapy to the pelvis, a temporary diverting colostomy is prudent.

Immediate postoperative complications include wound infection (most common), deep vein thrombosis, pulmonary embolus, pneumonia, and pelvic abscess. The mortality rate from cystectomy is low—2 per cent or less.

1291-C *(Campbell's, p. 2762)*

It has been suggested that repeated antibiotic bowel preparation within a two week period could result in an overgrowth of *Candida*, which could lead to sepsis and death after cystectomy. It is therefore recommended that when cystectomy is cancelled after the patient has already received an antibiotic bowel preparation, the operation should be delayed until the bowel recovers its normal flora, which takes at least 3 to 4 weeks. Alternatively, the second bowel preparation should be only mechanical (without oral antibiotics). In either case, the patient may benefit from preoperative oral antifungal agents.

1292-E *(Campbell's, p. 2762)*

The incision, exposure, timing, and extent of pelvic lymphadenectomy and the initial steps of the operation are the same as those described for radical cystectomy in the male.

The first structure encountered during incision of the lateral peritoneal reflection is the round ligament.

1293-B *(Campbell's, p. 2763)*

Following control of the lateral bladder pedicles bilaterally, a transverse incision is made in the posterior fornix of the vagina just above its junction with the rectum, thus entering the vaginal cavity. This maneuver is facilitated by upward retraction of the uterus and by a sponge on a sponge forceps placed into the vagina, all the way to the posterior fornix, and gently pushed cephalad. The sponge on a forceps in the vagina is of great help in dissecting and finding the vaginal vault and in preventing rectal and bladder injury. This is especially true in patients who have had a prior hysterectomy.

It is possible to perform a cystectomy without a vaginal approach; however, the risks of urethral tear and incomplete resection of the external urethral meatus are higher. The only possible advantage of avoiding the combined pelvic and vaginal approach is the diminished risk of contamination, and, therefore, infection.

1294-C *(Campbell's, p. 2765)*

The complications of radical cystectomy are similar for men and women (see the answer to question #1290). Complications specific to women include vaginal infections, prolonged vaginal drainage, vaginal bleeding from the suture line, vaginal contracture, and total loss of a functional vagina. Patients who develop vaginal contracture or shortening can be successfully managed with vaginal dilation. Reconstruction with skin grafts, flaps, or bowel segments is rarely needed.

1295-A *(Campbell's, pp. 2767–2768)*

Partial cystectomy, the resection of a segment of the bladder wall, is the ideal operation for localized benign lesions of the bladder that cannot be eliminated by transurethral resection alone, and for invasion of the bladder wall by tumors arising from adjacent organs such as the colon, cervix, uterus, and ovaries. The multicentric nature of transitional cell carcinoma makes the use of partial cystectomy for bladder cancer a controversial issue; however, the majority of partial cystectomies are being performed for invasive bladder cancer.

Partial cystectomy for invasive bladder cancer is an acceptable treatment option in patients with solitary tumors in the dome or posterior bladder wall who are elderly or who pose a significant surgical risk or in patients who refuse total cystectomy. Superficial transitional cell carcinoma in a bladder diverticulum that cannot be safely or completely resected transurethrally requires a partial cystectomy rather than a diverticulectomy alone. Patients with carcinoma in situ or mucosal dysplasia found on random biopsy samples should be advised against partial cystectomy.

The immediate complications of partial cystectomy are bleeding, extravasation, and infection. The late and more serious complications are a resultant small capacity bladder and pelvic and abdominal wall recurrences from tumor spillage. Treatment of small capacity bladders that are associated with very frequent voiding is augmentation cystoplasty.

1296-D *(Campbell's, pp. 2769–2770)*

Diverticula of the bladder are either congenital or secondary to bladder outlet obstruction. The majority do not require treatment; however, large diverticula that interfere with normal voiding or carry a large residual, which predisposes to recurrent infections or stone formation, require excision. As stated above, superficial transitional cell carcinoma in a bladder diverticulum that cannot be safely or completely resected transurethrally requires a partial cystectomy rather than a diverticulectomy alone. Treatment of bladder diverticula that are secondary to bladder outlet obstruction should always be preceded or accompanied by correcting the cause of the obstruction.

The major complication of bladder diverticulectomy is injury to the ureter, which can be avoided by catheterizing the ureter and freeing it up far away from the diverticulum before excising the latter. Bleeding and extravasation are uncommon.

1297-C, 1298-A, 1299-E *(Campbell's, pp. 2771–2773)*

Colovesical fistulas are the most common type of enterovesical fistula, and diverticular disease accounts for almost two thirds of the cases. Colon cancer causes about 20 per cent of colovesical fistulas and rare etiologies include Crohn's disease, radiation enteritis, trauma, bladder cancer, appendicitis, gynecologic tumors, tuberculosis, and actinomycosis.

The symptoms of enterovesical fistulas include urinary tract infection (95 per cent of patients), irritative voiding symptoms (up to 66 per cent), pneumaturia (63 per cent), fecaluria (43 per cent), and urine per rectum (<10 per cent).

A combination of procedures allows the diagnosis of enterovesical fistula and its underlying cause in the majority of cases. Intravenous urograms are not helpful. Cystograms allow diagnosis in only 34 per cent of cases, which is the same as that for barium enema studies. Computed tomography (CT) scans of the abdomen and pelvis have been the most accurate of all other imaging modalities. The typical CT findings in enterovesical fistulas are air in the bladder, focal bladder wall and bowel thickening and apposition, and extravesical soft tissue masses.

The accuracy of sigmoidoscopy or colonoscopy for diagnosis is only approximately 10 per cent; however, they are essential in every case of suspected colovesical fistula. Cystoscopy is much more accurate, showing changes suggestive of fistula in 77 per cent and allowing a definite diagnosis in 44 per cent of cases.

Once the diagnosis of fistula and its underlying causes are determined, a one-stage resection of the diseased organs and reparation of the fistula are the treatment of choice.

REFERENCES

1. Karamchandani, M.C., and West, C.F.: Vesicoenteric fistulas. Am. J. Surg., *147*:681, 1984.
2. Shatila, A.H., and Ackerman, N.B.: Diagnosis and management of colovesical fistulas. Surg. Gynecol. Obstet., *143*:71, 1976.

1300-E *(Campbell's, p. 2774)*

The indications for urethrectomy have been clarified. Previously, indications for urethrectomy included (1) multifocal tumors, (2) bladder neck tumors, (3) diffuse flat CIS, and (4) prostatic urethral involvement. Several studies have shown that the major risk factor for urethral recurrence following radical cystoprostatectomy is extension of tumor into the prostatic urethra, particularly when the tumor involves the prostatic stroma. In fact, prostatic urethral involvement appears to be the most compelling indication for simultaneous urethrectomy. Patients with multifocal tumors or CIS are candidates for orthotopic reconstruction of the bladder to the urethra, provided they are followed closely with urethral washing for cytology.

REFERENCE

1. Levinson, A.K., Johnson, D.E., and Wishnow, K.I.: Indications for urethrectomy in an era of continent urinary diversion. J. Urol., *144*:73, 1990.

1301-A *(Campbell's, p. 2778)*

The bulbomembranous urethra adjacent to the prostate is the segment of urethra most likely to be involved with recurrent tumor.

1302-A *(Campbell's, pp. 2782–2783)*

The pelvic diaphragm in the female consists of the levator ani and coccygeus muscle, which provide the major inferior support of the urethra, vagina, and rectum. The levator ani consists of the pubococcygeus, iliococcygeus, and ischiococcygeus muscles and as a unit pull the intrapelvic organs like a hammock. Fibers of the pubococcygeus muscles expand around the urethra and thus form its external sphincter components.

1303-E *(Campbell's, p. 2782)*

Several forces working in conjunction maintain normal continence in the female. These forces include the proper anatomic location of the sphincteric unit, the critical functional and anatomic urethral length, the coaptation of the urethral mucosal surface, and the increased urethral pressure generated by reflex pelvic contraction at the time of stress. Failure of one of the components of this delicate balance will not invariably produce stress incontinence because of the compensatory effect of the other components. On the other hand, urethral hypermobility contributes to the production of incontinence.

1304-B *(Campbell's, pp. 2783–2785)*

The urethropelvic ligaments provide the major support for the bladder neck and proximal urethra. This ligament is formed by the endopelvic fascia and fused to the periurethral fascia. The pubourethral ligament, also formed by the endopelvic fascia, supports and stabilizes the urethra and the anterior vaginal wall to the inferior aspect of the pubic bone; however, it does not contribute significant support to the bladder neck. The periurethral fascia is a fibrous structure that allows the attachment of the urethropelvic ligament to the tendinous part. The pubocervical fascia supports the bladder to the lateral pelvic wall superior to the levator plate. The cardinal ligament supports the uterus to the lateral pelvic wall and also facilitates the formation of cystoceles when they are lax.

1305-A *(Campbell's, p. 2787)*

The intrinsic urethral mechanism is a major contributor to the normal urinary continence mechanism. The layers of the urethra (which include the mucosa, submucosa, and smooth muscle) contribute individually to the continence mechanism. This mechanism is under hormonal control, and the lack of estrogen leads to atrophy of the mucosa and substitution of the vascular submucosa by fibrous tissue. Although commonly used, urethral pressure profilometry is nonspecific, poorly reproducible, and fraught with artifact.

1306-A *(Campbell's, pp. 2788–2789)*

A mixed type of stress urinary incontinence and urge incontinence is the most common type in incontinent females and constitutes roughly 55 per cent of the cases. Only 27 per cent of incontinent females exhibit a pure stress urinary incontinence profile. Several classification schemes of stress urinary incontinence have been described. The Raz classification divides stress incontinence into anatomic incontinence and intrinsic sphincter dysfunction incontinence based upon either the malposition of an intact sphincter unit versus malfunction of the sphincter with or without urethral hypermobility. Other classifications includes the McGuire and Blaivas types. Type III incontinence in the McGuire and Blaivas classifications correspond to intrinsic sphincter dysfunction incontinence in the Raz classification. Type I and type II stress incontinence in the McGuire classification demonstrate urethral closing pressures greater than 20 cm of water. Type I stress incontinence under the Blaivas classification occurs when the bladder neck and urethra open and descend less than 2 cm during stress with minimal or no cystocele. Anatomic incontinence accounts for roughly 90 to 95 per cent of stress urinary incontinence and results from the loss of pelvic support of the bladder and urethra. Intrinsic sphincter dysfunction results from damage to the sphincter through multiple prior operations, trauma, radiation, and neurogenic disorders.

1307-C *(Campbell's, pp. 2793–2794)*

Many treatment options for stress urinary incontinence are available. Conservative therapy is usually considered first line therapy. Kegel exercises exercise the pelvic musculature to improve urethral support and closure mechanisms, particular during stress maneuvers. Success rates with Kegel exercise vary depending upon the severity of incontinence. Biofeedback is a behavior modification technique designed to help patients gain sphincteric control as well as strengthening the pelvic floor and perineal muscles. Estrogen supplementation therapy improves the urethral sphincter mechanisms by stimulating the mucosal proliferation, improving mucosal coaptation, and enhancing urethral smooth muscle response to alpha-adrenergic stimulation. Estrogen supplements may be administered by mouth, dermal patch, injection, or vaginal cream. Alpha-adrenergic agonists such as phenylpropanolamine, ephedrine, and pseudoephedrine enhance urethral closure mechanisms by their direct action on the alpha receptors in the bladder neck. On the other hand, bladder relaxants such as anticholinergic medications, tricyclic antidepressants and prostaglandin inhibitors have no proven effectiveness in stress urinary incontinence and have no physiologic basis.

1308-E *(Campbell's, p. 2790)*

A change of the Q-tip angle of more than 35 degrees with straining indicates poor support of the bladder and urethra secondary to urethral hypermobility. The test is simple to administer but is very subjective and nonspecific with high false positive results.

1309-D *(Campbell's, p. 2791)*

A cystogram is an important adjuvant to the diagnostic evaluation for stress urinary incontinence. Anterior, posterior, oblique, and lateral views are obtained in an erect position in both a relaxing and a straining mode. Normally in a continent female, the bladder base is above the pubic ramus and pubic symphysis and usually will not descend more than 1 cm with stress maneuvers. A urethrotrigonal angle greater than 90 degrees on a true lateral view signifies funneling of the bladder neck. Funneling of the bladder neck is usually associated with anatomic stress incontinence. In patients with intrinsic sphincter dysfunction incontinence, the bladder neck is fixed and always open. Funneling of the bladder neck, however, is not pathognomonic for anatomic incontinence and can be found in patients with bladder instability, bladder fibrosis, and vaginal prolapse without incontinence. Urethral hypermobility can be demonstrated when the angle of inclination of the urethra to the vertical axis in an erect patient is greater than 35 degrees. Thus, the cystogram provides an excellent means to objectively assess anatomic defects.

1310-C *(Campbell's, p. 2795)*

The goal of surgery for anatomic incontinence is repositioning the bladder neck and the urethra to a high retropubic position. Various surgical approaches are available to perform this and include the Marshall-Marchetti-Krantz procedure, Burch colposuspension, Stamey needle suspension, Gittes needle suspension, Raz needle suspension, and Kelley plication. Periurethral collagen injection is utilized in the treatment of intrinsic sphincter dysfunction incontinence where the goal of surgery is coaptation, support, and compression of the damaged sphincteric unit.

1311-C *(Campbell's, pp. 2796–2797)*

The Marshall-Marchetti-Krantz procedure utilizes a retropubic approach to resuspend the urethra and bladder neck in a high retropubic position. Absorbable sutures are placed through the periurethral tissues and are anchored to the pubic bone. Because of the close proximity of the sutures to the urethra, postoperative urethral obstruction can be seen. Success rates with this procedure have been reported to be from 57 per cent to 95 per cent. However, a potential for osteitis pubis exists for this procedure. A concomitant cystocele cannot be simultaneously corrected when this procedure is performed. The Burch colposuspension utilizes absorbable sutures to anchor the perivaginal fascia and vaginal wall to Cooper's ligament.

1312-E *(Campbell's, pp. 2795–2797)*

The Burch colposuspension is another retropubic approach that allows reapproximation of the urethra and bladder neck in a high retropubic position and allows for correction of a concomitant cystocele. This procedure utilizes absorbable suture to tack the perivaginal fascia and vaginal wall to Cooper's ligament. The suspending sutures are placed laterally and thus the potential for urethral obstruction postoperatively is minimized. The anterior colporraphy or Kelly plication is used to treat cystoceles, and does not elevate the bladder neck and urethra in a high retropubic position. The Stamey and Gittes needle suspension and the Marshall-Marchetti-Krantz procedure correct the urethral and bladder neck hypermobility but do not correct a concomitant cystocele.

1313-D *(Campbell's, pp. 2798–2799)*

The Raz transvaginal needle suspension procedure is chosen for patients with anatomic stress incontinence due to urethral and bladder neck hypermobility with minimal or no cystocele. The procedure requires an incision in the anterior vaginal wall and detachment of the urethropelvic ligament from its attachment to the lateral pelvic wall in order to enter the retropubic space. The suspension sutures, which are of the nonabsorbable type, incorporate the urethropelvic ligaments, pubocervical fascia, and anterior vaginal wall and are anchored to the rectus fascia. Cystoscopy is performed during this procedure to rule out bladder and/or ureteral injury. Success rates for this procedure approach 94 per cent.

1314-A *(Campbell's, pp. 2801, 2804–2806)*

In the presence of intrinsic sphincter dysfunction, simple suspension of the bladder neck is unlikely to correct the problem, and urethral compression becomes necessary to achieve continence. Numerous techniques are available to achieve this and include: periurethral injection of fat, Teflon, or collagen; urethral slings including vaginal wall, rectus fascia, fascia lata, and synthetic materials; and artificial urinary sphincters. The four-corner bladder and bladder neck suspension procedure is a modification of the Raz transvaginal needle suspension operation and allows for the repositioning of the bladder neck in a high retropubic position and repairs moderate anterior vaginal wall prolapse with correction of cystoceles concomitantly.

1315-C *(Campbell's, p. 2806)*

Excessive bleeding intraoperatively can be controlled with packing of the retropubic space or with intravaginal inflation of the Foley catheter with approximately 50 to 60 ml of fluid. Since the vagina is a potentially contaminated space, perioperative antibiotic coverage is recommended for vaginal surgical procedures. The most common type of infection associated with vaginal surgery is a urinary tract infection. Injuries to the ureter include partial or complete tears and ligature of the ureter with suture or surgical clips. A partial ureteral tear is best treated with internal drainage, utilizing indwelling stents, or percutaneous methods, whereas a complete tear is best managed by primary repair. Urinary retention may be due to postoperative edema in the bladder or urethra, denervation, or a misplaced suture. Patients can be taught intermittent self catheterization if this problem persists postoperatively. Vaginal stenosis, which can be the cause of postoperative dyspareunia, is best prevented by avoiding excessive excision of the vaginal wall. Other complications of vaginal surgery include incontinence, postoperative pain, vaginal shortness, and nerve injury.

1316-C *(Campbell's, pp. 2807–2809)*

Rectoceles and perineal body laxity result from weakening of musculofascial support including the levator ani muscle complex and the pre- and pararectal fascia. The transvaginal approach can be used to repair the rectocele by reapproximating the prerectal and pararectal fascia in the midline over the rectocele and including the pubococcygeus muscle at the mid to distal third of the vaginal canal. The perineal laxity is corrected by reapproximating the deep and superficial transverse perineal muscles, bulbocavernosus muscle and levator ani complex with absorbable sutures in a horizontal mattress fashion. Rectal injury is a potential complication of this procedure and thus preoperative enemas and the use of a Deaver or Heaney retractor are recommended with this procedure.

1317-E *(Campbell's, pp. 2815–2816)*

In addition to a thorough history and physical examination, diagnostic studies are used to diagnose a urethral diverticulum. Urethroscopy with a zero degree lens may allow visualization of the orifice of a urethral diverticulum since the entire urethral lumen can be distended with constant water flow and bladder neck compression. The postvoid film of an intravenous urogram can also reveal a collection of contrast material in a urethral diverticulum. A VCUG study may delineate irregularity of the urethra suggestive of a urethral diverticulum. Positive pressure urethrography utilizing a Davis-Telinde or Trattner catheter can outline the sac of the diverticulum with the double balloon method. Other studies useful in the diagnosis of female urethral diverticula include pelvic ultrasound and urethral pressure profilometry. A cystometrogram is not usually included in the diagnostic work-up of a urethral diverticula.

1318-B *(Campbell's, pp. 2814–2815)*

The incidence of urethral diverticulum is between 1 and 6 per cent of all adult females. A racial prediliction is noted, with blacks affected in a ratio of 3.5 to 6:1 compared to whites. The average age at the time of diagnosis is approximately 40 years. Urethral diverticula can be either congenital or acquired. The majority of urethral diverticula are acquired and these are secondary to infections, parturition, iatrogenic injuries, urethral calculus, or a neurogenic bladder with high intravesical pressures on voiding. Congenital factors include Gardner's duct, ruptured vaginal cyst into the urethra, and nonunion of wolffian ducts. Up to 90 per cent of diverticula open into the mid or distal urethra. Although irritative voiding symptoms and hematuria occur in the majority of cases, the complaint most characteristic of urethral diverticulum is post micturition dribbling.

1319-D *(Campbell's, pp. 2817–2819)*

Recurrent urinary tract infections, severe pain, dyspareunia, frequency, urgency, and significant post-void dribbling are indications for surgical intervention in patients with a urethral diverticulum. Various methods are available to correct a urethral diverticulum and include a transvaginal excision technique. Endoscopic urethrotomy can also be performed to split the floor of the urethra from the meatus proximally to the diverticulum's orifice. Spence and Duckett have utilized marsupialization of the diverticulum to prevent recurrence, minimize operating time, and reduce blood loss. This technique is useful for diverticula in the distal one third of the urethra away from the intrinsic and external sphincter regions. Suprapubic catheter drainage may be an adjuvant to the other techniques; however, by itself it does not adequately treat a urethral diverticulum.

1320-A *(Campbell's, p. 2821)*

The most common cause of vesicovaginal fistula is gynecologic surgery, specifically hysterectomy. Other causes include obstetric trauma, radiation therapy, urologic surgery, and gastrointestinal surgery. Factors that predispose patients to the development of vesicovaginal fistulas include infection, ischemia, arteriosclerosis, diabetes mellitus, pelvic inflammatory disease, and tumor.

1321-A *(Campbell's, pp. 2820–2825)*

Total incontinence is characteristic of vesicovaginal fistulas. Cystoscopy, vaginoscopy, intravenous urography, retrograde pyelography, and VCUG are used to diagnose a vesicovaginal fistula. An initial trial of conservative therapy with bladder drainage is usually attempted first; however, surgical intervention is usually required. Estrogen replacement therapy is recommended since it results in improved vascular supply to the vaginal walls and improved turgor and thus may help in postoperative wound healing. Usually, a waiting period of 3 to 6 months is recommended prior to the actual surgical repair to allow inflammatory reactions to subside. However, with radiation therapy induced fistulas, a waiting period of 12 months is recommended prior to an attempt at surgical repair. Various approaches, either abdominal or vaginal, are available to repair a vesicovaginal fistula; however, basic principles such as the use of a layered closure with avoidance of overlapping suture lines and continuous uninterrupted postoperative urinary drainage are critical to prevent extravasation and distention with breakdown of suture lines. The closure can be reinforced with a Martius flap, myocutaneous gracilis muscle flap, peritoneal flaps, or rotational flaps of the entire labia and or gluteal skin.

1322-C *(Campbell's, pp. 2829–2830)*

Stress urinary incontinence is the most common cause of involuntary loss of urine in women. When carefully questioned, up to 50 per cent of normal nulliparous women will occasionally experience some stress urinary incontinence; however, this does not occur to a bothersome degree. A more exact definition for stress urinary incontinence would be the involuntary loss of urine through a normal urethra, caused by an increase in intra-abdominal pressure, which is of enough quantity to be socially embarrassing. Incontinence does not ordinarily accompany cystitis, although urgency can often be related to it. The other causes of incontinence are much less common. Stress urinary incontinence, nonobstructive detrusor instability, and women who lose urine but have no findings of stress incontinence or detrusor instability account for 95 per cent of cases of incontinence in women.

1323-D *(Campbell's, p. 2830)*

One third to two thirds of patients with surgically correctable stress incontinence will also have urgency incontinence. This should not be a contraindication to surgery, as most often both forms of incontinence are cured by elevation of the vesical neck. It is postulated that the urgency results as the urine flows into the proximal urethra as the bladder fills, causing an uncontrollable desire to urinate. When the bladder neck has fallen into a dependent position, this occurs much earlier than normal. Urgency incontinence may persist in the postoperative period, as well as occurring postoperatively in patients who did not have it preoperatively. This resolves in the majority of cases within a 6-month period of time. Some patients do have some long-standing urgency incontinence, and this can be controlled with anticholinergics, but this is not the majority of patients. In fact, Stamey had 2 out of 44 patients who had long-term urgency incontinence. Patients who have urgency preoperatively are more likely to have the sensation of urgency postoperatively and this is especially true in patients who are over the age of 65.

1324-B *(Campbell's, pp. 2832–2833)*

The demonstration of urinary incontinence when the patient has a full bladder is critical to the selection of surgical candidates. This can easily be done by having the patient cough while in the lithotomy position. Around 80 per cent of patients amenable to surgery will leak urine in this manner. Sometimes it is necessary to tilt them up into a 45 degree position, and another 10 per cent will leak at that time. The remaining 10 per cent can only be made to leak in the standing position. Stamey believes this simple test should be all that is necessary to diagnose surgically correctable incontinence. Other studies such as cystoscopy, cystometrograms, or radiologic studies should only be necessary in cases that are not straightforward. A positive Q-tip test demonstrates urethral hypermobility and a positive Bonney test demonstrates that with elevation of the bladder neck the leakage is prevented (this is the same as the Marshall-Marchetti test).

1325-E *(Campbell's, p. 2833)*

Trigonitis has in the past been the term used for the cystoscopic findings of a cobblestone or furry-appearing trigone in many women. These are actually just congenital inclusions of normal vaginal epithelium within the bladder which occurs in all women. Therefore, it does not exist as a pathologic entity. Urethritis cannot be diagnosed cystoscopically. Presence of urethral polyps are secondary to chronic bacteriuria and usually they go away when the urine is sterilized and no further infections occur.

1326-E *(Campbell's, pp. 2834–2835)*

Radiologic evaluation of stress urinary incontinence has greatly contributed to the understanding of surgically curable incontinence in females. However, it is rarely necessary to perform these studies except in complicated cases or to evaluate the efficacy of therapy.

A normal lateral cystogram is performed with the patient straining. Findings in a normal patient would include a high position of the urethrovesical junction behind the symphysis pubis, a flat and posteriorly directed base of the bladder, and a slightly posterior direction of the proximal urethra with a 90-degree posterior urethrovesical angle. It is not a voiding study, and therefore complete emptying is not necessary for a normal study.

1327-B *(Campbell's, p. 2835)*

The normal urethrovesical junction should be several centimeters above a line between the bottom of the sacrum and the bottom of the pubis. A endoscopic suspension of the vesical neck results in an average elevation of 5.5 cm. A Kelly plication only produces an elevation at most 1 cm. Therefore, the Kelly plication is an inadequate procedure except in cases of only minor incontinence. It is not recommended as an incontinence procedure in women.

1328-B *(Campbell's, pp. 2839–2841)*

The Stamey endoscopic vesical neck suspension has a high cure rate in patients with stress urinary continence. Because one third to two thirds of patients with stress urinary incontinence will also have a component of urgency incontinence, which resolves after vesical neck suspension, these patients are also good candidates for the Stamey suspension. Patients who have an acontractile bladder yet also stress urinary incontinence are candidates for vesical neck suspension as long as they understand that they will require intermittent catheterization the rest of their lives. Patients with an incompetent urethra or a "stove pipe" urethra are also candidates for the Stamey vesical neck suspension. The Dacron buttresses compress the urethra, resulting in a fairly good cure rate even for patients with an incompetent urethra. In patients who have pure urgency incontinence, it is contraindicated to do a vesical neck suspension as they will all continue to have incontinence and urethral obstruction can worsen the urgency incontinence.

1329-C *(Campbell's, pp. 2839–2840)*

Filling cystometry, flow studies, and urethral closure pressure measurements are generally not useful in the evaluation of patients with stress urinary incontinence. Patients with non-stress urinary incontinence have a higher maximum detrusor pressure during voiding when compared to patients with stress urinary incontinence. Unstable non-stress urinary incontinence patients void at slower flow rates than unstable stress urinary incontinence patients. These facts are compatible with the lower urethral resistance that is present in women with stress urinary incontinence, and therefore there is a smaller maximal detrusor pressure necessary to get the urine out and also a faster urinary flow rate due to less resistance in the urethra. Women who have stress urinary incontinence have lower maximal urethral closure pressures compared to healthy controls.

Urethral closure pressure declines dramatically with age. Anterior and posterior urethral closure pressures are about equal in normal patients and also in incontinent patients without stress urinary incontinence. Stress urinary incontinence patients have significantly decreased closure pressures in the posterior urethra compared to the anterior urethra. When the vesical neck is suspended, the posterior urethral closure pressure is doubled, making it equal to the anterior closure pressure.

1330-A *(Campbell's, p. 2843)*

The pubocervical fascia is the layer which forms the bulk of the suspending tissue. This is sometimes referred to as periurethral fascia and extends from the pubis to the cervix.

1331-D *(Campbell's, pp. 2843–2846)*

The Stamey needles should be passed through small suprapubic incisions, through the rectus fascia just posterior to and hugging the pubis. They should be just lateral to the urethrovesical junction. This can be assured by performing cystoscopy and gently moving the needle medially. This will result in an indentation in the urethral wall at the vesical neck. If the needle is passed through the wall of the urethra or into the bladder, it should be withdrawn and repositioned.

1332-D *(Campbell's, p. 2847)*

The suprapubic suspending sutures should be gently lifted and then tied under no tension. The bladder can be filled and you can test continence by applying suprapubic pressure with the suspending loops lifted gently. The bladder neck is seen visually to be narrowed after the sutures have been properly tied; however, the key is to tie them with no tension. Vaginal mucosa should be closed before tying the sutures as when the vesical neck is lifted, this incision is very difficult to expose to properly close. The average distance that the vesical neck is suspended is 5.5 cm; however, this should not guide the tying of the sutures.

1333-B *(Campbell's, pp. 2847–2849)*

Postoperatively, the patient should either have a suprapubic tube in place or be sent home on intermittent catheterization. They should wait for a strong urgency to void prior to initiating spontaneous voiding. Very few of these patients can void by the second to third postoperative day. Half of the patients are usually able to void by the seventh postoperative day and the suprapubic tube can be removed. In around 7 per cent of patients, more than 30 days were required before satisfactory voiding was achieved. In 1 to 2 per cent of patients, one of the sutures must be removed due to pain or infection. When these are removed for infection, the Dacron buttress should be removed as well as the suture. Removal of the suture can oftentimes be done under local anesthesia in the office. Success rate for the Stamey vesical neck suspension is around 91 per cent. The procedure can be performed more than once in a patient, and when a reoperation is done, the old

Dacron buttress should be left in place, and it will act as a reinforcement of the tissues.

1334-A *(Campbell's, pp. 2851)*

The contraindications for an open simple prostatectomy include a small, fibrous gland; carcinoma of the prostate; and prior prostatectomy in which most of the gland has previously been resected or removed and in which the planes are obliterated.

Over 90 per cent of the prostatectomies for benign hyperplasia are performed by transurethral resection of the prostate (TURP). When the obstructive tissue is estimated to weigh more than 50 g, consideration should be given to an open (suprapubic or retropubic) procedure. A smaller gland may, however, be best managed by open prostatectomy if one or more of the following conditions exist: large diverticula of the bladder that justify removal; large bladder calculi which are not amenable to fragmentation; coexisting urethral disease precluding simple transurethral instrumentation; or ankylosis of the hip preventing proper positioning for transurethral resection. Renal failure is not a contraindication for open prostatectomy; however, if the patient presents with urinary retention and an elevated serum creatinine level, one should delay surgery until renal function has stabilized.

1335-B *(Campbell's, pp. 2851–2852)*

Imaging of the prostate by transrectal ultrasound or magnetic resonance imaging may aid in assessing prostate size and possible lesions; however, it is not indicated in the evaluation of all patients who are to undergo open prostatectomy.

Cystoscopy should be performed on all patients to rule out unsuspected bladder tumor, bladder stone, or large diverticulum. In most cases, this can be delayed until the patient is under anesthesia just prior to surgery. The upper urinary tract should be evaluated to provide a baseline examination and to identify any lesions or unusually anatomic variations. Sonography of the upper urinary tract provides an excellent screening method for hydronephrosis and other suspected masses. An enema given the night prior to surgery reduces the morbidity associated with the rare occurrence of rectal injury. The transfusion of blood is required in approximately 15 per cent of patients who are undergoing open prostatectomy and the safest transfusion is autologous blood.

1336-D *(Campbell's, pp. 2852–2856)*

Following removal of the prostatic adenoma by the suprapubic route, bleeding frequently occurs in the 5 and 7 o'clock positions. The prostatic arteries enter the capsule and prostate at this level near the bladder neck. Suture ligature of these vessels is done even if there is no active bleeding.

The procedure does not involve total removal of the prostate because a tissue plane exists between the adenoma and the compressed true prostate, which is left intact. Vasectomy, which had previously been recommended in all prostatectomies to prevent postoperative epididymitis, is no longer routinely performed as this complication is now less commonly encountered. After the plane between the adenoma and the capsule of the prostate is developed, most of the remainder of the procedure is done bluntly by digital dissection. The urethra is firmly attached at the apex, however, and it is preferable to use scissors to sharply incise the urethra at this point. Traction should only be applied to the urethral foley when postoperative bleeding is excessive.

1337-D *(Campbell's, p. 2856)*

Excessive blood loss is the most common immediate complication encountered with suprapubic prostatectomy. Approximately 15 per cent of patients require blood transfusions. Point fulguration of bleeders in the fossa may provide hemostasis. Other methods described to control excessive bleeding intraoperatively include placement of a nylon purse-string suture around the vesicle neck, and plication of the posterior prostatic capsule.

Delayed bleeding, urethral stricture, and bladder neck contracture are all more commonly seen following TURP. Retrograde ejaculation is common following both TURP and suprapubic prostatectomy.

REFERENCES

1. Malament, M.: Maximal hemostasis in suprapubic prostatectomy. Surg. Gynecol. Obstet., *120*:1307, 1965.
2. O'Connor, V.J. Jr.: An aid for hemostasis in open prostatectomy: Capsular plication. J. Urol., *127*:448, 1982.

1338-B *(Campbell's, pp. 2852–2857)*

The retropubic approach offers a more anatomic exposure of the prostate compared to the more blind suprapubic approach. The urethra can be divided more accurately, reducing the risk of incontinence. The better visualization of the interior of the prostatic cavity allows for easier detection of residual adenoma and bleeding points.

1339-C *(Campbell's, pp. 2856–2863)*

After the dorsal vein complex and lateral pedicles have been ligated, a *transverse* capsulotomy is made 1.5 to 2 cm distal to the bladder neck. Although a longitudinal incision may have some advantages, it may extend through the prostatourethral juncture during enucleation, leaving the patient incontinent postoperatively. This dire complication does not occur with a transverse incision.

1340-A *(Campbell's, p. 2863)*

Retrograde ejaculation occurs in most but not all patients postoperatively and they should be informed of this possibility prior to surgery. The patients should also be informed of the possibility of impotence, which may affect 15 to 20 per cent. With improved understanding of the etiology of impotence following radical prostatectomy, it is hoped that impotence will result less commonly.

With control of the dorsal vein complex and lateral pedicles excessive postoperative bleeding should occur infrequently. Postoperative epididymitis is uncommon, but is seen more frequently in patients who have had long-term indwelling catheters for urinary retention. This complication can largely be avoided by prophylactic vasectomy at the time of surgery in these patients. Bladder neck contractures occur late in approximately 2 per cent of patients.

1341-C *(Campbell's, pp. 2865–2866)*

The prostate receives its arterial blood supply from the inferior vesical artery, which terminates in two large groups of prostatic vessels: the urethral and capsular groups. The urethral vessels enter the prostate at the posterolateral vesicoprostatic junction, providing arterial supply to the vesical neck and the periurethral portion of the gland. The capsular branches run along the pelvic sidewall in the lateral pelvic fascia and supply the outer portion of the prostate. The capsular vessels, both arteries and veins, provide the microscopic landmark that aids in the identification of the microscopic branches of the pelvic plexus that innervate the corpora cavernosi. The venous drainage of the prostate is into the Santorini plexus.

REFERENCES

1. Reiner, W.G., and Walsh, P.C.: An anatomical approach to the surgical management of the dorsal vein and Santorini's plexus during radical retropubic surgery. J. Urol., *121*:198–200, 1979.
2. Walsh, P.C., and Donker, P.J.: Impotence following radical prostatectomy: Insight into etiology and prevention. J. Urol., *128*:492, 1982.

1342-C *(Campbell's, p. 2867)*

The autonomic innervation of the pelvic organs and external genitalia arises from the pelvic plexus, which is formed by parasympathetic visceral efferent preganglionic fibers that arise from the sacral center (S2 to S4) and sympathetic fibers from the thoracolumbar center (T11 to L2). In humans, the pelvic plexus is located retroperitoneally beside the rectum, 5 to 11 cm from the anal verge, with its midpoint located at the level of the tip of the seminal vesicle.

REFERENCE

1. Schlegel, P., and Walsh, P.C.: Neuroanatomical approach to radical cystoprostatectomy with preservation of sexual function. J. Urol., *138*:1402, 1987.

1343-D *(Campbell's, pp. 2867–2869)*

The branches of the inferior vesical artery and vein that supply the bladder and prostate perforate the pelvic plexus. For this reason, ligation of the so-called lateral pedicle in its midportion not only interrupts the vessels but also transects the nerve supply to the prostate, urethra, and corpora converse.

The prostate is covered with two distinct and separate fascial layers: Denonvilliers' fascia and lateral pelvic fascia, also called prostatic fascia. Denonvilliers' fascia is located between the anterior wall of the rectum and the prostate. Microscopically, it is impossible to discern a "posterior" and an "anterior" layer to this fascia, therefore, to obtain an adequate surgical margin, one must excise this fascia completely.

Oelrich has demonstrated that the striated urethral sphincter with its surrounding fascia is a vertically oriented tubular sheath and not a pair of transverse planes. The external striated sphincter is more tubular and has broad attachments over the fascia of the prostate near the apex.

As stated above, the venous drainage of the prostate is into the Santorini plexus.

REFERENCES

1. Jewett, H.J., Eggleston, J.C., and Yawn, D.H.: Radical prostatectomy in the management of carcinoma of the prostate. Probable causes of some therapeutic failures. J. Urol., *107*:1034, 1972.
2. Oelrich, T.M.: The urethral sphincter muscle in the male. Am. J. Anat., *158*:229, 1980.

1344-E *(Campbell's, p. 2869)*

Surgery is deferred for 6 to 8 weeks following needle biopsy of the prostate and 12 weeks following transurethral resection of the prostate. These delays enable inflammatory adhesions or hematomas to resolve so that the anatomic relationships between the prostate and the surrounding structures are returned to a more normal state prior to surgery. This is especially important if one hopes to preserve the neurovascular bundles intraoperatively and to avoid rectal injury. During this waiting period, patients should be offered the opportunity to donate 3 units of blood for autotransfusion.

1345-B *(Campbell's, pp. 2869–2870)*

A spinal or epidural anesthetic seems to be associated with less blood loss and a lower frequency of pulmonary emboli.

Previously, when the vas deferens was routinely divided, some men complained of persistent testicular pain. If the vas deferens is not divided, the traction on the spermatic cord is absorbed by the vas deferens and persistent testalgia is rare. The lymphadenectomy is considered a staging and not a therapeutic procedure. The dissection is initiated along the external iliac vein on the same side as the most prominent clinical induration in the prostate. The lymphatics overlying the external iliac artery are preserved. The dissection proceeds inferiorly to the femoral canal where care is taken to ligate the lymphatic channels at the node of Cloquet. The medial extent of dissection is the obturator fossa and lymph nodes and the superior extent is usually the bifurcation of the common iliac artery.

REFERENCE

1. Peters, C., and Walsh, P.C.: Blood transfusion and anesthetic practice in radical retropubic prostatectomy. J. Urol., *134*:81, 1985.

1346-E *(Campbell's, p. 2871)*

The endopelvic fascia is entered where it reflects over the pelvic sidewall, well away from its attachments to the bladder and prostate. At the point where the fascia is incised, it is often transparent and reveals underlying levator ani musculature. The lateral venous plexuses traverse adjacent to the prostate and the lower portion of the bladder. Therefore, an incision in the endopelvic fascia too close to the bladder or prostate risks laceration of these structures with potential severe blood loss.

1347-A *(Campbell's, p. 2874)*

After the puboprostatic ligaments have been transected and the dorsal vein complex has been controlled and divided, the planes between the smooth musculature of the urethra and the striated sphincter is developed with sharp dissection. Umbilical tape is passed around the urethra. Care must be taken to avoid excessive traction on the urethra, which might disrupt the attachment of its smooth musculature to the striated sphincter and result in the delay of the return of urinary control.

1348-C *(Campbell's, pp. 2874–2875)*

When viewed laterally, this complex attaches to the apex of the prostate and Denonvillier's fascia. This entire complex is part of the extensive skeletal muscle sleeve of the external sphincter that attaches to the apex of the prostate.

Identification and precise division of this complex are most important in (1) obtaining adequate margins of resection for apical lesions, (2) identifying the correct plane on the anterior wall of the rectum to ensure that all layers of Denonvillier's fascia are excised, (3) avoiding blunt trauma to the neurovascular bundles, and (4) preserving urinary continence.

1349-D *(Campbell's, pp. 2876–2878)*

Under certain circumstances, it may be necessary to excise the lateral pelvic fascia and neurovascular bundles completely on one or both sides. These situations include (1) surgery on an impotent patient, (2) induration involving the lateral sulcus found either on preoperative physical examination or intraoperatively after opening the endopelvic fascia, and (3) fixation of the neurovascular bundle to the capsule of the prostate detected once the lateral pelvic fascia has been divided.

REFERENCES

1. Hatcher, P.A., and Oesterling, J.E.: Nerve-sparing procedures in urologic cancer surgery: Am. Overview. AVA Update Series. Vol. 12, Lesson 12, 1993.
2. Andriole, G.L.: Nerve Sparing Radical Retropubic Prostatectomy: Patient Selection and Techniques. AVA Update Series. Vol. 12, Lesson 13, 1993.

1350-A, 1351-C *(Campbell's, pp. 2882–2883)*

Radical retropubic prostatectomy is a procedure that is well tolerated with minimal morbidity and low mortality (0 to 1.7 per cent). The most common intraoperative problem during this procedure is hemorrhage, usually arising from the venous structures. Less common complications include obturator nerve injury (which should be repaired with very fine nonabsorbable sutures), ureteral injury (which should be repaired with ureteral reimplantation), and rectal injury.

Rectal injury is rare (1 to 9 per cent of cases), and usually occurs during apical dissection, when attempting to develop the plane between the rectum and Denonvillier's fascia. If a rectal injury occurs, the prostatectomy should be completed, the bladder neck should be reconstructed, and the sutures should be placed in the urethra. Before placing sutures through the bladder neck, the rectum should be closed in 2 layers after the anal sphincter has been dilated widely by an assistant. Interposition of omentum between the rectal closure and the vesicourethral anastomosis may reduce the possibility of a vesicourethral fistula. The wound should be irrigated with antibiotic solution, and the patient should be maintained on broad-spectrum antibiotics for both aerobic and anaerobic bacteria. If a patient has received prior radiotherapy, it would be prudent to perform a diverting colostomy.

REFERENCE

1. Borland, R.N., and Walsh, P.C.: Management of rectal injury during radical retropubic prostatectomy. J. Urol., *147*:905, 1992.

1352-B *(Campbell's, p. 2883)*

Thrombophlebitis and pulmonary embolism are two of the most common and potentially serious complications of radical retropubic prostatectomy, being noted in 3 to 12 per cent and 2 to 5 per cent, respectively. Recommended prophylactic measures have included intermittent compression devices on the lower extremities, minidose heparin, epidural anesthesia during surgery, and early postoperative ambulation.

1353-C *(Campbell's, p. 2883)*

Disruption of the urethrovesical anastomosis can lead to permanent incontinence. The catheter should be taped carefully to the thigh. The anchorage of the catheter should be examined each postoperative day. If the catheter comes out prematurely, one attempt to pass a smaller caliber catheter into the bladder should be made. If this is not successful on the first attempt, the patient should undergo cystoscopy and the catheter placed under direct vision.

1354-D *(Campbell's, p. 2883)*

Contracture of the bladder neck has been reported to occur in 3 to 12 per cent of cases, and it is usually caused by poor mucosa-to-mucosa apposition of the bladder to the urethra at the time of anastomosis. It can, however, also be caused by overzealous reconstruction of the bladder neck. The mucosal advancement procedure in reconstruction of the bladder neck had morbidly reduced this complication.

Bladder neck contractures usually respond to one or two dilations. If this fails, cold knife incision of the bladder neck at 12 o'clock usually resolves the problem.

REFERENCE

1. Surya, B.V., Provet, J., Johanson, K.E., and Brown, J.: Anastomotic strictures following radical prostatectomy: Risk factors and management. J. Urol., *143*: 755, 1990.

1355-B *(Campbell's, pp. 2883–2884)*

To achieve continence after radical retropubic prostatectomy, it is mandatory to avoid injury to the pelvic floor mechanism, to reconstruct the vesical neck so that it will provide a passive mechanism of continence, and to avoid stricture formation by coapting the bladder neck to the urethra accurately.

Following a radical prostatectomy, passive urinary control is maintained by the striated urethral sphincter. Age, weight of the prostate, prior transurethral resection of the prostate, pathologic stage, and preservation or wide excision of the neurovascular bundles have no significant influence on urinary continence. With the development of an anatomic approach to radical prostatectomy, urinary continence improved because the anterior component of the striated urethral sphincter/dorsal vein complex was preserved.

1356-B *(Campbell's, pp. 2884–2885)*

Today it is possible to preserve sexual function in many men undergoing radical retropubic prostatectomy. Factors identified to correlate with the return of sexual function include age, clinical and pathologic stage, and the preservation of the neurovascular bundle.

In men younger than age 50, potency was similar in those who had both neurovascular bundles preserved and those who had one neurovascular bundle widely excised. In those older than 50, sexual function was better in patients in whom both neurovascular bundles were preserved than in patients in whom one neurovascular bundle was excised. When the relative risk of postoperative impotence is adjusted for age, the risk of postoperative impotence is twofold greater if there is capsular penetration or seminal vesicle invasion or if one neurovascular bundle is excised.

REFERENCE

1. Quinlan, D.M., Epstein, J.I., Carter, B.S., and Walsh, P.C.: Sexual function following radical prostatectomy: Influence of preservation of neurovascular bundles. J. Urol., *145*:998, 1991.

1357-D *(Campbell's, pp. 2887–2888)*

The two most popular approaches for the surgical removal of a prostatic malignancy are radical retropubic prostatectomy and perineal prostatectomy. The perineal approach has the advantage of providing a relatively avascular field, good exposure for reconstruction of the vesicourethral anastomosis, and dependent post-operative drainage. Further, in the elderly patient, an intra-abdominal approach may compromise the patient's pulmonary function. The principal disadvantage of the perineal approach is that it does not afford simultaneous exposure of the pelvic lymphatic drainage; therefore, two incisions are necessary if the patient undergoing perineal prostatectomy is to have a staging lymphadenectomy. However, prostate-specific antigen levels can now be used to quite accurately predict the probability of lymphatic metastasis. Preservation of the anatomic innervation of the corporal vasculature may be more difficult through the perineum than through the retropubic approach.

REFERENCE

1. Jewett, J.H.: The case for radical perineal prostatectomy. J. Urol., *103*:195, 1970.

1358-D *(Campbell's, p. 2888)*

The patient should be assessed preoperatively to determine whether or not it is believed that the disease is confined to the prostate, since patients with obvious extraprostatic extension of disease are not candidates for radical perineal prostatectomy. Transrectal ultrasound to determine the extent of disease has not yet proved to be superior to careful digital examination. Preoperative cystoscopy is not warranted unless the patient has previously undergone a transurethral resection. Bowel preparation consists only of repeated enemas until return is clear, followed by a neomycin-containing enema given several hours prior to the patient's entry into the operating room. Oral laxatives and sterilization of the bowel with antibiotics are unnecessary.

1359-A *(Campbell's, p. 2897)*

Following division of superficial central muscles of the perineum, the rectal sphincter is visualized as an arch overlying the rectum. An anterior retractor is used to stretch the rectal sphincter superiorly. This maneuver helps identify the glistening fibers of the anterior rectal fascia, which are used as a guide to help gain entry to the prostate and prostatic apex. Failure to identify this anatomic landmark may cause the surgeon to carry dissection anteriorly, injuring either the bulbocavernosus muscle or the membranous urethra.

1360-B *(Campbell's, p. 2898)*

Vigorous venous bleeding may be encountered during dissection at the apex of the prostate or after division of the membranous urethra when the prostate is being separated from the bladder anteriorly and anterolaterally. Although one may be tempted to stop the dissection and control the venous bleeding, it is best to provide temporary control of the bleeding by pressure behind a curved narrow Deaver retractor until the prostate is separated from the bladder neck anteriorly. Once the prostate is separated, most of the venous bleeding ceases spontaneously.

1361-C *(Campbell's, p. 2898)*

A large median lobe may complicate the separation of the prostate from the posterior bladder neck. If the median lobe is pedunculated and can be delivered through the bladder neck into the operative field, the incision should be proximal to the lobe in such a manner that the bladder neck fibers are cut away sharply and the prostatic tissue is delivered into the operative field. If the median lobe cannot be delivered through the bladder neck into the operative field, it may be sharply amputated, to be removed following completion of the radical prostatectomy. This can be accomplished with little chance of seeding tumor, because the incidence of involvement of median lobe tissue by malignancy is minimal.

1362-B *(Campbell's, pp. 2898–2899)*

Urinary leakage from the incision usually stops. If the patient experiences leaking only when voiding, the leak is distal to the reconstructed bladder neck. In these instances, the Foley catheter is not replaced and the patient is instructed to void only seated. If the patient drains continually through the perineal incision, the catheter is replaced and the patient remains on catheter drainage. It is important that the Foley catheter be in the most dependent portion of the bladder.

1363-A, 1364-C *(Campbell's, p. 2899)*

Urinary incontinence may be divided into early and late incontinence. In the hands of surgeons skilled in radical prostatectomy, the actual incidence of incontinence is less than 2 per cent.

Early incontinence may be functional (due to residual inflammation from surgery) or mechanical (as a result of damage to the distal sphincteric mechanism or failure to adequately reconstruct the bladder neck).

The patient who presents with persistent incontinence usually has mechanical damage that was done at the time of surgery. This damage is most difficult to manage, and these patients usually have to undergo some form of artificial sphincter placement to establish continence. The scarring produced by the previous surgery usually requires that the artificial sphincter be placed around the bulb of the urethra.

1365-C *(Campbell's, pp. 2901–2902)*

Studies have shown that the chance of a 40-year-old man having a prostatectomy in his lifetime is roughly between 10 and 30 per cent. In addition, McPherson and associates (1992) noted that the incidence of prostatectomy per 100,000 was 264 in the United States, compared with 122 in England. The most common reasons for prostatectomy, found in 90 per cent of patients, are symptoms of prostatism—bladder outlet obstruction symptoms and bladder hyperreflexia symptoms. Multiple studies on the natural history of BPH and on indications for TURP reveal that 27 per cent of patients had the primary indication for surgery of acute urinary retention; however, it is impossible to predict who will have modest symptoms of prostatism and who will develop retention. Following TURP, over 80 per cent of patients will have improvement in symptoms and urinary flow rates.

1366-A *(Campbell's, pp. 2904, 2911)*

According to the AUA Cooperative Study (1989) the most common cause of death following TURP is sepsis, occurring in patients who were debilitated and had other systemic processes. The mortality rate in this study was 0.2 per cent. Prior to the AUA Cooperative Study, the most common cause of death was cardiovascular complication.

1367-B *(Campbell's, 5th Edition, p. 2815)*

The most common reasons for TURP are symptoms of prostatism (90 per cent); both bladder outlet obstruction symptoms (e.g., decrease in force of stream, hesitancy, straining to void, etc.) and bladder hyperreflexia symptoms (e.g., urgency, frequency, and nocturia) in the absence of significant postvoid residual and infection result from detrusor hyperreflexia (Turner-Warwick et al. 1973; Turner-Warwich 1973; Cote et al. 1981). This condition is initiated by stimulation of afferent sensory nerves entrapped or irritated by the enlarged prostate, evoking a detrusor response.

Bladder calculi are fairly uncommon in the United States and are usually associated with urinary stasis secondary to urinary obstruction in men. External sphincter dyssynergia is generally seen with suprasacral lesions. Detrusor areflexia can result from interruption of sacral reflex arcs, spinal shock after suprasacral spinal cord injury, and direct myogenic causes, such as urinary retention.

1368-D *(Campbell's, pp. 2904–2905)*

TURP may be performed with general anesthesia or an epidural, or a subdural spinal block, and Sinha and colleagues (1986) reported doing TURP with local anesthesia. Nielsen and coworkers (1987) noted no difference in blood loss between epidural or general anesthesia. McGowan and Smith (1980) confirmed this between spinal and general anesthesia, and the postoperative morbidity and mortality rates were not significantly different. However, there was a higher incidence of cardiac arrhythmias with general anesthesia.

1369-D *(Campbell's, pp. 2905–1906; Campbell's, 5th Edition, pp. 2816–2823)*

The TURP should begin with urethral calibration to prevent postoperative strictures from the use of resectoscope sheaths that are too large. Before proximal resection near the vesical neck is begun, the bladder should be moderately distended. This serves the dual purpose of helping to define the prostatovesical junction and pushing the anterior and lateral walls of the bladder out of the way, so that they are not inadvertently resected and possibly perforated. Proximal resection should be carried to the level of the circular fibers of the bladder neck. Deep resection or excessive cauterization should be avoided because it may lead to vesical neck contracture. The bladder should not be distended during resection of apical tissue so that the apical tissue projects into the prostatic fossa and is more easily resected.

1370-E *(Campbell's, pp. 2905–2910)*

During TURP, the most common area of damage to the external sphincter is at the 12 o'clock position. Frequently with the patient in the lithotomy position, the distal portion of the prostate is tilted cephalad making the external sphincter more susceptible at 12 o'clock. Most surgeons use a nonhemolytic irrigant, such as glycine, due to the risk of intravascular hemolysis with water. As mentioned previously, deep resection of the vesical neck frequently leads to vesical neck contracture. In cases of narrowing in the meatal postnavicular area, a dorsal internal urethrotomy may be performed. A generous ventral meatotomy often leads to splattering and/or errant direction of the urinary stream. During TURP, the resection is carried through the granular adenoma to the glistening white capsule.

1371-B *(Campbell's, p. 2911; Campbell's, 5th Edition, p. 2831)*

Arterial bleeding is controlled by electrocoagulation and the cardinal rule is to control arterial bleeding in one stage before moving to the next stage of resection. Persistent attempts at controlling venous sinus bleeding by electrocoagulation should not be made, because of intravasation of irrigant into the blood stream with such attempts. Venous bleeding can usually be controlled by proper placement of the urethral catheter.

1372-E *(Campbell's, pp. 2911–2912)*

Both intraoperative bleeding and the incidence of TUR syndrome are related to the size of the gland and length of surgery. They are significantly elevated in glands larger than 45 g and surgery longer than 90 minutes. The mortality rate of TURP has steadily declined and is presently 0.2 per cent.

The incidence of TUR syndrome is 2 per cent and this condition is characterized by mental confusion, nausea, vomiting, hypertension, bradycardia, and visual disturbances. Most of these cases can be managed with diuretics and observation. Penile erection during TURP may make surgery very difficult or impossible unless a perineal urethrostomy is performed. Some have used ketamine or intracorporal epinephrine in reducing penile erections.

1373-A *(Campbell's, p. 2912)*

TUR syndrome occurs in 2 per cent of patients and is felt to represent dilutional hyponatremia. Decreased serum osmolality is also noted. The risk is higher if the gland is greater than 45 g and the resection time is over 90 minutes. Most patients do not become symptomatic until the serum sodium concentration reaches 125 mEq/L and can be managed with diuretics and observation.

1374-C *(Campbell's, p. 2913)*

According to the AUA Cooperative Study, the most common problem in the postoperative period was failure to void, occurring in 6.5 per cent of patients. Half of these patients had hypotonic bladders. Patients who fail to void after a second trial should undergo cystoscopy to rule out residual adenoma and a cystometrogram should be performed. In patients with severely hypotonic bladders, catheter drainage may be required for 1 to 2 weeks, during which time bladder tone seems to return.

1375-B *(Campbell's, p. 2913)*

Vesical neck contracture occurs in 2.7 per cent of TURP patients and usually occurs within the first 4 to 6 weeks following surgery. Overresection or excessive cauterization of the vesical neck may lead to contracture. Classically, the patient has had a good urinary stream and then a marked reduction. Contracture is diagnosed endoscopically and can be treated by incising the neck with the Collings knife or cold knife urethrotome. Urethral stricture is slightly less common than vesical neck contracture and can usually be prevented by adequately calibrating the urethra preoperatively. Urethral stricture is related to the size of the gland and the length of resection time.

1376-C *(Campbell's, pp. 2915–1916; Campbell's, 5th Edition, p. 2815)*

Patients with significant symptoms, without prostate enlargement but with uroflow values suggesting outlet obstruction may be managed with transurethral incision of the prostate. The surgical technique is relatively simple, using a Collings knife to make incisions at the 5 o'clock and 7 o'clock positions. In addition, there is a decrease in retrograde ejaculation when compared to TURP. During the procedure, a biopsy of the prostate should be performed to ensure that carcinoma is not overlooked.

1377-D *(Campbell's, pp. 2918–2919)*

Most bladder calculi are the result of bladder outlet obstruction and infection. Therefore, in addition to removing the stone, the outlet obstruction should be corrected. A patient with a markedly enlarged gland and a large bladder calculus is certainly a candidate for an open procedure. The contraindications to EHL include large stones (>5 cm) and the necessity of doing an open prostatectomy. A large calculus is also not amenable to mechanical litholapaxy.

1378-E, 1379-C *(Campbell's, p. 2923)*

A laser generates a collimated, monochromatic beam of light with all of the photons in phase with one another. Generally, the tissue effects of a laser beam may be characterized as thermal, mechanical, or photochemical.

Most therapeutic laser effects depend on thermal transformation of light energy. Up to 60°C, only tissue warming occurs without irreversible cellular damage. Between 60 and 100°C, protein coagulation is observed, resulting in cell death but no loss of structural or architectural integrity of the tissue. Above 100°C, carbonization and vaporization occur.

A low-energy laser with a short pulse duration creates an optico-acoustic effect which can result in mechanical stone fragmentation. The effects are nonthermal and depend on absorption of the laser energy by the stone. Expansion of a plasma that is formed results in disruption of the stone.

Photosensitizers that are activated by light of a specific wavelength can result in cellular death from a photochemical effect. The photosensitizer most frequently used in clinical studies is hematoporphyrin derivative. The exact mechanism of cellular death is uncertain.

REFERENCES

1. Beason, R.C.: Hematoporphyrin derivative photodynamic therapy. *In* Smith, J.A. Jr. (Ed.): Laser in Urologic Surgery. Chicago, Year Book Medical Publisher, 1989, pp. 147–165.
2. Hofstetter, A., Frank, F., and Keiditsch, E.: Laser treatment of the bladder. Experimental and clinical results. *In* Smith, J.A. Jr. (Ed.): Lasers in Urologic Surgery. Chicago, Year Book Medical Publishers, 1989.

1380-E, 1381-B, 1382-B *(Campbell's, p. 2924)*

The active medium of a laser determines the wavelength of the emitted light. The active medium may be a gas (e.g., CO_2 or argon), liquid (e.g., rhodamine B), or solid (e.g., neodymium:YAG).

The CO_2 laser has a wavelength of 10,600 mm and penetrates to a depth of approximately 0.3 mm. It is rapidly absorbed by water and therefore is used for treatment of lesions of the external genitalia. It produces intense heat with vaporization of tissue.

The argon laser has a spectral emission between 488 and 514 mm and penetrates to a depth of 1.0 mm. It is poorly absorbed by water but is selectively absorbed by hemoglobin and melanin.

Over the last decade, the neodymium:YAG laser has been the most versatile and widely utilized laser in urologic surgery. It emits a wavelength of 1060 mm, produces tissue coagulation through protein denaturation, and penetrates to a depth of 5 mm. Minimal vaporization occurs.

A KTP laser has a wavelength of 532 mm, and produces tissue effects similar to those of an argon laser but with a higher power output. More vaporization but less coagulation occurs with a KTP laser than a neodymium:YAG laser.

The term pulsed-dye laser refers to a laser lithotriptor that employs pulsed output and an active medium of coumarin green. The fiber tip is placed in contact with a stone. Absorption of the laser energy by the stone forms a plasma that rapidly expands resulting in mechanical disruption of the stone with minimal thermal effect.

The term argon-dye laser usually refers to an argon-pumped laser, which uses rhodamine B dye as the active medium. The laser has little direct effect on tissue when applied alone.

1383-D *(Campbell's, pp. 2924–2925)*

Lasers have proven to be effective for treatment of condyloma accumination of the external genitalia. For typical, grossly visible condyloma acuminata, excellent results have been achieved with a CO_2, KTP-532, and a neodymium:YAG laser. When using a CO_2 laser, a power output of 3 to 5 watts generally is sufficient, resulting in vaporization of the lesion. Studies have shown that there may be viable DVA particles in the laser smoke plume, so vacuum smoke evacuators and special laser masks should be used.

With a neodymium:YAG laser, a power output of 15 to 20 watts will usually suffice. The lesion is treated until it undergoes a characteristic white discoloration.

The KTP-532 laser usually requires a power output of 7 to 9 watts when treating condyloma acuminata of the external genitalia. This laser may be preferred, because of its affinity for melanin, especially in black patients.

A major problem associated with condyloma acuminata is recurrence, and with microscopic subclinical lesions, the recurrence rate is high even after adequate destruction of detected lesions. Currently, laser therapy of aceto-white microscopic condyloma acuminata has not been found to decrease recurrence rates.

REFERENCE

1. Malloy, T.R., Zderic, S.A., and Carpiniello, V.L.: External genital lesions. *In* Smith, J.A., Jr. (Ed.): Lasers in Urologic Surgery. Chicago, Year Book Medical Publishers, 1989, pp. 23–35.

1384-B *(Campbell's, pp. 2925–2926)*

A laser is capable of providing effective local control for selected penile cancer. Patients chosen for primary laser therapy should have only superficially invasive tumors.

For tumor ablation, a neodymium:YAG laser is preferable; however, CO_2 laser excising of penile cancer has been reported.

REFERENCE

1. Smith, J.A. Jr., and Dixon, J.A.: Laser photoradiation in urologic surgery. J. Urol., *131*:655, 1984.

1385-C *(Campbell's, pp. 2927–2929)*

Partly because of the unsatisfactory results achieved with alternative therapy, lasers have been investigated in the treatment of benign urethral strictures. Since tissue vaporization occurs with minimal forward scatter of energy, a CO_2 laser would seem most appealing for treatment of urethral strictures. Practical considerations (e.g., rapid absorption of its energy by water) preclude the use of the CO_2 laser within the urethra. Gaseous distention of the urethra carries the hazard of air embolus, even with suprapubic venting.

The greatest experience with laser treatment of urethral strictures has been with the neodymium:YAG laser. Because minimal tissue vaporization occurs with a neodymium:YAG laser, dilation of the stricture is necessary to provide immediate symptomatic relief until tissue slough occurs. The most efficient way to increase the energy density of a neodymium: YAG laser and, thereby, improve the cutting effect, is through contact tips. However, several studies have led to the conclusion that laser therapy offers no advantages over cold knife urethrotomy for the treatment of most urethral strictures.

REFERENCE

1. Smith J.A. Jr.: Treatment of benign urethral strictures using a sapphire-tipped Nd:YAG laser. J. Urol., *142*: 1221, 1989.

1386-C *(Campbell's, p. 2930)*

Hemangioma of the bladder is a rare benign tumor that may occur as an isolated lesion or in association with cutaneous or visceral vascular malformations. Transurethral resection is inadvisable because of the possibility of excessive bleeding. The location of the lesion or diffuse bladder involvement may preclude segmental cystectomy. The poor tissue absorption of the neodymium:YAG laser wavelength produces an effective thermal coagulation and a characteristic lack of bleeding. Based on various reports, neodymium:YAG laser coagulation appears to be an effective method for treatment of bleeding from bladder hemangioma.

REFERENCE

1. Smith, J.A. Jr.: Laser treatment of bladder hemangioma. J. Urol., *143*:282, 1990.

1387-D *(Campbell's, p. 2932)*

An issue of paramount importance in treating cancer is tumor staging. In cases of bladder cancer in which adequate histologic material is important, a definitive transurethral resection with electrocautery should be performed. Primarily, patients are selected for laser therapy if they have previous histories of superficial, papillary transitional cell carcinomas of the bladder; normal or low-grade malignant cells on voided cytology examinations; and tumors that appear to be low grade on cystoscopic examination. If a cold-cup biopsy finding establishes the diagnosis of transitional cell carcinoma, a previous history of bladder cancer is not mandatory for confirmation. Partly because of staging considerations but also because of practical problems with large tumors, lesions to be treated should be limited to less than 2.5 cm.

Often when treating superficial lesions, general or regional anesthesia is unnecessary. In general, a power output of 35 to 40 watts is chosen, and laser energy is applied to the base of the tumor and the surrounding mucosa in continuous fashion. Treatment is maintained in a given area until a characteristic white discoloration indicative of adequate thermal necrosis is evident. This usually requires 2 to 3 seconds of energy application in a given area. Treatment of tumors overlying the ureteral orifice have not resulted in ureteral stricture. To date, sufficient data have not been reported to either support or refute the theory that recurrence rate is less after laser treatment than after electrocautery resection.

REFERENCE

1. Smith, J.A. Jr.: Bladder cancer. *In* Smith, J.A. Jr. (Ed.): Lasers in Urologic Surgery. Chicago, Year Book Medical Publishers, 1985, pp. 52–62.

1388-C *(Campbell's, p. 2933)*

By adhering to recommended techniques for the laser treatment of bladder cancer, thermal necrosis should extend to the deep lamina propria or superficial detrusor muscle. Excessive forward scatter of laser energy to adjacent organs is unlikely. However, several unpublished reports have been made of small bowel perforation after laser treatment of superficial bladder cancer. Therefore, caution should be maintained, especially when treating tumors on the "intraperitoneal" portion of the bladder and when previous pelvic surgery or irradiation has caused adhesions between small bowel and the bladder dome.

1389-B *(Campbell's, pp. 2937–2938)*

Photodynamic therapy (PDT) defines a methodology that involves photosensitization of cells with subsequent destruction by application of light of a specific wavelength. Preferential destruction of malignant cells occurs by the selective retention of the photosensitizer within the target cells or by the specific direction of the light to the affected areas.

Several photosensitizer are known to exist but hematoporphyrin derivative (HPD) has been used most often clinically. HPD is cleared from most tissues within a few hours after systemic administration. However, the drug is retained in liver, spleen, kidneys, and skin as well as in malignant and dysplastic cells. Retention within malignant cells is measurable for several days.

Usually, 630 mm light from an argon laser has been preferred for PDT, and it has been shown to penetrate tissue up to 1 cm. The exact mechanism of cellular death is uncertain; however, it has been postulated that slight oxygen production caused by irradiation of dihematoporphyria esters is responsible for the toxic effects of PDT on cells.

Although the optimal time for delivery of laser energy after drug administration has not been determined, most studies have reported 48 to 72 hours. The laser fiber is introduced into the bladder through a cystoscope, and difficulty exists in maintaining the fiber tip in the center of the bladder. Optimal positioning is determined by visual inspection as well as by ultrasound guidance.

Postoperatively, patients usually experience irritative voiding symptoms which can persist for several weeks until bladder healing occurs. It is imperative that the patient be cautioned to stay out of direct sunlight for a minimum of 6 weeks. Retention of the drug within the skin places the patient at risk for severe sunburn even with limited exposure.

Although good response rates have been reported with PDT, it remains an investigational procedure with limited clinical data available.

REFERENCES

1. Benson, R.C. Jr.: Hematoporphyrin derivative photodynamic therapy. *In* Smith, J.A. Jr. (Ed.): Lasers in Urologic Surgery. Chicago, Year Book Medical Publishers, 1989, pp. 147–165.
2. Nseyo, U.O., Dougherty, T.J., and Sullivan, L.: Photodynamic therapy in management of resistant lower urinary tract carcinoma. Cancer, *12*:3113, 1987.

1390-A, 1391-B *(Campbell's, pp. 2938–2939)*

The term pulsed-dye laser generally refers to lasers that utilize coumarin green dye. When excited, this dye generates a wavelength of 504 nm that is well absorbed by the yellow color of most calculi but poorly absorbed by body tissues.

The laser fiber may be employed with a rigid or flexible ureteroscope. When the calculus is visualized, the laser fiber is placed in direct contact with the stone. The laser beam is fired at a discharge rate of 5 Hz. Higher frequencies may impair the surgeons' visual field because of the light flash. The laser energy is absorbed by the stone which results in the formation of a "plasma" bubble on the surface of the stone. This expansion bubble of a column of electrons mechanically disrupts the stone along stress lines.

The pulsed-dye laser has proved to be effective in the treatment of ureteral calculi. Even if the probe is inadvertently fired on the ureteral mucosa, no discernible damage is done. The greatest risk of ureteral injury comes from the ureterscopy itself.

The most easily fragmented calculi are those of struvite and calcium oxalate dihydrate. Cystine and pure calcium oxalate monohydrate stones are more resistant to fragmentation.

REFERENCES

1. Dretler, S.P.: Urinary Stone Fragmentation: Clinical application. *In* Smith, J.A. Jr. (Ed.): Lasers in Urologic Surgery. Chicago, Year Book Medical Publishers, 1989, pp. 126–137.
2. Watson, G.M., Murray, S., Dretler, S.P., and Parrish, J.A.: The pulsed-dye laser for fragmenting urinary calculi. J. Urol., *138*:195, 1987.

1392-E *(Campbell's, pp. 2939–2940)*

A milliwatt CO_2 laser has been utilized for vasovasostomy. The theoretical advantages that have been discussed are increased patency, decreased sperm granuloma, the ability to perform the laser weld rapidly, and minimal local tissue resection. Laser-assisted vascular anastomosis has been promising, and many of its principles are applicable to vasovasostomy; however, studies have failed to demonstrate any increase in pregnancy rates as compared to the standard technique of vasovasostomy.

REFERENCE

1. Shanberg, A., Tansey, L., Baghdassarian, R., et al.: Laser-assisted vasectomy reversed: Experience in 32 patients. J. Urol., *143*:528, 1990.

1393-D *(Campbell's, p. 2942)*

The seminal vesicle is strictly a male organ with no female homologue and develops as a dorsal lateral bulbous swelling of the distal mesonephric duct at approximately 13 fetal weeks. Congenital absence of the seminal vesicle does occur and lack of a vas deferens does not necessarily imply absence of the seminal vesicles. It has also been shown that 50 per cent of ectopic ureters in males join the posterior urethra, whereas 30 per cent join the seminal vesicle. It is also true that cystic fibrosis patients commonly do not have vas deferens or seminal vesicles.

REFERENCES

1. Arey, L.B.: The urinary system. Developmental Anatomy. Philadelphia, W.B. Saunders Co., 1965, p. 313.
2. Brewster, S.F.: The development and differentiation of human seminal vesicles. J. Anat., *143*:45, 1985.
3. Gorden, H.L., and Kessler, R.: Ectopic ureter entering the seminal vesicle associated with renal dysplasia. J. Urol., *108*:389, 1972.
4. Goldstein, M., and Schlossberg, S.: Men with congenital absence of the vas deferens often have seminal vesicles. J. Urol., *140*:85, 1988.
5. Kaplan, E., Shawachman, H., Perlmutter, A.D., et al.: Reproductive failure in men with cystic fibrosis. N. Engl. J. Med., *279*:65, 1968.

1394-D *(Campbell's, pp. 2942–2944)*

The normal adult seminal vesicle is 5 to 10 cm in length, 3 to 5 cm in diameter, and does have a volume capacity of 13 ml on average. The right seminal vesicle is also known to be slightly larger than the left in one third of men. The size of both glands does decrease with age. The blood supply to the seminal vesicle is from the vesiculodeferential artery, which is a branch of the umbilical artery. Occasionally, the inferior vesical artery provides a communicating vessel. Innervation to the seminal vesicles is through adrenergic fibers from the hypogastric nerve.

REFERENCES

1. Redman, J.F.: Anatomy of the genitourinary system. *In* Gillenwater, J.Y., Grayhack, J.T., Howards, S.S., and Duckett, J.W. (Eds.): Adult and Pediatric Urology. St. Louis, Mosby Year Book, 1991, p. 134.
2. Braithwaite, J.L.: The arterial supply of the male urinary bladder. Br. J. Urol., *24*:64, 1952.
3. Mawhinney, M.G.: Male accessory sex organs and androgen action. *In* Lipschultz, L.I., and Howards, S.S. (Eds.): Infertility of the Male. New York, Churchill Livingstone, 1983, p. 135.

1395-A *(Campbell's, p. 2944)*

Male vesicle secretions are known to contain primarily carbohydrates such as fructose. In addition, these secretions also contain prostaglandins E, A, B, and F and coagulation factor. Alpha-tocopherol is vitamin E and is not reported to be among seminal vesicle secretions. D-Sorbitol is a precursor to D-fructose and may possibly be present in seminal vesicle secretion; however, it is not reported.

REFERENCES

1. Tauber, P.F., Zaneveld, L.J.D., Propping, D., et al.: Components of human split ejaculate. J. Reprod. Fertil., *43*:249, 1975.
2. Tauber, P.F., Zaneveld, L.J.D., Propping, D., et al.: Components of human split ejaculate II. Enzymes and proteinase inhibitors. J. Reprod. Fertil., *46*:165, 1976.

1396-C *(Campbell's, p. 2944)*

The seminal vesicle is responsible for the majority of the volume of ejaculate and therefore a low semen volume would be an indication of absence of the seminal vesicles. The seminal vesicles do produce secretions rich in carbohydrate, primarily fructose, and lack of fructose or carbohydrate in ejaculate would again indicate absence of the seminal vesicle. Finally, the seminal vesicle secretion also contains coagulation factor responsible for the initial coagulation of semen. Liquefaction of semen would indicate absence of the coagulation factor and imply absence of the seminal vesicle. The sperm count would not necessarily be related to the seminal vesicle secretion.

1397-D *(Campbell's, pp. 2944–2946)*

Antegrade vasography is highly successful in evaluating duct obstruction. Vasography, however, does not provide accurate demonstration of pathology of the seminal vesicles in patients with tumors, vesiculitis, or cysts. Transrectal ultrasound has become one of the most accurate methods of evaluating the seminal vesicle. Ultrasound can be used to successfully identify seminal vesicle aplasia and atrophy as well as cyst formation. Additionally, solid tumors can be detected and seminal vesicle calcification seen which may be an indication of infection such as bilharziasis. However, inflammatory conditions which may involve the seminal vesicle cannot be differentiated by ultrasound and these include both chronic prostatourethritis and prostatodynia. Primary tumors within the seminal vesicle are readily seen on CT as an enlarged vesicle with a higher attenuation number in the area of tumor than that in the normal seminal vesicle. However, CT scanning cannot distinguish between benign and malignant tumors and cannot routinely distinguish between primary and secondary tumors, although obliteration of tissue planes between seminal vesicle and other organs is an indication of a secondary tumor. With magnetic resonance imaging, T1-weighted images of the seminal vesicles are of low signal intensity and T2-weighted images are of higher intensity and this is thought to be due to the secretions contained within. Hemorrhagic cysts within the seminal vesicles have high intensity signals on both T1- and T2-weighted images. MRI of the seminal vesicles adequately portrays solid tumors; however, benign and malignant lesions cannot be distinguished from each other.

REFERENCES

1. Dunnick, N.R., Ford, K., Osborne, D., et al.: Seminal vesiculography: Limited value in vesiculitis. Urology, *20*:454, 1982.
2. King, B.F., Hattery, R.R., Lieber, M.M., et al.: Seminal vesicle imaging. Radiographics, *9*:653, 1989.
3. Littrup, P.J., Lee, F., McLeary, R.D., et al.: Transrectal US of the seminal vesicles and ejaculatory ducts: Clinical correlations. Radiology, *168*:625, 1988.
4. Sussman, S.K., Dunnick, N.R., Silverman, P.M., and Cohan, R.H.: Case report: carcinoma of the seminal vesicle: CT appearance. J. Comput. Assist. Tomogr., *10*:519, 1986.
5. Sue, D.E., Chicola, C., Brant-Zawadzki, M.N., et al.: MR imaging in seminal vesiculitis. J. Comput. Assist. Tomogr., *13*:662, 1989.

1398-E *(Campbell's, pp. 2947–2948)*

In the third world, tuberculosis and schistosomiasis do remain common causes of seminal vesicle masses, abscesses, and calcifications. However, infection of the seminal vesicles is an uncommon problem in the United States. Bacterial infections of the seminal vesicles found in industrialized nations are commonly caused by colonic flora and thought to be secondarily due to bacterial prostatitis. Bacterial seminal vesiculitis can be treated successfully with antibiotics in most cases. However, in the case of recurrent septicemia due to infection of the seminal vesicle, surgical excision of the infected vesicle is appropriate therapy. Glandular congestion of the seminal vesicle is not a term that is used in describing the radiographic findings of the seminal vesicle. Transrectal needle aspiration followed by antibiotic therapy is appropriate treatment for an infected seminal vesicle cyst or seminal vesicle abscess; however, this is not reported as standard treatment for simple seminal vesiculitis.

1399-D *(Campbell's, p. 2948)*

Few primary tumors of the seminal vesicles have been reported to date. Small tumors often lack symptoms. With adenocarcinoma, tumors are often discovered at the time of local extension into the prostate and bladder and/or rectum. Hematospermia is not reported as a common presenting complaint. These tumors commonly occur over the age of 50. Serum carcinoembryonic antigen levels may be elevated. Serum markers for prostate cancer including prostate-specific antigen (PSA) and prostatic acid-phosphatase (PAP) are normal. Pathology of the most common primary carcinoma of the seminal vesicle shows a muscin-producing papillary or anaplastic carcinoma that may contain lipofuscin.

REFERENCES

1. Benson, R.C. Jr., Clark, W.R., and Farrow, G.M.: Carcinoma of the seminal vesicle. J. Urol., *132*:483, 1984.
2. Mostofi, F.K., and Price, E.B.: Tumors of the seminal vesicle. *In* Mostofi, F.K., and Price, E.B. (Eds.): Tumors of the Male Genital System. Washington, D.C., Armed Forces Institute of Pathology, 1973, p. 259.
3. Tanaka, T., Takeuchi, T., Oguchi, K., et al.: Primary adenocarcinoma of the seminal vesicle. Hum. Pathol., *18*:200, 1987.

1400-C *(Campbell's, p. 2948)*

Benign primary tumors of the seminal vesicle include papillary adenoma, cyst adenoma, fibroma, and leiomyoma. Primary malignant tumors of the seminal vesicle include the papillary adenocarcinoma, leiomyosarcoma or hemangiosarcoma. Cystic teratoma is not reported among tumors of the seminal vesicles.

1401-A *(Campbell's, p. 2948)*

Malignancies metastatic to the seminal vesicle are more common than primary seminal vesicle malignancies, and include transitional cell carcinoma in situ, adenocarcinoma of the prostate, lymphoma, and rectal carcinoma. Adenocarcinoma of the vas deferens is not reported.

REFERENCES

1. Jakse, G., Putz, A., and Hofstadter, F.: Carcinoma in situ of the bladder extending into the seminal vesicles. J. Urol., *137*:44, 1987.
2. Mostofi, F.K., and Price, E.B.: Tumors of the seminal vesicle. *In* Mostofi, F.K., and Price, E.B. (Eds.): Tumors of the Male Genital System. Washington, DC, Armed Forces Institute of Pathology, 1973, p. 259.
3. Ro, J.Y., Ayala, A.G., el-Naggar, A., and Wishnow, K.I.: Seminal vesicle involvement by in situ and invasive transitional cell carcinoma of the bladder. Am. J. Surg. Pathol., *11*:951, 1987.

1402-B *(Campbell's, p. 2949)*

Small seminal vesicle cysts obstructing ejaculatory ducts or causing local symptoms should undergo an initial attempt at a transperineal or transrectal ultrasound guided aspiration. When this attempt is not successful because the cyst recumulates, consideration could be given to reaspiration with injection of a sclerosing solution such as tetracycline. When these approaches are not successful and the cyst or abscess is adjacent to the prostate and in the proximal seminal vesicle, it may be possible to unroof the cavity with a deep transurethral resection into the prostatic tissue just distal to the bladder neck at the 5 or 7 o'clock positions. When aspiration of cysts or transurethral resection are not successful, small cysts may be managed with transperineal excision. Large lesions may require an anterior paravesicle approach. Marsupialization of large cysts to the bladder is not reported as therapy for symptomatic seminal vesicle cysts.

REFERENCES

1. Frye, K., and Loughlin, K.: Successful transurethral drainage of bilateral seminal vesicle abscesses. J. Urol., *139*:1323, 1988.
2. Honnens de Lichtenberg, M., and Hvidt, V.: Transurethral, transprostatic incision of a seminal vesicle cyst. Scand. J. Urol. Nephrol., *23*:303, 1989.

1403-E *(Campbell's, p. 2950)*

The transperineal, transcoccygeal and transvesical approaches should be prepared preoperatively with complete bowel preparation including a mechanical preparation as well as an oral antibiotic regimen including neomycin/erythromycin. A prophylactic systemic antibiotic of choice is administered immediately before surgery. Blood loss expected from seminal vesicle surgery depends on the surgical approach. One to two units should be prepared for those involving perineal or transcoccygeal approaches and 2 to 3 units for anterior approaches. Present recommendations for prevention of deep vein thrombosis include use of intermittent compression stockings. However, minidose heparin is not recommended unless the patient has history of venous stasis, varices, or thromboembolic disease. Certainly, full preoperative heparinization is not recommended.

1404-A *(Campbell's, pp. 2950–2951)*

With the transperineal approach the incision in Denonvilliers' fascia is made either transversely, just above the level of the base of the seminal vesicles on the prostate or vertically when attempting to save the neurovascular bundle responsible for potency. Dissection at the base of the seminal vesicle is enhanced by posterior traction on a Lowsley tractor which is placed through the urethra into the bladder. This elevates the prostate and places tension on Denonvilliers' fascia. The seminal vesicle of concern is dissected out at the base of the prostate, a right angle clamp placed around the seminal vesicle, and 2-0 sutures used to ligate the stump of the seminal vesicle directly on the prostate. It is not necessary to dissect the seminal vesicle out before ligating the entry into the prostate. If this is done, the operation is made more difficult and lengthy. The vascular bundle is encountered approximately 1 cm from the distal tip of the seminal vesicle. Drainage of the seminal vesicle bed is recommended.

REFERENCE

1. Weldon, V.E., and Tavel, F.R.: Potency-sparing radical perineal prostatectomy: Anatomy, surgical technique and initial results. J. Urol., *140*:559, 1988.

1405-B *(Campbell's, pp. 2951–2952)*

The transvesical approach to seminal vesicle surgery begins with a midline extraperitoneal suprapubic incision. The space of Retzius is opened. The bladder is opened longitudinally and a Deaver retractor placed inside the dome to place the open bladder on stretch. Although not necessary, it is preferable to place long No. 8 feeding tubes in the ureters at this point to help with definition of the orifices and to help identify the subtrigonal ureters in order to prevent their injury. A vertical incision is then made through the trigone on the posterior midline approximately 5 cm in length. A transverse incision in this region might injure the ureters and is not employed. A transverse incision could be employed just above the bladder neck but this is not preferred. For completion of the procedure, suprapubic cystostomy is optional. The transvesical approach is more prone to blood loss and ureteral injury than other approaches. However, rectal laceration is much less likely.

1406-C *(Campbell's, p. 2952)*

The paravesicle approach to seminal vesicle surgery is commonly used when a large unilateral cyst is present which lies lateral to the bladder. This approach is also useful in children when a nephroureterectomy may be contemplated. This approach is not necessarily chosen for smaller unilateral seminal vesicle cysts. A midline suprapubic incision or Pfannestiel incision is made into the extraperitoneal space. The bladder is dissected away from the lateral pelvic side wall on the affected side. The vas deferens is then identified and placed on tension. The vas is followed down to the base of the bladder where the seminal vesicle cyst or mass should be readily identified. The bladder is drained with a Foley catheter and this facilitates the development of the plane between the bladder and the cyst. As dissection proceeds, the bladder is progressively rolled medially and the cyst or mass of the seminal vesicle is dissected away from the bladder laterally. Both the inferior and the superior vesicle arteries may be sacrificed without concern. When the prostate is approached, one must be concerned when dissecting lateral to the seminal vesicle as the neurovascular bundle is in this region. The seminal vesicle is ligated and divided at the prostate base using a 2-0 absorbable suture.

1407-E *(Campbell's, p. 2952)*

With the retrovesicle approach to seminal vesicle surgery, a midline suprapubic incision is made into the peritoneal space. The bladder is drained. The reflection of the peritoneum over the rectum at the posterior bladder wall is then incised transversely. The bladder is then elevated from the back of the rectum progressively until the ampullae of the vasa and the tips of the seminal vesicles are observed. This approach is thought to be useful for excision of small bilateral seminal vesicle cysts or benign masses.

1408-D *(Campbell's, pp. 2952–2955)*

The transcoccygeal approach is not a common choice due to fear of rectal injury. The patient is positioned prone and in a relative jackknife position. An L-shaped incision is employed from midway on the sacrum and angled at the tip of the coccyx down to the gluteal cleft within 3 cm of the anus. Gluteal layers are then moved aside and the rectosigmoid is then dissected carefully from the underside of the sacrum. Use of an O'Connor sheath and finger in the anus does help in the development of the correct plane. The lateral wall of the rectum is dissected medially from the levator ani muscle until the prostate is encountered. On identification of the prostate, dissection is directed superiorly to the base of the prostate along the midline and this should reveal the ampullae of the vasa and lateral to these the seminal vesicles. Removal of the affected seminal vesicle proceeds as noted in the other approaches. A Penrose drain is placed and the wound closed in layers.

1409-C *(Campbell's, p. 2957)*

A, B, and D are correct statements. While full-thickness skin grafts do revascularize more slowly, they actually resist contraction due to the presence of the reticular dermis. Split-thickness skin grafts have much of the reticular dermis removed and therefore undergo contraction routinely.

1410-D *(Campbell's, pp. 2961–2963)*

All are true except D. The primary lymphatic drainage of the penis coalesces behind the corona dorsally and travels beneath Buck's fascia, terminating mostly in the deep (not superficial) inguinal lymph nodes. Some lymphatics go to the presymphyseal nodes and then onto the external (not internal) iliac lymph nodes.

1411-B *(Campbell's, p. 2967)*

All are true except B. There is typically a hooded dorsal prepuce (not ventral). There is typically no or minimal ventral prepuce.

1412-D *(Campbell's, pp. 2967, 2970)*

Urinary diversion is not currently recommended for uncomplicated hypospadias repair. A distal urethral stent is usually left in place for distal hypospadias. Urinary diversion may be simply and effectively achieved by placing a feeding tube/stent through the urethra or placing a long stent into the bladder to allow drainage.

1413-B *(Campbell's, pp. 2967–2970)*

All mucosal/urethral closure should be with small-gauge absorbable suture in an inverting (not everting) fashion. Inverting the mucosal edges decreases the incidence of fistula as well as avoiding overlapping suture lines.

1414-A *(Campbell's, pp. 2970–2971)*

B, C, D, and E are true statements. VCUG frequently will not demonstrate a urethral diverticulum. Retrograde urethrogram and cystoscopy/urethroscopy are more effective at demonstrating a urethral diverticulum. In females, a special catheter may be required to occlude the bladder neck and external meatus while an opening in the urethral catheter is used to fill the urethra with contrast.

1415-D *(Campbell's, pp. 2973–2978)*

Bladder closure and bladder neck reconstruction should be accomplished prior to the penile and urethral reconstruction. At times (E) urethral construction must be delayed if a cavernosa dermal graft is placed to avoid overlapping a dermal graft with the urethral graft. Such a relationship may decrease the ability of one or both grafts to survive due to poor nutrition from the graft bed.

1416-C *(Campbell's, pp. 2979–2981)*

With severe genital burns, early urinary diversion is important. A primary suprapubic tube may be inserted while initial debridement/evaluation proceeds. The corporal bodies cannot be replaced and have very good vascularity. Therefore, less aggressive debridement is reasonable with the corporal bodies. If the urethra is partially or totally destroyed, a perineal urethrostomy may be better than long-term suprapubic drainage.

1417-B *(Campbell's, pp. 2982–2983)*

Chlamydia and ureaplasma have not been shown to be linked to urethral stricture disease at this time.

1418-C *(Campbell's, pp. 2983–2990)*

With full thickness involvement of the corpora spongiosum, urethral dilatation and visual internal urethrotomy are unlikely to provide a good long-term functional result. An island flap is frequently useful when long segments of urethra must be repaired, but with only a 1- (in this case) to 3-cm lesion, the urethra can generally be mobilized adequately to allow primary end-to-end anastomosis. The split thickness graft is not routinely used for urethral reconstruction due to its tendency for contraction, but full-thickness graft patches are very versatile and can be used for even long strictures if there is not full severe scarring of the spongiosum.

1419-A *(Campbell's, p. 3034)*

As in almost all of medicine, the patient's history is the most important factor in diagnosis. Careful questioning regarding the onset of erectile dysfunction, the presence of early morning erections, the ability to have erections with different sexual partners or with masturbation provides clues to whether the patient's problem is primarily psychogenic or organic.

1420-D *(Campbell's, p. 3035)*

Diabetes mellitus is commonly associated with erectile dysfunction; 35 to 50 per cent of diabetic patients will be impotent. Both vascular and neurologic complications of diabetes have been thought to be involved in erectile dysfunction.

1421-C *(Campbell's, p. 3036)*

Antihypertensives can act both centrally and peripherally to cause erectile dysfunction. Drugs such as the alpha-adrenergic receptor blockers and vasodilators may cause erectile dysfunction by reducing systolic blood pressure and thereby decreasing blood flow through the arteriosclerotic arteries often found in hypertensive patients.

1422-E *(Campbell's, pp. 3036–3037)*

Patients with psychogenic impotence usually have normal nocturnal erections during REM sleep, whereas patients with organic impotence often do not demonstrate nocturnal erections. Accuracy is not 100 per cent, however, because some patients with psychologic abnormalities may experience sleep disorders with absence of REM sleep, and some organic causes of impotence do not interfere with erections during sleep. Lack of complete accuracy coupled with the high cost and complexity have tended to limit use of this test to situations where maximum information is necessary, such as medicolegal conflicts.

1423-D *(Campbell's, p. 3037)*

Visual sexual stimulation testing, monitoring penile erections during patient exposure to videotaped erotic material, has been used as a simpler and less expensive test than nocturnal penile testing to distinguish psychogenic from organic impotence.

1424-A *(Campbell's, p. 3038)*

Biothesiometry involves testing the sensory perception threshold to a vibratory stimulation applied to the penis. Patients with sensory loss will not detect vibratory stimulation at the low end of the scale. These patients may be candidates for more detailed neurologic evaluation.

1425-B *(Campbell's, p. 3041)*

A low LH level is found in patients with hypogonadotropic hypogonadism, whereas patients with an elevated LH level have hypergonadotropic hypogonadism due to testicular failure.

1426-B *(Campbell's, p. 3041)*

Serum testosterone varies widely in normal men related to periodic secretion of luteinizing hormone. Peak levels are usually in the morning.

1427-E *(Campbell's, p. 3041)*

Elevated prolactin, from a pituitary microadenoma, chronic renal failure, drugs, or idiopathic causes, acts to decrease serum testosterone by interfering with LH secretion, and also blocks peripheral action of testosterone.

1428-D *(Campbell's, pp. 3041–3042)*

The inability to consistently measure flow in the cavernosa artery as opposed to the dorsal or spongiosal arteries limits usefulness of the penile-brachial index. It is flow in the cavernosal arteries exclusively that is physiologically important.

1429-A *(Campbell's, p. 3042)*

A skilled operator is necessary to get consistently accurate results with duplex ultrasound; the high expense of the equipment is another limiting factor.

1430-C *(Campbell's, p. 3043)*

The cavernosa artery occlusion pressure is obtained in the dynamic state by simultaneously measuring systolic arterial pressure and monitoring pulsatile flow through the cavernosa artery using Doppler ultrasound while infusing saline into the corpora cavernosa. When intracavernosal pressure exceeds the cavernosa artery perfusion pressure, Doppler ultrasound will show cessation of flow in the cavernosa artery. A normal cavernosa artery occlusion pressure is not more than 35 mm Hg below systolic pressure.

1431-D *(Campbell's, p. 3044)*

As with all diagnostic techniques involving pharmacologic-induced erections, it must be remembered that anxiety can prevent the full relaxation of corporal smooth muscle necessary to obtain a full erection and activate the veno-occlusive mechanism.

1432-A *(Campbell's, p. 3050)*

Gravity pharmacocavernosometry is performed by obtaining a pharmacologically induced erection with full smooth muscle relaxation and infusing saline by gravity. In the normal individual the intracavernosal pressure will approximate the infusion pressure of the saline and only a small volume of saline will be infused. This test is less complex than pump cavernosometry.

1433-C *(Campbell's, pp. 3040, 3052)*

Impotence leads to performance anxiety and a vicious cycle of repeated failure. Anxiety causes increased levels of circulating catecholamines, which interfere with the full corporal smooth muscle relaxation necessary for erection.

1434-D *(Campbell's, p. 3053)*

Testosterone therapy, usually with an intramuscular preparation such as testosterone enanthate, is indicated only after consistently low serum testosterone is documented on at least several tests.

1435-E *(Campbell's, pp. 3041, 3053, 3057)*

Hyperprolactinemia causes sexual dysfunction by decreasing serum testosterone and blocking its peripheral action. Bromocriptine is a medical therapy for microadenoma. Alternatively, hyperprolactinemia due to microadenoma may be treated surgically.

1436-A *(Campbell's, pp. 3054–3055)*

A penile diameter equal to or greater than that obtained with a physiologic erection can be produced by a vacuum constriction device, possibly because of blood trapped in extracorporeal tissue.

1437-C *(Campbell's, p. 3055)*

Venous leakage prevents normal erection even when increased blood flow is induced by pharmacologic agents. The long-acting smooth muscle relaxation caused by these agents can produce an erection even in patients with arterial insufficiency.

1438-C *(Campbell's, p. 3061)*

Persistent penile pain after prosthetic surgery may be a sign of infection. An elevated white blood cell count or sedimentation rate may suggest infection, but in some cases prosthesis removal may be necessary for diagnosis.

1439-D *(Campbell's, p. 3061)*

Decreased sensation in patients with paraplegia or diabetes mellitus predisposes to prosthesis erosion.

1440-E *(Campbell's, p. 3063)*

Young men with discrete lesions due to pelvic or perineal trauma involving the pudendal or penile arteries are the best candidates for vascular reconstructive surgery.

1441-B *(Campbell's, pp. 3063, 3065)*

The Virag procedure involves anastomosing the inferior epigastric artery to a segment of the deep dorsal vein of the penis after ligating it proximally and distally. Conceptually, this supplies blood to the erectile tissue by retrograde flow through the emissary veins.

1442-C *(Campbell's, p. 3036)*

Patients in whom cavernosography demonstrates leakage through the spongiosum have only rarely benefitted from venous surgery. Patients with a generalized abnormality of corporal tissue compliance and venous leakage from all areas of the corpora cavernosa are also unlikely to benefit from venous surgery.

1443-E *(Campbell's, p. 3071)*

The distal corpus cavernosum is most susceptible to fibrotic changes after prolonged priapism; a proximal shunt may be necessary to reestablish venous drainage in such cases.

1444-A *(Campbell's, pp. 3073–3074)*

In the male, the lymphatics of the prepuce and penile skin converge in the dorsum of the penis and coalesce into several trunks which separate to terminate bilaterally in the superficial inguinal nodes, particularly the superomedial group. The lymphatics decussate at the base of the penis accounting for unilateral and, on occasion, bilateral regional node involvement.

All the lymphatics of the glands initially converge in the frenulum. Drainage from this point is usually to the superficial inguinal lymph nodes; however, alternate pathways that terminate in nodes of the deep inguinal, external iliac, or hypogastric region have been discussed.

The corporal bodies are drained by lymphatic trunks that terminate in lymph nodes of the superficial and deep inguinal and also the external iliac regions.

The lymphatics draining the distal urethra pass to the superficial inguinal lymph nodes, and those draining the bulbomembranous and prostate urethra terminate in the obturator and medial external iliac nodes.

In the female, the lymphatics of the proximal urethra course to the external iliac, hypogastric, and obturator nodes. Lymphatic channels of the distal urethra and meatus communicate freely with glandular lymphatics and course toward the mons pubis to terminate in the superomedial group of the superficial inguinal nodes. Inguinal metastases may be seen, therefore, from distal urethral cancers.

REFERENCES

1. Riveros, M., et al.: Lymphadenography of the dorsal lymphatics of the penis. Cancer, *20*:2026, 1967.
2. Sen. A., et al.: Study of the lymphatic drainage from the growth in the penis by radioactive colloidal gold. Ind. J. Cancer, *4*:295, 1967.

1445-C *(Campbell's, p. 3074)*

The pattern of progression of a particular malignancy can vary with its histology and can have an impact on specific therapeutic considerations. Adenocarcinoma of the female urethra generally arises from the proximal urethra or periurethral glands and tends to be a locally aggressive and highly metastatic lesion. Squamous cell carcinoma may involve the entire female urethra or may be localized to the distal third. The distal squamous carcinoma tends to remain localized and amenable to surgical cure by distal urethrectomy.

Secondary transitional cell carcinoma generally involves the urethra as a manifestation of bladder carcinoma. Routine en bloc urethrectomy in the male at the time of cystectomy for transitional cell carcinoma removes current/future sites of tumor formation and may improve local control by obviating tumor cell spillage with transection of the membranous urethra. Total en bloc urethrectomy is routinely included as part of a radical cystectomy in the female patient.

1446-D *(Campbell's, p. 3074)*

The therapeutic alternatives in carcinomas of the penis and of the male and female urethra are varied and depend on the extent of the disease. Radiotherapy for penile cancer has obvious psychologic and cosmetic advantages over surgery, particularly for invasive lesions. Many forms of delivery have been successfully applied. Whereas local control increases with external beam therapy compared with mould techniques, morbidity increases as well. Pretreatment circumcision and generous meatotomy are mandatory to minimize acute inflammatory complications, such as phimosis, paraphimosis, and balanitis. Therapy is more morbid if there is associated infection. Tumor persistence after irradiation is much more common than new tumor formation. Locally recurrent carcinomas range from 10 to 50 per cent, depending on lesion size, depth of invasion, and radiation technique.

Time to regression of penile cancer treated with irradiation may be prolonged. With palpable inguinal adenopathy, a more expedient form of primary therapy is appropriate (i.e., surgery).

REFERENCES

1. Grabstald, H., and Kelley, C.D.: Radiation therapy for penile cancer. Urology, *15*:575, 1980.
2. Pointon, R.C.: Carcinoma of the penis: External beam therapy. Proc. R. Soc. Med., *68*:779, 1975.

1447-C, 1448-B *(Campbell's, pp. 3075–3076)*

Invasive penile cancer not suitable for irradiation, local excision, or micrographic surgery by virtue of its size, location, depth, or degree of invasion is best managed by total or partial penectomy. Attainment of a 2 cm gross tumor margin affords excellent local control. Penile length sufficient to permit upright and directable micturition may be retained after partial penectomy. At least 3 cm of a residual proximal shaft should be available for consideration of this technique. Total penectomy is necessary when adequate tumor margin precludes conservative resection.

REFERENCE

1. Dean, A.L.: Conservative amputation of the penis for carcinoma. J. Urol., *68*:374, 1952.

1449-C *(Campbell's, p. 3076)*

Successful local control by partial penectomy depends on division of the penis 2 cm proximal to the gross tumor extent. After the lesion is excluded by a towel or surgical glove and a tourniquet is applied to the base of the penis, the skin is incised circumferentially, and the cavernous bodies are divided sharply to the urethra. The urethra is dissected distally to attain a 1-cm distal redundancy. After the corpora are secured by opposing the margins of Buck's fascia, the tourniquet is removed, and hemostasis is obtained. The urethra is then spatulated in both its dorsal and ventral surfaces. A skin-urethra anastomosis is performed by using 3-0 or 4-0 absorbable suture. A small urinary catheter is placed and a light dressing applied. Both may be removed on the following day.

1450-B *(Campbell's, p. 3077)*

The inguinal lymph nodes are divided into superficial and deep groups, which are anatomically separated by the deep fascia of the thigh—the fascia lata. The superficial group of nodes is situated in the deep layer of the superficial fascia of the thigh, and drains to the two or three deep inguinal nodes that lie along the femoral vessels within the femoral sheath. The node of Cloquet is the most cephalad of this deep group and is situated within the femoral canal (medial to the femoral vein). The sentinel lymph node is part of the superficial inguinal group. Virchow's node is part of the supraclavicular lymphatic chain.

REFERENCE

1. Daseler, E.H., et al.: Radical excision of the inguinal and iliac lymph glands. Surg. Gynecol. Obstet., *87*: 679, 1948.

1451-D *(Campbell's, p. 3078)*

The femoral nerve lies deep to the iliacus fascia and supplies motor function to the pectineus, quadriceps femoris, and sartorius muscles. In addition, this nerve provides cutaneous sensation to the anterior thigh and should be preserved during inguinal lymph node dissection. The hamstring muscles of the thigh (biceps, semimembranosus, semitendinosus) are supplied by the sciatic nerve.

1452-C *(Campbell's, p. 3078)*

The femoral triangle, the area that contains the pertinent lymphatic groups, is bounded by the inguinal ligament superiorly, the sartorius laterally, and the adductor longus medially. The floor of the triangle is composed of the pectineus medially and the iliopsoas laterally.

1453-C, 1454-E *(Campbell's, p. 3078)*

Approximately 30 to 60 per cent of patients with penile carcinomas present with palpable inguinal lymphadenopathy. After treatment of the primary lesion and resolution of the lymphadenitis, half of these patients will have metastatic deposits at node dissection. The likelihood of metastatic disease within palpable adenopathy is increased when the primary lesion is sizable, high grade, or when it shows stromal, vascular, or lymphatic invasion.

Approximately 5 to 20 per cent of patients with initially uninvolved nodes will have positive nodes at prophylactic lymphadenectomy.

At initial diagnosis, if positive nodes are detected ipsilaterally, metastases are present contralaterally in 60 per cent of cases. When regional disease has been proved by biopsy, surgical dissection of the ilioinguinal lymph nodes should follow. For penile cancer, if metastatic adenopathy is present in either groin at the time of presentation, bilateral regional node dissections should be done in view of the high incidence of bilateral deposits in this setting. However, if the regional nodes are judged initially free of disease, the delayed appearance of metastatic adenopathy should prompt ipsilateral dissection alone.

REFERENCES

1. Ekstrom, T., and Edsmyr, F.: Cancer of the penis. Acta Chir. Scand., *115*:25, 1958.
2. Johnson, D.E.: Carcinoma of the penis. Urology, *1*: 404, 1973.
3. Thompson, I.M., and Fair, W.R.: Penile carcinoma. AVA Update Series, Vol. 9, Lesson 1, 1990.

1455-A *(Campbell's, pp. 3078–3079)*

The sentinel lymph node has been suggested to be the primary "landing" site of regional lymph nodes most likely to be first involved by metastatic penile cancer. This node is located at the saphenofemoral junction (two fingerbreadths lateral and inferior to the pubic tubercle) between the superficial external pudendal and superficial epigastric veins. When the superior medial superficial inguinal node is negative, all other groin nodes are usually negative at dissection; when only one node is positive, it is usually the sentinel node; and when multiple nodes are positive, the sentinel node is always positive as well. However, patients with negative sentinel node biopsy findings have developed extensive regional metastases.

REFERENCES

1. Cabanas, R.M.: An approach for the penile carcinoma. Cancer, *39*:456, 1977.
2. Perinetti, E., et al.: Unreliability of sentinel lymph node biopsy for staging penile carcinoma. J. Urol., *124*:334, 1980.

1456-E, 1457-D *(Campbell's, pp. 3080–3081)*

A 6-week interval following treatment of the penile lesion allows for reduction of any inflammatory component of the regional adenopathy and minimizes the incidence of wound infection.

For cases that require bilateral dissection, an oblique or elliptic, incision below and parallel to the inguinal ligament is preferred because these incisions, comprised of thick skin flaps reduce problems of skin necrosis. Addition of a lower midline extraperitoneal incision allows access to the pelvic nodes.

After the superficial and deep inguinal nodes have been dissected and removed, the sartorius muscle is mobilized from its origin at the anterior superior iliac spine and either transposed or rolled medially to cover the femoral vessels. Its origin is sutured to inguinal ligament superiorly, and its margins are sutured to the muscles of the thigh adjacent to the femoral vessels.

Primary closure of the inguinofemoral dissection is usually possible with minimal or no further mobilization of the excision margins. When circumstances demand a particularly large area of inguinal soft tissue sacrifice, primary closure utilizing scrotal skin rotating flaps may suffice. With extensive defects, coverage by a myocutaneous flap is preferred. Scrotal rotational flaps or myocutoneous flaps are preferable to primary closure under tension.

The groin dissection is usually drained by a suction catheter placed through a stab wound inferiorly. Light dressings or collodium are applied. Efforts should be made to minimize lymph flow during initial postoperative period (i.e., bed rest for at least 5 days, elevation of foot of bed, and thigh-high stockings). Postoperative anticoagulation has been recommended to decrease the risk of thrombophlebitis, but may increase the risk of prolonged lymphatic drainage, infection, and lymphocele.

REFERENCES

1. Sogani, P.C., et al.: Lymphocele after pelvic lymphadenectomy for urologic cancer. Urology, *17*:39, 1981.
2. Whitmore, W.F. Jr., and Vagaiwala, M.R.: A technique of ilioinguinal lymph node dissection for carcinoma of the penis. Surg. Gynecol. Obstet., *159*:573, 1984.

1458-B *(Campbell's, p. 3082)*

The modified groin dissection differs from the standard dissection in that (1) the skin incision is shorter; (2) the node dissection is limited, excluding regions lateral to the femoral artery and caudal to the fossa ovalis; (3) the saphenous veins are preserved; and (4) the transposition of the sartorius muscle is eliminated. The medial margin of the dissection is the adductor longus muscle; the lateral margin is the femoral artery. This limited lymphadenectomy was proposed for patients with clinically negative nodes or with equivocally or minimally enlarged nodes.

REFERENCE

1. Catalona, W.J.: Modified inguinal lymphadenectomy for carcinoma of the penis with preservation of saphenous vein: Techniques and preliminary results. J. Urol., *140*:306, 1988.

1459-D *(Campbell's, p. 3084)*

Urethral tumors at the meatus are simply excised. The entire urethra should be assessed. Transurethral resection can be effective therapy for low-grade and superficial lesions of the penile or prostatic urethra. For isolated lesions of similar low grade and stage, a segmented urethrectomy with reanastomosis has occasionally been successful. Invasive lesions of the distal penile urethra are surgically managed by partial penectomy.

With proximal urethral lesions or large genital tumors extensively involving the perineum, additional soft tissue clearance is recommended to maximize local control. In addition to en bloc cystectomy, excision of the pubic arch or its subsymphysical segment has been utilized as a surgical adjunct in these circumstances.

REFERENCE

1. Bracken, R.B.: Exenterative surgery for posterior urethral cancer. Urology, *19*:248, 1982.

1460-C *(Campbell's, p. 3085)*

The incidence of metastatic inguinal adenopathy from distal male urethral cancers is about 50 to 60 per cent. In contradistinction to penile primary lesions, there is little inflammation associated with these lesions. Clinical adenopathy in this setting is a highly reliable sign of metastasis. Therapeutic dissection has been successful, but there is no documented advantage to prophylactic surgery.

Although the treatment of inguinal and pelvic metastases from urethral cancer is primarily surgical, the overall results are poor. The surgical procedure required is the standard ilioinguinal lymphadenectomy.

REFERENCE

1. Ray, B., et al.: Experience with primary carcinoma of the male urethra. J. Urol., *117*:591, 1977.

1461-A *(Campbell's, p. 3085)*

The potential multifocal nature of transitional cell carcinoma places the entire urothelium at risk in the patient with bladder cancer. The prostatic and penile urethra is uncommonly involved at the time of cystectomy. Therefore, the entire urethra from the mebranous portion to the meatus, is generally not removed with the specimen. Because this urothelium remains at risk, close follow-up with urethral washing for cytology, flow cytometry, and biopsy (if necessary) is required at 3- to 4-month intervals for at least 5 years. The incidence of subsequent severe epithelial atypia or frank in situ urethral carcinoma is estimated at 12.5 per cent in male patients in whom urethrectomy was not performed prophylactically during total cystectomy for bladder cancer.

REFERENCE

1. Schellhammer, P.F., and Whitmore, W.F. Jr.: Transitional cell carcinoma of the urethra in men having cystectomy for bladder cancer. J. Urol., *115*:56, 1976.

1462-B *(Campbell's, p. 3087)*

The urethral branches for the internal pudendal arteries are isolated, ligated, and divided as they enter the bulb at 4 and 8 o'clock, just inferior to the perineal membrane.

REFERENCE

1. Herr, H.W.: Urethrectomy. *In* Glenn, J.F. (Ed.): Urologic Surgery, 3rd ed. Philadelphia, J.B. Lippincott Co., 1983.

1463-A, 1464-D *(Campbell's, pp. 3087–3088)*

The therapy of urethral carcinoma in the female is based primarily on tumor extent and to a lesser degree on histologic type. The diagnosis of a urethral carcinoma requires biopsy and histopathologic confirmation.

For small, exophytic, and well-differentiated lesions of the external meatus or distal third of the urethra, circumferential local excision of the distal urethra and adjacent portions of the anterior vaginal wall can be accomplished.

For entire or proximal urethral invasive lesions, cystourethrectomy (anterior exenteration), including a wide margin of vagina, and in some cases the entire vagina, is required. For bulky female urethral lesions, and/or local recurrences, an extended excision may be necessary.

Groin dissection is reserved for the patient who presents initially with histologically confirmed regional lymph nodes without distant metastases or one who subsequently demonstrates lymph node involvement. Groin dissections in the female are performed in a fashion identical to that in the male for penile cancer.

REFERENCE

1. Johnson, D.E., and O'Connell, J.R.: Primary carcinoma of the female urethra. Urology, *21*:42, 1983.

1465-C *(Campbell's, pp. 3090–3092)*

The majority of patients with testicular cancer present with a painless lump in the scrotum. Scrotal ultrasound is over 90 per cent sensitive and specific for the diagnosis of a solid testis mass; however, when ultrasound is inconclusive, inguinal exploration and biopsy are indicated. Ultrasound is an unnecessary expense for the patient with unequivocal examination findings.

Blood for serum human chorionic gonadotropin-beta subunit (B-HCG), alpha-fetaprotein (AFP), and lactate dehydrogenase (LDH) determinations should be drawn prior to orchiectomy when a testis tumor is suspected.

Little controversy exists about the role of radical inguinal orchiectomy in the treatment of primary testicular cancer. The inguinal approach avoids interruption of the scrotal lymphatics, and allows complete removal of the spermatic cord up to the internal ring.

Early placement of a clamp versus the cord avoids any potential tumor spread via veins or lymphatics during the subsequent mobilization of the testis.

The vas should be ligated separately with 3.0 silk or controlled with a hemoclip. The internal ring is obliterated with a No. 1 polyglycolic acid (PGA) suture.

The most serious complication of orchiectomy is bleeding from the spermatic cord stump. Therefore, the ligated cord should be carefully inspected prior to allowing it to retract into the retroperitoneum.

REFERENCE

1. Gottesman, J.E.: Radical Inguinal Onchiectomy. *In* Crawford, E.D., and Das, S. (Eds.): Current Genitourinary Cancer Surgery. Philadelphia, Lea & Febiger, 1990, p. 319.

1466-C, 1467-C *(Campbell's, pp. 3092–3093)*

The urologist must occasionally treat patients who have undergone transcrotal biopsies or orchiectomies of testicular cancer. Most workers argue that a full hemiscrotectomy or prophylactic inguinal node dissection is no longer necessary in this situation. The following management is recommended:

1. In Stage A seminoma, prophylactic retroperitoneal radiation should be extended to include the hemiscrotum and ipsilateral inguinal nodes.
2. In Stage A nonseminoma, the previous scrotal incision should be excised at the time of retroperitoneal lymph node dissection. The remaining stump of the spermatic cord must also be completely removed.
3. If an observation protocol for Stage A nonseminoma is considered, the cord and scrotal incision should be excised as a separate procedure. Inguinal nodes must also be monitored for metastases.
4. In advanced disease treated with full-dose platinum-based chemotherapy, no further treatment of the scrotum is probably necessary. The inguinal nodes and scrotum should be carefully examined at each follow-up visit.

REFERENCE

1. Giguere, J.K., Stablein, D.M., Spaulding, J.T., et al.: The clinical significance of unconventional orchiectomy approaches in testicular cancer: A report from the testicular cancer intergroup study. J. Urol., *139*: 1225, 1988.

1468-A *(Campbell's, p. 3093)*

A patient with advanced testicular cancer occasionally presents with severe or even life-threatening complication. Others may have the tissue diagnosis already established from the biopsy of a metastatic focus. In these cases, it may be in the best interest of the patient to proceed directly to immediate chemotherapy without orchiectomy.

It is important in these patients that eventual inguinal orchiectomy be carried out, even if a complete response from chemotherapy is achieved. In a patient with normal testes by both palpation and ultrasound throughout the course of treatment, who is believed to have extragonodal germ cell malignancy, the testes may be left in place and monitored carefully at follow-up visits. If the retroperitoneal disease localizes to one side, however, it has been recommended to remove the ipsilateral testis at the time of lymphadenectomy.

REFERENCE

1. Clavo, F., Hodson, N., Barrett, A., and Peckham, M.J.: Chemotherapy of primary (in situ) testicular tumors: Response in advanced metastatic disease. Br. J. Urol., *55*:560, 1983.

1469-E *(Campbell's, p. 3093)*

It is of importance that the diagnosis of pure seminoma be made only after step sectioning of the testis. The significance of the findings of elevated serum marker levels in the presence of pure seminoma has been an area of some controversy. Most investigators agree that any elevation of AFP, which is normally produced by embryonal tumor cells, should be considered a hallmark of occult nonseminomatous disease.

Elevation of B-HCG has been reported in 8 to 40 per cent of pure seminomas. Very high levels of B-HCG (less than 200 MIU/ml) almost certainly reflect occult metastatic nonseminomatous elements, but lower levels do not exclude them. Therefore, it is recommended that a patient with a primary pure seminoma and B-HCG more than 20 MIU/ml, or a patient with a lower B-HCG level but no identifiable syncitiotrophoblastic giant cells in the testis, be treated as having nonseminoma.

REFERENCE

1. Pritchett, T.R., Skinner, D.G., Selser, S.F., and Kern, W.H.: Seminoma with elevated human chorionic gonadotropin: The case for retroperitoneal lymph node dissection. Urology, *25*:244, 1985.

1470-D *(Campbell's, pp. 3093–3094)*

Whitmore documented that tumors that extend outside the testis parenchyma to invade the tunica albuginea, rete testis, epididymis, or spermatic cord (stage T2 to T4) are associated with a higher risk of metastatic disease. Additional histologic features that appear to correlate with a higher risk of metastatic disease include predominant embryonal cell type or undifferentiated tumor and the presence of vascular or lymphatic invasion. The presence of yolk sac elements had a protective effect in one study, but this was not confirmed in others.

REFERENCES

1. Whitmore, E.F. Jr.: Germinal testis tumors: Guest overview. In Skinner, D.G. (Ed.): Urological Cancer. New York, Grave and Stratton, 1983, p. 335.
2. Freedman, L.S., Jones, W.G., Peckham, M.J., et al.: Histopathology in the prediction of relapse of patients with stage I testicular teratoma treated by orchidectomy alone. Lancet, 2:295, 1987.

1471-E *(Campbell's, p. 3094)*

The basic staging work-up currently includes serum tumor markers (AFP, hCG-β, and LDH) before and after orchiectomy, chest radiography, and abdominal and pelvic CT scans. Although whole-lung tomography and chest CT scan have been helpful, they have not been shown to alter initial therapy.

REFERENCE

1. Richie, J.P.: Diagnosis and staging of testicular tumors. *In* Skinner, D.G., and Lieskovsky, G. (Eds.): Diagnosis and Management of Genitourinary Cancer. W.B. Saunders Co., Philadelphia, 1988, p. 498.

1472-B, 1473-A *(Campbell's, pp. 3095–3096)*

Considerable controversy exists over the role of bipedal lymphangiogram (LAG). In the case of a planned node dissection, little information is to be gained over that available from CT scan, and the use of LAG prior to entrance into a surveillance protocol is also controversial.

The accuracy of magnetic resonance imaging (MRI) in detecting retroperitoneal adenopathy appears to be no better than CT scanning.

Results are now available from surveillance protocols. Consistently, 25 to 35 per cent of patients eventually develop metastatic disease, and importantly, a few experience recurrences 2 to 4 years after diagnosis. Approximately 50 to 75 per cent of recurrences in patients in surveillance protocols occur in the retroperitoneum, compared with less than 1 per cent in patients following lymph node dissection.

REFERENCES

1. Fossa, S.D., Stenevig, A.E., Lien, H.H., et al.: Nonseminomatous testicular cancer clinical stage I: prediction of outcome by histopathological parameters. A multivariate analysis. Oncology, *46*:297, 1989.
2. Wishnow, K.I., Johnson, D.E., and Tenney, D.M.: Are lymphangiograms necessary before placing patients with nonseminomatous testicular tumors on surveillance? J. Urol., *141*:1133, 1989.
3. Foster, R.S., and Donohue, J.P.: Nerve-sparing RPLND. AVA update series, Vol. 12, Lesson 15, 1993.

1474-B, 1475-E *(Campbell's, p. 3096)*

As the cure rate for low-stage nonseminoma surpassed 90 per cent, concern became focused on the morbidity of treatments. As interest rose in the surveillance of patients with low-stage nonseminoma, surgeons focused on developing a limited node dissection that could preserve ejaculation. Most investigators agree that the most important area to preserve is the hypogastric plexus overlying the aorta and sacrum below the origin of the inferior mesenteric artery. Some workers have advocated dissecting out the postganglionic nerve fibers of the lumbar sympathetic chain, which course anteriorly over the aorta and fuse into multiple common trunks. This approach reportedly achieves preservation of ejaculation in up to 100 per cent of cases.

REFERENCE

1. Donohue, J.P., Foster, R.S., Rowland, R.G., et al.: Nerve-sparing retroperitoneal lymphadenectomy with preservation of ejaculation. J. Urol., *144*:287, 1990.

1476-D *(Campbell's, p. 3097)*

Approximately 10 per cent of patients thought to suffer clinical stage A disease will be found to have grossly positive nodes at surgery. When enlarged or indurated nodes are discovered at surgery, the decision must be made whether or not to extend the limits of dissection. If positive nodes are discovered near the origin of the inferior mesenteric artery, it is necessary to extend the dissection over the lower aorta and down the contralateral common iliac artery. However, when positive nodes are located only superiorly, preservation of the lower aortic area can be attempted. In probable stage II B disease, however, the dissection should be extended to the contralateral side with full mobilization of the aorta and vena cava.

REFERENCES

1. Fung, C.Y., Kalish, L.A., Brodsky, G.L., et al.: Stage I nonseminomatous germ cell testicular tumor: Prediction of metastatic potential by primary histopathology. J. Clin. Oncol., 6:1467, 1988.
2. Foster, R.S., and Donohue, J.P.: Nerve-sparing RPLND. AMA Update Series. Vol. 12, Lesson 15, 1993.

1477-C *(Campbell's, p. 3099)*

The risk of tumor recurrence following node dissection alone is 37 to 49 per cent for pathologic stage II A and II B combined. This risk can be decreased to 0 to 15 per cent with adjuvant chemotherapy regimens. Adjuvant chemotherapy is recommended for all patients with stage II B disease, and those patients with stage II A disease can be treated with observation or adjuvant chemotherapy after their node dissections.

REFERENCE

1. Williams, S.D., Stablein, D.M., Einhorn, L.H., et al.: Immediate adjuvant chemotherapy versus observation with treatment at relapse in pathological stage II testicular cancer. N. Engl. J. Med., *317*:1433, 1987.

1478-B *(Campbell's, p. 3100)*

The two popular approaches to the retroperitoneum are the thoracoabdominal and transabdominal incisions. The thoracoabdominal approach provides superb exposure to the upper retroperitoneum, with the renal hilum essentially in the center of the field. This approach is crucial in patients with advanced disease who may require a thorough suprahilar dissection. In most patients, the dissection can be performed outside the peritoneal cavity, reducing the risk of postoperative ileus and late bowel obstruction, which is approximately 3 per cent in transabdominal surgery.

The transabdominal approach, however, offers a faster opening and closure of the incision and is a more familiar procedure to most surgeons. Exposure to the hilum can be achieved but requires mobilization of the pancreas and spleen, resulting in a higher risk of pancreatitis than with the thoracoabdominal approach. No need exists to enter the chest cavity, decreasing the potential complications related to atelectasis and accumulation of pleural fluid. In low-stage disease, the choice between the two approaches primarily reflects the training of the surgeon.

1479-C *(Campbell's, p. 3100)*

An incision is usually made over the bed of the eighth or ninth rib from the midaxillary line to the midepigastrium. It is then carried down as a paramedian incision.

REFERENCE

1. Skinner, D.G., and Lieskovsky, G.: The thoracoabdominal approach for management of nonseminomatous germ cell tumors of the testis. (Movie). 1984. Available by request from Norwich Eaton, Inc.

1480-B *(Campbell's, p. 3102)*

In full bilateral RPLND, the dissection is carried to the medial aspects of both ureters. This tissue represents the lateral limit of dissection and should be clipped with hemoclips.

REFERENCE

1. Wise, P.G., and Scandino, P.T.: *In* Skinner, D.G., and Lieskovsky, G. (Eds.): Diagnosis and Management of Genitourinary Cancer. Philadelphia, W.B. Saunders Co., 1988, p. 779.

1481-C, 1482-A, 1483-D *(Campbell's, p. 3105)*

The most common intraoperative complications of RPLND result from damage to one of the major vascular structures (i.e., aorta, vena cava, or main renal artery). Aortic and vena caval injuries can usually be repaired with sutures. Damage to the main renal artery should be repaired if possible. If a small polar vessel is ligated or injured, it is best left alone. Hypertension appears to be extremely rare in such instances.

Distal ureteral injury during dissection is best repaired by ureteroneocystostomy, and mid or proximal ureteral injury can be repaired by primary ureteroureterostomy over an internal stint.

The most common long-term complication of full bilateral RPLND is anejaculation.

REFERENCES

1. Donohue, J.P.: Complications of lymph node dissection. *In* Marshall, F.F. (Ed.): Urologic Complications: Medical and Surgical, Adult and Pediatric. Chicago, Year Book Medical Publishers, 1986, p. 281.
2. Richie, J.P.: Complications of Retroperitoneal Lymph Node Dissection. AUA Update Series, Vol. 12, Lesson 16, 1993.

1484-B *(Campbell's, p. 3106)*

During the transabdominal approach for RPLND, the inferior mesenteric vein is divided between ligatures to facilitate mobilization of the mesentery of the left colon.

REFERENCE

1. Donohue, J.P., Rowland, R.G., and Bihrle, R.: Transabdominal retroperitoneal lymph node dissection. *In* Skinner, D.G., and Lieskovsky, G. (Eds.): Diagnosis and Management of Genitourinary Cancer. Philadelphia, W.B. Saunders Co., 1988, p. 802.

1485-C *(Campbell's, p. 3107)*

Interest has been evolving in attempting to improve on the 50 to 75 per cent preservation of ejaculation, which is attainable with template-type limited dissections. The nerve-sparing node dissection involves the early identification for the postganglionic fibers emanating from the lumbar ganglia at L1 to L4, which course anteriorly over the aorta and coalesce into multiple trunks, forming the hypogastric plexus. This technique reliably results in close to 100 per cent preservation of ejaculation.

REFERENCE

1. Donohue, J.P., Foster, R.S., Rowland, R.G., et al.: Nerve-sparing retroperitoneal lymphadenectomy with preservation of ejaculation. J. Urol., *144*:287, 1990.

1486-E *(Campbell's, p. 3108)*

Mature teratoma in the retroperitoneum generally is not eradicated by chemotherapy and has a tendency for persistent growth over many years. Therefore, it is recommended that all patients with teratomatous elements in the primary tumor undergo lymphadenectomy at the time of least disease (e.g., shortly after finishing chemotherapy).

REFERENCE

1. Logothetis, C.J., Samuels, M.L., Trimdade, A., and Johnson, D.E.: The growing teratoma syndrome. Cancer, *50*:1629, 1982.

1487-B *(Campbell's, p. 3109)*

The management of residual bulk tumor following chemotherapy remains controversial. Viable tumor cells are discovered in the residual mass in 0 to 42 per cent of patients, depending in part on the size of the residual mass.

All series have relatively small numbers, and it has not been proven that resection of residual masses translates into a survival advantage; however, current policy, after primary chemotherapy, is to surgically resect any residual retroperitoneal mass greater than 3.0 cm. Masses less than 3.0 cm are observed with CT scan every 3 months the first year, and every 6 months the second and third years.

REFERENCES

1. Donohue, J.P., Roth, L.M., Zachary, J.M., et al.: Cytoreductive surgery for metastatic testis cancer. Tissue analysis of retroperitoneal masses after chemotherapy. J. Urol., *127*:111, 1982.
2. Schultz, S.M., Einhorn, L.H., Conces, D.J. Jr., et al.: Management of postchemotherapy residual mass in patients wit advanced seminoma: Indiana University experience. J. Urol. Oncol., *7*:1497, 1989.

1488-D, 1489-B *(Campbell's, pp. 3109–3110)*

Patients who have been exposed to chemotherapy require special attention to prepare them for retroperitoneal node dissection. The white blood cell and platelet counts must be at normal levels prior to surgery. Patients exposed to bleomycin should have a pulmonary function evaluation. The anesthesiologist must be advised about the need to maintain low inspired oxygen and low crystalloid replacement intraoperatively and postoperatively. Goldfinger and Schweizer associated the pulmonary toxicity seen after bleomycin use with increased inspired oxygen and overhydration. The patient should, therefore, be ventilated with room air (FIO_2 of 0.21) and never have the inspired FIO_2 to exceed 25 per cent. Also, for hydration, colloid is preferred over crystalloid.

Patients requiring a postchemotherapy node dissection, especially those with significant retroperitoneal mass, are best approached by a thoracoabdominal incision.

REFERENCES

1. Goldfinger, P.L., and Schweizer, O.: The hazards for anesthesia and surgery in gleomycin treated patients. Semin. Oncol., *6*:121, 1979.
2. Richie, J.P.: Complications of Retroperitoneal Lymph Node Dissection. AUA Update Series, Vol. 12, Lesson 16, 1993.

1490-E *(Campbell's, p. 3110)*

In these cases of advanced disease persisting after primary chemotherapy, the ipsilateral ureter is often encased in the tumor mass. This ureter should be dissected out early to allow the surgeon to decide if it can be salvaged. If the ureter is damaged during the dissection, or if it cannot be separated from the tumor, a nephrectomy should be preformed with the dissection, provided that the patient has a normal contralateral kidney.

1491-C *(Campbell's, pp. 3115–3116)*

A testis biopsy is indicated in patients with azoospermia who have testes that appear normal and palpable vas deferens. FSH should also be normal. The biopsy is done to rule out azoospermia from obstruction versus primary seminiferous tubular failure. Azoospermia with small firm testes and elevated FSH is seen in Klinefelter's patients and a karyotype would be indicated first. Prior to the induction of in vitro fertilization with aspirated epididymal sperm, a testis biopsy should be obtained.

Testis biopsy is best performed in an open manner. The biopsy should be taken from the upper pole (medial or lateral aspect) as it is less likely to injure any major branches of the testicular artery running superficially under the tunica albuginea in these areas. The samples should be placed into special solutions for evaluation and should not be placed into formalin.

1492-E *(Campbell's, pp. 3116–3119)*

When a man has had a prior inguinal operation and obstruction is suspected, the exploration should be done through the inguinal incision. If there is no obstruction found, then the testis can be pulled up through this incision and a vasogram performed. The vas is usually opened at the junction of the straight and convoluted portions of the vas. After the cut is made, any fluid is placed on a slide and examined for sperm. If there is no sperm present, then irrigating with 0.1–.2 ml of saline or Ringer's solution can be performed; if there is no sperm in that fluid, then epididymal obstruction is confirmed. The patency of the seminal vesicle portion of the vas can be determined by injecting saline. Methylene blue could also be injected and the bladder catheterized, and if a blue color is present, then the segment is patent. If sperm is found in the fluid, then distal obstruction is suspected. A No. 3 whistletip ureteral catheter could be gently passed toward the seminal vesicle if the vas is dilated. If it reaches the inguinal ring without resistance then a vasogram can be performed using 50 per cent water-soluble contrast. Both vas can be injected at the same time and a Foley catheter should be placed into the bladder and pulled tightly against the bladder neck so that contrast does not reflux into the bladder and obscure the view of the vasograms. If there is obstruction at the ejaculatory ducts, then transurethral resection is indicated.

Vasography should not be directed toward the epididymis and testis as the high pressure could injure the epididymis and cause secondary obstruction.

1493-D *(Campbell's, p. 3119)*

When examination of vasal fluid reveals absence of sperm and the seminal vesicle end of the vas is confirmed to be patent, then epididymal obstruction is presumed, and a vasoepididymostomy is in order. If the vasal fluid does contain many sperm and the vasogram is also normal, then retrograde ejaculation, lack of emission, or vas aperistalsis could be the cause of the azoospermia. A postejaculatory urine should be spun down in all patients with azoospermia to rule out retrograde ejaculation.

1494-A *(Campbell's, pp. 3121–3123)*

The no-scalpel technique was developed in China. There is a greatly reduced incidence of hematoma, infection, and pain with this technique. It takes a while to learn, but once mastered it results in 40 per cent less time to do the procedure as well. The failure rate is equal to other vasectomy techniques. The lower complication rate of this technique has made vasectomy more appealing.

1495-B *(Campbell's, pp. 3123–3124)*

The incidence of recanalization is determined by the technique used to occlude the ends of the vas as well as the length of the vas that is removed. Removing long segments of the vas obviously decreases the rate of recanalization. Suture ligature is commonly used to tie off both ends of the vas. This may result in necrosis and sloughing of the cut end distal to the suture and result in sperm granuloma. If both ends slough, then recanalization is more common. The failure rate is between 1 to 5 per cent when sutures alone are used for occlusion. Using hemoclips on each end decreases the failure rate to less than 1 per cent. This is because a clip applies more even pressure and there is less ischemia. By cauterizing the lumen with a needle cautery, which is just powerful enough to destroy the mucosa and not the entire wall of the vas, the failure rate can be reduced to less than 0.5 per cent. Putting the two cut ends in different fascial layers is thought to decrease the failure rate, although no controlled studies have been performed. When a vasectomy is done with open ends then the failure rate has been found anywhere from 7 to 50 per cent. Two semen specimens 4 to 6 weeks apart are essential to assure that the vasectomy has been effective and that the sperm count has dropped to zero. Recanalization usually occurs early.

1496-E *(Campbell's, pp. 3124–3125)*

Experience of the surgeon is the single most important factor relating to complication rates of a vasectomy. Studies have shown that the complication rates are much higher for surgeons performing few vasectomies per year compared to those performing many per year. Hematoma is one of the most common complications, with an average incidence of around 2 per cent. Infection is also relatively common (3.4 per cent rate). Sperm granulomas are present in approximately 10 to 30 per cent of men who undergo vasectomy reversals but are only symptomatic with pain in 0.1 to 3 per cent of patients. There are no significant systemic effects in the long-term period that are directly attributed to vasectomy. Epididymal obstruction can often occur secondary to high intravasal back pressure. This pressure is not transmitted to the seminiferous tubules; therefore, spermatogenesis is usually normal postvasectomy. Chronic testicular pain is reported in about 1 in 10,000 patients. Antisperm antibodies are frequently seen but their significance is uncertain.

1497-C *(Campbell's, pp. 3126–3127)*

The best incision for a vasovasostomy is a high vertical scrotal incision. The vas should be identified and the obstructed segment and any sperm granulomas resected. The vas should be mobilized (2 to 3 cm) on either side of the vasectomy site and the vascularity preserved. The vas can be freed up into the inguinal canal bluntly with the finger if additional length is needed. An additional 4 to 6 cm in length can be gained by freeing the convoluted vas from its attachments to the epididymal tunic and then allowing the testis to drop upside-down. If further length is needed, then the floor of the canal can be cut and the vas rerouted under the floor. With all these combinations, up to 12-cm gaps can be bridged.

The vas should be cut and then the end examined for presence of fluid. A glass slide should touch the surface and then be examined for sperm with the addition of two drops of saline. If no sperm are seen, then the lumen should be gently cannulated with a 24-gauge angiocatheter and a small amount of saline injected and examined for the presence of sperm.

If no sperm are present on washings and no fluid is present, then vasoepididymostomy should be performed. If sperm are present with tails, then vasovasostomy should be performed. If there is white milky fluid without sperm present and no evidence of epididymal obstruction, then vasovasostomy should be performed. If there is evidence of epididymal obstruction with white milky fluid, then vasoepididymostomy should be performed. If there is clear fluid without any sperm and no evidence of obstruction, then vasovasostomy should be performed. Up to 60 per cent of men with bilateral absence of sperm in the vasal fluid will ultimately have sperm in their ejaculate and 31 per cent will go on to achieve "successful fertilization."

1498-A *(Campbell's, pp. 3127–3130)*

Success of vasovasostomy is dependent upon accurate mucosa to mucosa approximations, leakproof/tension-free anastomosis, good blood supply, healthy mucosa and muscularis, and good atraumatic anastomotic technique. The testicular side lumen is often dilated three to four times that of the abdominal side lumen. When this is the case, a two-layered anastomosis is preferable. If the lumens have similar diameters, then a one-layer anastomosis may be satisfactory. When sperm leak, they cause an inflammatory reaction which decreases the success rate of vasovasostomy. In situations where there is a unilateral inguinal obstruction along with an atrophic testicle on the opposite side, then a crossed vasovasostomy should be performed. Unilateral obstruction or aplasia of the inguinal vas or the ejaculatory duct with contralateral obstruction of the epididymis is also best managed with crossed vasovasostomy. It is much more preferable to perform one good anastomosis then two anastomoses that have a much lower chance to stay patent.

1499-C *(Campbell's, p. 3131)*

When sperm is found in the vasal fluid on at least one side at the time of surgery, sperm can be found in the ejaculate in 98 per cent of men. Late obstruction will occur in 5 to 10 per cent of these men after 2 years. Pregnancy occurs in 50 to 60 per cent of couples followed for at least 2 years.

1500-A *(Campbell's, pp. 3131–3132)*

Sperm motility and the capacity to fertilize increase as the sperm progress through the length of the epididymis. When the epididymis is shortened, then the epithelium will adapt so that some sperm will become functional. During epididymal surgery, however, the greatest length of epididymis should be preserved to result in best sperm quality. Anastomoses are easier to perform in the distal regions because of the thicker wall. Blood supply is very rich to the epididymis from the testicular vessels superiorly and the deferential vessels inferiorly. Deferential vessels usually come off of a branch of the inferior vesical artery. The spermatic cord vessels enter at the junction of the middle and upper thirds of the testis, medial to the epididymis.

The efferent ducts of the testis are superior to the vascular pedicle.

1501-D *(Campbell's, p. 3132)*

The most common solid epididymal mass is an adenomatoid tumor. These are benign. Malignant epididymal tumors are very rare. Evaluation of a solid epididymal mass should be performed through a standard inguinal incision. The cord should be clamped and the testis can be examined and cooled prior to opening tunica vaginalis and inspecting the lesion. If it can be confirmed to be benign, then local excision with salvage of the testis may be performed.

1502-E *(Campbell's, pp. 3132–3133)*

End-to-end vasoepididymostomy is useful when the epididymal tubules are not dilated, which is seen often when the epididymis is obstructed by sperm granulomas. When the obstruction is distal (near the vasoepididymal junction), then the diameter of the epididymis is narrower and more closely matches that of the vas deferens, a situation well-suited to an anastomosis. When vasal length is compromised (which commonly occurs after a vasectomy), the epididymis can be dissected off the testis and flipped up, providing an additional 5 cm of length. Congenital epididymal obstruction usually results in dilated epididymal tubules and is better managed with an end-to-side anastomosis. Proximal obstruction of the epididymis also is better managed with end-to-side vasoepididymostomy, as the epididymis is usually dilated.

1503-B *(Campbell's, p. 3135)*

The appearance of sperm in the ejaculate after a vasoepididymostomy is seen in 50 to 70 per cent. Twenty-five per cent of those will scar down and result in azoospermia again. Overall pregnancy rates are between 15 and 30 per cent after vasoepididymostomy. They are higher the more distal the anastomosis performed on the epididymis, because the sperm have a better chance to become motile and functional. Vasovasostomy pregnancy rates are between 50 and 60 per cent.

1504-A *(Campbell's, pp. 3135–3136)*

Ejaculatory duct obstruction is suspected in patients who have severe oligospermia or azoospermia with palpable vas deferens. Semen volume is low and the semen fructose level is either negative or low. Testis biopsies show normal spermatogenesis. The FSH is normal. Vasovasography can confirm the obstruction, and the recommended treatment is transurethral resection of the ejaculatory duct. Transrectal ultrasound can be diagnostic. Sperm will be seen in the semen of about 50 per cent of patients after ejaculatory duct resection; however, reports of pregnancy are rare. If azoospermia persists, then obstruction of the epididymis should be considered and possible vasoepididymostomy performed.

1505-B *(Campbell's, pp. 3137–3138)*

In obstructed systems, sperm can be aspirated for use in in vitro fertilization programs. Although sperm have better motility in the distal epididymis under normal circumstances, when obstruction is present parodoxically, it is better in the proximal epididymis. Blood has a very detrimental effect on the ability of sperm to fertilize. Techniques to aspirate sperm should be done under the microscope in a manner to avoid contamination with blood.

1506-C *(Campbell's, p. 3141)*

With microsurgical varicocelectomy, the internal spermatic vein is ligated. All external spermatic and cremasteric veins are also ligated. The transcrotal collaterals running in the gubernaculum are also divided. This leaves only the vasal vein as collateral venous return from the testis.

1507-D *(Campbell's, pp. 3139–3144)*

Hydroceles after varicocele repair are due to ligation of lymphatics during the procedure. The average incidence is around 7 per cent. Half of these will become large enough to warrant surgical repair. They can occur after any of the approaches except for radiographic occlusion techniques and they have not been seen with the microsurgical high inguinal varicocelectomy technique.

1508-C *(Campbell's, pp. 3139–3145)*

Varicocele recurrence can occur with any of the repairs discussed. A retroperitoneal approach ties off only the internal spermatic vein. Recurrence rates are around 15 per cent usually due to presence of peritoneal, inguinal, or retroperitoneal collaterals. Cremasteric veins can also be a cause of recurrence as well as external spermatic veins. The incidence of recurrence is higher in children, with rates of between 15 and 45 per cent. Inguinal approach will allow access to the external spermatic vein and the cremasteric veins and the gubernacular veins. Inguinal varicocelectomy has a recurrence rate of 9 per cent. Subinguinal microscopic techniques are associated with a 6 per cent recurrence. Microsurgical high inguinal varicocelectomy when done properly results in only a 0.6 per cent recurrence rate. Radiographic occlusion techniques have recurrence rates as low as 4 per cent and as high as 11 per cent. Laparoscopic techniques have recurrence rates comparable to those seen with open retroperitoneal repairs.

1509-A *(Campbell's, p. 3145)*

Varicocelectomy produces a significant improvement in semen parameters in 60 to 80 per cent of men. However, pregnancy rates average only around 35 per cent. Varicoceles are found in 15 per cent of normal men. They are seen in 35 per cent of men with primary infertility and up to 85 per cent of men with secondary infertility. There is a greater improvement in semen parameters when large varicoceles are repaired and also when varicoceles are repaired in kids.

1510-D *(Campbell's, p. 3147)*

The most common complication of hydrocelectomy is hematoma formation. Meticulous hemostasis and drainage of the scrotum can help decrease the incidence. All the other choices are well-known complications of hydrocelectomy, although less common.